Cocaine and Other Stimulants

ADVANCES IN BEHAVIORAL BIOLOGY

Recent Volumes in this Series

Volume 10 • NEUROHUMORAL CODING OF BRAIN FUNCTION
Edited by R. D. Myers and René Raúl Drucker-Colín • 1974

Volume 11 • REPRODUCTIVE BEHAVIOR
Edited by William Montagna and William A. Sadler • 1974

Volume 12 • THE NEUROPSYCHOLOGY OF AGGRESSION
Edited by Richard E. Whalen • 1974

Volume 13 • ANEURAL ORGANISMS IN NEUROBIOLOGY
Edited by Edward M. Eisenstein • 1975

Volume 14 • NUTRITION AND MENTAL FUNCTIONS
Edited by George Serban • 1975

Volume 15 • SENSORY PHYSIOLOGY AND BEHAVIOR
Edited by Rachel Galun, Peter Hillman, Itzhak Parnas, and Robert Werman • 1975

Volume 16 • NEUROBIOLOGY OF AGING
Edited by J. M. Ordy and K. R. Brizzee • 1975

Volume 17 • ENVIRONMENTS AS THERAPY FOR BRAIN DYSFUNCTION
Edited by Roger N. Walsh and William T. Greenough • 1976

Volume 18 • NEURAL CONTROL OF LOCOMOTION
Edited by Richard M. Herman, Sten Grillner, Paul S. G. Stein, and Douglas G. Stuart • 1976

Volume 19 • THE BIOLOGY OF THE SCHIZOPHRENIC PROCESS
Edited by Stewart Wolf and Beatrice Bishop Berle • 1976

Volume 20 • THE SEPTAL NUCLEI
Edited by Jon F. DeFrance • 1976

Volume 21 • COCAINE AND OTHER STIMULANTS
Edited by Everett H. Ellinwood, Jr. and M. Marlyne Kilbey • 1977

Cocaine and Other Stimulants

Edited by
Everett H. Ellinwood, Jr.
and
M. Marlyne Kilbey
Duke University Medical School

PLENUM PRESS · NEW YORK AND LONDON

Library of Congress Cataloging in Publication Data

Main entry under title:

Cocaine and other stimulants.

(Advances in behavioral biology; v. 21)
"Proceedings of a conference on contemporary issues in stimulant research held at Duke University Medical Center, Durham, North Carolina, November 10-12, 1975."
Includes indexes.
1. Cocaine—Physiological effect—Congresses. 2. Amphetamine—Physiological effect—Congresses. 3. Neuropsychopharmacology—Congresses. 4. Stimulants—Congresses. I. Ellinwood, Everett H. II. Kilbey, M. Marlyne. [DNLM: 1. Stimulation, Chemical—Congresses. 2. Cocaine—Pharmacodynamics—Congresses. QC113 C748c 1975]
QP921.C7C59 615'.785 76-47488
ISBN-13: 978-1-4684-3089-9 e-ISBN-13: 978-1-4684-3087-5
DOI: 10.1007/978-1-4684-3087-5

Proceedings of a Conference on Contemporary Issues
in Stimulant Research held at Duke University Medical Center,
Durham, North Carolina, November 10—12, 1975

Softcover reprint of the hardcover 1st edition 1977

A Division of Plenum Publishing Corporation
227 West 17th Street, New York, N.Y. 10011

Acknowledgments

Material from many of the chapters in this book was presented at a conference on contemporary issues in stimulant research held at Duke University Medical Center, November 10-12, 1975. The conference was supported by Grant DA 01262-01 from the National Institute on Drug Abuse and a contribution from the Hoechst Corporation.

We thank Steven S. Szara and Michael E. Rolnick of the National Institute on Drug Abuse for their assistance in the initial planning of the conference. We also thank Sally Moorer, who administered the grant and proofread all of the manuscripts; Janet Benoit, who was responsible for arranging and assisting in many aspects of the conference; and Slater Raymond, who coordinated the preparation of the manuscripts. The following persons typed the manuscripts: Jane Culver, Nancy Glenn, Phil Hall, and Nancy Rosebaugh, and their efforts are greatly appreciated.

Contents

COCAINE: 1884-1974

Craig Van Dyke and Robert Byck

Yale University School of Medicine

333 Cedar Street, New Haven, Connecticut 06510

Cocaine, because of its unique properties as a local anesthetic, is still widely used in medicine some one hundred years after its introduction to Europe as a panacea. Karl Koller's discovery of the local anesthetic action of cocaine defined its legitimate medical usage. Today, cocaine is a drug of abuse that has dramatically increased in popularity. It is reported to produce an intense euphoria 3-5 minutes after intranasal application and thereby has gained the reputation of being the "champagne of drugs."

Despite its popularity both as a therapeutic agent and a drug of abuse, research on cocaine in both of these areas has been limited since the early 1900's. Freud (1884) and more recently Woods and Downs (1974) summarized the available information on cocaine. This review concentrates on the psychopharmacological effects of cocaine and is intended to provide a background upon which to view cocaine research during 1975, the results of which are presented in this volume.

HISTORY

Since pre-Columbian times Peruvian Indians have chewed coca leaves as a central nervous system stimulant, but it wasn't until the 1500's that the leaves were introduced to Europe by explorers returning from Peru. Gardeke in 1855 was the first to extract the active ingredient of coca leaves, calling it *erythroxylon*, and five years later Niemann isolated the alkaloid naming it *cocaine* (Byck, 1974). Von Anrep (1880) first studied the pharmacological effects of cocaine; however, Aschenbrandt (1883) and Freud (1884) were the first to describe cocaine's effect on the central nervous system (euphoria and a decrease in fatigue) and Koller (1884) discovered its ability to produce local anesthesia. Soon after Koller's discovery cocaine gained wide acceptance as a local and regional anesthetic. Cocaine was also the first effective treatment for nasal congestion associated with seasonal allergies. By the end of the 19th and the beginning of the 20th centuries cocaine attained great popularity, was contained in proprietary medications, and was advocated as a cure for opium, morphine, and alcohol habits.

As cocaine gained in popularity, society became alarmed over its addictive potential and mythical effects on human behavior, especially the reputed aggressive and sexual behavior of certain minority groups. Because of this, governments began to restrict its use as early as 1897 and by the early 1900's it was coming under strict regulations (Musto, 1973). Most of these regulations were linked to laws on morphine and opium, an association which persists to the present time.

The early history of cocaine is presented in Cocaine Papers: Sigmund Freud edited by R. Byck (1974); in the classical Peru, History of Coca by W. Mortimer (1901, reprinted 1974); and The American Disease by D. Musto (1973).

CHEMISTRY

Cocaine is one of several alkaloids present in the leaves of the plant *Erythroxylon Coca.* The total alkaloidal content of the leaves is from 0.6 to 1.8 percent (Ritchie and Cohen, 1975). Chemically it is benzoylmethylecgonine, an ester of benzoic acid and a nitrogen containing base, methylecgonine. The pharmaceutical preparation is the hydrochloride salt. Its structural formula is:

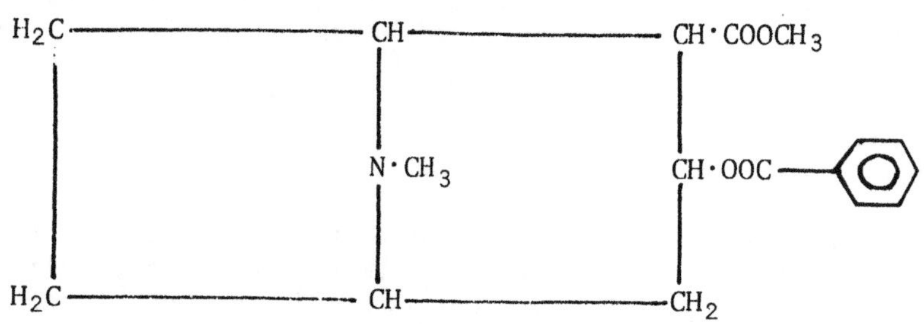

ABSORPTION, DISTRIBUTION, AND FATE

Cocaine rapidly achieves high concentrations in plasma after intravenous injection but its rate of absorption after intramuscular subcutaneous, or topical administration is probably limited by its vasoconstrictive effect. Data on the plasma concentration of cocaine following different routes of administration in dogs is presented by Woods, McMahon, and Seevers (1951a). Since cocaine is applied topically in most clinical situations, research in animals focused on this route of administration. Adriani and Campbell (1958), using the method of Woods, Cochin, Fornefeld, McMahon, and Seevers (1951b), reported that blood concentrations following the topical application of cocaine to mucous membranes closely simulated rapid intravenous injection, with peak blood concentrations 1/3 to 1/2 that obtained by the intravenous route. Adriani (1960) found that cocaine was absorbed more rapidly from the trachea than from the pharynx and was readily absorbed through the alveoli if nebulized into particles three microns or less in diameter. Cocaine was not absorbed through intact skin and was reputedly not absorbed from the bladder unless the mucous membrane was inflamed. All of these results, however, must be interpreted with caution since sensitive assays for cocaine have only recently become available.

In man, it was not clear whether the absorption of cocaine by topical application to mucous membranes was a function of the concentration of the solution or the total dose of cocaine applied. For years many clinicians observed that higher concentrations were less toxic than more dilute solutions. They attributed this to the vasoconstriction's being more intense with the more concentrated solutions and thus slowing absorption. However, Mayer (1924), in his review of fatalities from local anesthetics, cautioned against the more concentrated solutions of cocaine, feeling that they were more toxic. Adriani and Campbell (1958) attempted to clarify this issue by measuring cocaine blood concentrations after applying the same total dose of cocaine in solutions of different percent concentrations. Their results indicated that the peak blood concentrations were a function of the total dosage of cocaine applied rather than the concentration of the solution. It may be that the fatalities reported by Mayer were the result of larger total dosages of cocaine, not the more concentrated solutions.

Absorption of cocaine by the oral route of administration is limited by gastric hydrolysis (Ritchie and Cohen, 1975). Woods et al. (1951b) reported greatly reduced blood concentrations and a shorter sojourn in the blood after the oral administration of cocaine (15mg/kg) in dogs. Nevertheless, the central stimulant effects of chewing coca leaves have been utilized by man for centuries. Post, Gillin, Wyatt, and Goodwin (1974) noted psychopharmacological effects in man after cocaine was administered orally in dosages of 200 mg.

Occasional deaths in humans have also been reported following the ingestion of large doses of cocaine (Mattison, 1891; Bose, 1913).

The distribution of cocaine in humans is unknown. Woods et al. (1951b) studied the distribution of intravenous cocaine in dogs and concluded that cocaine had a much greater affinity for tissues than for plasma. After 1 to 2 hours most cocaine was concentrated in the spleen, liver, and kidneys. Nayak, Misra, and Mulé (1974) found significant levels of cocaine in the brains of rats following parenteral administration.

The more rapid the rate of detoxification or elimination, the lower cocaine's systemic toxicity. Cocaine is a complex ester and is hydrolyzed more slowly in humans than is procaine (Adriani & Campbell, 1956; Adriani, 1960). Most hydrolysis of cocaine has been thought to occur in the liver with the major urinary metabolite in man being benzoylecgonine (Ritchie & Cohen, 1975). In rabbits cocaine was shown to be hydrolyzed in the plasma by a specific, cocainesterase (Glick and Glaubach, 1941; Blaschko, Himms, and Strömblad, 1955). There is evidence in rabbits that, with repeated dosages of cocaine, the rate of metabolism of cocaine by the liver decreases with time. These rabbits developed increasing sensitivity to the toxic effects of cocaine over the duration of the experiment (Yamamoto, Mikami, and Kurogochi, 1953). In humans, it is unclear whether cocaine is hydrolyzed in the plasma or whether chronic administration affects its metabolism by the liver.

Small amounts of cocaine are eliminated unchanged in the urine of humans. Usually this accounts for less than 20 percent of the total dose, but in a case report of a fatal overdose (McIntyre, 1936) 54 percent of an 800 mg dose was excreted unchanged in 12 hours. The increased proportion of unchanged cocaine in the urine probably resulted from a limited ability to metabolize such a large dose of cocaine. Fish and Wilson (1969) studied the urinary excretion of cocaine in a chronic user of cocaine and diacetylmorphine. The amount of cocaine base excreted unchanged in the urine was pH dependent and, as expected, was highest when the urine was acidic.

TOXICOLOGY

Table I lists fatal dosages of cocaine by various routes of administration in animals. Early studies on this subject are cited by Hirschfelder and Bietu (1932). In general cocaine is more toxic in species with more highly developed central nervous systems (Nielsen and Higgins, 1923). Death from cocaine has been attributed to a direct effect on the heart, to depression of the respiratory and vasomotor centers, to hyperthermia, or to convulsions (Tatum, Atkinson, and Collins, 1925; Knoefel, Herwick, and Loevenhart, 1930; Hirschfelder and Bieter, 1932; Steinhaus and Tatum, 1950; Hardinge and Peterson, 1964). Feinberg (1886) noted that decerebration raised the tolerance of animals to cocaine, while in guinea pigs submucosal injection of the palate was much more toxic than other parenteral routes (Suzuki, Fukazawa, Yano, and Sakai, 1968).

Very little information is available on the safe dosage of cocaine in man. Numerous authors have pointed out the great individual variation in the response of human beings to cocaine. Table II lists the fatal dosages reported for cocaine in humans by various routes of administration. Harrison (1911) gave himself 300 mg intravenously in a 2 percent solution without serious adverse effects. Post, Kotin, and Goodwin (1974) administered cocaine intravenously in doses from 2.5 to 25 mg in depressed patients. Pulse and blood pressure increased but there were no serious adverse effects. Although there are many reports of the subcutaneous use of cocaine, occasionally in doses up to 1080 mg (Hammond, 1885), it has also been reported that doses as low as 22 mg have caused severe toxic reactions and death (Scheppegrell, 1898). Sollman (1917) and Ritchie and Cohen (1975) estimated a 1200 mg lethal dose in man though the basis for this is not clear.

Even less information is available, in either the scientific literature or from individuals who abuse cocaine, about safe dosages after topical application. Cocaine in doses up to 300 mg is commonly applied to mucous membranes as a local anesthetic in surgical procedures. Concentrations of 2 to 10 percent are used or the total dose required is dissolved on a cotton applicator (i.e., cocaine paste or mud). Few serious adverse effects are reported. However, Orr and Jones (1968) reported on a series of patients who were treated with 3 ml of 5 percent (150 mg) aqueous cocaine hydrochloride applied topically for laryngoscopy. Mean heart rate increased from 97 to 120/min, mean blood pressure increased, and seven of the 20 patients developed cardiac arrhythmias, including bigeminal rhythms and multiple ectopic ventricular contractions.

ALLERGIC REACTIONS

Allergic reactions to cocaine are extremely rare; and, to our knowledge, the literature does not contain a single case report of an anaphylactic reaction to cocaine. Most studies indicate that symptoms arising from use of cocaine are toxic manifestations, not allergic reactions (Mayer, 1924; Adriani, 1960).

PERIPHERAL ACTIONS

Cocaine is a drug with a complex set of actions in the periphery. First, it is a local anesthetic; second, it potentiates the actions

TABLE I

FATAL DOSAGE OF COCAINE IN ANIMALS (mg/kg)

Specie	Reference	Oral	Intra-nasal	Intra-tracheal	Intra-vesical	Subcu-taneous	Intraperi-toneal	Intra-venous
RAT	Nielsen and Higgins (1923)					370		
	Schmitz and Loevenhart (1924)					250		
MOUSE	Schmitz and Loevenhart (1924)					150		
	Shriver and Long (1971)						68	12.5
RABBIT	Nielsen and Higgins (1923)					200		12
	Schmitz and Loevenhart (1924)					90		
	Tatum, Atkinson, and Collins (1925)					100		
	Knoefel, Herwick and Loevenhart (1930)					100		
	Astrom and Persson (1961)		50	30	310			15

TABLE I (Cont.)

FATAL DOSAGE OF COCAINE IN ANIMALS (mg/kg)

Specie	Reference	Oral	Intra-nasal	Intra-tracheal	Intra-vesical	Subcu-taneous	Intraperi-toneal	Intra-venous
DOG	Nielsen and Higgins (1923)					45		
	Tatum, Atkinson and Collins (1925)					26.7		
CAT	Egglesten and Hatcher (1919)							15 (rapid)
	Ross (1923)							12.8 (rapid)
	Nielsen and Higgins (1923)	40				50		15 (rapid)
	Schmitz and Loevenhart (1924)					30		
	MacGregor (1939)							
	(a) Decerebrate preparation							77 (slow)
	(b) Spinal preparation							57.5 (slow)
MONKEY (Macacus Rhesus)	Tatum and Collins (1926)					< 30		

TABLE II

FATAL DOSAGE OF COCAINE IN MAN

Oral	
Mattison (1891)	1300 mg
	1430 mg
Bose (1913)	800 mg
Submucosal (Dental Extraction)	
Mattison (1891)	65 mg
Scheppegrell (1898)	22 mg
	260 mg
Subcutaneous	
Mattison (1891)	225 mg
Mayer (1924)	100 mg
Schumaker (1941)	2500 mg
per Urethra	
Mattison (1891)	800 mg
Mayer (1924)	160 mg
	400 mg
per Rectum	
Bose (1913)	1430 mg

of sympathomimetic amines; and, third, it may have sympathomimetic actions of its own. The explanation of some of these actions has been elucidated only recently while other actions remain mysterious.

Local Anesthetic Action

Cocaine is a non-synthetic local anesthetic and, in low concentrations, produces conduction block without depolarizing the nerve membrane (Bishop, 1932). Cocaine inhibits sodium and potassium exchange in nerve fibers and competes with calcium at the site that controls membrane permeability (Wiedmann, 1955; Ritchie and Greengard, 1966; Blaustein and Goldman, 1966; Strichartz, 1973). This is consistent with the current view of how local anesthetics block conduction in nerves (Taylor, 1959; Ritchie and Cohen, 1975).

It is an effective and widely used local anesthetic that has the advantage of causing vasoconstriction. When applied to the peripheral nerve, cocaine blocks the small nerve fibers first and the larger fibers last and is effective in terminal sensory fibers in concentrations as low as 0.02 percent (Gasser and Erlanger, 1929). There is one report (Ritter, 1910) of intravenous cocaine's being used to produce general anesthesia in dogs.

Sympathomimetic Action

Fröhlich and Loewi (1910) first reported that cocaine sensitized blood vessels, the iris, and the bladder, but not the salivary glands, to the effects of circulating epinephrine (E). Torda (1943) found that cocaine potentiated the effects of norepinephrine (NE), while Tatum (1920) noted that it potentiated the vasoconstrictor effects of electrical stimulation of the cervical and splanchnic sympathetic nerves. The explanation for these sympathomimetic actions is still unclear. Some authors indicate that cocaine blocks NE reuptake; others attribute its action to release of NE from the sympathetic nerve terminals. Still others hypothesize a direct action of cocaine on adrenergic receptors.

In evaluating the following studies in animals, it must be kept clearly in mind that current methodology does not allow isolation of the adrenergic receptors. Many of the compounds (e.g., phenoxybenzamine) used in these experiments on the sympathetic nervous system are not specific and bind to many other receptors besides adrenergic receptors. A further limitation in many of the animal studies is that cocaine is used in much higher dosages (10 to 100 mg/kg) and in concentrations as high as 10^{-5} to 10^{-4}M; whereas, in man, cocaine rarely, if ever, is used in dosages greater than 5 mg/kg or reaches a concentration greater than 10^{-6}M.

The most widely accepted theory of cocaine's sympathomimetic action is that it blocks uptake of amines into the sympathetic nerve terminals and thereby allows higher concentrations of amine to interact with the physiological receptor site. In a number of tissues, cocaine has been demonstrated to inhibit the uptake of NE and E and to elevate the blood concentrations of NE (Lawrence, Morton, and Tainter, 1942; Torda, 1943; Whitby, Hertting, and Axelrod, 1960; Muscholl, 1961; Hertting, Axelrod, and Whitby, 1961). Trendelenberg (1959) also reported that the increased response of blood pressure to NE after cocaine administration could be fully explained by the delayed inactivation of NE. In skeletal muscle, uterus (Wurtman Axelrod, and Patter, 1964), and heart (Eisenfeld, Axelrod, and Krakoff 1967; Simmonds and Gillis, 1968) cocaine did not block the extraneuronal uptake of NE by tissue.

If the uptake hypothesis for cocaine's action is correct, the administration of cocaine should sensitize an effector organ much more to an amine that is taken up rapidly than to one with slow uptake The d-isomers of NE and E are less rapidly taken up by the nerve terminals than the corresponding l-isomers. The relative rates of uptake are: l-NE > l-E > the d-isomers. Cocaine increases the sensitivity of the nictitating membrane of the spinal cat to these amines by factors of 23, 5, and 2.5, respectively (Trendelenberg, 1966). Cocaine does not potentiate the effects of isoproterenol, an amine which is not retained by tissues (Maxwell, Daniel, Sheppard, and Zimmerman, 1962). This correlation of rate of uptake with degree of supersensitivity to the amines after cocaine is in agreement with the uptake theory.

Cocaine, unlike other local anesthetics, inhibits the vasopressor action of tyramine (Tainter and Chang, 1926; MacGregor, 1939). In 1931, Burn and Tainter coined the phrase "the cocaine paradox" to characterize the seemingly inconsistent findings of cocaine's increasing the sensitivity to E while decreasing the sensitivity to tyramine in a number of sympathetic effector systems. Over the next 30 years, experimental findings led to a possible explanation of this paradox which is consistent with the reuptake hypothesis of cocaine's action. Tyramine is an indirectly acting sympathomimetic amine and its action of releasing NE from sympathetic nerve endings can be inhibited by cocaine (Fleckenstein and Stöckle, 1955; Lindmar and Muscholl, 1961). Trendelenburg (1961a) and Furchgott, Kirpekar, Rieker, and Schwab (1963) theorized that the "cocaine paradox" could be explained by cocaine's blocking in a competitive fashion both the uptake of NE and of tyramine by the presynaptic nerve.

Sympathetic denervation experiments lend further evidence that cocaine supersensitivity is a result of blocked uptake of NE. Trendelenburg (1963) reviewed the two qualitatively different types (i.e., decentralization and denervation) of supersensitivity to NE that follows the denervation of the nictitating membrane of the cat. The denervation type of supersensitivity was both qualitatively and quantitatively similar to the supersensitivity produced by cocaine. In 1966 Trendelenburg concluded that both denervation supersensitivity and cocaine supersensitivity were the result of impaired uptake of NE.

In addition to blocking reuptake, cocaine may also release NE from sympathetic nerve terminals (Campos, Stitzel, and Slideman, 1963; Teeters, Koppanyi, and Cowan, 1963; Maengwyn-Davies and Koppanyi, 1966). As NE-releasing and the NE-sensitizing effects of cocaine appeared in the same concentration range, cocaine-induced supersensitivity is difficult to evaluate. Pretreatment with reserpine (which eliminated the NE releasing effect), however, produced reliable values for the cocaine-induced supersensitivity. Furchgott et al. (1963) and Trendelenburg (1968) concluded from their work with reserpinized atria that cocaine was able to release small amounts of NE from minor storage sites (i.e., sites either not affected by reserpine or replenishable by exogenous NE) and that this process was insignificant in comparison to cocaine's ability to block reuptake of NE.

Whether cocaine has a direct effect on adrenergic receptors is much less clear. Cocaine produced supersensitivity to catecholamines in the isolated human placenta (van Euler, 1938), a preparation with little or no sympathetic innervation. Maxwell, Westila, and Ackhardt (1966) using aortic strips demonstrated that with a 30 percent block of reuptake (i.e., 30 percent reduction in binding rate) there was no increase in the response to NE. In the range of 30 to 70 percent block of reuptake, the response to NE was an increasing function of the percent of reuptake blocked by cocaine. Cocaine could lead to a further increase in response to NE without further block of reuptake. Similarly, Kalsner and Nickerson (1969), working with the same preparation, were able to assess potentiation and rate of amine inactivation separately. Cocaine slowed the inactivation of NE and also potentiated NE; however, the correlation between these two factors was poor and the delay in inactivation was inadequate to account for the potentiation. These investigators suggested that the most likely explanation for the potentiation of NE by cocaine was a direct effect on the muscle cells of the aortic strips.

Others (Lewis and Miller, 1966; Green and Fleming, 1967, and 1968) challenged the theory that cocaine produced supersensitivity to endogenous amines by having a direct action on adrenergic receptors and altering its affinity for NE. Innes and Mailhot (1973) tested the affinity of the alpha adrenergic receptor for NE by determining the ability of NE to protect against block by phenoxybenzamine. The degree of protection should depend on the affinity of the alpha receptor for NE. Cocaine (in doses that produce supersensitivity in isolated spleen strips) did not increase the protection of the alpha receptor given by NE against the block by phenoxybenzamine. In addition, if the theory that cocaine has a direct effect on adrenergic receptors is correct, then it should potentiate the response to NE in smooth muscle devoid of adrenergic nerve terminals. However, experiments performed on vascular smooth muscle (Somlyo, Woo, and Somlyo, 1965; Bevan and Verity, 1967; de la Lande, Freqin, Waterson, and Canell, 1967), in nictitating membrane (Langer, Draskoczy, and Trendelenburg, 1967; Tsai, Denham, and McGrath, 1968), and in spleen (Green and Fleming, 1968) indicated that, when adrenergic nerve terminals had completely degenerated after surgical sympathectomy, cocaine did not potentiate the response to NE. These data suggest that cocaine does not potentiate NE by a direct action on smooth muscle.

In summary, the sympathomimetic action of cocaine seems to be primarily related to its ability to block reuptake of NE. Evidence that it releases NE from sympathetic nerve endings or has a direct action on the adrenergic receptor is not as convincing and indicates that, if these actions do exist, they occur at higher concentrations of cocaine and are of minor importance.

Cholinomimetic Action

Cocaine does not usually sensitize smooth muscle to acetylcholine. However, it has been reported to sensitize the cat's nictitating membrane to acetylcholine (Rosenblueth, 1932; Thompson, 1958; Koppanyi and Feeney, 1959). Trendelenburg (1961b) found that cocaine did not produce a shift of the whole dose response curve of acetylcholine, but only increased the response to small concentrations. This was unlike its action of shifting the whole dose response curve for NE. The shift in the dose response curve for acetylcholine represented a case of additive synergism of endogenous NE and acetylcholine similar to the additive action of E and acetylcholine on the nictitating membrane (Morison and Acheson, 1938). In contrast, denervation of the nictitating membrane produced a true supersensitivity to acetylcholine (i.e., shift in the whole dose response curve). Cocaine, which mimics denervation with sympathomimetic substances, fails to mimic denervation in the case of acetylcholine.

CENTRAL ACTIONS

Up until now this review has considered cocaine's action in the periphery. Even less is known about its action in the central nervous system. As an example, it is unclear whether cocaine blocks the reuptake of NE in the central nervous system (Glowinski and Axelrod, 1965). In rat brain (Fuxe, Hamberger, and Malmfors, 1967; Fekete and Borsy, 1971), slices of brain cortex (Ross and Renyi, 1966, 1967), and synaptic vesicles (Segawa, Kuruma, Takatsuka, and Takagi, 1968), cocaine blocked the uptake of Serotonin (5-HT), dopamine, and tyramine. In synaptosomal preparations, cocaine also decreased the uptake of tryptophan and decreased the activity of tryptophan hydroxylase (Knapp and Mandell, 1972).

PERIPHERAL EFFECTS

The effect of cocaine on each organ system may well be a combination of its local anesthetic action and its potentiation of sympathomimetic amines. The relative balance of these two different and, in many cases, opposing actions depends on the specie and organ system involved and on the systemic concentration of cocaine.

Eye

Cocaine applied topically to the eye or administered parenterally produces mydriasis (Schultz, 1898). Except in very high concentrations, which produce cycloplegia (Koppanyi, 1930), the dilated pupil maintains its light reflex and ability to respond to parasympathetic stimulation (Schultz, 1898; Anitschkow and Sarubin, 1928). The mydriasis following topical application has been attributed to paralysis of the smooth muscle fibers of the iris (Kuroda, 1915), but a more likely explanation is that it results from the sensitization of the sympathetic nervous system (Frölich and Loewi, 1910). There is now considerable evidence that the mydriasis produced by cocaine requires an intact sympathetic nervous system (Limbourg, 1892; Schultz, 1898; Gold, 1924; Koppanyi, 1928).

Smooth Muscle

The action of cocaine on non-vascular smooth muscle has been investigated in the past in a number of isolated tissues. It appears that low systemic concentrations of cocaine stimulate while higher concentrations inhibit the rhythm and tone of smooth muscle in the stomach, the small intestine, the uterus (Kuroda, 1915), the urinary bladder, and the vas deferens (Waddell, 1917).

Striated Muscle

For many years it was known that inhabitants of Peru chewed coca leaves to improve their physical performance at high altitudes. Others (Aschenbrandt, 1883; Freud, 1884; Luco, Eyzaguirre, and Perez, 1948) noted that cocaine reduced fatigue and allowed increased muscular work at sea level. Guttierrez-Noriega (1944) reported that chronic administration of cocaine to dogs improved their exercise tolerance. Much of this effect was attributed to cocaine's stimulation of skeletal muscle and its ability to reduce muscular fatigue.

In contrast, other investigators (von Anrep, 1880; Kobert, 1882; Berthold, 1885) reported either no effect or a decrease in contractions following cocaine. Kubota and Macht (1919) studied the effect of cocaine on excised muscle. Dilute solutions of cocaine (0.01 to 0.5 percent) had no effect while, in concentrations of 1 percent, it depressed the excitability and contractility of the striated muscle. Of the metabolic products of cocaine, ecgonine was a powerful depressant, while benzoylecgonine was mildly depressant. MacGregor (1939) found that cocaine reduced the strength of contractions in skeletal muscle when the muscle was stimulated by the nerve or when there was direct stimulation of the muscle after complete degeneration of the motor nerves. Cocaine also antagonized the contractions of denervated skeletal muscle to the intravenous injection of acetylcholine or nicotine. He suggested that cocaine reduced skeletal muscle contractility and excitability by its local anesthetic action on the motor nerve and the muscle itself and theorized that the stimulating effect of cocaine on muscular work was not the result of its action on striated muscle but, rather, the effect of stimulating the central nervous system.

Blood Vessels

It is a common clinical observation that cocaine constricts blood vessels when it is applied topically (Kuroda, 1915); but, in high systemic concentrations, cocaine may produce vasodilation (Kober 1882; Kuroda, 1915). For cocaine to produce sustained vasoconstriction, the sympathetic nervous system must be intact (Tatum, 1920; Crosby, 1939). Cocaine has no direct stimulating effect on aortic strips; but, in the presence of sufficient cocaine, the response to NE is potentiated. Cocaine in more concentrated solutions than 5×10^{-5}M does not result in further increase in the tone of the strips, and occasionally decreases the tone (Furchgott, 1955; Maxwell et al., 1962). In evaluating experiments of cocaine's effect on arterial vessels, it must be remembered that adrenergic nerve terminals are not distributed throughout the entire tissue as they are in other sympathetically innervated organs (Falck, 1962; Norberg and Hamberger, 1964; de la Lande and Waterson, 1967).

Heart

Cocaine has a mixture of both positive and negative ionotropic effects on the heart (Kuroda, 1915; MacGregor, 1939). Furchgott et al. (1963) studied the effects of cocaine on the left atria of guinea pigs and cats. Alone, cocaine produced no increase in contractile strength in normal cat atria, but it often did in normal guinea pig atria at concentrations of 10^{-5}M. This was interpreted as cocaine's having an ability to release NE in the guinea pig atria. Cat atria were much more sensitive to the depressing action of cocaine; and, at 10^{-5}M cocaine, a concentration well tolerated by guinea pig atria, cat atria exhibited a marked decrease in contractile force (partly due to conduction blocks) as well as an increase in the threshold for electrical stimulation. In both cat and guinea pig atria, cocaine at 10^{-6}M potentiated the effect of NE on contractile strength, while it antagonized the effect of tyramine. Cocaine also potentiated the ionotropic effect of sympathetic nerve stimulation in isolated rabbit atria (Huković, 1959).

Just as cocaine has a mixed ionotropic effect, it also appears to have both positive and negative chronotropic effects (Kuroda, 1915; MacGregor, 1939; Tsai et al., 1968). Cocaine potentiated the effects of NE and antagonized the effects of tyramine on the rate of contraction of spontaneously beating isolated guinea pig atria (Holtz, Osswald, and Stock, 1960). Trendelenburg's study in 1968 revealed that cocaine had three separate actions on the pacemaker of the isolated guinea pig atria: it released NE, caused supersensitivity to NE (by blocking reuptake), and it slowed spontaneous rate (this slowing was unmasked if the atria were pretreated with reserpine or exposed to propranolol or both). The resulting positive and negative chronotropic effects tended to mask each other since the dose response curves for all three actions were quite similar.

CENTRAL EFFECTS

As mentioned earlier, the mechanism of action of cocaine on the central nervous system is unknown. Cocaine may well have both a local anesthetic and sympathomimetic action on the central nervous system. Many feel that it is a central nervous system stimulant and has the ability to overcome the effects of fatigue. It is unclear whether cocaine is a stimulant or depressant of the central nervous system. Certainly it increases activity, increases respiratory rate, and stimulates vomiting. However, in large doses, it leads to depression of the medullary centers with hypotension and death from respiratory or cardiac arrest. It may well be that the spectrum of cocaine's effects on the central nervous system reflect varying degrees of depression. The apparent stimulating effects may represent depression of inhibitory neurons, while both the anticonvulsant properties (Tanaka, 1955) and the convulsant properties may indicate varying degrees of central nervous system depression. Finally, in evaluating cocaine's effects on the central nervous system, it should be stressed that cocaine's acute effects often differ from its chronic effects. For example, dosages of cocaine that do not produce convulsions following acute administration may produce convulsions after chronic administration (Gutierrez-Noriega and Zapata-Ortiz, 1944).

Electroencephalogram

In animals cocaine increased the multiple unit activity of the reticular formation (Wallach and Gershon, 1971) and produced desynchronization and an arousal effect on the electroencephalogram. The arousal effect was maintained when the brain stem was sectioned at the level of the middle pons but was abolished when the section was placed at the boundary between the pons and mesencephalon (Lux and Schmidt, 1964). The electroencephalographic pattern and clinical picture of cocaine-induced seizures in rats closely resembled temporal lobe epilepsy with the acute convulsive dose being 50 ± 5 mg/kg. At higher dosages the convulsions were often preceded by marked agitation, ataxia, or opisthotonus (Eidelberg, Lesse, and Gault, 1963).

Even less information is available on the seizure activity of cocaine in man. Stevens et al. (1969) gave 80 to 100 mg of cocaine by nasal insufflation to a patient with epilepsy. The patient had electrodes implanted in his temporal lobes from which slow high voltage (300 microvolts) spike and wave discharges were recorded, but there was no clinical evidence of seizures.

Body Temperature

Cocaine is known to increase activity and body temperature in animals (Barbour and Marshall, 1931; Barbour and Gilman, 1934; Dews, 1953). Peterson and Hardinge (1967) studied the effect of ambient temperature, grouping, and activity on cocaine toxicity in mice. Increasing the ambient temperature increased the number of mice dying probably as a result of less rapid heat loss. Grouping increased the activity and toxicity while exercise increased body temperature and toxicity of the mice treated with cocaine. In their study, death resulted either from hyperthermia or convulsions.

Psychological

For many years cocaine was known as a powerful stimulant of man's central nervous system. It was reputed to produce a brief euphoria and to reduce fatigue and was tried as an antidepressant by Freud (1884) and by Post et al. (1974). In higher doses or with chronic use, cocaine was reported to produce a psychosis characterized by clear sensorium; paranoid delusions; tactile, auditory and visual hallucinations; and stereotyped behavior. The psychosis resembled that induced by amphetamines and was quite similar to paranoid schizophrenia (Lewin, 1924; Snyder, 1972). Despite this, its effects on the central nervous system are poorly documented. It is a major drug of abuse but its addictive qualities are poorly described. The development of tolerance or a true withdrawal syndrome after chronic use has not been conclusively demonstrated. In fact, there is evidence of increasing sensitization to cocaine with repeated use, perhaps secondary to a decreased rate of metabolism, to an accumulation of the drug, or to alterations within the central nervous system. Much of the conflicting information about cocaine's psychological effect may represent differences in specie, dosage, and route and schedule of administration amongst the many animal studies.

Appetite

Cocaine has an anorexic effect in animals and humans (Freud, 1884; Balster and Schuster, 1973). Whether this is the sole cause of impaired growth rates in animals at high dosages is unclear. Downs and Eddy (1932) reported no effect on the growth rate of dogs that received daily injections of cocaine (50 mg/kg) by the subcutaneous route and no effect on the growth rates of growing rats that received cocaine (20 to 30 mg/kg) intraperitoneally. However, the rats had their growth rates impaired by repeated injections of cocaine in a dose of 75 mg/kg/day.

Self-administration

Cocaine can alter behavior that is maintained by other reinforcers (i.e., median forebrain bundle stimulation or food delivery) or it may act as a reinforcer itself. Animals can be easily trained to self-administer cocaine on a chronic basis. Downs and Woods (1974) compared the effects of codeine and cocaine as reinforcers for responding in rhesus monkeys. Cocaine was a more effective reinforcer of lever-pressing behavior than was codeine; the maximum response rate for cocaine was over 3½ times greater than the maximum response rate for codeine.

Alterations in the reinforcing schedule and treatment with other drugs can affect the rate of self-administration of cocaine in animals. There was an inverse relationship between the dosage per injection and the frequency of intravenous self-administration (Pickens and Thompson, 1968). Increasing the duration of cocaine infusion while the dose remained constant produced a change in the response rate which was similar to decreasing the unit dosage (Balster and Schuster, 1973). Animals that were self-administering cocaine tended to limit their daily access to cocaine in such a way as to maintain drug intake at a stable level. Wilson and Schuster (1972) demonstrated that pretreatment with chlorpromazine led to a significant increase in the frequency of self-administration of cocaine, but they were unable to determine a specific cause for this. Pretreatment with d-amphetamine or imipramine produced a dose-related decrease in cocaine self-administration. Morphine sulfate and pentobarbital had no effect on the self-administration of cocaine except when they were given in very high dosages that disrupted grooming and exploratory behaviors. In a related experiment, Hoffmeister and Goldberg (1973) looked at the effect of a number of drugs on the self-administration of cocaine in cocaine-dependent rhesus monkeys. Morphine sulfate, d-amphetamine, and cocaine injections maintained the self-administration behavior; however, chlorpromazine injections markedly suppressed self-administration behavior, while saline and imipramine produced responses in which there was a gradual decrease in the response rates.

Stereotypy

Cocaine can produce hyperactive behavior in animals and, in high doses, can produce stereotypic behavior. The latter behavior, characterized by repetitive movements, such as grooming or turning, may actually represent many different behaviors and may represent the action of cocaine on different pathways and neurotransmitters. Chlorpromazine and reserpine diminished the hyperactivity while atropine increased the hypermotility induced by cocaine. Other drugs, such as propranolol, morphine sulfate, and methysergide, had no effect on the behavioral toxicity of cocaine (Hatch and Fischer, 1972). Cocaine stereotypy can be blocked by reserpine and haloperidol but was only partially blocked when catecholamine synthesis was interrupted by alpha-methyl-para-tyrosine (Willner, Samach, Angrist, Wallach, and Gershon, 1970; Wallach and Gershon, 1972).

Tolerance and Withdrawal

There are conflicting reports as to whether or not tolerance develops from chronic cocaine use. At the turn of the century it was observed in man that chronic users might take 6 to 8 gm/day without serious toxicity. Whether this represented tolerance or individual resistance to cocaine was not clear. Experiments with the chronic administration of cocaine in animals did not demonstrate any tolerance and, in fact, there was evidence of increasing sensitivity to the effects of cocaine. This was characterized by hyperactivity, hyperthermia, and a decrease in the minimal convulsive and lethal dosages (Tatum and Seevers, 1929; Gutierrez-Moriega and Ortiz, 1944).

The early studies of the chronic administration of cocaine to animals failed to demonstrate a withdrawal syndrome. Post et al. (1974) did demonstrate REM rebound in humans following the sudden cessation of cocaine that had been administered by the oral route. Clearly, much work needs to be done in defining whether tolerance develops to cocaine and whether a true withdrawal syndrome results following the discontinuation of cocaine after chronic administration

CONCLUSION

As can be seen from this review many people have investigated the effects of coca leaves and cocaine in animals, yet much remains in understanding cocaine's central actions and its effect on behavior. Over the past year numerous investigators have begun to define these issues and to investigate the acute effects of cocaine in man. This chapter has been intended to provide a background upon which to judge this new information.

ACKNOWLEDGMENTS

This research was supported in part by the Burroughs-Wellcome Fund and by National Institute on Drug Abuse contract ADM 45-74-164.

We are grateful to Mary Ahern for typing and editorial assistance.

REFERENCES

Adriani, J.: The clinical pharmacology of local anesthetics, Clin. Pharmac. Ther. 1, 645-673 (1960).

Adriani, J. and Campbell, D.: Fatalities following topical application of local anesthetics to mucous membranes, J. Am. med. Ass. 162, 1527-1530 (1956).

Adriani, J. and Campbell, D.: The absorption of topically applied tetracaine and cocaine, Laryn. 68, 65-72 (1958).

Anitschkow, S.V. and Sarubin, A.A.: Über die Lokalisation der sensibilisierenden Wirkung des Kokains auf die Pupille, Arch. exp. Path. Pharmak. 131, 376-382 (1928).

Aschenbrandt, T.: Die physiologische Wirkung und Bedeutung des Cocain auf den menschilichen Organismus, Dt. med. Wschr. 50, 730-732 (1883).

Astrom, A. and Persson, N.H.: The toxicity of some local anesthetics after application on different mucous membranes and its relation to anesthetic action on the nasal mucosa of the rabbit, J. Pharmac. exp. Ther. 132, 87-90 (1961).

Balster, R.L. and Schuster, C.R.: Fixed interval schedule of cocaine reinforcement: Effect of dose and infusion duration, J. Exp. Analysis Behav. 20, 119-129 (1973).

Barbour, H.G. and Gilman, A.: Heat regulation and water exchange. XVII. The regulation of serum osmotic pressure to the onset of fever, J. Pharmac. exp. Ther. 50, 277-285 (1934).

Barbour, H.G. and Marshall, H.T.: Heat regulation and water exchange. XII. The underlying mechanism of fever as illustrated by cocaine poisoned rabbits, J. Pharmac. exp. Ther. 43, 147-162 (1931).

Berthold, E.: Zur Physiologischen Wirkung des Cocain, Zentbl. med. Wiss. 146 (1885).

Bevan, J.A. and Verity, M.A.: Sympathetic nerve-free vascular muscle J. Pharmac. exp. Ther. 157, 117-124 (1967).

Bishop, G.H.: Action of nerve depressants on potential, J. cell. comp. Physiol. 1, 177-194 (1932).

Blaschko, H., Himms, J.M., and Strömblad, B.C.R.: The enzyme hydrolysis of cocaine and alpha-cocaine, Br. J. Pharmac. 10, 442-444 (1955).

Blaustein, M.P. and Goldman, D.E.: Competitive action of calcium and procaine on lobster axon, J. gen. Physiol. 49, 1043-1063 (1966).

Bose, C.: Cocaine poisoning, Br. med. J. 1, 16-17 (1913).

Burn, J.H. and Tainter, M.L.: An analysis of the effect of cocaine on the actions of adrenaline and tyramine, J. Physiol. 71, 169-193 (1931).

Byck, R.: Cocaine Papers: Sigmund Freud. New York: Stonehill Publishing Co., 1975.

Campos, H.A., Stitzel, R.E., and Shideman, F.E.: Actions of tyramine and cocaine on catecholamine levels in subcellular fractions of the isolated cat heart, J. Pharmac exp. Ther. 141, 290-300 (1963).

Crosby, W.H.: The vasoconstrictor action of cocaine, J. Pharmac. exp. Ther. 65, 150-155 (1939).

de la Lande, I.S., Frewin, D., Waterson, J., and Canell, V.: Factors influencing supersensitivity to noradrenaline in the isolated perfused artery: Comparative effects of cocaine, denervation and serotonin, Circulation Res. 21, 177-181 (1967).

de la Lande, I.S. and Waterson, J.G.: Site of action of cocaine on the perfused artery, Nature 214, 313-314 (1967).

Dews, P.B.: The measurement of the influence of drugs on voluntary activity in mice, Br. J. Pharmac. Chemother. 8, 46-48 (1953).

Downs, A.W. and Eddy, N.B.: The effect of repeated doses of cocaine on the dog, J. Pharmac. exp. Ther. 46, 195-198 (1932a).

Downs, A.W. and Eddy, N.B.: The effect of repeated doses of cocaine on the rat, J. Pharmac. exp. Ther. 46, 199-200 (1932b).

Downs, D.A. and Woods, J.H.: Codeine- and cocaine-reinforced responding in rhesus monkeys: Effects of dose on response rates under a fixed-ratio schedule, J. Pharmac. exp. Ther. 191, 179-188 (1974).

Eggleston, C. and Hatcher, R.A.: A further contribution to the pharmacology of the local anesthetics, J. Pharmac. exp. Ther. 13, 433-487 (1919).

Eidelberg, E., Lesse, H., and Gault, F.P.: An experimental model of temporal lobe epilepsy: Studies of the convulsant properties of cocaine. In: EEG and Behavior. Glaser, G.H., Ed., pp. 272-283. New York: Basic Books, 1963.

Eisenfeld, A.J., Axelrod, J., and Krakoff, L.: Inhibition of the extra-neuronal accumulation and metabolism of norepinephrine by adrenergic blocking agents, J. Pharmac. exp. Ther. 156, 107-113 (1967).

Falck, B.: Observations on the possibilities of the cellular localization of monoamines by a fluorescence method, Acta physiol. Scand. 56, 1-25 (1962).

Feinberg, J.: Zur Cocainwirkung, Berl. klin. Wschr. 23, 52-54 (1886).

Fekete, M. and Borsy, J.: Chlorpromazine-cocaine antagonism: Its relation to changes of dopamine metabolism in the brain, Eur. J. Pharmacol. 16, 171-175 (1971).

Fish, F. and Wilson, W.D.C.: Excretion of cocaine and its metabolites in man, J. Pharm. Pharmac. 21, 135S-138S (1969).

Fleckenstein, A. and Stöckle, D.: Zum Mechanismus der Wirkungs-Verstärkung und Wirkungs-Abschwächung sympathomimetischer amine durch Cocaine und andere Pharmaka, Archs. exp. Path. Pharmak. 224, 401-415 (1955).

Freud, S.: Uber Coca, Zentbl. Ther. 2, 289-314 (1884).

Frölich, A. and Loewi, O.: Über eine Steigerung der Adrenalinempfindlichkeit durch Cocaine, Archs. exp. Path. Pharmak. 62, 159-169 (1910).

Furchgott, R.F.: The pharmacology of vascular smooth muscle, Pharmac Rev. 7, 183-265 (1955).

Furchgott, R.F., Kirpekar, S.M., Rieker, M., and Schwab, A.: Actions and interactions of norepinephrine, tyramine and cocaine on aortic strips of rabbit and left atria of guinea pig and cat, J. Pharmac. exp. Ther. 142, 39-58 (1963).

Fuxe, K., Hamberger, B., and Malmfors, T.: The effect of drugs on accumulation of monoamines in tubero-infundibular dopamine neurons, Eur. J. Pharmacol. 1, 334-341 (1967).

Gasser, H.S. and Erlanger, J.: Role of fibre size in establishment of nerve block by pressure or cocaine, Am. J. Physiol. 88, 581-591 (1929).

Glick, D. and Glaubach, S.: The occurrence and distribution of atropinesterase, and the specificity of tropinesterases, J. gen. Physiol. 25, 197-205 (1941).

Glowinski, J. and Axelrod, J.: Effects of drugs on the uptake, release and metabolism of ^{3}H-norepinephrine in the rat brain, J. Pharmac. exp. Ther. 149, 43-49 (1965).

Gold, H.: The seat of the mydriatic action of cocaine, J. Pharmac. exp. Ther. 23, 365-372 (1924).

Green, R.D. and Fleming, W.W.: Agonist-antagonist interactions in the normal and supersensitive nictitating membrane of the spinal cat, J. Pharmac. exp. Ther. 156, 207-214 (1967).

Green, R.D. and Fleming, W.W.: Analysis of supersensitivity in the isolated spleen of the cat, J. Pharmac. exp. Ther. 162, 254-262 (1968).

Gutierrez-Noriega, C.: Accion de la Cocaina sobre la Resistencia a la Fatiga en el Perro, Revta Med. exp. 3, 329-340 (1944).

Gutierrez-Noriega, C. and Ortiz, V.Z.: Cocainismo Experimental. I. Toxicologia General, Acostumbramiento y Sensibilizacion, Revta Med. exp. 3, 279-306 (1944).

Hammond, W.A.: Coca, Tri. med. Soc. Va. 212-226 (1885).

Hardinge, M.G. and Peterson, D.I.: Effect of forced exercise on body temperature and amphetamine toxicity, J. Pharmac. exp. Ther. 145, 47-51 (1964).

Harrison, P.W.: Intravenous use of cocaine, Boston med. surg. J. 114, 151 (1911).

Hatch, R.C. and Fischer, R.: Cocaine-elicited behavior and toxicity in dogs pretreated with synaptic blocking agents, morphine, or diphenylhydantoin, Pharmac. Res. Commun. 4, 383-392 (1972).

Hertting, G., Axelrod, J., and Whitby, G.: Effect of drugs on the uptake and metabolism of H^3-norepinephrine, J. Pharmac. exp. Ther. 134, 146-153 (1961).

Hirschfelder, A.D. and Bieter, R.N.: Local anesthetics, Physiol. Rev. 12, 190-282 (1932).

Hoffmeister, F. and Goldberg, S.R.: A comparison of chlorpromazine, imipramine, morphine and d-amphetamine self-administration in cocaine-dependent rhesus monkeys, J. Pharmac. exp. Ther. 187, 8-14 (1973).

Holtz, P., Osswald, W., and Stock, K.: Über die Beeinflussung der Wirkungen Sympathicomimetischen amine durch Cocain und Reserpin, Archs. exp. Path. Pharmak. 239, 14-28 (1960).

Huković, S.: Isolated rabbit atria with sympathetic nerve supply, Br. J. Pharmac. Chemother. 14, 372-376 (1959).

Innes, I.R. and Mailhot, R.: Effect of cocaine on the affinity of α-adrenoceptors for noradrenaline, Br. J. Pharmac. 48, 139-143 (1973).

Kalsner, S. and Nickerson, M.: Mechanism of cocaine potentiation of responses to amines, Br. J. Pharmac. 35, 428-439 (1969).

Knapp, S. and Mandell, A.J.: Narcotic drugs: Effects on the serotonin biosynthetic systems of the brain, Science 177, 1209-1211 (1972).

Knoefel, P.K., Herwick, R.P., and Loevenhart, A.S.: The prevention of acute intoxication from local anesthetics, J. Pharmac. exp. Ther. 39, 397-411 (1930).

Kobert, E.R.: Ueber den Einfluss Verschiedener pharmakologischer Agentien auf die Muskelsubstanz, Arch. exp. Path. Pharmak. 15, 22-80 (1882).

Koller, C.: Über die Verwendung des Cocain zur Anästhesierung am Auge, Weiner med. Wschr. 34, Nos. 43 and 44 (1884).

Koppanyi, T.: Action of sympathomimetic drugs on pupil of guinea pig, Proc. Soc. exp. Biol. Med. 26, 80 (1928).

Koppanyi, T.: Studies on pupillary reactions in tetrapods. VII. Sympathetic actions of cocaine, procaine and pilocarpine, J. Pharmac. exp. Ther. 38, 113-119 (1930).

Koppanyi, T. and Feeney, G.C.: Newly found action of cocaine, Science 129, 151-152 (1959).

Kubota, S. and Macht, D.I.: Concerning the action of local anesthetic on striated muscle, J. Pharmac. exp. Ther. 13, 31-44 (1919).

Kuroda, M.: On the action of cocaine, J. Pharmac. exp. Ther. 7, 423-439 (1915).

Langer, S.Z., Draskoczy, P.R., and Trendelenburg, U.: Time course on the development of supersensitivity to various amines in the nictitating membrane of the pithed cat after denervation or decentralization, J. Pharmac. exp. Ther. 157, 255-273 (1967).

Lawrence, W.S., Morton, M.C., and Tainter, M.L.: Effects of cocaine and sympathomimetic amines on humoral transmission of sympathetic nerve actions, J. Pharmac. exp. Ther. 75, 219-225 (1942).

Lewin, L.: Phantastica, Narcotic and Stimulating Drugs, Their Use and Abuse. New York: E.P. Dutton and Co., 1931.

Lewis, J.E. and Miller, J.W.: The use of tritiated phenoxybenzamine for investigating receptors, J. Pharmac. exp. Ther. 154, 46-55 (1966).

Limbourg, P.: Kritische und experimentelle Untersuchungen die Irisbewegungen und über den Einfluss von Giften auf dieselben, besonders des Cocaine, Arch. exp. Path. Pharmak. 30, 93-125 (1892).

Lindmar, R. and Muscholl, E.: Die Wirkung von Cocain, Guanethidin, Reserpin, Hexamethonium, Tetracain und Psicain auf die Noradrenaline-Freisetzung aus dem Herzen, Arch. exp. Path. Pharmak. 242, 214-227 (1961).

Luco, J.V., Eyzaguirre, C., and Perez, F.: Effects of amphetamine and cocaine on neuromuscular function, J. Pharmac. exp. Ther. 93, 261-272 (1948).

Lux, H.D. and Schmidt, G.: Hirnelektrische Untersuchungen ueber die Wirkungen von Cocain und Pseudococain, Naunyn-Schmiedeberg's, Arch. exp. Path. Pharmak. 246, 452-468 (1964).

MacGregor, D.F.: The action of procaine and of cocaine on mammalian skeletal muscle, J. Pharmac. exp. Ther. 66, 350-365 (1939).

Maengwyn-Davies, G.D. and Koppanyi, T.: Cocaine tachyphylaxis and effects on indirectly-acting sympathomimetic drugs in the rabbit aortic strip and in splenic tissue, J. Pharmac. exp. Ther. 154, 481-492 (1966).

Mattison, J.B.: Cocaine poisoning, Med. surg. Rep. Boston Cy. Hosp. 65, 645-650 (1891).

Maxwell, R.S., Daniel, A.I., Sheppard, H., and Zimmerman, J.H.: Some interactions of guanethedine, cocaine, methylphenidate and phenylalkylamines in rabbit aortic strips, J. Pharmac. exp. Ther. 137, 31-38 (1962).

Maxwell, R.A., Wastila, W.B., and Eckhardt, S.B.: Some factors determining the response of rabbit aortic strips to dl-norepinephrine-7-H^3 hydrochloride and the influence of cocaine, guanethidine and methylphenidate on these factors. J. Pharmac. exp. Ther. 151, 253-261 (1966).

Mayer, E.: The toxic effects following the use of local anesthetics, J. Am. med. Ass. 82, 876-885 (1924).

McIntyre, A.R.: Renal excretion of cocain in a case of acute cocain poisoning, J. Pharmac. exp. Ther. 57, 133 (1936).

Morison, R.S. and Acheson, G.H.: A quantitative study of the effects of acetylcholine and adrenalin on the nictitating membrane, Am. J. Physiol. 121, 149-156 (1938).

Mortimer, W.G.: Peru History of Coca, The Divine Plant of the Incas, with an Introductory Account of the Incas and of the Andean Indians of Today. New York: J.H. Vail and Co., 1901.

Muscholl, E.: Effect of cocaine and related drugs on the uptake of noradrenaline by heart and spleen, Br. J. Pharmac. Chemother. 16, 352-359 (1961).

Musto, D.F.: The American Disease: Origins of Narcotic Control. New Haven: Yale University Press, 1973.

Nayak, P.K., Misra, A.L., and Mulé, E.J.: Physiologic disposition and metabolism of [^{3}H]-cocaine in the rat, Fed. Proc. 33, 527 (1974).

Nielsen, C. and Higgins, J.A.: Safety of local anesthetics, with particular reference to cocaine and butyn, J. Lab. clin. Med. 8, 440-453 (1923).

Norberg, K-A. and Hamberger, B.: The sympathetic adrenergic neuron, Acta Physiol. Scand. 63(238), 1-42 (1964).

Orr, D. and Jones, I.: Anaesthesia for laryngoscopy, Anaesthesia 23, 194-202 (1968).

Peterson, D.I. and Hardinge, M.G.: The effect of various environmental factors on cocaine and ephedrine toxicity, J. Pharm. Pharmac. 19, 810-814 (1967).

Pickens, R. and Thompson, T.: Cocaine-reinforced behavior in rats: Effects of reinforcement magnitude and fixed-ratio size, J. Pharmac. exp. Ther. 161, 122-129 (1968).

Post, R.M., Gillin, J.C., Wyatt, R.J., and Goodwin, F.K.: The effect of orally administered cocaine on sleep of depressed patients, Psychopharmacologia 37, 59-66 (1974).

Post, R.M., Kotin, J., and Goodwin, F.K.: The effects of cocaine on depressed patients, Am. J. Psychiat. 131 (5), 511-517 (1974).

Ritchie, J.M. and Cohen, P.J.: Local anesthetics. In: The Pharmacological Basis of Therapeutics. Goodman, L.S. and Gilman, A., Eds., 5th edition, pp. 379-403. New York: Macmillan, 1975.

Ritchie, J.M. and Greengard, P.: On the mode of action of local anesthetics, Ann. Rev. Pharmacol. 6, 405-430 (1966).

Ritter, C.: Total anaesthesia by injection of cocain into the veins (Abstract) J. Am. med. Ass. 54, 822 (1910).

Rosenblueth, A.: The action of certain drugs on the nictitating membrane, Am. J. Physiol. 100, 443-446 (1932).

Ross, E.L.: Toxicity of cocain as influenced by rate of absorption and presence of adrenalin, J. Lab. clin. Med. 8, 656-661 (1923).

Ross, S.B. and Renyi, A.L.: Uptake of some tritiated sympathomimetic amines by mouse brain cortex slices in vitro, Acta Pharmac. Tox. 24, 297-309 (1966).

Ross, S.B. and Renyi, A.L.: Accumulation of tritiated 5-hydroxytryptamine in brain slices, Life Sci. 6, 407-1415 (1967).

Scheppegrell, W.: The abuse and dangers of cocaine, Med. News, N.Y. 73, 417-422 (1898).

Schmitz, H.L. and Lovenhart, A.S.: A comparative study of the local anesthetic properties of P-amino benzoyl di-iso-propyl amino ethanol hydrochloride ("isocaine"), cocaine, procaine and butyn, J. Pharmac. exp. Ther. 24, 167-177 (1924).

Schultz, P.: Ueber die Wirkungsweise der Mydriaca und Miotica, Arch. Psyiol. 23, 47-74 (1898).

Schumacker, H.B., Jr.: Reactions to local anesthetic agents. II. A clinical report, Surgery, 134-144 (1941).

Segawa, T., Kuruma, I., Takatsuka, K., and Takagi, H.: The influences of drugs on the uptake of 5-hydroxytryptamine by synaptic vesicles of rabbit brain stem, J. Pharm. Pharmac. 20, 800-801 (1968)

Shriver, D.A. and Long, J.P.: A pharmacologic comparison of some quaternary derivatives of cocaine, Archs. int. Pharmacodyn. Thér. 189, 198-208 (1971).

Simmonds, M.A. and Gillis, C.N.: Uptake of normetanephrine and norepinephrine by cocaine-treated rat heart, J. Pharmac. exp. Ther. 159, 283-289 (1968).

Snyder, S.H.: Catecholamines in the brain as mediators of amphetamine psychosis, Arch. gen. Psychiat. 27, 169-179 (1972).

Sollman, T.: A Manual of Pharmacology. Pp. 251-291. Philadelphia: W.B. Saunders, 1917.

Somlyo, A.V., Woo, C-Y., and Somlyo, A.P.: Responses of nerve-free vessels to vasoactive amines and polypeptides, Am. J. Physiol. 208, 748-753 (1965).

Steinhaus, J.E. and Tatum, A.L.: An experimental study of cocaine intoxication and its treatment, J. Pharmac. exp. Ther. 100, 351-361, (1950).

Stevens, J.R., Mark, V.H., Erwin, F., Pacheco, P., and Suematsu, K.: Deep temporal stimulation in man, long latency, long lasting psychological changes, Arch. Neurol. 21, 157-169 (1969).

Strichartz, G.R.: The inhibition of sodium currents in myelinated nerve by quaternary derivatives of lidocaine, J. gen. Physiol. 62, 37-57 (1973).

Suzuki, Y., Fukazawa, H., Yano, U., and Sakai, M.: Study on shock resulting from stimulation of the palatine area by cocaine and its prophylaxis in guinea pigs, Keijo J. Med. 17, 217-228 (1968).

Tainter, M.L. and Chang, D.K.: The antagonism of the pressor action of tyramine by cocaine, J. Pharmac. exp. Ther. 30, 193-207 (1926).

Tanaka, K. (introduced by Goodman, L.S.): Anticonvulsant properties of procaine, cocaine, adiphenine and related structures, Proc. Soc. exp. Biol. Med. 90, 192-195 (1955).

Tatum, A.L.: A study of the action of cocaine on the splanchnic and cervical sympathetic neuromuscular mechanisms, J. Pharmac. exp. Ther. 16, 109-123 (1920).

Tatum, A.L., Atkinson, A.J., and Collins, K.H.: Acute cocaine poisoning, its prophylaxis and treatment in laboratory animals, J. Pharmac. exp. Ther. 26, 325-335 (1925).

Tatum, A.L. and Collins, K.H.: Acute cocaine poisoning and its treatment in the monkey (Macacus Rhesus), Arch. int. Med. 38, 405-409 (1926).

Tatum, A.L. and Seevers, M.H.: Experimental cocaine addiction, J. Pharmac. exp. Ther. 36, 401-410 (1929).

Taylor, R.E.: Effect of procaine on electrical properties of quid axon membrane, Am. J. Physiol. 196, 1071-1078 (1959).

Teeters, W.R., Koppanyi, T., and Cowan, F.F.: Cocaine tachyphylaxis, Life Sci. 7, 509-518 (1963).

Thompson, J.W.: Studies on the responses of the isolated nictitating membrane of the cat, J. Physiol. 141, 46-72 (1958).

Torda, C.: Effect of cocaine on the inactivation of epinephrine and sympathin, J. Pharmac. exp. Ther. 78, 331-335 (1943).

Trendelenburg, U.: The supersensitivity caused by cocaine, J. Pharmac. exp. Ther. 125, 55-65 (1959).

Trendelenburg, U.: Modification of the effect of tyramine by various agents and procedures, J. Pharmac. exp. Ther. 134, 8-17 (1961a).

Trendelenburg, U.: The action of acetylcholine on the nictitating membrane of the spinal cat, J. Pharmac. exp. Ther. 135, 39-44 (1961b).

Trendelenburg, U.: Supersensitivity and subsensitivity to sympathomimetic amines, Pharmac. Rev. 15, 225-276 (1963).

Trendelenburg, U.: I. Mechanisms of supersensitivity and subsensitivity to sympathomimetic amines, Pharmac. Rev. 18, 629-640 (1966).

Trendelenburg, U.: The effect of cocaine on the pacemaker of isolated guinea pig atria, J. Pharmac. exp. Ther. 161, 222-231 (1968).

Tsai, T.H., Denham, S., and McGrath, W.R.: Sensitivity of the isolated nictitating membrane of the cat to norepinephrine and acetylcholine after various procedures and agents, J. Pharmac. exp. Ther. 164, 146-157 (1968).

van Euler, U.S.: Action of adrenaline, acetylcholine and other substances on nerve-free vessels (human placenta), J. Physiol., Lond. 93, 129-143 (1938).

von Anrep, B.: Ueber die physiologische Wirkung des Cocain, J. Med. Chir. Pharmac., Brux. 70, 373-377 (1880).

Waddell, J.A.: The effects of strychnine, cocaine, and quinine on the vas deferens, J. Pharmac. exp. Ther. 9, 279-286 (1917).

Wallach, M.B. and Gershon, S.: A neuropsychopharmacological comparison of d-amphetamine, L-dopa and cocaine, Neuropharmacol. 10, 743-752 (1971).

Wallach, M.B. and Gershon, S.: The induction and antagonism of central nervous system stimulant-induced stereotyped behavior in the cat, Eur. J. Pharmacol. 18, 22-26 (1972).

Weidmann, S.: Effects of calcium ions and local anesthetics on electrical properties on purkinje fibres, J. Physiol., Lond. 129, 568-582 (1955).

Whitby, L.G., Hertting, G., and Axelrod, J.: Effect of cocaine on the disposition of noradrenaline labelled with tritium, Nature 187, 604-605 (1960).

Willner, J.H., Samach, M., Angrist, B.M., Wallach, M.B., and Gerson, S.: Drug-induced stereotyped behavior and its antagonism in dogs, Commun. behav. Biol. 5, 135-141 (1970).

Wilson, M.D. and Schuster, C.R.: The effects of chlorpromazine on psychomotor stimulant self-administration in the rhesus monkey, Psychopharmacologia 26, 115-126 (1972).

Woods, J.H. and Downs, D.A.: The psychopharmacology of cocaine, prepared for the National Commission on Marihuana and Drug Abuse, 1974.

Woods, L.A., Cochin, H., Forenfeld, E.J., McMahon, F.G., and Seevers, M.H.: The estimation of amines in biological materials with critical data for cocaine and mescaline, J. Pharmac. exp. Ther. 101, 188-199 (1951a).

Woods, L.A., McMahon, F.G., and Seevers, M.H.: Distribution and metabolism of cocaine in the dog and rabbit, J. Pharmac. exp. Ther. 101, 200-204 (1951b).

Wurtman, R.J., Axelrod, J., and Patter, L.T.: The disposition of catecholamines in the rat uterus and the effect of drugs and hormones, J. Pharmac. exp. Ther. 144, 150-155 (1964).

Yamamoto, I., Mikami, K., and Kurogochi, Y.: The enzymic breakdown of cocaine by the rabbit liver, Jap. J. Pharmac. 3, 39-49 (1953).

NEURAL SUBSTRATES MEDIATING AMPHETAMINE RESPONSES

Susan D. Iversen

Department of Psychology

Downing Street, Cambridge, England

In a range of species amphetamine produces highly characteristic changes in behaviour. Rats have been studied most intensively, and in this species low doses (1.5mg/kg) of d-amphetamine induce a persistent running or locomotor behaviour. Higher doses (5mg/kg) lead to a disruption of motor behaviour, described as stereotyped, in which elements of the normal motor repertoire, such as sniffing, rearing, licking, biting and gnawing, are repeated in both abnormal order and frequency. In practical terms these behaviours are easy to quantify; and, very largely for this reason, amphetamine has often been selected as the "model" drug in experiments designed to elucidate the modes of action of stimulants.

The interest in amphetamine is strengthened by the observation in man that, as well as general stimulatory action, large doses of the drug also induce stereotyped behaviour. As in the rat, the behavioural elements which are repeated abnormally tend to be those with a high normal probability of occurrence in that individual: in other words behaviours which by choice, habit or social convention are favoured by that individual. Rylander (1969) has described these phenomena in Swedish Preludin addicts and coined the term punding. The behaviours are clearly motor. Individuals pace back and forth and move their mouths from side to side. More highly organized patterns of motor behaviour are also seen. Women sort their handbags again and again, or tidy up their flats whether they need tidying or not. Individuals with a mechanical bent dismantled and put together again complicated machines, for example, clocks. In man, stereotypy is associated with chronic drug usage and, as Ellinwood (1967) pointed out, is seen only in addicts who develop a more generalised psychosis which shows a virtually identical clinical picture to that seen in paranoid schizophrenia. The striking similarity of the behavioural responses in animals and man encourages the view that in studying amphetamine we shall learn more of the basic mechanisms essential for stimulant action in the brain.

For almost as long as it has been known that there are catecholamine neurotransmitters in the brain, it has been surmised that amphetamine interacts with them. Accumulated evidence (Glowinski and Baldessarini, 1966) indicates that amphetamine influences the uptake, release, and metabolism of brain noradrenaline (NA) and dopamine (DA). Amphetamine interacts with both NA and DA, and the majority of biochemical and pharmacological tools for manipulating brain levels of amines also influences, at least to a degree, both neurotransmitters. It has proved difficult, therefore, with neuropharmacological approaches, to determine if one or other of the amines plays a more central role in the mediation of the behavioural effects of the drug. Our approach to this problem was dictated by the discovery that NA and DA are localized to different forebrain projections (Fig. 1).

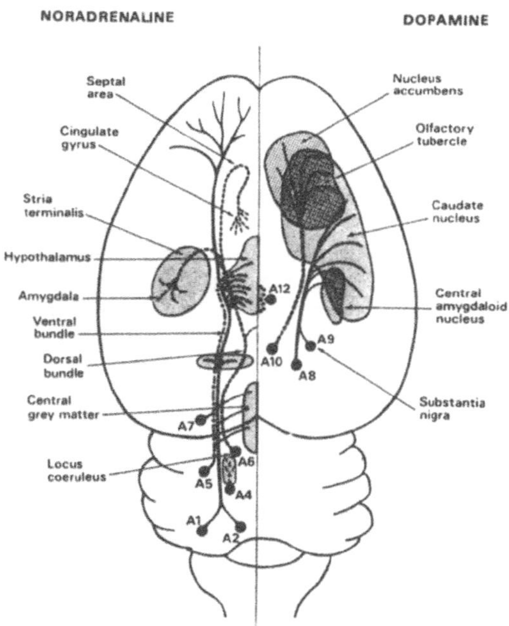

Fig. 1. Horizontal representation of ascending NA and DA pathways in the rat brain. Modified from Ungerstedt (1971).

These findings made it possible, with lesion techniques, to search for the critical sector of the catecholamine forebrain innervation essential for the behavioural effects of amphetamine. The original interest in the DA systems was dictated by the straightforward observation that two of the most characteristic effects of amphetamine, notably locomotor stimulation and stereotypy, are motor behaviours; and, therefore, likely to involve parts of the nervous system associated with the control of movement. The innervation of the striatum by DA neurones arising from the substantia nigra (SN: cell groups A8 and 9) provided the initial focus for our studies.

METHODS

6-OHDA Lesion Technique

Some workers have used electrolytic lesions to destroy the amine-containing pathways. More recently, we have favoured the intracerebral injection of 6-hydroxydopamine (6-OHDA) to achieve selective damage of amine pathways. 6-OHDA is taken up by a high affinity uptake mechanism, and destroys NA- and DA-containing neurones. It is usually injected into brain regions containing the cell bodies of the amine neurones or their terminal innervations but is also taken up by axons traversing a site of local injection and can be effectively administered by intra-ventricular injection. Intraperitoneal pretreatment of the animal with pargyline before the lesion increases the uptake of 6-OHDA into both DA and NA neurones and results in more complete damage to both amine systems. Pretreatment with desipramine (DMI) may be used to protect NA neurones from the effects of 6-OHDA (Breese and Traylor, 1971), as it is known to inhibit specific uptake processes in NA but not DA neurones. Our particular surgical technique involves the injection of 6-OHDA in doses of 8μg in 2μl of injection fluid, infused at 1μl/min through a 30 gauge cannula at stereotaxically-defined sites in the brain. The merits of various doses of 6-OHDA and injection volumes have been extensively argued (Agid, Javoy, Glowinski, Bovet, and Sotelo, 1973; Sotelo, Javoy, Agid, and Glowinski, 1973). We select our particular dosage as one which achieves the maximum damage of amine neurones associated with a minimal amount of non-specific damage at the injection site.

Behavioural Testing

At various times after 6-OHDA lesions, the response of the animals were tested to drugs which are known, or thought, to interact with amine receptors in the brain. Locomotor activity is measured in a bank of wire cages, each with two horizontal photocell beams along the long axis. The cages were contained in a room which was masked with white noise and maintained at 22°C. Non-cumulative recordings of photocell beam interruptions were taken every 10 min in each experimental session. Prior to any drug manipulations the animals were habituated to the photocell cages for 30 min and spontaneous locomotor activity was recorded. Following amphetamine administration locomotor activity was recorded for 2 hr, and following apomorphine it was recorded for 90 min. Beam interruptions by locomotor activity are reliably recorded. However, stereotypy is inconsistently recorded and may yield high or low counts depending on the physical location of the rat in relation to the photocell and the amount of concurrent locomotor activity. It is, therefore, important to combine photocell recording of amphetamine responses with direct observation. Accordingly the nature of the response being repeated and the degree of repetition were assessed by means of a rating scale, previously developed from observations of the behaviour of normal rats exposed to increasing doses of amphetamine.

0 - asleep or stationary
1 - active
2 - predominantly active with bursts of stereotyped sniffing or rearing
3 - stereotyped activity, predominantly sniffing and rearing over a large area of the cage
4 - stereotyped behaviour maintained in one location, usually directed to the floor of the cage
5 - stereotyped behaviour in one location with bursts of gnawing or licking
6 - continual gnawing or licking of the cage bars

Stereotypy ratings for each animal were made immediately after the number of photocell beam interruptions for the preceding 10 min had been recorded.

RESULTS

The Early 6-OHDA Lesion Studies

In 1972 Creese and Iversen reported that bilateral 6-OHDA lesions to the substantia nigra (cell groups A8 and 9 in Fig. 1) markedly attenuated intense forms of stereotyped behaviour normally induced by iproniazid treatment followed by 5mg/kg d-amphetamine. The lesions resulted in an 85-90% loss of striatal DA as assessed by a radiochemical tyrosine hydroxylase assay (Hendry and Iversen, 1971). Disappointingly, the lesion did not attentuate the locomotor stimulation induced by 1.5mg/kg d-amphetamine. Indeed, during the first hour after the drug, when the maximum stimulation is observed in normal rats, the SN-lesioned rats showed an enhanced response (Fig. 2). It was true that during the second hour the response in the SN-lesioned animals was reduced but, it was argued, this second hour after a dose of 1.5mg/kg d-amphetamine, rats characteristically continue to show running behaviour; but this is associated with the milder forms of stereotypy, principally rearing and sniffing. This combination of behaviours tends to sustain the high number of photocell interruptions recorded during the second hour after the drug. It was argued that the lower counts recorded in the SN-lesioned rats reflected an attenuation of the normal stereotypy pattern seen at this dose and was thus in keeping with the results obtained with the higher dose of amphetamine. In retrospect it seems that this interpretation may be questioned. Sniffing and rearing, the responses which are commonly stereotyped after low doses of amphetamine, appear not to be mediated via the striatal DA system (Kelly, Seviour, and Iversen, 1975) but by the neural substrate serving locomotor behaviour. It seems more likely

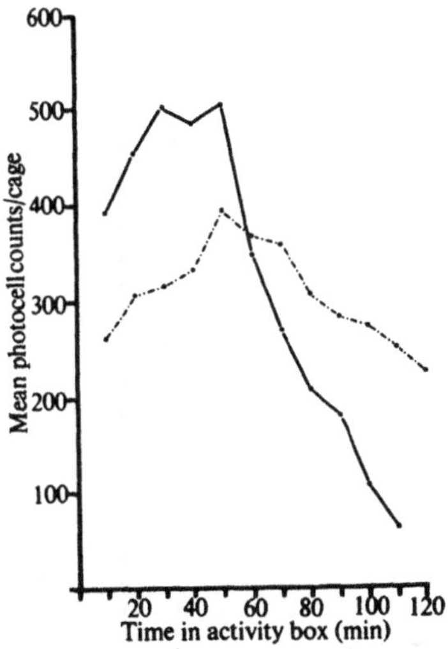

Fig. 2. Mean locomotor response to 1.5mg/kg d-amphetamine in rats with bilateral 6-OHDA lesions to the substantia nigra and sham controls. The responses were averaged for three test sessions on different days and the saline response subtracted. ●——● , lesions in S. nigra; ●----● , controls.

that the partial lesion to the forebrain DA systems mediating locomotor behaviour results in supersensitivity of the post synaptic receptor and leaves the remaining terminals more readily depleted by indirect acting sympathomimetic amines, such as amphetamine. These two factors may explain the initially enhanced response to amphetamine followed by a more rapid decrease of the behavioural response as the damaged terminal sites are depleted of their remaining DA content.

Subsequently Creese was able to show that a virtually total lesion of the forebrain DA system (as indicated by a striatal tyrosine hydroxylase value of 0.4% of control levels) resulted in blockade of both the locomotor stimulation and the intense forms of stereotyped responding normally induced by high doses of amphetamine (Fig. 3) (Creese and Iversen, 1975).

Further Localization of Amphetamine Effects

At this time we noted findings of Pijnenburg and van Rossum (1973): that DA injected directly into the nucleus accumbens (NAS) induced locomotor behaviour, but intrastriatal injections did

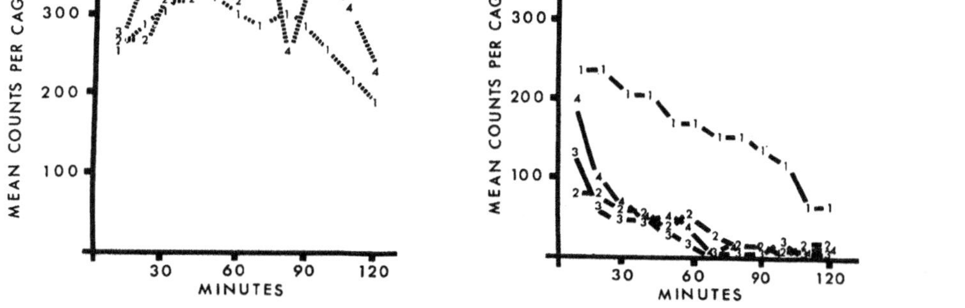

Fig. 3. Mean photocell beam interruptions/10 min for the sham-operated and the 7 complete SN-lesioned rats to 1.5mg/kg d-amphetamine recorded on days 3, 14, 22 and 33 postoperation. The characteristic locomotor activity response to amphetamine was abolished in the SN-lesioned rats.

not. This made us consider the possible pattern of forebrain DA loss we had induced with total SN lesions. A successful lesion to the SN (cell groups A8 and 9) probably also involved the origins of mesolimbic DA systems in the nearby A10 neurones. To prove this point, it was decided to selectively damage bilaterally the DA terminals in either the nucleus accumbens (NAS), a principal terminal site of the mesolimbic DA projection, or the caudate nucleus. In rats with these selective 6-OHDA lesions it has been possible to demonstrate a dissociation of drug induced locomotor stimulation and intense amphetamine-induced stereotyped behaviour (Kelly et al., 1975). At 14 days after surgery, NAS lesions prevented the locomotor response and associated rearing and sniffing seen after 1.5 mg/kg d-amphetamine (Fig. 4, left). It could be suggested that this combination of behavioural elements normally mediates investigative behaviour in the rat. At the same time DA agonists, such as apomorphine, induced a greatly enhanced amount of these behaviours (Fig. 4, right). By contrast, the caudate lesions prevented the intense forms of stereotypy (such as licking, biting, gnawing) induced by 5mg/kg of amphetamine. Under our testing conditions

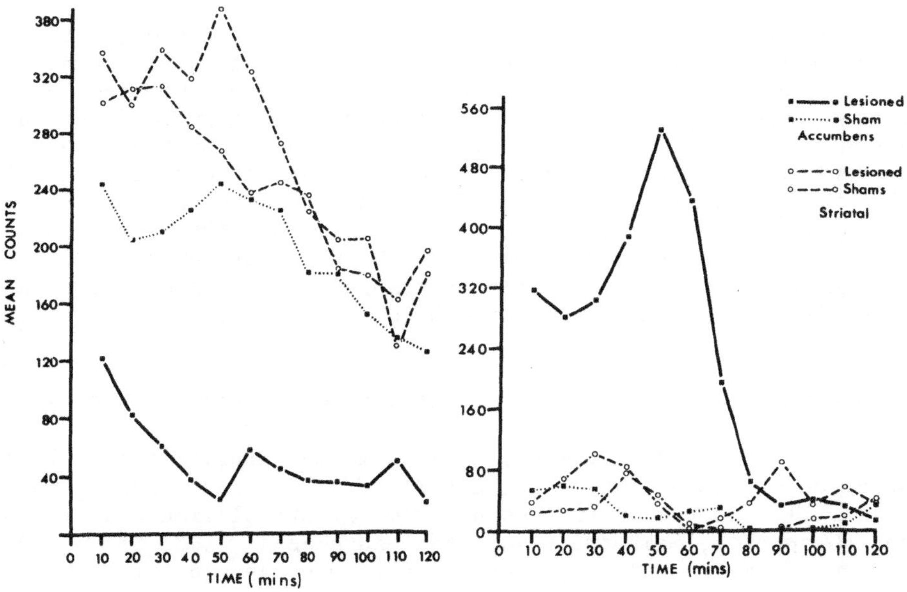

Fig. 4. Left: Locomotor activity response to 1.5mg/kg d-amphetamine on postoperative day 14. Mean photocell beam interruptions per 10 min for caudate and nucleus accumbens 6-OHDA lesioned rats and their sham-operated controls. Right: Locomotor activity response to 1.0mg/kg apomorphine on postoperative day 10: mean photocell beam interruptions per 10 min for caudate and nucleus accumbens 6-OHDA lesioned rats and their sham-operated controls.

these behavioural elements were persistently directed to the floor of the cage.

Does NA Play Any Role in Amphetamine Stimulation?

Biochemical and neuropharmacological approaches have provided equivocal evidence for a role of NA in one or other apsect of psychomotor stimulation. Lesion studies are unequivocal. Direct bilateral lesions to either the dorsal or ventral NA bundles did not block either locomotor response or stereotyped behaviour induction by amphetamine (Creese and Iversen, 1975). We, therefore, had no reason to believe that the results in NAS-lesioned animals could be attributed to the 89% loss of cortical NA observed in those animals (Kelly et al., 1975). However, if the NAS-lesioned preparation was to be a model of any general value for studying drugs which interacted with DA receptors, it was essential to produce a NAS-lesioned preparation without this unwanted NA loss. Peter Kelly achieved this by pretreating the rats with pargyline and DMI i.p. 30 min before the NAS lesion was made.

A summary of these biochemical results is presented in Table 1. In both the pargyline and pargyline + DMI pretreated animals, the locomotor response to 1.5mg/kg d-amphetamine was blocked to the same degree and the response to apomorphine enhanced (Iversen and Kelly, 1975). The DA depletion was virtually identical in the two preparations, whereas NA depletion was prevented by the additional DMI pretreatment. It is therefore reasonable to ascribe the blocked amphetamine response to loss of DA rather than NA. The fact that NA neurones can be protected by DMI pretreatment, which is known to inhibit a high affinity membrane uptake process, speaks further for the selectivity of the 6-OHDA lesion technique.

The Effect of Lesions to Amine Pathways on Cocaine Responses

Cocaine, like amphetamine, is a stimulant drug. It has similar biochemical effects, inhibiting uptake of amines and stimulating release. It induces in rats both locomotor stimulation and stereotypy (Groppetti, Sambott, Biazi, and Mantegazza, 1973; Simon, 1973). Furthermore, in man it also induces excitement and in large doses results in stereotyped responding as a part of a more generalized psychosis (Snyder, 1972).

We have tested cocaine responses in several of our preparations. Firstly, Creese and Iversen (1975) found that the locomotor response to 20mg/kg of cocaine was markedly attenuated after total lesions to the SN (Fig. 5). More recently, Kelly tested the NAS-lesioned rats with 20mg/kg cocaine. Both the pargyline <u>and</u> pargyline + DMI

TABLE 1

Effect of Pargyline or Pargyline + DMI Pretreatment on DA and NA Depletion Produced by 6-OHDA Lesions to the NAS

GROUP	DOPAMINE (μg/g)			NORADRENALINE (μg/g)
	Olfactory tubercle	Nucleus accumbens	Striatum	Forebrain
Sham (n = 6)	5.97 ± 0.45	7.90 ± 0.63	8.86 ± 0.74	0.27 ± 0.04
Parg. 6-OHDA (n = 7)	1.58 ± 0.44**(26)	0.71 ± 0.26**(9)	7.05 ± 0.37*(80)	0.04 ± 0.01**(15)
Parg. DMI 6-OHDA (n = 5)	1.25 ± 0.74**(21)	0.57 ± 0.39**(7)	7.93 ± 1.48(90)	0.26 ± 0.04(96)

*$p \leq 0.025$, **$p \leq 0.001$ compared to sham

Figures in parentheses indicate the values of the lesioned animals as a percentage of those of the controls. DA and NA levels were measured with a radio enzymatic method (Cuello, Hiley, and Iversen, 1973).

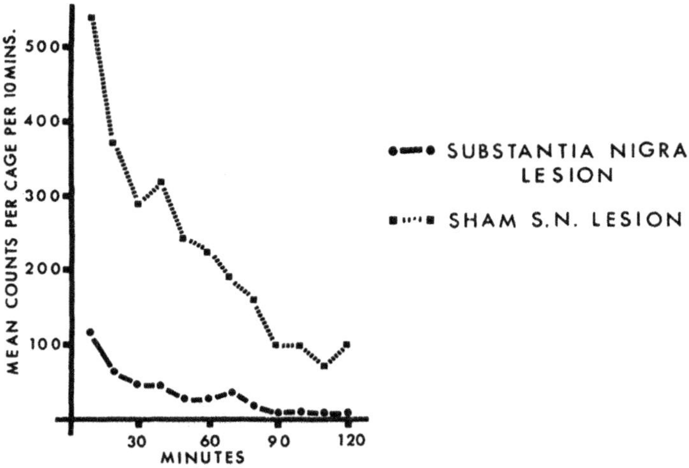

Fig. 5. Mean photocell beam interruptions/10 min for the 7 complete SN-lesioned rats and sham-operated controls to 20mg/kg cocaine.

pretreated NAS-lesioned groups showed a significant block of the cocaine response (Fig. 6). Thus, again, we can argue that DA rather than the NA loss is the likely explanation for these results in the NAS preparation. The absolute scores and the degree of attenuation of the cocaine response obtained with the SN and the NAS lesions are strikingly similar, again suggesting that the damage to the mesolimbic DA system is the common feature of these two lesion techniques resulting in the blockage of stimulant motor effects. Thus the effects of cocaine and amphetamine on motor behaviour are attenuated by the same patterns of DA depletion suggesting that both of these stimulants interact with the same neural substrate.

Practical Implications of Localization Studies

DA synaptic interactions clearly play a central role in stimulant activity. The localization of the DA synapses mediating the various aspects of stimulant activity is of both academic and practical interest. Stimulant-induced psychosis in man resembles certain forms of paranoid schizophrenia (Snyder, 1972) and the most effective anti-schizophrenic or anti-psychotic drugs are potent DA receptor blocking agents. Clearly DA antagonists will interact

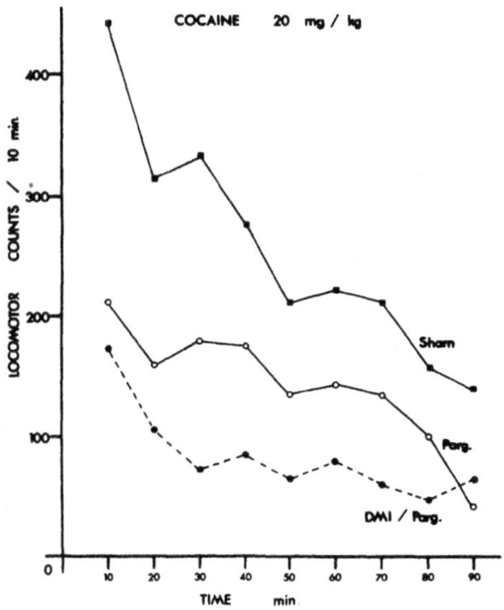

Fig. 6. Mean photocell beam interruptions/10 min Pargyline + 6-OHDA NAS lesions, Pargyline + DMI NAS lesions and sham-operated controls to 20mg/kg cocaine. N = 6 in each group.

with all DA receptors but it is now suggested that differently located DA receptors may vary in their responsiveness to certain classes of anti-dopaminergic drugs.

Unilateral damage to the nigro-striatal pathways in the rat results in a preparation which shows stereotyped circling to one or other direction depending on whether the intact DA terminals or the contralateral supersensitive receptors are stimulated by sympathomimetic amines (Ungerstedt and Arbuthnott, 1970). This model system provided a useful way of quantifying the classical DA antagonists, such as chlorpromazine; the more recently developed butyrophenones, such as haloperidol, spiroperidol and pimozide; and the very potent DA antagonists of the thiozanthene class, such as α-flupenthixol (Kelly and Miller, 1975). However, the novel antipsychotic clozapine and the phenothiazine thioridazine were unable to block circling behaviour. Both of these neuroleptics have anti-muscarinic (Anden and Stock, 1973; Miller and Hiley, 1974) as well as anti-dopaminergic properties, and it is suggested that the additional anti-muscarinic effects on the striatum prevent the DA antagonist action resulting in the predicted behavioural effect (Kelly and Miller, 1975).

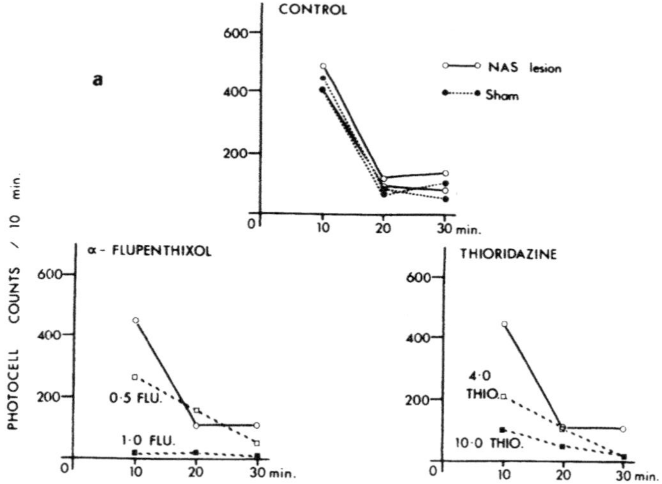

Fig. 7a. Spontaneous locomotor activity during 30 min habituation in NAS-lesioned and sham-operated controls (upper graph) compared with habituation in same animals after treatment with 0.5 and 1.0mg/kg α-flupenthixol (bottom left) and 4.0 and 10.0mg/kg thioridazine (bottom right).

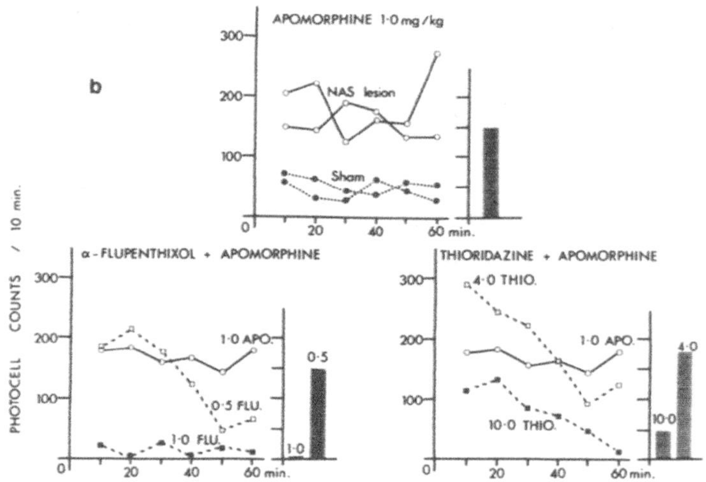

Fig. 7b. Locomotor response to 1.0 mg/kg apomorphine in NAS-lesioned and sham-operated controls (upper graph) run on two independent days during the series of drug treatments. The effects of α-flupenthixol and thioridazine on the apomorphine response in NAS-lesioned animals are shown in the lower figures. The bars to the right of the figures indicate the mean stereotypy rating seen at the peak of the apomorphine response.

We have begun to explore the supersensitive NAS preparation as a model system for comparing and quantifying DA antagonist action. The ability of various neuroleptics to block the enhanced response to apomorphine has been studied. In these experiments a group of NAS-lesioned rats prepared by Dr. Kelly were used. They had been pretreated with pargyline and DMI before the NAS lesion was made and at assay were found to have the NAS DA terminals depleted to 18% of control values. Our usual behavioural methods were used to obtain these results and the rats were injected i.p. with the neuroleptics 2 hr before the 30 min habituation run. Apomorphine (1μg/kg) was then given and behaviour measured for 1 hr.

So far, it appears that the typical and novel antipsychotics behave in this system in an equivalent manner. Although thioridazine and clozapine induce only minimal catalepsy and weakly antagonize amphetamine-induced stereotypy (Costall and Naylor, 1975), they, and the typical neuroleptics, markedly reduce spontaneous locomotor activity (Fig. 7 left). Furthermore, if these drugs are used to block the supersensitive response of the NAS preparation to apomorphine, then again all the neuroleptics are found to be capable of blocking the locomotor response (Fig. 7 right).

These results, although of a preliminary nature, suggest that the mesolimbic DA preparation may be a useful one for identifying neuroleptic agents with potential antipsychotic activity. The currently favoured anti-schizophrenia drugs, like thioridazine and clozapine, do not produce extrapyramidal side effects in patients (Cole and Clyde, 1961; Burki, Ruck, Asper, Baggiolini, and Stille, 1973). Presumably, their antimuscarinic effects on the striatum counter their anti-dopaminergic action. If this reasoning is correct, their antipsychotic action must be mediated by effects on DA receptors outside the striatum. The mesolimbic DA terminals are an obvious site of such an action.

REFERENCES

Agid, Y., Javoy, F., Glowinski, J., Bovert, D. and Sotelo, C.: Injection of 6-hydroxydopamine into the substantia nigra of the rat. II. Diffusion and specificity, Brain Res. 58, 291-301 (1973).

Anden, N.E. and Stock, G.: Effect of clozapine on the turnover of dopamine in the corpus striatum and in the limbic system, J. Pharm. Pharmac. 25, 346-348 (1973).

Breese, G.R. and Traylor, T.D.: Depletion of brain noradrenaline and dopamine by 6-hydroxydopamine, Br. J. Pharmacol. 42, 88-89 (1971).

Burki, H.R., Rush, W., Asper, H., Baggiolini, N. and Stille, G.: Pharmakologische und neurochemische wirkungen von clozapin. Neue Gesichtspunkte in der medikamentosen Behandlung der Schizophrenie, Schweiz. med. Wschr. 103, 1716-1724 (1973).

Cole, J.O. and Clyde, D.J.: Extrapyramidal side effects and clinical response to the phenothiazines, Revue Can. Biol. 20, 565-574 (1961).

Costall, B. and Naylor, R.J.: Detection of the neuroleptic properties of clozapine, sulpiride and thioridazine, Psychopharmacologia 43, 69-74 (1975).

Creese, I. and Iversen, S.D.: Amphetamine response after dopamine neurone destruction, Nature New Biol. 238, 247-248 (1972).

Cuello, A., Hiley, R. and Iversen, L.L.: Use of catechol-O-methyltransferase for the enzyme radiochemical assay of dopamine, J. Neurochem. 21, 1337-1340 (1973).

Ellinwood, E.H.: Amphetamine psychosis: I. Description of the individuals and process, J. nerv. ment. Dis. 144, 273-283 (1967).

Glowinski, J. and Baldessarini, R.J.: Metabolism of norepinephrine in the central nervous system, Pharmac. Rev. 18, 1201-1238 (1966).

Groppetti, A., Zambotti, F., Biazzi, A. and Mantegazza, P.: Amphetamine and cocaine on amine turnover. In: Frontiers in Catecholamine Research. Usdin, E. and Snyder, S.H., Eds., pp. 917-925. Oxford: Pergamon Press, 1973.

Hendry, I.A. and Iversen, L.L.: Effect of nerve growth factor and its antiserum on tyrosine hydroxylase activity in mouse superior cervical sympathetic ganglion, Brain Res. 29, 159-162 (1971).

Iversen, S.D. and Kelly, P.H.: The use of 6-hydroxydopamine (6-OHDA) techniques for studying the pathways involved in drug-induced motor behaviours. In: Chemical Tools in Catecholamine Research. New York: Elsevier, in press.

Kelly, P.H. and Miller, R.J.: The interaction of neuroleptic and muscarinic agents with central dopaminergic systems, Br. J. Pharmacol. 54, 115-121 (1975).

Kelly, P.H., Seviour, P.W. and Iversen, S.D.: Amphetamine and apomorphine responses in the rat following 6-OHDA lesions of the nucleus accumbens septi and corpus striatum, Brain Res. 94, 507-522 (1975).

Miller, R.J. and Hiley, C.R.: Antimuscarinic properties of neuroleptic drugs and drug induced parkinsonism, Nature, Lond. 248, 596-597 (1974).

Pijnenburg, A.J.J. and van Rossum, J.M.: Stimulation of locomotor activity following injection of dopamine into the nucleus accumbens, J. Pharm. Pharmac. 25, 1003-1005 (1973).

Rylander, G.: Clinical and medico-criminological aspects of addictions to central stimulating drugs. In: Abuse of Central Stimulants. Sjoquist, F. and Tottie, M., Eds., pp. 251-273. New York: Raven Press, 1969.

Simon, P.: Psychopharmacological profile of cocaine. In: Frontiers of Catecholamine Research. Usdin, E. and Snyder, S.H., Eds., pp. 1043-1044. Oxford: Pergamon Press, 1973.

Snyder, S.H.: Catecholamines in the brain as mediators of amphetamine psychosis, Arch. gen. Psychiat. 27, 169-179 (1972).

Sotelo, C., Javoy, F., Agid, Y. and Glowinski, J.: Injection of 6-hydroxydopamine in the substantia nigra of the rat. I. Morphological study, Brain Res. 58, 269-290 (1973).

Ungerstedt, U.: Stereotaxic mapping of the monoamine pathway in the rat brain, Acta Physiol. Scand. 83, Suppl. 367, 49-68 (1971).

Ungerstedt, U. and Arbuthnott, G.: Quantitative recording of rotational behaviour in rats after 6-OH dopamine lesions of the rat nigrostriatal dopamine system, Brain Res. 24, 486-493 (1970).

MESOLIMBIC AND EXTRAPYRAMIDAL SITES FOR THE MEDIATION OF STEREOTYPED BEHAVIOUR PATTERNS AND HYPERACTIVITY BY AMPHETAMINE AND APOMORPHINE IN THE RAT

Brenda Costall and Robert J. Naylor

Postgraduate School of Studies in Pharmacology

University of Bradford, Bradford, West Yorkshire, England

In small laboratory animals, amphetamine and amphetamine-like drugs induce a spectrum of behavioural changes characterised mainly by stereotyped behaviour and an increase in activity (Randrup and Munkvad, 1967). These behavioural changes have been the centre of many studies to determine the site of action of amphetamine-like agents in the brain. These studies have basically employed the brain lesion technique, assuming that disruption of a discrete area essentially required to mediate a certain behavioural effect will lead to an abolition of that behaviour, and the intracerebral injection technique to induce the behaviour from the "essential" area. This approach would appear correct and logical but has, instead of clarifying hypotheses on the site of amphetamine action, led to massive confusion in the literature. However, a careful review of the data would indicate that most discrepancies are in definitions and methodology. It is, therefore, our intention in this chapter to examine the literature related to the site of stimulant drug action in the brain, with particular reference to amphetamine and apomorphine and the stereotyped behaviour patterns and hyperactivity induced by these agents in the rat, in an attempt to clarify many of the discrepancies in the available data and to formulate acceptable hypotheses on cerebral sites mediating the effects of stimulant drugs. We make one basic assumption, that amphetamine and apomorphine mediate their behavioural effects via cerebral dopamine, but in so doing we do not exclude a role for other neurotransmitter substances.

DEFINITION OF "STEREOTYPED BEHAVIOUR"

In early studies the stereotyped behaviour patterns of "sniffing, licking, biting, or gnawing" induced by amphetamine and related agents in the rat were tacitly assumed to represent a single expression of drug action (Fog, 1972). Recent work, however, has clearly indicated that there are at least two distinct components of stereotyped behaviour. At lower doses, amphetamine induces a behaviour characterised entirely by repetitive head and limb movements and sniffing, but as the dose is increased, biting/gnawing/licking become apparent and eventually dominate (Costall and Naylor, 1974). This could be considered in terms of increased stimulation of the same receptor sites, but that the two behaviours are distinct was clearly indicated by the introduction of agents that could preferentially induce one or the other component. Thus, amantadine, phenylethylamine, and piribedil will induce sniffing and repetitive head and limb movements but even very large doses fail to induce the intense gnawing syndrome (Braestrup, Anderson, and Randrup, 1975; Costall and Naylor, 1973a, 1975a). Conversely, the behaviour induced by (-)N-n-propylnorapomorphine is characterised almost entirely by stereotyped gnawing and biting (Costall, Naylor, and Neumeyer, 1975a). Further, the two stereotypic components can be differentiated pharmacologically (amantadine inhibits the biting component; α-methylparatyrosine inhibits the sniffing; see Costall and Naylor, 1975a; Cox and Tha, 1973; and Hackman, Pentikäinen, Neuroven, and Vapaatalo, 1973) and by lesions of the different dopamine-containing nuclei of the extrapyramidal and mesolimbic areas (see Table 1). Therefore, the basic essential of any study on stereotyped behaviour is the selection of suitable doses and a clear definition of the nature of the behaviour recorded.

THE ROLE OF THE NEOSTRIATUM IN THE MEDIATION OF STEREOTYPED BEHAVIOUR PATTERNS

Results of studies attempting to ablate the neostriatum by surgical means are varied. This may simply reflect variations in size of the lesion since the remaining tissue could retain some functional capacity (see Glick, 1976). In order to induce more "specific" lesions of this area, we have recently employed the 6-hydroxydopamine technique.

The injection of 16 μg 6-hydroxydopamine into the "centre" or "head" of the neostriatal complex, which caused falls in neostriatal dopamine content of 55-65%, significantly reduced or abolished the gnawing, biting, and licking components of amphetamine stereotypy (Fig. 1). The maximum inhibition was recorded between the 4th and 10th postoperative days but after this time the biting response

TABLE 1

Differentiation of the Sniffing and Biting Components of the Stereotypic Effects of d-Amphetamine and Apomorphine by Electrolesions of Extrapyramidal and Mesolimbic Nuclei

	Lesion location									
	Caudate-putamen		Globus pallidus		Central amygdaloid nucleus		Tuberculum olfactorium		Nucleus accumbens	
	Sniffing	Biting	Sniffing	Biting	Sniffing	Biting	Sniffing	Biting	Sniffing	Biting
Apomorphine	0	0	R/A	R/A	0	R/A	R/A	R/A	R/A	0
d-Amphetamine	0	0	R/A	R/A	0	R/A	R/A	0	0	0

0 = no effect; R/A = reduction or abolition depending on dose and time after surgery
See also Costall and Naylor (1973a, 1974).

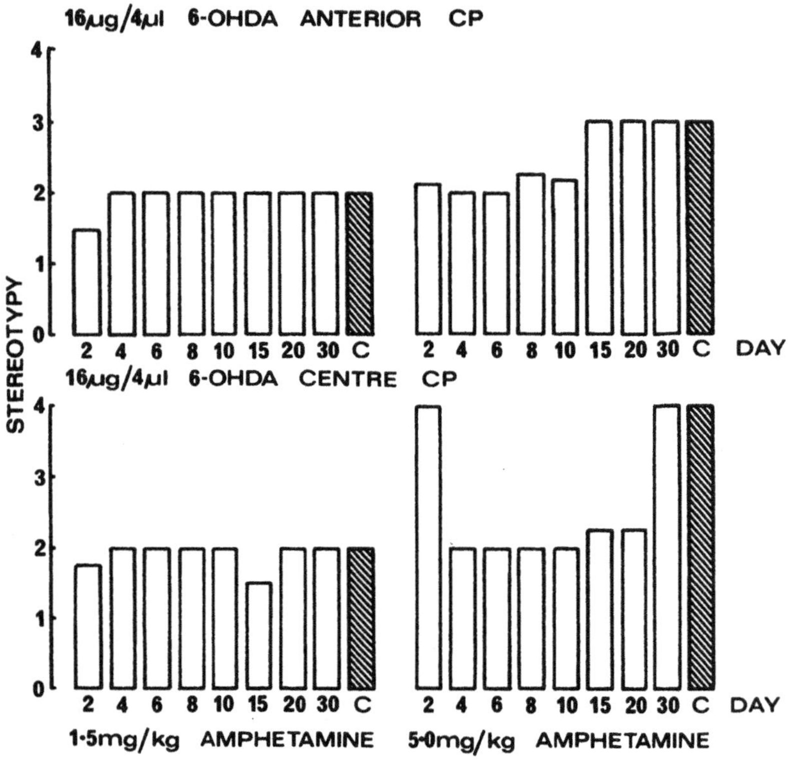

Fig. 1. Changes in the stereotyped behaviour patterns induced by d-amphetamine after the bilateral injections of 16 μg/4 μl 6-hydroxydopamine (4 μg/1 μl over 4 min) into the centre of the caudate-putamen (Ant. 8.0, Vert. + 1.5, Lat. ± 3.0) or into the anterior portion of the caudate-putamen (Ant. 9.0, Vert. + 1.5, Lat. ± 2.5) (De Groot, 1959). Stereotyped behaviour was assessed on Days 2-30 following the injections on a simple system: 0 = no stereotypy; 1 = periodic sniffing; 2 = continuous sniffing; 3 = periodic biting; 4 = continuous biting. 1.5 mg/kg d-amphetamine was selected as a dose inducing reliable score 2 sniffing behaviour and 5.0 mg/kg as a dose normally inducing continuous biting scored 5 (see control values, C, hatched columns). Each value given is the mean of responses from 6-12 rats. Standard errors are within 14% of the means. The injections of 6-hydroxydopamine into the centre of the caudate-putamen depleted striatal dopamine by 55%, but did not significantly reduce dopamine levels in the tuberculum olfactorium, nucleus accumbens, or central amygdaloid nucleus. The 6-hydroxydopamine lesions of the anterior caudate-putamen reduced striatal dopamine by 65%, but also reduced dopamine in the nucleus accumbens by 40%, although dopamine levels in the tuberculum olfactorium and amygdala were not significantly reduced. Details of the biochemistry are forthcoming (Costall, Marsden, Naylor, and Pycock, unpublished data).

again developed and it is tempting to suggest that this is indicative of the compensatory capacity of the brain. It is emphasised that at no time were the stereotyped sniffing and head and limb movements reduced by these lesions.

Kelly, Seviour, and Iversen (1975b) and Creese and Iversen (1974) have recorded similar results following the injection of 8 μg 6-hydroxydopamine into the caudate-putamen. In their studies the biting and licking responses to amphetamine were attenuated by this lesion although sniffing and rearing still developed. These authors conclude that dopamine in the caudate-putamen is essential for amphetamine to induce "intense stereotypy"; we suggest that this intense stereotypy may be more precisely termed the biting/licking component of the stereotypic response to amphetamine. Asher and Aghajanian (1974) also report an abolition of the biting/licking response to amphetamine after the injection of 40 μg 6-hydroxydopamine into the head of the caudate-putamen while, again, animals continued to exhibit "marked sniffing activity in conjunction with their exploratory activities" (p. 8). But these authors did not categorise this sniffing behaviour as stereotyped and concluded that amphetamine stereotypy is mediated in total via the dopamine projection to the head of the caudate nucleus.

From these data it may be argued that a greater depletion of neostriatal dopamine is required to inhibit the sniffing response than to inhibit biting. However, we have found that injections of up to 64 μg 6-hydroxydopamine into the caudate-putamen failed to inhibit sniffing; and injections of 6-hydroxydopamine into the substantia nigra, which markedly reduce the striatal dopamine content, also fail to reduce sniffing behaviour even though biting is abolished (Creese and Iversen, 1972; Fibiger, Fibiger, and Zis, 1973). As such, the results obtained using the 6-hydroxydopamine technique indicate that a nigrostriatal dopamine projection is essentially concerned with the amphetamine biting and licking syndrome but not with the stereotyped sniffing response.

In contrast to these studies many authors have found that electrolesions of the neostriatum fail to reduce the intensity of any component of amphetamine stereotypy (Costall and Naylor, 1974; Divac, 1972; Neill, Boggan, and Grossman, 1974; Yehuda and Wurtman, 1975). It would appear improbable that this failure reflects the inability of electrolesions to deplete striatal dopamine for, in many experiments, the extent of the lesions was greater than when using 6-hydroxydopamine. Similar difficulties underlie an explanation of the failure of electrolytic nigral lesions to reduce amphetamine stereotypy (Costall, Naylor, and Olley, 1972b; Iversen, 1971; Simpson and Iversen, 1971). While Creese and Iversen (1975) and Price and Fibiger (1974) have pointed out how unsuccessful this lesion procedure is with respect to striatal dopamine depletion, others have shown that electrolesions of the substantia nigra can produce reliable, extensive, and far more selective depletions of striatal dopamine than the 6-hydroxydopamine technique (Costall et al., 1975a; Faull and Laverty, 1969; Koob, Balcom, and Meyerhoff, 1975). We have no explanation as to why an electrolesion of the substantia nigra which produces an 80% fall in striatal dopamine fails to reduce amphetamine stereotypy, whereas a fall of 50% induced by intrastriatal 6-hydroxydopamine is effective. Further, it is difficult to appreciate why, if amphetamine is initiating its biting response at a striatal site, the intrastriatal administration of amphetamine fails to elicit this behaviour (Costall, Naylor, and Olley, 1972a; Costall, Naylor, and Pinder, 1974) when intrastriatal dopamine can itself induce biting (Costall et al., 1974; Fog and Pakkenberg, 1971) and, presumably, amphetamine is acting via dopamine in this brain area.

While amphetamine is generally considered to act via presynaptic dopamine mechanisms, apomorphine is thought to mediate its stereotypic effects via a direct stimulation of dopamine receptors, again, within the neostriatum (Fuxe and Ungerstedt, 1970). However, similarly to amphetamine, electrolesions of the caudate-putamen have failed to reduce apomorphine stereotypy (Costall and Naylor, 1973c; Divac, 1972; Wolfarth, 1974; Wolfarth, Grabowska, Lacki, Dulska, and Antkiewicz, 1973). If this reflects the incomplete nature of the destruction, with functional receptor sites remaining, then why have electrolesions of the substantia nigra (which may deplete striatal dopamine by at least 70%, but presumably leave all receptor sites intact) been shown to reduce apomorphine stereotypy? (Baum, Etevenon, Piarroux, Simon, and Boissier, 1971; Costall et al., 1972b). Further, if the concept of dopamine receptors developing supersensitivity after 6-hydroxydopamine lesions is correct, then why have many workers found difficulty in demonstrating a supersensitivity to apomorphine after such lesions? For example, the gross manipulation of cerebral catecholamines by intraventricular injections of 6-hydroxydopamine has produced varying effects: Schoenfeld and Uretsky (1972) abolished apomorphine gnawing by this treatment (even an exceptionally large dose of 10 mg/kg was ineffective), although they observed a "modified stereotypy" that consisted of rats "running back and forth and 'wall climbing'" (p. 116). Since the dose required to produce a "modified stereotypy" was only half that required to produce a stereotyped response in normal animals, the authors rather surprisingly concluded that the dopamine receptor is more sensitive to apomorphine as a consequence of 6-OHDA treatment. In a similar experiment Jalfre and Haefely (1971) concluded that the doses of apomorphine that produced compulsive gnawing in 6-hydroxydopamine-treated rats were not different from those required in control rats (although there was actually a clear trend for apomorphine to be less effective in the 6-hydroxydopamine-lesioned rats), but they also noted that the 6-hydroxydopamine-treated rats were drastically excited at doses which failed to modify the behaviour of normal rats. Creese and Iversen (1973), however, using neonatal rats, showed an increased sensitivity to both the locomotor and stereotypic activity of apomorphine.

Similar difficulties have been encountered in studies using more discrete locations of 6-hydroxydopamine. Ungerstedt (1971) has reported that rats injected with 6-hydroxydopamine into the substantia nigra (a procedure which is now known to disrupt mesolimbic as well as extrapyramidal dopamine systems) developed a "furious compulsive gnawing . . . far more violent than after the same dose [5 mg/kg] of apomorphine administered to a normal animal" (p. 108). However, with the use of this supramaximal stereotypic dose, it is difficult to accept Ungerstedt's interpretation that "the operated animals were more sensitive to apomorphine than normal animals" (p. 111), which he attributed to a supersensitivity of the denervated receptor. Creese and Iversen (1975) have also placed 6-hydroxydopamine into the substantia nigra and have stated that "the substantia nigra-lesioned rats were behaviourally supersensitive to apomorphine" (p. 419), although the increased sensitivity was <u>not</u> of the main component of the apomorphine behavioural syndrome, the biting or gnawing, but was almost entirely limited to a more restricted sniffing or rearing activity. In contrast, Loew and Vigouret (1975) have <u>reduced</u> apomorphine stereotypy by 6-hydroxydopamine lesions of the nigra.

Injections of 6-hydroxydopamine into the striatum have been equally unsuccessful. Asher and Aghajanian (1974) concluded that apomorphine produced the "normal" stereotyped responses after neostriatal injections of 6-hydroxydopamine. Creese and Iversen (1974, 1975) report that similar lesions exaggerated the stereotyped response to apomorphine but the increase in response was very small and indicated as a more restricted sniffing behaviour. Further, we have shown that injections of 6-hydroxydopamine into the anterior portion or centre of the caudate-putamen not merely failed to enhance any component of apomorphine stereotypy, but the anterior injections temporarily reduced the biting response to 1 mg/kg s.c. apomorphine, a dose just sufficient to induce a maximal effect in normal rats (the doses used by the above workers were inappropriate to demonstrate this effect). Also, the biting response to intrastriatal apomorphine (Costall et al., 1974; Ernst and Smelik, 1966; Fuxe and Understedt, 1970) was not enhanced in rats that had been previously subjected to intrastriatal 6-hydroxydopamine (Costall and Naylor, unpublished observations).

We consider that the studies of Ungerstedt (1971), Schoenfeld and Uretsky (1972), Jalfre and Haefely (1971), and Creese and Iversen (1973) indicate that 6-hydroxydopamine treatment alters the nature of the response to apomorphine (i.e., increased locomotion, sniffing, aggression) but does not lead to the development of supersensitivity of those dopamine receptors that mediate the major component of the apomorphine effect, the biting response. Such studies would thus question the assumption that it is neostriatal dopamine receptors that primarily become supersensitive after 6-hydroxydopamine since those components of the apomorphine behaviour that are enhanced after 6-hydroxydopamine are now known to be mediated to a large extent via mesolimbic dopamine mechanisms. Further, a consideration of these findings in terms of dopamine alone may be misleading. Using the circling model, we have shown that 6-hydroxydopamine can not only render a dopamine-containing area more sensitive to dopamine itself, but can cause changes in the receptor specificity such that a typical dopamine response may be induced by other neurotransmitter substances that are normally inactive in this respect, in particular by noradrenaline and 5-hydroxytryptamine (Costall, Naylor, and Pycock, in press, b) (Table 2). Both these neurotransmitters have been shown to play a critical role in the actions of amphetamine and apomorphine, and it is important to note that, in all the studies reporting supersensitivity to apomorphine after 6-hydroxydopamine, this lesion also lowered forebrain noradrenaline levels. In our own studies (Fig. 2) we have also found that a marked increase in sensitivity to the biting response of apomorphine is observed when the 6-hydroxydopamine location leads to changes in noradrenaline as well as in dopamine, for example, locations in the lateral hypothalamus to interrupt the medial forebrain bundle and just anterior to the substantia nigra.

THE ROLE OF THE PALEOSTRIATUM IN THE MEDIATION OF STEREOTYPED BEHAVIOUR PATTERNS

The importance of the paleostriatum, as distinct from the neostriatum, for the induction of stereotyped responses has been emphasised by a number of experiments carried out in these laboratories. First, discrete electrolesions of the globus pallidus have been shown to markedly reduce or abolish all components of the stereotyped behaviour induced by many dopamine agonists, including amphetamine and apomorphine (Costall and Naylor, 1975c). It has been argued that these results simply reflect a deafferentation of the striatum (Randrup, Munkvad, and Scheel-Krüger, 1973), and certainly a vast number of fibres passing to and from the caudate do traverse the area of the pallidum, but the pallidal tissue itself is very sensitive to intracerebrally applied drug, and apomorphine and amphetamine are more potent in this area than in the neostriatum itself in inducing stereotyped biting responses (Bergmann, Chaimovitz, Pasternak [Na'or], and Ramu, 1974; Costall et al., 1972a; Ernst and Smelik, 1966). Further, 6-hydroxydopamine applied to the paleostriatum has been shown to cause marked changes in stereotyped biting behaviour (Fig. 3). These injections initially enhanced the stereotypic effects of both apomorphine and amphetamine but, after the 6th to 8th postoperative days, the biting normally induced by both

TABLE 2

Changes in Sensitivity and Specificity of Responses to Unilateral Intrastriatally Administered Drug after Unilateral 6-Hydroxydopamine Lesion of the Medial Forebrain Bundle in the Lateral Hypothalamus

Intrastriatal Injection	Dose (μg/1 μl)	Contralateral asymmetry/circling (scored)			
		6-OHDA lesion		No lesion	
Dopamine	100	(8/8)	2-3	(8/8)	1
	50	(3/8)	2-3	(0/8)	0
	25	(0/8)	0	(0/8)	0
Apomorphine	25	(8/8)	1-3	(0/8)	0
	12.5	(6/8)	1-2	(0/8)	0
Noradrenaline	100	(8/8)	2-3	(0/8)	0
	50	(8/8)	2-3	(0/8)	0
	25	(8/8)	2-3		
	12.5	(7/8)	2-3		
	6.25	(2/8)	3		
5-Hydroxy-tryptamine	100	(8/8)	3	(0/8)	0
	50	(8/8)	2-3	(0/8)	0
	25	(8/8)	2-3		
	12.5	(0/8)	0		

Asymmetries/circling were scored on the system 0 = no asymmetry/circling; 1 = periodic holding of the head and neck to contralateral side, contralateral movements of body when disturbed; 2 = constant holding of head and neck to contralateral side, contralateral circling when disturbed; 3 = intense twisting of head and body to contralateral side, periods of spontaneous contralateral circling.
The number of rats responding is shown in parentheses.

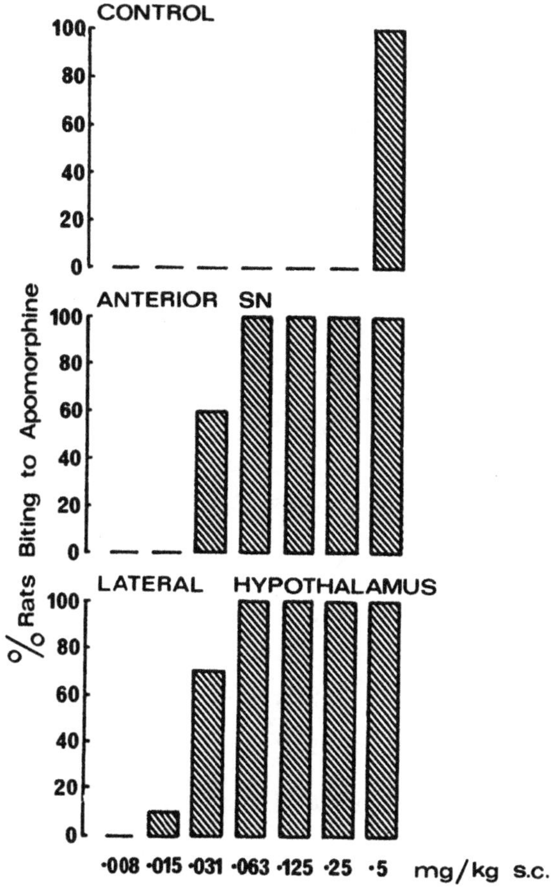

Fig. 2. Increased sensitivity to the biting component of the stereotyped behaviour induced by apomorphine after bilateral 6-hydroxydopamine injections into the medial forebrain bundle in the lateral hypothalamus (Ant. 4.6, Vert. -2.7, Lat. ± 1.9) and anterior to the substantia nigra (SN) (Ant. 3.0, Vert. -2.7, Lat. ± 2.0) (De Groot, 1959). 6-Hydroxydopamine was delivered as a 2 µg/1 µl solution at a rate of 1 µl/min for a total of 8 µg (details of technique are forthcoming [Costall, Marsden, Naylor, and Pycock, unpublished data]). The increased sensitivity to apomorphine developed over the first 7-8 postoperative days. Results were determined on the 10th-24th postoperative days. Each value is the mean of 10-15 determinations. Standard errors are less than 10% of the means. The injection of 6-hydroxydopamine into the lateral hypothalamus depleted striatal and limbic dopamine by approximately 80% and 60% respectively, while similar injections anterior to the substantia nigra depleted striatal dopamine by about 70% and limbic dopamine by 40%. Details of the biochemistry are forthcoming (Costall, Marsden, Naylor, and Pycock, unpublished data).

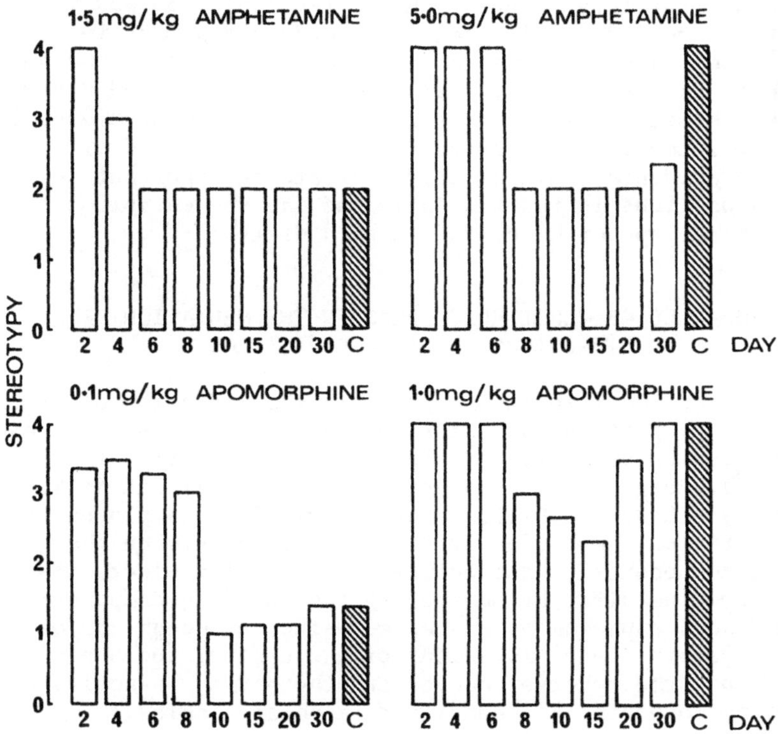

Fig. 3. Changes in the stereotyped behaviour patterns induced by apomorphine and d-amphetamine after bilateral 6-hydroxydopamine lesions of the globus pallidus (8 μg/4 μl, Ant. 7.0, Vert. 0, Lat. ± 3.0) (De Groot, 1959). Stereotyped behaviour was assessed on Days 2-30 following lesion using the system shown on Fig. 1. 0.1 mg/kg s.c. apomorphine and 1.5 mg/kg i.p. d-amphetamine were selected as doses which reliably induced the sniffing component of stereotypy, and 1.0 mg/kg s.c. apomorphine and 5.0 mg/kg i.p. d-amphetamine as doses inducing the biting component (see control values, C, hatched columns). Each value given is the mean of responses from 6-12 rats. Standard errors are less than 12% of the means. The 6-hydroxydopamine injection depleted striatal dopamine by 40% but did not significantly reduce the dopamine content of the tuberculum olfactorium, nucleus accumbens, or amygdala. Details of the biochemistry are forthcoming (Costall, Marsden, Naylor, and Pycock, unpublished data).

drugs was abolished, although sniffing still developed. It is improbable that these changes induced by intrapallidal 6-hydroxydopamine are due to changes in neostriatal dopamine since, although striatal dopamine levels were reduced, the depletion was much less than that recorded for injections of 6-hydroxydopamine into the striatum itself and which failed to produce such clear and persistent effects as the intrapallidal injections. Loew and Vigouret (1975) have similarly shown that intrapallidal 6-hydroxydopamine reduces the intensity of stereotyped behaviour induced by apomorphine. The evidence would clearly indicate an important role for the globus pallidus in the modulation of the stereotypic activities of amphetamine, apomorphine, and related drugs.

THE ROLE OF MESOLIMBIC AREAS IN THE MEDIATION OF STEREOTYPED BEHAVIOUR PATTERNS

A role for the mesolimbic system in the mediation of stereotyped behaviour patterns has been advanced on the basis of results from brain lesion and intracerebral injection experiments (Butterworth, Poignant, and Barbeau, 1975; Costall and Naylor, 1973c, 1974, 1975b; McKenzie, 1972). Electrolytic lesions placed in the mesolimbic regions have clearly differentiated between the sniffing and biting components of stereotypy. Thus, while electrolesions of the tuberculum olfactorium abolish the sniffing component of the effects of both amphetamine and apomorphine, although the biting components persist, electrolesions of the central nucleus of the amygdala cause the reverse changes and the biting is abolished while the sniffing component is unmodified (also see Table 1).

The differential roles of the mesolimbic nuclei has been confirmed by recent studies in which lesions were induced by the direct application of 6-hydroxydopamine to discrete mesolimbic areas. Similarly to electrolesions, 6-hydroxydopamine lesions of the amygdala markedly reduced or abolished the biting/licking component of the amphetamine response but failed to reduce the sniffing components (Fig. 4). However, the 6-hydroxydopamine lesions also reduced the apomorphine response in a similar manner to the electrolesions, and the primary effect was a clear and persistent reduction in the intensity of the biting response (Fig. 4). Unless 6-hydroxydopamine is exerting some direct neurotoxic effect on the dopamine receptors or postsynaptic structures, this result would suggest that apomorphine may normally exert its effects, at least in part, by indirectly stimulating dopamine receptors. This is not a novel concept, but has been forwarded on several other occasions to explain changes in an apomorphine response (Costall and Naylor, 1973b).

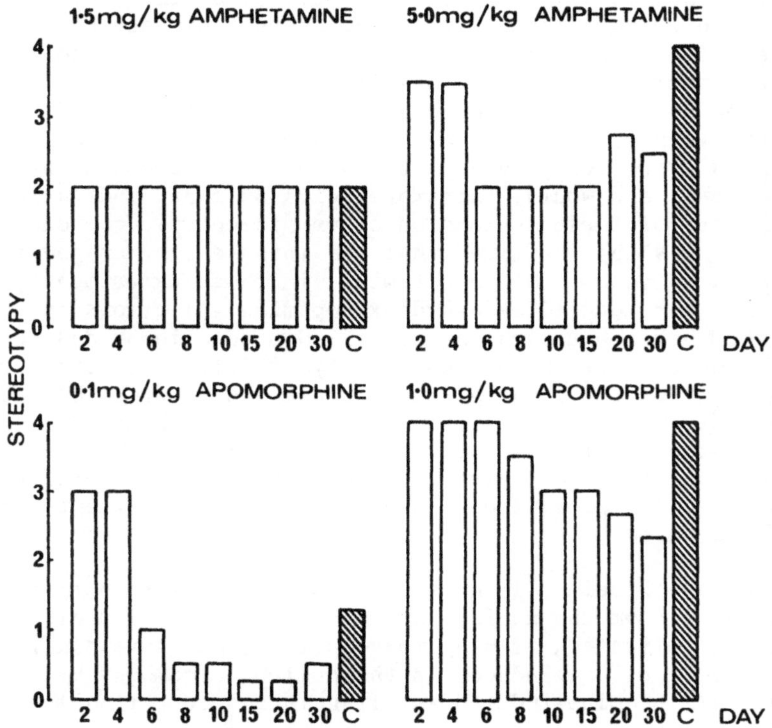

Fig. 4. Changes in the stereotyped behaviour patterns induced by apomorphine and d-amphetamine after bilateral 6-hydroxydopamine lesions of the nucleus amgydaloideus centralis (8 μg/4 μl, Ant. 6.0, Vert. -1.75, Lat. ± 4.0) (De Groot, 1959). Stereotyped behaviour was assessed on Days 2-30 using the scoring system shown on Fig. 1. Doses of stereotypic agent were selected as those inducing sniffing (0.1 mg/kg apomorphine and 1.5 mg/kg d-amphetamine) or biting (1.0 mg/kg apomorphine and 5.0 mg/kg d-amphetamine) (see control values, C, hatched columns). Each value given is the mean of responses from 6-12 rats. Standard errors are less than 15% of the means. The 6-hydroxydopamine injection depleted the dopamine content of the amygdala by approximately 90% while causing no significant reductions in the dopamine content of the striatum, tuberculum olfactorium, or nucleus accumbens. Details of the biochemistry are forthcoming (Costall, Marsden, Naylor, and Pycock, unpublished data).

Asher and Aghajanian (1974) have used the 6-hydroxydopamine lesion technique to investigate the relevance of the nucleus accumbens and tuberculum olfactorium to the stereotypic actions of amphetamine. Their lesions failed to modify the amphetamine response and it was concluded that the "mesolimbic dopamine pathway does not appear to be necessary for amphetamine-induced stereotypy" (p. 1). However, in these studies the authors based their conclusions on observations using 10 mg/kg amphetamine which induces an intense biting response and would, therefore, give no clear indication as to the effects of these lesions on other stereotypic components. Kelly et al. (1975b) confirmed that the intense stereotyped activity induced by a large dose of amphetamine, in these experiments, 5 mg/kg, was not reduced by 6-hydroxydopamine injections into the nucleus accumbens; but these authors also used a lower dose of 1.5 mg/kg amphetamine which induced only "sniffing stereotypy" and this component of the amphetamine response was shown to be reduced by the 6-hydroxydopamine lesions. However, the 6-hydroxydopamine injected in these latter studies not only depleted dopamine from the nucleus accumbens but also from the tuberculum olfactorium which the electrolytic lesion studies have shown to be important for the sniffing response.

In our own studies, we have been able to more selectively deplete dopamine from the nucleus accumbens or tuberculum olfactorium by discrete application of 6-hydroxydopamine, and have confirmed that, when lesions are induced in the nucleus accumbens by this technique, amphetamine-induced sniffing is reduced or abolished, although similar lesions in the tuberculum olfactorium only reduce this component during the acute stage (Figs. 5 and 6). Neither lesion modified the biting induced by amphetamine but both significantly potentiated this component of the apomorphine behaviour (Figs. 5 and 6).

The importance of the tuberculum olfactorium for the mediation of stereotyped responses has been further emphasised by intracerebral injection studies. Both dopamine and apomorphine injected into this area are able to elicit stereotyped sniffing and biting responses (Butterworth et al., 1975; Costall and Naylor, 1975b; Costall et al., 1975a), which are enhanced when injections are made after 6-hydroxydopamine lesion of the area (Costall and Naylor, unpublished observations).

However, in contrast to the tuberculum olfactorium, there is little evidence to suggest a major role for the nucleus accumbens in mediating stereotyped responses in the normal situation. Thus, electrolesions of this area have been shown to cause little or no change in the stereotypic activities of the dopamine agonists, with the exception of reducing the minor, sniffing component of the apomorphine effect (Costall and Naylor, 1973c, 1974, 1975c). Dopamine

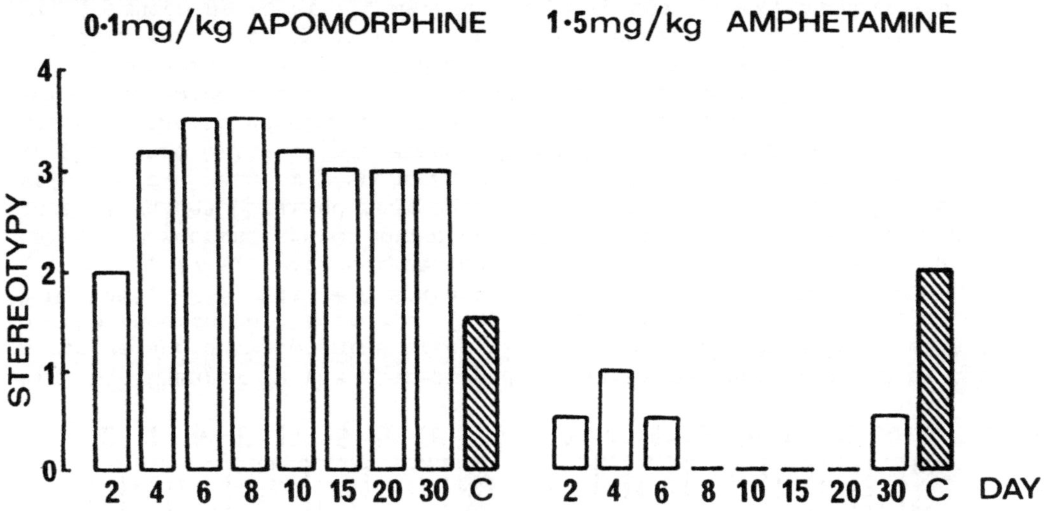

Fig. 5. Changes in the stereotyped behaviour patterns induced by apomorphine and d-amphetamine after bilateral 6-hydroxydopamine lesions of the nucleus accumbens (8 μg/4 μl, Ant. 9.4, Vert. 0, Lat. ± 1.6) (De Groot, 1959). Stereotyped behaviour was assessed on Days 2-30 using the scoring system shown on Fig. 1. Hatched columns represent control values obtained from normal and sham-operated animals (C). Each value is the mean of responses from 6-12 rats. Standard errors are less than 14% of the means. The 6-hydroxydopamine injection caused an approximate 75% depletion of dopamine from the nucleus accumbens and reduced the dopamine content of the tuberculum olfactorium by about 25%. There were no significant reductions in the dopamine content of the striatum or amygdala. Details of the biochemistry are forthcoming (Costall, Marsden, Naylor, and Pycock, unpublished data).

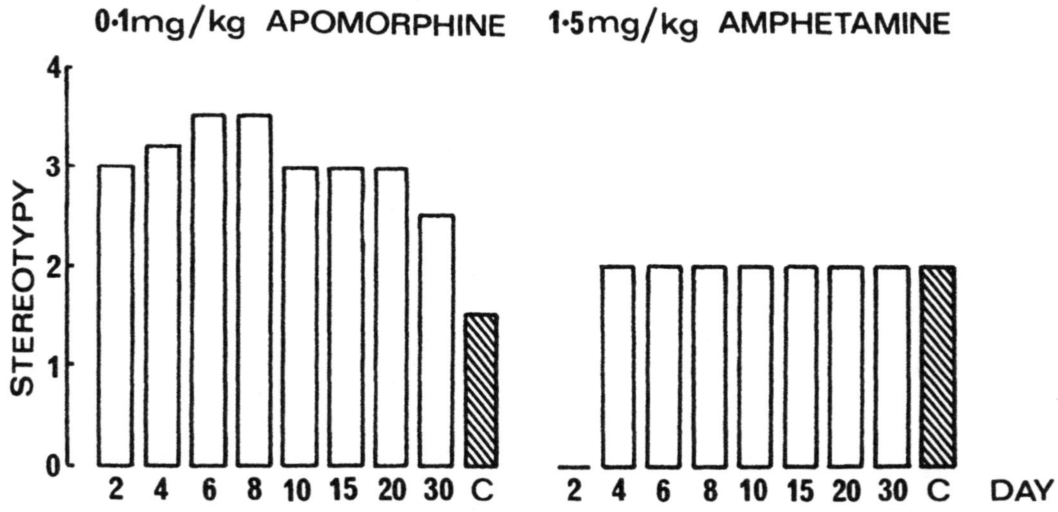

Fig. 6. Changes in the stereotyped behaviour patterns induced by apomorphine and d-amphetamine after bilateral 6-hydroxydopamine lesions of the tuberculum olfactorium (two injections each of 8 μg/4 μl at Ant. 9.0, Vert, -2.5, Lat. ± 2.5 and Ant. 10.0, Vert. -1.8, Lat. ± 2.0) (De Groot, 1959). Stereotyped behaviour was assessed on Days 2-30 using the scoring system shown on Fig. 1. Hatched columns represent control values obtained from normal and sham-operated rats (C). Each value is the mean of responses from 6-12 rats. Standard errors are in the range 0-11% of the means. The 6-hydroxydopamine injections depleted the tuberculum olfactorium of approximately 80% of its normal dopamine content, and the nucleus accumbens of 25% of its normal dopamine content. The dopamine levels in the striatum and amygdala were not significantly reduced. Details of the biochemistry are forthcoming (Costall, Marsden, Naylor, and Pycock, unpublished data).

injected directly into this area may induce sniffing behaviour, but in extensive studies we have never observed biting after injections of dopamine into the accumbens (Costall, Naylor, and Pinder, in press, a; Pijnenberg and van Rossum, 1973; Pijnenberg, Honig, and van Rossum, 1975). Also, apomorphine applied to the accumbens is virtually without effect (Pijnenberg, Honig, van der Heyden, and van Rossum, 1976): sniffing may develop in a small proportion of animals but the biting that is occasionally observed is of a very periodic nature (Costall, Naylor, and Neumeyer, 1975b). Other aporphines are more effective in this respect and (-)N-n-propylnorapomorphine, in particular, has been shown to cause biting after intra-accumbens administration although, again, the sniffing response is inconsistent (Costall et al., 1975b). It is therefore possible that, after 6-hydroxydopamine lesion of the nucleus accumbens, the dopamine receptor sensitivity and specificity may be modified to accommodate apomorphine. However, even after this lesion, although the responses to peripherally administered apomorphine are enhanced, we have still failed to elicit more than a periodic biting from the intra-accumbens injection of apomorphine (Costall and Naylor, unpublished observations). We believe that, of the mesolimbic areas, the integrity of the tuberculum olfactorium is most critical for the development of apomorphine stereotypy. The central amygdaloid nucleus also appears important, but the nature of its involvement is uncertain since we have failed to induce responses from this area by the direct injection of drugs either before (Costall and Naylor, 1975b) or after 6-hydroxydopamine lesion (Costall and Naylor, unpublished observations). Certainly, the degree of involvement of the different areas may differ for other dopamine agonists and, not surprisingly, areas shown to be important for the stereotypic activity of a drug may not necessarily be the same as those involved with mediating its effect on locomotor activity.

THE ROLE OF EXTRAPYRAMIDAL AND MESOLIMBIC AREAS IN THE MEDIATION OF HYPERACTIVITY

Both extrapyramidal and mesolimbic regions are now known to play important roles in the modulation of the hyperactivity induced by amphetamine. However, virtually all initial studies on amphetamine hyperactivity concentrated on the neostriatum, and certainly this would appear to be a suitable substrate since Costa, Groppetti, and Naimzada (1972) and Aylmer, Steinberg, and Webster (1975) showed an association between an increase in locomotor activity and an acceleration of striatal dopamine turnover. Nevertheless, brain lesion studies have clearly indicated the limitations of considering the amphetamine response purely in terms of neostriatal or nigroneostriatal function. Thus, Naylor and Olley (1972) reported that extensive neostriatal electrolesions failed to reduce amphetamine hyperactivity and they concluded that the nigro-striatal dopamine system is not essential for this effect. This conclusion is supported by the observations that electrolesions of the substantia nigra, which selectively deplete striatal dopamine (Costall, Marsden, Naylor, and Pycock, unpublished observations), fail to reduce amphetamine hyperactivity (Costall and Naylor, 1973d) and by more recent studies showing a similar failure of 6-hydroxydopamine lesions of the neostriatum (Asher and Aghajanian, 1974; Creese and Iversen, 1974; Costall, Marsden, Naylor, and Pycock, unpublished observations; Kelly, Miller, and Neumeyer, 1975a). However, there are conflicting reports as to the effects of intranigral 6-hydroxydopamine: Creese and Iversen (1972) and Brook and Iversen (1975) have failed to reduce amphetamine hyperactivity by these lesions (reflecting an inadequate disruption of the nigrostriatal system?), while both Creese and Iversen (1975) and Roberts, Zis, and Fibiger (1975) have shown that amphetamine hyperactivity is reduced by intranigral 6-hydroxydopamine and have suggested that the amphetamine response is dependent on the functional integrity of the nigrostriatal dopamine system. However, these conclusions were based on the erroneous premise that intranigral 6-hydroxydopamine selectively disrupts the nigrostriatal dopamine system, when, in fact, such injections are now known to reduce mesolimbic as well as striatal dopamine (a factor now accepted by both Iversen and Fibiger). We consider that the reduced amphetamine hyperactivity recorded in the above two experiments may be more reasonably attributed to an interruption of the mesolimbic dopamine input. There are several studies that lead us to this conclusion. First, electrolesions placed in the rostral hypothalamus to selectively interrupt the mesolimbic dopamine input markedly reduce or abolish amphetamine hyperactivity (Costall and Naylor, 1974). Second, injections of 6-hydroxydopamine into the nucleus accumbens reduce the hyperactivity induced after peripheral administration of amphetamine (Fig. 7) (Iversen, Kelly, Miller, and Seviour, 1975; Kelly et al., 1975b), and, even more important, the hyperactivity induced by injections of amphetamine into the nucleus accumbens is far more intense than that observed after neostriatal injections (Costall et al., in press, a; Pijnenberg and van Rossum, 1973; Pijnenberg et al., 1975) and is attenuated by prior injection of 6-hydroxydopamine into the same nucleus (Costall and Naylor, unpublished observations).

Although the nucleus accumbens plays an important role in mediation of the amphetamine response, we would wish to emphasise that this involvement is not exclusive. Amphetamine can evoke a modest locomotor response from the neostriatum (Costall et al., 1972a; Costall et al., 1974; Fuxe and Ungerstedt, 1970), and hyperactivity also results from injections into the tuberculum olfactorium (Costall and Naylor, unpublished observations; Pijnenberg et al., 1976). However, the nature of the involvement of these two areas is uncertain for lesion of either area, by electrolytic means or by

6-hydroxydopamine, fails to reduce amphetamine hyperactivity. Conversely, 6-hydroxydopamine lesions of the tuberculum olfactorium may actually enhance the amphetamine response (Fig. 8). This latter observation initially appears paradoxical, but we suggest that this enhancement reflects the ability of amphetamine to release dopamine from the remaining and functional nerve terminals on to receptive structures of enhanced sensitivity. This is supported by the observation that, if amphetamine is injected directly into the tuberculum olfactorium after 6-hydroxydopamine lesion of the area, an enhanced response to amphetamine is recorded (Costall and Naylor, unpublished observations).

An elucidation of the extrapyramidal and mesolimbic sites at which apomorphine is able to modify activity has proven more difficult. An initial and serious drawback to our own studies was the failure of peripherally administered apomorphine to induce a hyperactivity response that could be distinguished from control values. While a number of workers have reported the development of hyperactivity to apomorphine (Maj, Grabowska, and Gajda, 1972; Iversen et al., 1975), we remain unconvinced as to its validity for a number of reasons. First, why has it proven so difficult to demonstrate a relationship between the dose of apomorphine and the intensity of the response? Second, an even more surprising observation is the failure of Maj and colleagues (1972) to demonstrate a reduction in hyperactivity responding as the intensity of stereotyped behaviour increased with increasing dosage. This latter anomaly possibly reflects the inadequacies of the recording system: when using photocells for recording activity, it is essential to constantly monitor stereotyped behaviour in order to differentiate recordings of these movements from increased locomotor responses.

The most valuable data on the sites at which apomorphine may induce hyperactivity have been gained from intracerebral injection studies. Since the neostriatum, nucleus accumbens, and tuberculum olfactorium have assumed particular importance as sites for amphetamine activity, studies on apomorphine have also tended to concentrate on these regions. However, apomorphine injections into the caudate-putamen fail to initiate hyperactivity (Costall et al., 1974) and intrastriatal 6-hydroxydopamine fails to render the area more sensitive to this effect of apomorphine when administered peripherally (Asher and Aghajanian, 1974; Creese and Iversen, 1974; Costall, Marsden, Naylor, and Pycock, unpublished observations; Kelly et al., 1975b) or directly into the striatum (Costall and Naylor, unpublished observations). Thus, there is no evidence available to suggest that apomorphine may normally increase activity by an effect in the striatum.

In contrast, Iversen et al. (1975) have shown an enhancement of the locomotor response to apomorphine after injection of 6-hydroxydopamine into the area of the nucleus accumbens, and these

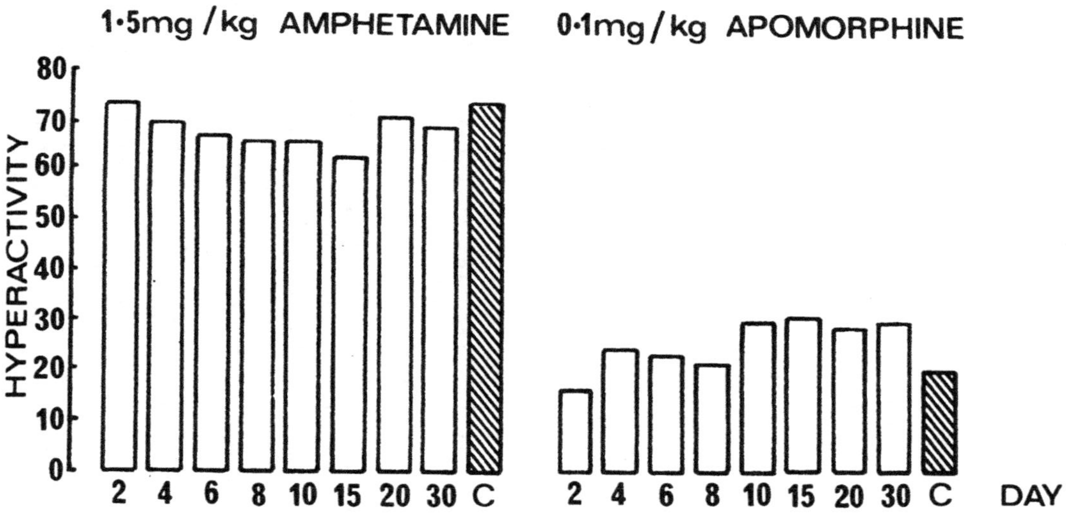

Fig. 7. Modification of the hyperactivity responses to d-amphetamine and apomorphine after bilateral 6-hydroxydopamine lesions of the nucleus accumbens (see Fig. 5 legend). Hyperactivity was measured in photocell cages on Days 2-30 following lesion. Values presented are the mean responses of 6-12 animals measured as the number of interruptions of the light beam occurring within a 5 min period. Hatched columns (C) represent control responses of normal and sham-operated rats. Standard errors are in the range 8-18% of the means. The biochemistry of these lesions is indicated in Fig. 5 legend.

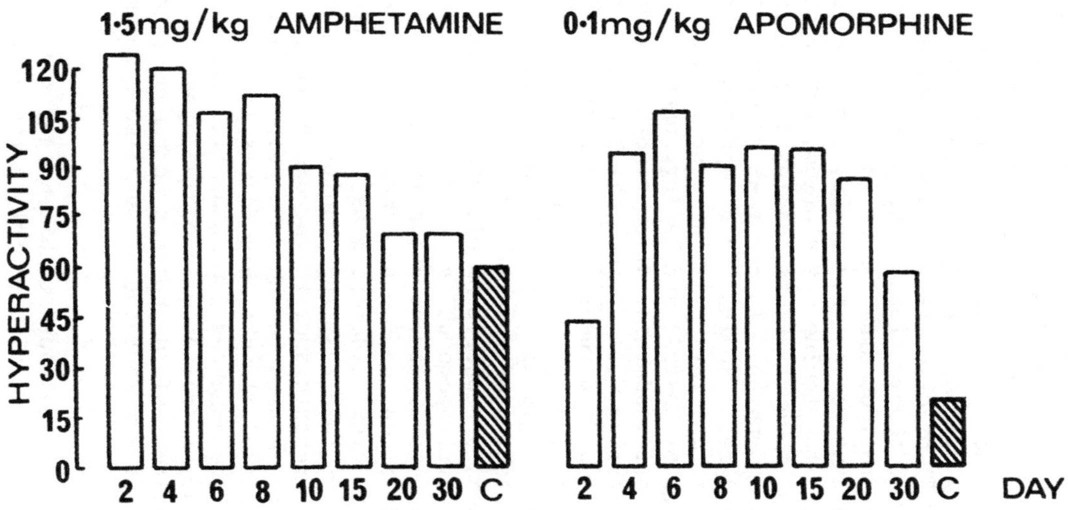

Fig. 8. Modification of the hyperactivity responses to amphetamine and apomorphine after bilateral 6-hydroxydopamine lesions of the tuberculum olfactorium (see legend Fig. 6). Hyperactivity was assessed in cages fitted with photocells and is presented as the number of interruptions of the light beam occurring during each 5 min period. Animals were constantly observed to differentiate hyperactivity counts from those caused purely by repetitive stereotyped movements and values presented are considered to represent "true" activity counts. Hatched columns represent control values (C). Each value is the mean of responses from 6-12 rats obtained on Days 2-30 after surgery. Standard errors are in the range 9-16% of the means. The biochemistry of these lesions is indicated in Fig. 6 legend.

authors have concluded that this enhanced response to apomorphine results from its action on supersensitive dopamine receptors within the nucleus accumbens (also see Iversen, 1976). Nevertheless, we would question a primary accumbens site for this action of apomorphine: first, because apomorphine injections into the nucleus accumbens of normal rats fail to increase their locomotor activity (Costall et al., 1975b; Pijnenberg et al., 1975); and second, even more important, because in our hands the discrete injection of 6-hydroxydopamine into the nucleus accumbens (which causes minimal changes in dopamine content of the tuberculum olfactorium) does not result in enhanced activity responses to apomorphine when administered peripherally (Fig. 7) or directly into the accumbens (Costall and Naylor, unpublished observations). We particularly qualify the extent of the 6-hydroxydopamine lesion induced in our own studies for the very important reason that there is good evidence to suggest a major role for the tuberculum olfactorium, rather than the nucleus accumbens, in modulation of events leading to an increase in the activity response to apomorphine. In contrast to observations at the nucleus accumbens, the direct application of apomorphine to the tuberculum olfactorium of normal rats will increase locomotor activity (Pijnenberg et al., 1976; Costall and Naylor, unpublished observations), and the prior administration of 6-hydroxydopamine into the tuberculum olfactorium will enhance the hyperactivity induced by apomorphine injections into the same area (Costall and Naylor, unpublished observations); and, further, apomorphine will induce hyperactivity in these animals after peripheral administration. Therefore, there is a clear need to differentiate between effects in the nucleus accumbens or tuberculum olfactorium when reference is made to the action of apomorphine. Iversen and colleagues (1975) failed to make this differentiation in their studies when the 6-hydroxydopamine injections caused an almost equally severe dopamine depletion in the tuberculum olfactorium as in the nucleus accumbens. Therefore, it is possible that the results they attributed to changes in the dopamine receptors of the accumbens could equally have been attributed to changes in the tuberculum olfactorium. In later studies, Kelly et al. (1975b) take this factor into account, and subsequent work refers to the enhanced locomotor activity observed after the peripheral administration of dopamine agonists to rats with 6-hydroxydopamine lesions of the nucleus accumbens (and tuberculum olfactorium) as an effect mediated at mesolimbic dopamine receptors (Kelly, 1975).

However, it is important to point out at this stage, that, although we would forward the tuberculum olfactorium as the primary site of action of apomorphine, we have no evidence for extending this to the aporphines in general for, although intra-accumbens apomorphine is virtually void of any effect on activity, (-)N-n-propylnorapomorphine can evoke a hyperactivity after similar injection, albeit a small effect in normal animals (Costall et al., 1975b).

Thus, changes in the accumbens may contribute to the enhanced hyperactivity recorded by Kelly et al. (1975a) for (-)N-n-propylnorapomorphine after their 6-hydroxydopamine lesions of the nucleus accumbens/tuberculum olfactorium region.

Irrespective of the precise role each dopamine containing area is considered to play in the development of drug-induced locomotor activity, it is apparent that more than one dopamine-containing area is capable of influencing the response, and it is reasonable to expect that all systems must act in concert for the final expression of a meaningful behaviour. Compensatory changes in one system(s) may be expected to reduce the adverse effects caused by dysfunction in another and may, for example, partly explain the gradual resumption of amphetamine hyperactivity after 6-hydroxydopamine lesion of the nucleus accumbens (see Fig. 7). In addition, dopamine mechanisms within the nucleus accumbens may modify their own intrinsic activity.

In this review we have been primarily concerned with the neostriatum, nucleus accumbens septi, and tuberculum olfactorium as areas of the extrapyramidal and mesolimbic systems that are considered most important for the control of drug-induced hyperactivity. However, the nucleus amygdaloideus centralis and the paleostriatum have both been shown to modulate the stereotypic activity of amphetamine and related drugs; they must, therefore, be considered as possible sites at which these drugs can also modify activity. We have already pointed out that a site of stereotypic activity may not necessarily be a site at which the same drug may modulate locomotor activity, and results of studies on the nucleus amygdaloideus centralis emphasise this view. Thus, while lesions of this area can abolish stereotyped biting responses, they fail to modify amphetamine-induced hyperactivity. 6-Hydroxydopamine lesions of this nucleus also fail to modify activity; and injections of dopamine into the area, either before or after 6-hydroxydopamine lesions, fail to increase activity (Costall and Naylor, 1975b, unpublished observations). In contrast, the critical role of the paleostriatum in modulating stereotyped responses has been extended to hyperactivity, although the nature of its role in this behaviour is more difficult to evaluate. Certainly, the most marked hyperactivity recorded in our 6-hydroxydopamine lesion studies was from rats with 6-hydroxydopamine lesions of the globus pallidus treated with amphetamine (Fig. 9). These marked increases in activity have also been shown to occur after electrolytic lesions of the pallidum (Naylor and Olley, 1972). It is conceivable that, in both types of lesion experiment, the hyperactivity may result from dopamine denervation within the globus pallidus or associated areas, but the lack of an enhanced response to apomorphine would indicate that a "supersensitivity" of dopamine receptors does not occur in this nucleus.

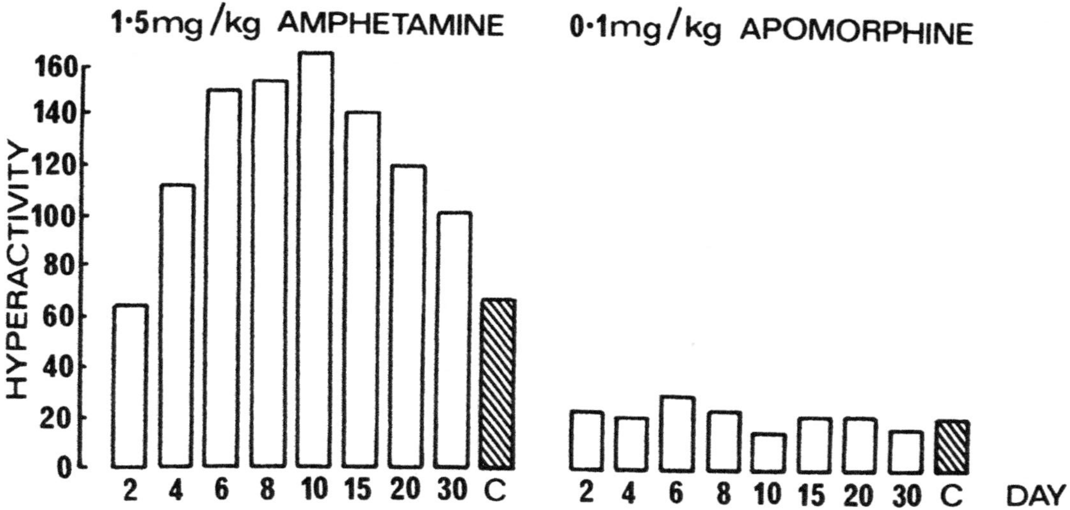

Fig. 9. Modification of the hyperactivity responses to d-amphetamine and apomorphine after bilateral 6-hydroxydopamine lesions of the globus pallidus (see the legend to Fig. 3 for dose of 6-hydroxydopamine, coordinates, and biochemical effects of the lesions). Hyperactivity was measured in photocell cages on Days 2-30 following lesion. Values presented are the mean responses of 6-12 animals measured as the number of interruptions of the light beam occurring within a 5 min period. Hatched columns (C) represent control responses obtained from normal and sham-operated rats. Standard errors are less than 17% of the means.

As in experiments on stereotyped behaviour, the globus pallidus has been largely overlooked in hyperactivity studies as being secondary in importance to the neostriatum, but the data so far available would suggest that, for both behavioural states, the globus pallidus warrants more intensive investigation as a site itself for the action of amphetamine and related drugs.

ACKNOWLEDGMENTS

This work was supported by the Medical Research Council.

The biochemical estimations following 6-hydroxydopamine lesions presented in this manuscript were carried out by Dr. C.J. Pycock, Department of Neurology, Institute of Psychiatry, London. Miss M.Y. Green gave excellent technical assistance throughout the behavioural studies.

REFERENCES

Asher, I.M. and Aghajanian, G.K.: 6-Hydroxydopamine lesions of olfactory tubercles and caudate nuclei: Effect on amphetamine-induced stereotyped behaviour in rats, Brain Res. 82, 1-12 (1974).

Aylmer, C.G.G., Steinberg, H., and Webster, R.A.: Dopamine and drug-induced hyperactivity in rats, Br. J. Pharmacol. 55, 293P (1975).

Baum, E., Etevenon, P., Piarroux, M-C. Simon, P., and Boissier, J.R.: Modifications compartmentales et pharmacologiques obtenues chez le rat après lésion bilatérale de la substance noir, J. Pharmacol. 2, 423-434 (1971).

Bergmann, F., Chaimovitz, M., Pasternak (Na'or), V., and Ramu, A.: Compulsive gnawing in rats after implantation of drugs into the ventral thalamus. A contribution to the mechanism of morphine action, Br. J. Pharmacol. 51, 197-205 (1974).

Braestrup, C., Anderson, H., and Randrup, A.: The monoamine oxidase B inhibitor deprenyl potentiates phenylethylamine behaviour in rats without inhibition of catecholamine metabolite formation, Eur. J. Pharmacol. 34, 181-189 (1975).

Brook C. and Iversen, S.D.: Changed eating and locomotor behaviour in the rat after 6-hydroxydopamine lesions to the substantia nigra, Neuropharmacol. 14, 95-105 (1975).

Butterworth, R.F., Poignant, J.-C., and Barbeau, A.: Apomorphine and ET-495 in rats - biochemical and pharmacological studies, Adv. Neurol. 9, 307-326 (1975).

Costa, E., Groppetti, A, and Naimzada, M.K.: Effects of amphetamine on the turnover rate of brain catecholamines and motor activity, Br. J. Pharmacol. 44, 742-751 (1972).

Costall, B. and Naylor, R.J.: The site and mode of action of ET-495 for the mediation of stereotyped behaviour in the rat, Naunyn-Schmiedebergs Arch. exp. Path. Pharmak. 278, 117-133 (1973a).

Costall, B. and Naylor, R.J.: On the mode of action of apomorphine, Eur. J. Pharmacol. 21, 350-361 (1973b).

Costall, B. and Naylor, R.J.: The role of telencephalic dopaminergic systems in the mediation of apomorphine-stereotyped behaviour, Eur. J. Pharmacol. 24, 8-24 (1973c).

Costall, B. and Naylor, R.J.: The role of the substantia nigra in the locomotor stimulant action of amphetamine, Br. J. Pharmacol. 49, 29-36 (1973d).

Costall, B. and Naylor, R.J.: Extrapyramidal and mesolimbic involvement with the stereotypic activity of d- and l-amphetamine, Eur. J. Pharmacol. 25, 121-129 (1974).

Costall, B. and Naylor, R.J.: Neuropharmacological studies on D145 (1, 3-dimethyl-5-aminoadamantan), Psychopharmacologia 43, 53-61 (1975a).

Costall, B. and Naylor, R.J.: The behavioural effects of dopamine applied intracerebrally to areas of the mesolimbic system, Eur. J. Pharmacol. 32, 87-92 (1975b).

Costall, B. and Naylor, R.J.: Actions of dopaminergic agonists on motor function, Adv. Neurol. 9, 285-297 (1975c).

Costall, B., Naylor, R.J., and Neumeyer, J.L.: Differences in the nature of the stereotyped behaviour induced by aporphine derivatives in the rat and in their actions in extrapyramidal and mesolimbic brain areas, Eur. J. Pharmacol. 31, 1-16 (1975a).

Costall, B., Naylor, R.J., and Neumeyer, J.L.: Dissociation by the aporphine derivatives of the stereotypic and hyperactivity responses resulting from injections into the nucleus accumbens septi, J. Pharm. Pharmac. 27, 875-877 (1975b).

Costall, B., Naylor, R.J., and Olley, J.E.: Stereotypic and anti-cataleptic activities of amphetamine after intracerebral injections, Eur. J. Pharmacol. 18, 83-94 (1972a).

Costall, B., Naylor, R.J., and Olley, J.E.: The substantia nigra and stereotyped behaviour, Eur. J. Pharmacol. 18, 95-106 (1972b).

Costall, B., Naylor, R.J., and Pinder, R.M.: Design of agents for stimulation of neostriatal dopaminergic mechanisms, J. Pharm. Pharmac. 26, 753-762 (1974).

Costall, B., Naylor, R.J., and Pinder, R.M.: Characterisation of the mechanisms for hyperactivity induction from the nucleus accumbens by phenylethylamine derivatives, Psychopharmacologia, in press, a.

Costall, B., Naylor, R.J., and Pycock, C.: Non-specific supersensitivity of striatal dopamine receptors after 6-hydroxydopamine lesion of the nigro-striatal pathway, Eur. J. Pharmacol., in press, b.

Cox, B. and Tha, S.J.: Effects of amantadine and l-dopa on apomorphine and d-amphetamine induced stereotyped behaviour in rats, Eur. J. Pharmacol. 24, 96-101 (1973).

Creese, I. and Iversen, S.D.: Amphetamine response in the rat after dopamine neurone destruction, Nature new Biol. 238, 247-248 (1972).

Creese, I. and Iversen, S.D.: Blockage of amphetamine induced motor stimulation and stereotypy in the adult rat following neonatal treatment with 6-hydroxydopamine, Brain Res. 55, 369-382 (1973).

Creese, I. and Iversen, S.D.: The role of forebrain dopamine systems in amphetamine induced stereotyped behaviour in the rat, Psychopharmacologia 39, 345-357 (1974).

Creese, I. and Iversen, S.D.: The pharmacological and anatomical substrates of the amphetamine response in the rat, Brain Res. 83, 419-436 (1975).

De Groot, J.: The rat forebrain in stereotaxic coordinates, Verh. K. ned. Akad. Wet. 52, 11-39 (1959).

Divac, I.: Drug induced syndromes in rats with large, chronic lesions in the corpus striatum, Psychopharmacologia 27, 171-178 (1972).

Ernst, A.M. and Smelik, P.G.: Site of action of dopamine and apomorphine on compulsive gnawing behaviour in rats, Experientia 22, 837-838 (1966).

Faull, R.L.M. and Laverty, R.: Changes in dopamine levels in the corpus striatum following lesions in the substantia nigra, Expl Neurol. 23, 332-340 (1969).

Fibiger, H.C., Fibiger, H.P., and Zis, A.P.: Attenuation of amphetamine-induced motor stimulation and stereotypy by 6-hydroxydopamine in the rat, Br. J. Pharmacol. 47, 683-692 (1973).

Fog., R.: On stereotypy and catalepsy: Studies on the effect of amphetamines and neuroleptics in rat, Acta Neurol Scand. 48, Suppl. 50 (1972).

Fog., R. and Pakkenberg, H.: Behavioural effects of dopamine and p-hydroxyamphetamine injected into corpus striatum of rats, Expl Neurol. 31, 71-86 (1971).

Fuxe, K. and Ungerstedt, U.: Histochemical, biochemical and functional studies on central monoamine neurons after acute and chronic amphetamine administration. In: Amphetamines and Related Compounds. Costa, E. and Garattini, S., Eds., pp. 257-288. New York: Raven Press, 1970.

Glick, S.D.: Behavioral effects of amphetamine in brain damaged animals: Problems in the search for sites of action. In: Cocaine and Other Stimulants. Ellinwood, E.H. and Kilbey, M.M., Eds. New York: Plenum Press, 1976.

Hackman, R., Pentikäinen, P., Neuroven, R.J., and Vapaatalo, H.: Inhibition of apomorphine gnawing compulsion by amantadine, Experientia 29, 1524-1525 (1973).

Iversen, S.D.: The effect of surgical lesions to frontal cortex and substantia nigra on amphetamine responses in rats, Brain Res. 31, 295-311 (1971).

Iversen, S.D.: Neural substrates mediating amphetamine responses. In: Cocaine and Other Stimulants. Ellinwood, E.H. and Kilbey, M.M., Eds. New York: Plenum Press, 1976.

Iversen, S.D., Kelly, P.H., Miller, R.J., and Seviour, P.: Amphetamine and apomorphine responses in the rat after lesion of mesolimbic or striatal dopamine neurones, Br. J. Pharmacol. 54, 244P (1975).

Jalfre, M. and Haefely, W.: Effects of some centrally acting agents in rats after intraventricular injections of 6-hydroxydopamine. In: 6-Hydroxydopamine and Catecholamine Neurons. Malmfors, T. and Thoenen, H., Eds., pp. 333-346. Amsterdam: North Holland Publishing Company, 1971.

Kelly, P.H.: Action of LSD on supersensitive mesolimbic dopamine receptors, Br. J. Pharmacol. 55, 291P (1975).

Kelly, P.H., Miller, R.J., and Neumeyer, J.L.: Effect of aporphine alkaloids on central dopamine receptors, Br. J. Pharmacol. 54, 271P (1975a).

Kelly, P.H., Seviour, P.W., and Iversen, S.D.: Amphetamine and apomorphine responses in the rat following 6-OHDA lesions of the nucleus accumbens septi and corpus striatum, Brain Res. 94, 507-522 (1975b).

Koob, G.F., Balcom, G.J., and Meyerhoff, J.L.: Dopamine and norepinephrine levels in the nucleus accumbens, olfactory tubercle and corpus striatum following lesions to the ventral tegmental area, Brain Res. 94, 45-55 (1975).

Loew, D.M. and Vigouret, J.M.: Mechanisms involved in the effect of apomorphine on the extrapyramidal system of the rat, Naunyn-Schmiedebergs Arch. exp. Path. Pharmak. 287, R10 (1975).

Maj, J., Grabowska, M., and Gajda, L.: Effect of apomorphine on motility in rats, Eur. J. Pharmacol. 17, 208-214 (1972).

McKenzie, G.M.: Role of the tuberculum olfactorium in stereotyped behaviour induced by apomorphine in the rat, Psychopharmacologia 23, 212-219 (1972).

Naylor, R.J. and Olley, J.E.: Modification of the behavioural changes induced by amphetamine in the rat by lesions in the caudate nucleus, the caudate-putamen and the globus pallidus, Neuropharmacol. 11, 91-99 (1972).

Neill, D.B., Boggan, W.O., and Grossman, S.P.: Behavioural effects of amphetamine in rats with lesions in the corpus striatum, J. comp. physiol. Psychol. 86, 1019-1030 (1974).

Pijnenberg, A.J.J. and van Rossum, J.M.: Stimulation of locomotor activity following injection of dopamine into the nucleus accumbens, J. Pharm. Pharmac. 25, 1003-1005 (1973).

Pijnenberg, A.J.J., Honig, W.M.M., and van Rossum, J.M.: Effects of antagonists upon locomotor stimulation induced by injection of dopamine and noradrenaline into the nucleus accumbens of nialamide-pretreated rats, Psychopharmacologia 41, 175-180 (1975).

Pijnenberg, A.J.J., Honig, W.M.M., van der Heyden, J.A.M., and van Rossum, J.M.: Effects of chemical stimulation of the mesolimbic dopamine system upon locomotor activity, Eur. J. Pharmacol. 35, 45-58 (1976).

Price, M.T.C. and Fibiger, H.C.: Apomorphine and amphetamine stereotypy after 6-hydroxydopamine lesions of the substantia nigra, J. Pharmacol. 29, 249-252 (1974).

Randrup, A. and Munkvad, I.: Stereotyped activities produced by amphetamine in several animal species and man, Psychopharmacologia 11, 300-310 (1967).

Randrup, A., Munkvad, I., and Scheel-Krüger, J.: Mechanisms by which amphetamines produce stereotypy, aggression and other behavioural effects. In: Psychopharmacology, Sexual Disorders and Drug Abuse. Ban, T.A., Boissier, J.R., Gessa, G.J., Heimann, H., Hollister, L., Lehmann, H.E., Munkvad, I., Steinberg, H., Sulser, F., Sundwall, A., and Vinar, O., Eds., pp. 659-673. Amsterdam: North Holland Publishing Company, 1973.

Roberts, D.C.S., Zis, A.P., and Fibiger, H.C.: Ascending catecholamine pathways and amphetamine induced locomotor activity: Importance of dopamine and apparent non-involvement of norepinephrine, Brain Res. 93, 441-454 (1975).

Schoenfeld, R. and Uretsky, N.: Altered response to apomorphine in 6-hydroxydopamine-treated rats, Eur. J. Pharmacol. 19, 115-118 (1972).

Simpson, B.A. and Iversen, S.D.: Effects of substantia nigra lesions on the locomotor and stereotypy responses to amphetamine, Nature new Biol. 230, 30-32 (1971).

Ungerstedt, U.: Adipsia and aphagia after 6-hydroxydopamine induced degeneration of the nigro-striatal dopamine system, Acta Physiol. Scand., Suppl. 367, 95-122 (1971).

Wolfarth, S.: Reactions to apomorphine and spiroperidol of rats with striatal lesions: The relevance of kind and size of the lesion, Pharmac. Biochem. Behav. 2, 181-186 (1974).

Wolfarth, S.M., Grabowska, M., Lacki, M., Dulska, E., and Antkiewicz, L.: The action of apomorphine in rats with striatal lesions, Activitas nerv. sup. 15, 132 (1973).

Yehuda, S. and Wurtman, R.J.: Dopaminergic neurons in the nigrostriatal and mesolimbic pathways: Mediation of specific effects of d-amphetamine, Eur. J. Pharmacol. 30, 154-158 (1975).

BEHAVIORAL EFFECTS OF AMPHETAMINE IN BRAIN DAMAGED ANIMALS: PROBLEMS IN THE SEARCH FOR SITES OF ACTION

Stanley D. Glick

Department of Pharmacology, Mount Sinai School of Medicine, CUNY, New York, N.Y. 10029

Many investigators have studied brain lesion-induced changes in sensitivity to the behavioral effects of amphetamine (i.e., dl-amphetamine, d-amphetamine, methamphetamine) in animals. The majority of these studies have been concerned with determining a site or sites of action of amphetamine. It has usually been assumed (though not necessarily correctly) that damage to a site of action will decrease or abolish an effect of the drug. Although such an approach is seemingly straightforward, there have been a large number of contradictory reports, with "decreases", "no effects", and "increases" in sensitivity to amphetamine sometimes reported to follow lesions in the same brain region. Based on methodological considerations, an attempt will be made in this review to resolve some of this confusion. In addition, evidence that amphetamine enhances an intrinsic asymmetry in nigro-striatal function will be discussed. This action, it will be proposed, may be responsible for normal variations among animals in drug sensitivity before as well as after lesions.

AMPHETAMINE-INDUCED ANOREXIA

Brobeck, Larsson, and Reyes (1956), on the basis of electrophysiological findings, first suggested that the anorexic effect of amphetamine might be due to direct stimulation of a ventromedial hypothalamic satiety center. The results of subsequent lesion studies appeared to refute this hypothesis. Stowe and Miller (1957), Reynolds (1959), and Epstein (1959) all reported that ventromedial hypothalamic lesions made rats hypersensitive to the anorexic effect of amphetamine. However, Sharp, Neilson, and Porter

(1962) reported that ventromedial hypothalamic lesions made cats less sensitive to the anorexic effect of amphetamine and interpreted their results as being consistent with the Brobeck et al. hypothesis. In contrast to all previous studies, Kennedy and Mitra (1963) reported that rats with ventromedial hypothalamic lesions were less sensitive to the anorexic action of amphetamine during the early postoperative period of hyperphagia but more sensitive to amphetamine during the later postoperative period of static obesity. More recently, rats with ventromedial hypothalamic lesions have been found to be normally sensitive to amphetamine-induced anorexia (Wishart and Walls, 1973). These discrepancies might be reconcilable in terms of denervation supersensitivity (Trendelenburg, 1963). Although there is no definitive evidence that denervation supersensitivity (post-synaptic) develops in the central nervous system (Sharpless, 1975), there are many findings (e.g., Ungerstedt, 1971; Glick, Greenstein, and Zimmerberg, 1972) consistent with its occurrence; and, at least for heuristic purposes, the concept is useful when trying to interpret a diverse body of data (Glick, 1974). In the present context, it might be expected that there would be time-dependent changes in drug sensitivity if ventromedial hypothalamic lesions partially damaged a system affected by amphetamine. Early after surgery, animals might be less sensitive to amphetamine; whereas, at later postoperative intervals, when supersensitivity of remaining tissue had occurred, there might be increased anorexic sensitivity. Exactly this pattern of results occurred in the study by Kennedy and Mitra (1963); since the time-course of changing sensitivity would depend upon lesion size, the results of all of the other studies might be explicable on this basis. Recent findings (Kapatos and Gold, 1973; Ahlskog and Hoebel, 1973; Gold, 1973; Glick, Greenstein, and Waters, 1973) have indicated that ventromedial hypothalamic hyperphagia occurs as a consequence of damage to a ventral ascending noradrenergic bundle (Ungerstedt, 1971) passing through the ventromedial hypothalamus And hyperphagic rats with lesions in this bundle have been reported to be less sensitive to amphetamine-induced anorexia (Ahlskog and Hoebel, 1973). In view of amphetamine's effects on norepinephrine metabolism, it would appear reasonable to speculate that changing sensitivity to amphetamine-induced anorexia in rats with ventromedial hypothalamic lesions is mediated by denervation supersensitivity in a noradrenergic pathway.

Results with lateral hypothalamic lesions have been less ambiguous. In four studies (Carlisle, 1964; Russek, Rodriquez-Zendejas, and Teitelbaum, 1973; Fibiger, Zis, and McGreer, 1973; Blundell and Leshem, 1974), it has been reported that rats which had recovered from the aphagia and adipsia following lateral hypothalamic lesions were less sensitive to the anorexic effect of amphetamine, although sensitivity returned to normal by 20 weeks after surgery in the Blundell and Leshem study. The lesions in the latter study appear, however, to have been smaller than those in the other studies. Despite the degree of consistency among these studies, recent findings concerning the etiology of the aphagic and adipsic syndrome following lateral hypothalamic lesions suggest another site of action mediating amphetamine-induced anorexia. There have been several reports (e.g., Ungerstedt, 1971; Oltmans and Harvey, 1972; Marshall and Teitelbaum, 1973; Fibiger et al., 1973; Stricker and Zigmond, 1974; Neill and Linn, 1975) that bilateral lesions of the dopaminergic nigro-striatal system in the rat produce the same or very similar aphagic and adipsic syndrome as previously described for lateral hypothalamic lesions (Teitelbaum and Epstein, 1962). And nigral lesions have been found to decrease sensitivity to amphetamine's anorexic effect (Fibiger et al., 1973). Because nigro-striatal fibers course through the medial part of the internal capsule and because the internal capsule lies adjacent to the lateral hypothalamus, most lesions intended for the lateral hypothalamus produce some damage to nigro-striatal fibers. The lateral hypothalamic syndrome appears, to some extent, to be a nigro-striatal syndrome. In view of amphetamine's effects on dopamine metabolism, it is likely that amphetamine induces anorexia at least partially as a result of an action in the corpus striatum. The fact that a lesion of the ventral ascending noradrenergic bundle and a lesion of the dopaminergic nigro-striatal pathway can each diminish amphetamine-induced anorexia but neither lesion can abolish amphetamine-induced anorexia suggests that both catecholaminergic systems are involved.

AMPHETAMINE-INDUCED STEREOTYPY

High doses of amphetamine induce stereotypy in most species of animals including man. In the rat, amphetamine-induced stereotypic behaviors include rearing, gnawing, crouching and sniffing. Although much neurochemical evidence has indicated that these effects of amphetamine are mediated by a dopaminergic action or actions in the corpus striatum (e.g., Scheel-Krüger and Randrup, 1967; Taylor and Snyder, 1970), the results of lesion studies have been inconsistent. In several studies, it has indeed been found, as would be expected, that bilateral lesions of the substantia nigra or corpus striatum diminish or abolish amphetamine-induced stereotypy (Fog, Randrup, and Pakkenberg, 1970; Naylor and Olley, 1972; Creese and Iversen, 1972; Fibiger, Fibiger, and Zis, 1973; Neill, Boggan, and Grossman, 1974; Creese and Iversen, 1974; Price and Fibiger, 1974; Creese and Iversen, 1975). However, in other studies, such lesions have been found to produce no change in sensitivity (Simpson and Iversen, 1971; Iversen, 1971; Divac, 1972; Costall, Naylor, and Olley, 1972a; Costall and Naylor, 1974); and recently it has been reported that a unilateral caudate lesion potentiates amphetamine-induced stereotypy (Yehuda and Wurtman,

1975). All of these results may be reconcilable in terms of lesion size. That is, it appears that only lesions which produce large (greater than 80%) depletions of dopamine in the striatum will block amphetamine-induced stereotypy (Price and Fibiger, 1974; Creese and Iversen, 1975). Smaller lesions may be ineffective or potentiate amphetamine's effects because remaining nigro-striatal terminals are hyperactive (Agid, Javoy, and Glowinski, 1973) and because partially denervated dopamine receptors become supersensitive (Ungerstedt, 1971; Mishra, Gardner, Katzman, and Makman, 1974).

AMPHETAMINE-INDUCED ROTATION

Unilateral lesions of the nigro-striatal system cause rats and mice to rotate or turn in circles toward the side of the lesion. This rotational behavior is potentiated by amphetamine and can be induced by amphetamine long after animals have recovered from the tendency to rotate spontaneously (e.g., Ungerstedt and Arbuthnott, 1970; Ungerstedt, 1971; Christie and Crow, 1971; Crow, 1971; Marsden and Guldberg, 1973; Von Voigtlander and Moore, 1973). Rotation is presumed to reflect an imbalance in nigro-striatal function on the two sides of the brain: animals rotate contralateral to the more active nigro-striatal pathway (e.g., Arbuthnott and Crow, 1971; Zimmerberg and Glick, 1974). Amphetamine apparently enhances the imbalance by acting predominantly on the intact side, e.g., releasing dopamine from intact nigro-striatal nerve endings. Although there is general agreement that an asymmetry in striatal dopaminergic function is of primary importance for rotation, there is evidence, although controversial, for modulation of rotation by noradrenergic (Marsden and Guldberg, 1973), cholinergic (Anden and Bedard, 1971; Costall, Naylor, and Olley, 1972b: Muller and Seeman, 1974), and serotonergic (Neill, Grant, and Grossman, 1972; Costall and Naylor, 1974) mechanisms. Interpretation of rotation data may sometimes be confounded by two methodological problems: (1) Some investigators measure rotation by subjective visual observation only. Because the latter can often produce unrepresentative and erroneous results, it is preferable to utilize an automated rotometer which distinguishes complete 360° rotations from incomplete oscillatory turns (e.g., Greenstein and Glick, 1975). (2) It has been established that normal rats will also rotate following the administration of amphetamine and other drugs eliciting rotation in lesioned rats (Jerussi and Glick, 1974, 1975). This rotation appears to be related to a normal and intrinsic asymmetry in dopaminergic nigro-striatal function (Zimmerberg, Glick, and Jerussi, 1974; Glick, Jerussi, Waters, and Green, 1974). The magnitude of rotation following a unilateral nigro-striatal lesion will depend upon whether the lesion is in the side ipsilateral or contralateral to the preoperative direction of rotation (Jerussi and Glick, 1975). Table 1 shows this effect for d-amphetamine in rats with unilateral caudate lesions (Fleisher and Glick, unpublished results). If the preoperative direction and magnitude of rotation are not considered (as they frequently are not), erroneous conclusions may be reached with regard to the kind of magnitude of effect produced by a lesion. For example, although it has been reported that unilateral lesions of the olfactory tubercle result in amphetamine-induced rotation (Yehuda and Wurtman, 1975), such lesions were found to have no effect when postoperative rotation data were compared to preoperative data (Fleisher and Glick, 1975).

AMPHETAMINE-INDUCED LOCOMOTOR STIMULATION

There is considerable controversy concerning the mechanism of amphetamine's stimulant effect on locomotor activity. There are two major opposing views, each based on many neurochemical findings. The views differ according to whether they attribute primary importance to amphetamine's dopaminergic or noradrenergic action (e.g., Thornburg and Moore, 1973). The results of lesion studies in rodents have been remarkably inconsistent. Both hypersensitivity (Iversen, 1971; Creese and Iversen, 1972; Costall and Naylor, 1973) and hyposensitivity (Simpson and Iversen, 1971; Iversen, 1971; Costall and Naylor, 1973; Creese and Iversen, 1975) to amphetamine have been reported to occur after lesions of the

Table 1

Mean Net Rotations (± S.E.) Per Hour Elicited by d-Amphetamine (1.0 mg/kg) Before and After Unilateral Lesions of the Caudate Nucleus Either Ipsilateral or Contralateral to the Pre-Operative Direction of Rotation

	Pre-Operative	Post-Operative*
Ipsilateral (N = 6)	43.8 ± 9.9	220.4 ± 54.5
Contralateral (N = 9)	53.7 ± 18.0	107.1 ± 23.0

*difference between ipsilateral and contralateral groups significant at $p < 0.05$ (t test); there was no significant difference pre-operatively ($p > 0.1$).

substantia nigra. Similarly, lesions of the corpus striatum have been found to have no effect (Naylor and Olley, 1972; Creese and Iversen, 1974; Neill, Boggan and Grossman, 1974), diminish (Glick and Marsanico, 1974), or increase (Neill, Ross, and Grossman, 1974) sensitivity to amphetamine-induced locomotor stimulation. Again, many of these discrepant findings may be reconcilable in terms of denervation supersensitivity. For example, Costall and Naylor (1973) reported that rats with nigral lesions were less sensitive to amphetamine early (1-2 days) after surgery but more sensitive at later (1-2 weeks) times. This kind of time-course is exactly what one would expect if the lesions were incomplete and if denervation supersensitivity occurred. Creese and Iversen (1975) have reached a similar interpretation and have shown that the striatum must be depleted of dopamine by more than 90% in order to abolish the locomotor response to amphetamine.

There have been several studies concerned with changes in amphetamine-induced locomotor stimulation after lesions of the frontal cortex in rats. Adler (1961) initially reported that rats with bilateral ablations of frontal cortex became increasingly sensitive to this effect of amphetamine with increasing time following surgery. Adler interpreted his results as being consistent with the occurrence of denervation supersensitivity. Frontal cortical lesions were supposed to have denervated subcortical structures; amphetamine presumably released catecholamines from remaining input to such structures whereby supersensitive post-synaptic receptors were activated. However, Lynch, Ballantine, and Campbell (1969, 1971) subsequently found that amphetamine hypersensitivity in frontal rats gradually disappeared with increasing time following surgery, while Glick (1970), Iversen, Wilkinson, and Simpson (1971), and Iversen (1971) reported data compatible with Adler's. The conflicting results were eventually attributed to a testing artifact. In the Lynch et al. experiments, rats were well habituated to their test cages prior to drug administration whereas, in all of the other studies, there was no prior habituation. When tested a month after surgery, amphetamine hypersensitivity in frontal rats was found to be minimal if a long period of habituation preceded testing with the drug (Glick, 1972). Thus testing variables which alter the baseline rate of activity may profoundly influence the kind of drug-lesion interaction observed.

EFFECTS ON OPERANT BEHAVIOR: DOSE-RELATED CONSIDERATIONS

In most behavioral situations in which very complete dose-response curves for amphetamine have been determined, inverted U or inverted J functions have generally been found (e.g., Glick and Muller, 1971). Low doses will facilitate and high doses will depress performance; the exact doses which produce each of these effects may vary tremendously depending upon the task and particular testing parameters affecting the rate of baseline behavior (Kelleher and Morse, 1968). These non-monotonic effects of amphetamine in normal animals may, occasionally, make it difficult to decipher changes in drug sensitivity after a lesion. For example, in early studies, rats, mice and monkeys having lesions of the frontal cortex were found to be less sensitive to the depressant effects of amphetamine on various learned tasks (Glick and Jarvik, 1970; Glick, 1971; Glick, Nakamura, and Jarvik, 1971). These results contrasted sharply with the results, reviewed above, of increased sensitivity of frontal rats to the activity stimulant effect of amphetamine. The apparent discrepancy was subsequently attributed to incomplete sampling of the whole amphetamine-dose response curve. Figure 1 shows the effects of d-amphetamine on fixed interval 15 second bar-pressing performance before and 6-8 weeks after ablation of frontal cortex in rats. After surgery, the whole dose-response curve is higher but less so at higher doses; this finding indicated that hypersensitivity occurs to all actions of d-amphetamine, but more to the facilitatory action than to the depressant action (Glick and Marsanico, 1974). In comparison, lesions of the caudate nucleus shift the whole amphetamine dose-response curve in parallel, to the left or to the right, respectively, depending upon whether the lesions are small or large (Figure 2). The latter difference between small and large lesions have been correlated with whether or not, respectively, near complete recovery of function occurs; the data suggested that, following small lesions which damage some nigro-striatal fibers, supersensitivity of the remaining caudate to remaining nigral input may develop whereas, following large lesions, d-amphetamine is less potent because its site of action has been excessively damaged (Glick, 1975). Thus in addition to amphetamine-induced anorexia, stereotypy, rotation, and activity enhancement, amphetamine-induced effects on operant behavior seem to be mediated, at least in part, via an action or actions in the striatum.

DEGREE OF STRIATAL ASYMMETRY AND INDIVIDUALITY

As mentioned earlier, amphetamine appears to induce rotation in normal rats as a result of potentiating an intrinsic asymmetry between left and right nigro-striatal systems. The dopamine contents of normal left and right striata have been found to differ by about 15%. Following the administration of d-amphetamine (20 mg/kg), the dopamine contents of left and right striata differ by approximately 25% and rats rotate contralateral to the side containing the higher level of dopamine (Glick et al., 1974; also, see Glick, Jerussi, and Zimmerberg, in press, for a review of many other rotation studies in normal animals). Other data have

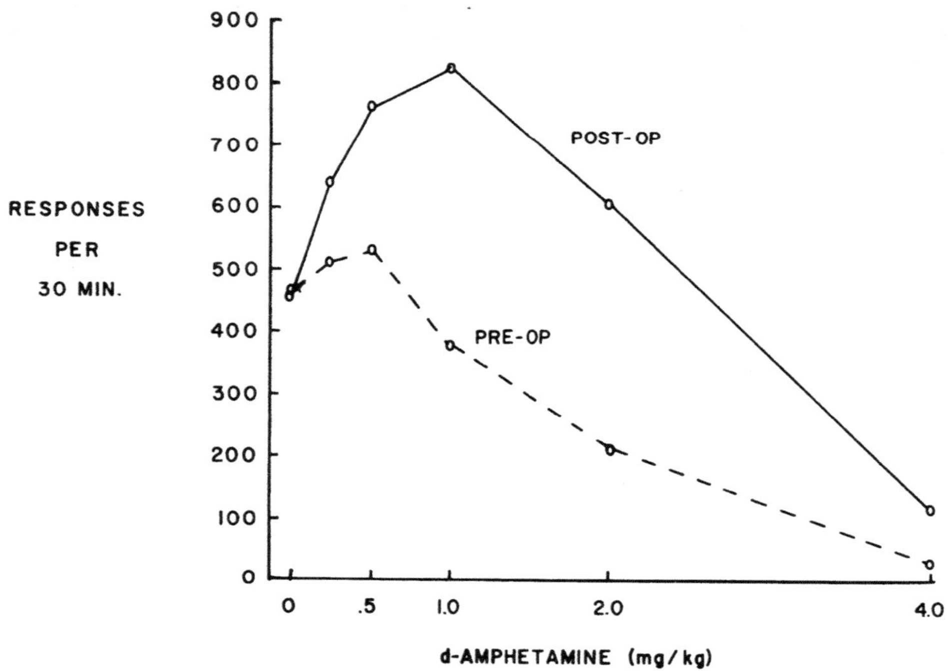

Fig. 1. Preoperative and postoperative (6-8 weeks after surgery) d-amphetamine dose-response curves for frontal rats (mean results for 4 rats; data derived from Glick and Marsancico, 1974).

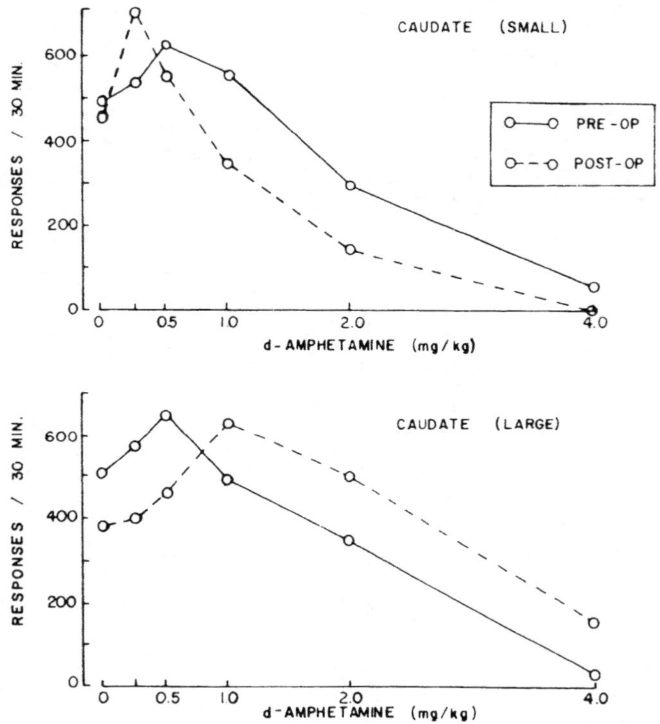

Fig. 2. Preoperative and postoperative (6-8 weeks after surgery) d-amphetamine dose-response curve for rats with either small (1-1½ mm in diameter) or large (2¼-2 3/4 mm in diameter) lesions of the caudate nuclei (mean results for 4 rats; from Glick, 1975). Reproduced by permission of Academic Press.

indicated that this striatal dopamine asymmetry is related not only to rotation but to spatial behavior in general. Initially, this was suggested by the finding that rats trained to bar-press in a two-lever operant chamber had stable side preferences which were correlated in direction with d-amphetamine-induced rotation (Glick and Jerussi, 1974). Subsequently, after a T-maze test to determine side preferences, dopamine levels were found to be significantly higher in the striata contralateral to rats' side preferences than in the ipsilateral striata (Zimmerberg et al., 1974).

Further studies have been concerned with examining possible associations of side preferences with behaviors not obviously spatial in nature. The relationship between side preferences and DRL (differential reinforcement of low rates) 16 second timing performance in rats is particularly interesting in this regard. Baseline rates of responding are normally inversely correlated with the strength of side preferences for the left or right lever in the two-lever operant chamber; lower rates and better timing performance are associated with greater preferences. Between successive lever-presses, rats have been observed to conduct characteristic stereotyped patterns of motor behavior which appear to be associated with side preferences. These and other results have suggested that motor feedback functions as a counting mechanism in normal timing behavior and that side preferences facilitate the stereotyped programming of motor patterns used in timing (Glick, Cox, and Greenstein, 1975). The effects of d-amphetamine on timing performance are related to its effects on side preferences. Amphetamine impairs timing performance when it decreases side preferences and facilitates or has no effect on timing performance when it increases side preferences (Figure 3). A similar relationship has been observed in the case of unilateral caudate lesions. Such lesions increase or decrease side preferences, respectively, when placed in the caudate nucleus ipsilateral or contralateral to the preoperative bias. The ipsilateral lesions facilitate timing performance and the contralateral lesions impair timing performance (Figure 4). Thus, individual variations in responsiveness of rats to amphetamine and to lesions may be attributable, at least in part, to interactions with side preferences and, presumably, striatal asymmetry (Glick and Cox, 1976).

The relationship of side preferences and amphetamine-induced rotation to locomotor activity has been examined in mice (Glick, Zimmerberg, and Greenstein, in press). As shown in Table 2, there are significant inverse correlations between strength of side preferences and locomotor activity and between net rotations and locomotor activity following amphetamine. More active mice, both normally and after d-amphetamine, have lower indices of behavioral laterality than less active mice. To the extent that side preferences and rotation are manifestations of

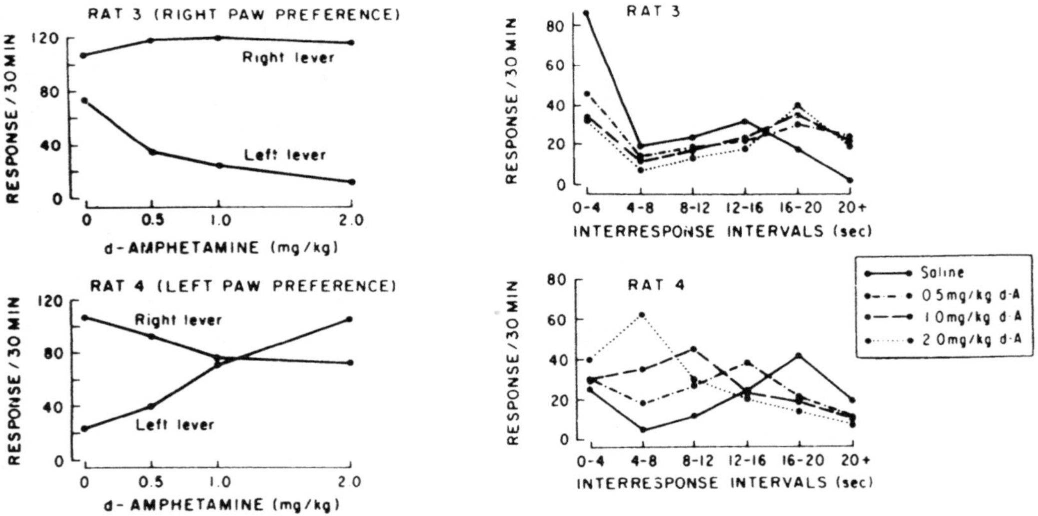

Fig. 3. DRL rate data (left) and inter-response time distributions (right) of two rats following saline or d-amphetamine. Note that d-amphetamine increases the side lever preference and facilitates the timing performance of Rat 3 and decreases the side lever preference and impairs the timing performance of Rat 4 (from Glick, Cox, and Greenstein, 1975). Reproduced by permission of North Holland Publishing Company.

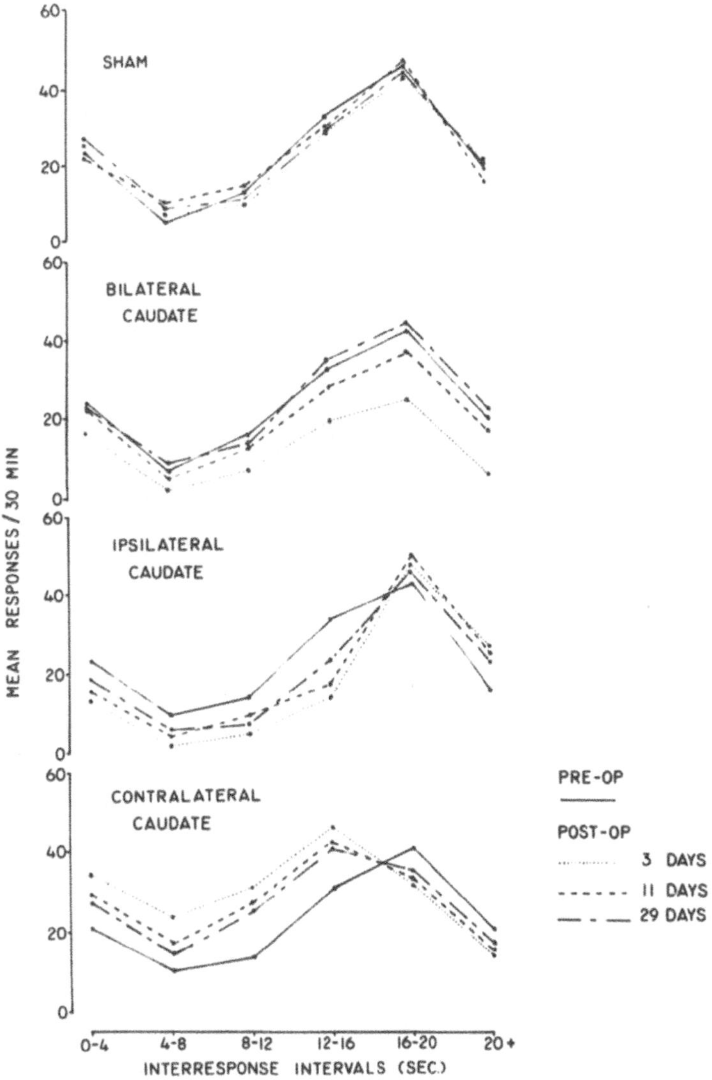

Fig. 4. Effects of caudate lesions on DRL inter-response time distributions (mean results for 6 rats per group). Preoperative side preferences were approximately 80%. Ipsilateral lesions increased preferences to about 90% and facilitated timing performances whereas contralateral lesions decreased preferences to about 70% and impaired timing performance. Bilateral lesions had no significant effects other than a transient overall decrease in response rates (from Glick and Cox, in press). Copyright 1976 by the American Psychological Association. Reprinted by permission.

TABLE 2

Correlation of Spontaneous Side Preferences with Normal Locomotor Activity (Group 1)*, and Amphetamine-induced Rotation with Amphetamine-enhanced Locomotor Activity (Group 2)*

	Means ± S.D.			Regression Coefficient (r)
	Side Pref. (%)	Net Rotation	Activity	
Group 1	74.6 ± 17.2	--	2347 ± 339	-0.57**
Group 2	--	114.9 ± 43.7	3372 ± 472	-0.64**

*Each group received two behavioral tests, with two weeks between tests. Group 1 (N = 24) was tested for side preferences in the T-maze and for locomotor activity in the photocell box. Group 2 (N = 16) was tested for d-amphetamine-induced rotation and locomotor activity following d-amphetamine (5.0 mg/kg in both tests).

**Significant correlation at $p < 0.01$, t test

(From Glick, Zimmerberg, and Greenstein, in press, by permission of Elsevier Scientific Publishing Company.)

striatal asymmetry, these correlations suggest individual differences in locomotor activity may be attributable to different degrees of striatal asymmetry. Effects on striatal asymmetry can not account, however, for overall group changes in activity following drug treatment. For all mice, d-amphetamine both increases locomotor activity and induces rotation, even though the increase in locomotor activity is less in those mice that rotate more. While amphetamine-induced rotation is related to an increase in the striatal dopamine asymmetry (Glick et al., 1974), amphetamine-induced stimulation of locomotor activity is probably related to release of dopamine *per se* in both striata (e.g., Thornburg and Moore, 1973). Perhaps an intrinsic symmetry between nigro-striatal pathways sets a maximal limit to the total amount of dopamine available for release in both striata. The greater the asymmetry, the lower the maximal limit and, since the dopamine-releasing action of amphetamine depends on the rate of neuronal firing (Von Voigtlander and Moore, 1973), the less potent amphetamine would be in activating the system as a whole. It might then be expected--as is, in fact, the case--that individual differences in sensitivity to the activity stimulant effect of amphetamine would in turn depend upon individual differences in baseline activity (Glick and Milloy, 1973). In attempting to generalize, it might be speculated that degree of striatal asymmetry is, overall, a major determinant of individuality. Needless to say, much additional research will be required to substantiate this hypothesis.

ACKNOWLEDGMENT

This work was supported by NIMH grant MH25644 and NIDA Research Scientist Development Award (Type 2) DA70082.

REFERENCES

Adler, M.W.: Changes in sensitivity to amphetamine in rats with chronic brain lesions. J. Pharmac. exp. Ther. 134, 204-211 (1961).

Agid, Y., Javoy, F., and Glowinski, J.: Hyperactivity of remaining dopaminergic neurons after partial destruction of the nigro-striatal dopaminergic system in the rat. Nature new Biol. 245, 150-151 (1973).

Ahlskog, J.E., and Hoebel, B.G.: Overeating and obesity from damage to a noradrenergic system in the brain. Science 182, 166-169 (1973).

Anden, N., and Bedard, P.: Influences of cholinergic mechanisms on the function and turnover of brain dopamine. J. Pharm. Pharmac. 23, 460-462 (1971).

Arbuthnott, G.W., and Crow, T.J.: Relation of contraversive turning to unilateral release of dopamine from the nigrostrial pathway in rat. Expl. Neurol. 30, 484-491 (1971).

Blundell, J.E., and Leshem, M.B.: Central action of anorexic agents: Effects of amphetamine and fenfluramine in rats with lateral hypothalamic lesions. Eur. J. Pharmacol. 28, 81-88 (1974).

Brobeck, J.R., Larsson, S., and Reyes, E.: A study of electrical activity of the hypothalamic feeding mechanism. J. Physiol. 132, 358-364 (1956).

Carlisle, H.J.: Differential effects of amphetamine on food and water intake in rats with lateral hypothalamic lesions. J. comp. Physiol. Psychol. 58, 47-54 (1964).

Christie, J.E., and Crow, T.J.: Turning behavior as an index of the action of amphetamines and ephedrines on central dopamine-containing neurons. Br. J. Pharmac. 43, 658-667 (1971).

Costall, B., Naylor, R.J., and Olley, J.E.: The substantia nigra and stereotyped behavior. Eur. J. Pharmacol. 18, 95-106 (1972a).

Costall, B., Naylor, R.J., and Olley, J.E.: Catalepsy and circling behaviour after intra-cerebral injections of neuroleptic, cholinergic and anticholinergic agents into the caudate-putamen, globus pallidus, and substantia nigra of rat brain. Neuropharmacology 11, 645-663 (1972b).

Costall, B. and Naylor, R.J.: The role of the substantia nigra in the locomotor stimulant action of amphetamine. Br. J. Pharmac. 49, 29-36, (1973).

Costall, B. and Naylor, R.J.: Stereotyped and circling behaviour induced by dopaminergic agonists after lesions of the midbrain raphe nuclei. Eur. J. Pharmacol. 29, 206-222 (1974).

Creese, I. and Iversen, S.D.: Amphetamine response in rat after dopamine neuron destruction. Nature new Biol. 238-247-248 (1972).

Creese, I. and Iversen, S.D.: The role of forebrain dopamine system in amphetamine induced stereotyped behavior in the rat. Psychopharmacologia 39, 345-357 (1974).

Creese, I. and Iversen, S.D.: The pharmacological and anatomical substrates of the amphetamine response in the rat. Brain Res. 83, 419-436 (1975).

Crow, T.J.: The relationship between lesion site, dopamine neurons, and turning behavior in the rat. Exptl. Neurol. 32, 247-255 (1971).

Divac, I.: Drug-induced syndrome in rats with large, chronic lesions in the corpus striatum. Psychopharmacologia 27, 272-278 (1972).

Epstein, A.: Suppression of eating and drinking by amphetamine and other drugs in normal and hyperphagic rats. J. comp. Physiol. Psychol. 52, 37-45 (1959).

Fibiger, H.C., Fibiger, H.P., and Zis, A.P.: Attenuation of amphetamine-induced motor stimulation and stereotypy of 6-hydroxydopamine in the rat. Br. J. Pharmac. 47, 683-692 (1973).

Fibiger, H.C., Zis, A.P., and McGreer, E.G.: Feeding and drinking deficits after 6-hydroxydopamine administration in the rat: Similarities to the lateral hypothalamic syndrome. Brain Res. 55, 135-148 (1973).

Fleisher, L.N. and Glick, S.D.: A telencephalic lesion site for d-amphetamine-induced contralateral rotation in rats. Brain Res. 96, 413-417 (1975).

Fog, R., Randrup, A., and Pakkenberg, H.: Lesions in corpus striatum and cortex of rat brains and the effect on pharmacologically induced stereotyped, aggressive and cataleptic behaviour. Psychopharmacologia 18, 346-356 (1970).

Glick, S.D.: Changes in sensitivity to d-amphetamine in frontal rats as a function of time: Shifting of the dose-response curve. Psychon. Sci. 19, 57-58 (1970).

Glick, S.D.: Changes in amphetamine sensitivity following frontal cortical damage in rats and mice. Eur. J. Pharmacol. 20, 352-356 (1972).

Glick, S.D.: Changes in drug sensitivity and mechanisms of functional recovery following brain damage. In: Plasticity and Recovery of Function in the Central Nervous System. Stein, D.G., Rosen, J.A. and Butter, N., Eds., pp. 339-372, New York: Academic Press, 1974.

Glick, S.D.: Recovery of function and changes in sensitivity to amphetamine following caudate lesions in rats. Behav. Biol. 13, 239-244 (1975).

Glick, S.D. and Cox, R.D.: Differential effects of unilateral and bilateral caudate lesions on side preferences and timing behavior in rats. J. comp. Physiol. Psychol. (in press).

Glick, S.D., Cox, R.D., and Greenstein, S.: Relationship of rats' spatial preferences to effects of d-amphetamine on timing behaviour. Eur. J. Pharmacol. 33, 173-182 (1975).

Glick, S.D., Greenstein, S., and Zimmerberg, B.: Facilitation of recovery after lateral hypothalamic damage by prior ablation of frontal cortex. Nature new Biol. 239, 187-188 (1972).

Glick, S.D. and Jarvik, M.E.: Differential effects of amphetamine and scopolamine on matching performance of monkeys with lateral frontal lesions. J. comp. Physiol. Psychol. 73, 307-313 (1970).

Glick, S.D. and Jerussi, T.P.: Spatial and paw preferences in rats: Their relationship to rate-dependent effects of d-amphetamine. J. Pharmac. exp. Ther. 188, 714-725 (1974).

Glick, S.D., Jerussi, T.P., Waters, D.H., and Green, J.P.: Amphetamine-induced changes in striatal dopamine and acetylcholine levels and relationship to rotation (circling behavior) in rats. Biochem. Pharmacol. 23, 3223-3225 (1974).

Glick, S.D., Jerussi, T.P., and Zimmerberg, B.: Behavioral and neuropharmacological correlates of nigro-striatal asymmetry in rats. In: Lateralization in the Nervous System. Harnad, S., Ed. New York: Academic Press, in press.

Glick, S.D. and Marsanico, R.G.: Shifting of the d-amphetamine dose-response curve in rats with frontal cortical ablations. Psychopharmacologia 36, 109-115 (1974).

Glick, S.D. and Milloy, S.: Rate-dependent effects of d-amphetamine in mice: Possible relationship to paradoxical amphetamine sedation in minimal brain dysfunction. Eur. J. Pharmacol. 24, 266-268 (1973).

Glick, S.D. and Muller, R.U.: Paradoxical effects of low doses of d-amphetamine in rats. Psychopharmacologia 22, 396-402 (1971).

Glick, S.D., Nakamura, R.K., and Jarvik, M.E.: Recovery of function following frontal brain damage in mice: Changes in sensitivity to d-amphetamine. J. comp. Physiol. Psychol. 76, 454-459 (1971).

Glick, S.D., Waters, D.H., and Milloy S.: Depletion of hypothalamic norepinephrine by food deprivation and interaction with d-amphetamine. Res. Comm. Chem. Path. Pharmac. 6, 775-778 (1973).

Glick, S.D., Zimmerberg, B., and Greenstein, S.: Individual differences among mice in normal and amphetamine-enhanced locomotor activity: Relationship to behavioral indices of striatal asymmetry. Brain Res. (in press).

Gold, R.M.: Hypothalamic obesity: The myth of the ventromedial nucleus. Science 182, 488-490 (1973).

Greenstein, S. and Glick, S.D.: An improved automated apparatus for recording rotation in rats or mice. Pharmac. Biochem. Behav. 3, 507-510 (1975).

Iversen, S.D.: The effect of surgical lesions to frontal cortex and substantia nigra on amphetamine responses in rats. Brain Res. 31, 295-311 (1971).

Jerussi, T.P. and Glick, S.D.: Amphetamine-induced rotation in rats without lesions. Neuropharmacology 13, 283-286 (1974).

Jerussi, T.P. and Glick, S.D.: Apomorphine-induced rotation in normal rats and interaction with unilateral caudate lesion. Psychopharmacologia 40, 329-334 (1975).

Kapatos, G. and Gold, R.M.: Evidence for ascending noradrenergic mediation of hypothalamic hyperphagia. Pharmac. Biochem. Behav. 1, 81-87 (1973).

Kelleher, R.T. and Morse, W.H.: Determinants of the specificity of behavioral effects of drugs. Ergebn. Physiol. 60, 1-56 (1968).

Kennedy, G.C. and Mitra, J.: The effect of d-amphetamine on energy balance in hypothalamic obese rats. Br. J. Nutr. 17, 569-573 (1963).

Lynch, G.S., Ballantine, P., and Campbell, B.A.: Potentiation of behavioral arousal after cortical damage and subsequent recovery. Exp. Neurol. 23, 195-206 (1969).

Lynch, G., Ballantine, P., and Campbell, B.A.: Differential rates of recovery following frontal cortical lesions in rats. Physiol. Behav. 7, 737-741 (1971).

Marsden, C.A. and Guldberg, H.C.: The role of monoamines in rotation induced or potentiated by amphetamine after nigral raphe and mesencephalic reticular lesions in the rat brain. Neuropharmacology 12, 195-211 (1973).

Marshall, J.F. and Teitelbaum, P.: A comparison of the eating in response to hypothermic and glucoprivic challenges after nigral 6-hydroxydopamine and lateral hypothalamic electrolytic lesions in rats. Brain Res. 55, 229-233 (1973).

Mishra, R.K., Gardner, E.L., Katzman, R., and Makman, M.H.: Enhancement of dopamine-stimulated adenylate cyclase activity in rat caudate after lesions in substantia nigra: Evidence for denervation supersensitivity. Proc. Nat. Acad. Sci. 71, 3883-3887 (1974).

Muller, P. and Seeman, P.: Neuroleptics: Relation between cataleptic and anti-turning action, and role of the cholinergic system. J. Pharm. Pharmac. 26, 981-984 (1974).

Naylor, R.J. and Olley, J.E.: Modification of the behavioral changes induced by haloperidol in the rat by lesions in the caudate nucleus, the caudate-putamen and global pallidus. Neuropharmacology 11, 81-89 (1972).

Neill, D.B., Boggan, W.O., and Grossman, S.P.: Behavioral effects of amphetamine in rats with lesions in the corpus striatum. J. comp. Physiol. Psychol. 86, 1019-1030 (1974).

Neill, D.B., Grant, L.D., and Grossman, S.P.: Selective potentiation of locomotor effects of amphetamine by midbrain raphe lesions. Physiol. Behav. 9, 655-657 (1972).

Neill, D.B. and Linn, C.L.: Deficits in consummatory responses to regulatory challenges following basal ganglia lesions in rats. Physiol. Behav. 14, 617-624 (1975).

Oltmans, G.A. and Harvey, J.A.: LH syndromes and brain catecholamine levels after lesions of the nigrostriatal bundle. Physiol. Behav. 8, 69-78 (1972).

Price, M.T. and Fibiger, H.C.: Apomorphine and amphetamine stereotypy after 6-hydroxydopamine lesions of the substantia nigra. Eur. J. Pharmacol. 29, 240-252 (1974).

Reynolds, R.W.: The effect of amphetamine on food intake in normal and hypothalamic hyperphagic rats. J. comp. Physiol. Psychol. 52, 682-684 (1959).

Russek, M., Rodriguez-Zendejas, A.M., and Teitelbaum, P.: The action of adrenergic anorexigenic substances on rats recovered from lateral hypothalamic lesions. Physiol. Behav. 10, 329-333 (1973).

Scheel-Krüger, J. and Randrup, A.: Stereotype hyperactive behaviour produced by dopamine in the absence of noradrenaline. Life Sci. 6, 1389-1394 (1967).

Sharp, J.C., Neilson, H.C., and Porter, P.B.: The effect of amphetamine upon cats with lesions in the ventromedial hypothalamus. J. comp. Physiol. Psychol. 55, 198-200 (1962).

Sharpless, S.K.: Supersensitivity-like phenomena in the central nervous system. Fed. Proc. 34, 1990-1997 (1975).

Simpson, B.A. and Iversen, S.D.: Effects of substantia nigra lesions on the locomotor and stereotypy responses to amphetamine. Nature new Biol. 230, 30-32 (1971).

Stowe, F.R. and Miller, A.T.: The effect of amphetamine on food intake in rats with hypothalamic hyperphagia. Experientia 13, 114-115 (1957).

Stricker, E.M. and Zigmond, M.J.: Effects on homeostasis of intraventricular injections of 6-hydroxydopamine in rats. J. comp. Physiol. Psychol. 86, 973-994 (1974).

Taylor, K.M. and Snyder, S.H.: Amphetamine: Differentiation by d and l isomers of behavior involving brain norepinephrine or dopamine. Science 168, 1487-1489 (1970).

Teitelbaum, P. and Epstein, A.: The lateral hypothalamic syndrome: Recovery of feeding and drinking after lateral hypothalamic lesions. Psychol. Rev. 69, 74-90 (1962).

Thornburg, J.E. and Moore, K.E.: The relative importance of dopaminergic and noradrenergic neuronal systems for the stimulation of locomotor activity induced by amphetamine and other drugs. Neuropharmacology 12, 853-866 (1973).

Trendelenburg, U.: Supersensitivity and subsensitivity to sympathomimetic amines. Pharmac. Rev. 14, 225-277 (1963).

Ungerstedt, U.: Postsynaptic supersensitivity after 6-hydroxydopamine induced degeneration of the nigro-striatal dopamine system. Acta physiol. Scand., Suppl. 367,69-93 (1971).

Ungerstedt, U. and Arbuthnott, G.W.: Quantitative recording of rotational behavior in rats after 6-hydroxydopamine lesions of the nigro-striatal dopamine system. Brain Res. 24, 485-493 (1970).

Von Voigtlander, P.E. and Moore, K.E.: Involvement of nigro-striatal neurons in the vivo release of dopamine by amphetamine, amantadine and tyramine. J. Pharm. exp. Ther. 184, 542-552 (1973).

Wishart, T.B. and Walls, E.K.: The effects of anorexic doses of dextro-amphetamine on the ventromedial-hypothalamic hyperphagic rat. Can. J. Physiol. Pharmac. 51, 354-359 (1973).

Yehuda, S. and Wurtman, R.J.: Dopaminergic neurons in the nigro-striatal and mesolimbic pathways: Mediation of specific effects of d-amphetamine. Eur. J. Pharmacol. 30, 154-158 (1975).

Zimmerberg, B. and Glick, S.D.: Rotation and stereotype during electrical stimulation of the caudate nucleus. Res. Comm. Chem. Path. Pharmac. 8, 195-196 (1974).

Zimmerberg, B., Glick, S.D. and Jerussi, T.P.: Neurochemical correlate of a spatial preference in rats. Science 185, 623-625 (1974).

BASIC CONSIDERATIONS ON THE ROLE OF CONCERTEDLY WORKING DOPAMINERGIC, GABA-ERGIC, CHOLINERGIC AND SEROTONERGIC MECHANISMS WITHIN THE NEO-STRIATUM AND NUCLEUS ACCUMBENS IN LOCOMOTOR ACTIVITY, STEREOTYPED GNAWING, TURNING AND DYSKINETIC ACTIVITIES

A. R. Cools

Department of Pharmacology

Geert Grooteplein N. 21, Nijmegen, The Netherlands

INTRODUCTION

In man there seems to exist an unmistakable correlation between central dopaminergic activity and psychomotor diseases such as Parkinson's disease, Huntington's chorea, tardive dyskinesias and some psychotic disorders (Barbeau, Doshey and Spiegel, 1965; Barbeau and McDowell, 1969; Barrett, Yahr, and Duvoisin, 1970; Calne, 1970; Crane, 1968a-b; Fog and Pakkenberg, 1970; Klawans, 1969, 1970, 1973; Klawans, Ilahi, and Shenker, 1970; La Plante and St. Laurent, 1973; Papeschi, 1972; Randrup and Munkvad, 1972; Stevens, 1973; Weil-Malherbe and Szara, 1971; Wyatt, Fermini, and Davis, 1971).

Today an enormous list of articles, reviews and books is devoted to studies dealing with the therapeutic efficacy of dopaminergic agents such as L-DOPA and neuroleptics in the treatment of psychomotor diseases and psychosis. Despite the initial enthusiasm about the clinical application of these substances, it appears that neurologists and psychiatrists are too often confronted with treatment failures: apart from the fact that these agents just improve some symptoms in some patients, they often elicit unwanted side-effects. At least two reasons for the lack of success in this respect can be mentioned. First, the drugs used are not potent and/or selective enough. Second, the therapeutic approach either to correct a hypoactive dopaminergic system in all patients with Parkinson's disease or to correct a hyperactive dopaminergic system in all patients with spontaneously occurring psychoses is not always the right starting point. Though there is little doubt about the role of a dysfunctioning, nigro-neostriatal dopaminergic pathway and/or a dysfunctioning striatum in psychomotor disorders, it is also beyond any doubt that other neurotransmitters are involved. As Barbeau has aptly stated in his excellent paper on the biology of the striatum (Barbeau, 1973): "it is outdated to look at any one system, such as the nigrostriatal dopaminergic pathway, as acting alone. The resulting clinical manifestations of a defect in this pathway involve, in addition to akinesia, the interplay of GABA-ergic, cholinergic, and serotonergic systems translated into rigidity, postural difficulties, and tremor" (p.346).

The purpose of this article is an attempt to increase our scientific insight into the basic mechanisms involved in the pathophysiology of psychomotor diseases by reviewing the very recent literature dealing with the interaction of these neurotransmitters within the striatum of animals and by offering new data and ideas about their role in stereotyped behavior, oro-facial-lingual dyskinesias, turning and motility in cats and rats. It is believed that these data offer experimental support to the idea of Barbeau (1973) that: "a completely new outlook on the management of these illnesses is now permitted."

At present, the experimental work dealing with the behavioral function of the neurotransmitters occurring within the striatum can be divided into two broad types:

1) studies on the behavioral effects triggered by extracerebrally administered drugs known to penetrate specific parts of the brain;
2) studies on the behavioral effects triggered by intracerebrally administered drugs.

Furthermore, the following subclasses can be discerned: a) behavioral studies dealing with the effects of drugs upon syndromes previously induced; most often, the so-called apomorphine or dexamphetamine stereotypy, the catalepsy induced by neuroleptics, the carbachol-induced tremor, and experimentally induced turning or circling movements are used in this type of research; and b) behavioral studies dealing with the effects of drugs in animals showing normal behavior.

Although studies belonging to the first-mentioned subclass are very useful for understanding certain biochemical and pharmacological aspects of the mechanisms of action of drugs, they seldom offer insight into the function of neurotransmitters within specific brain areas. Since it is my purpose to focus attention on the role of neurotransmitters within the striatum and adjacent structures, studies dealing with the effects of striatally applied substances in non-pretreated animals are especially considered below. Studies with rats, however, confront us with a large number of confusing data; at present, they do not permit us to put forward clear-cut conclusions. However, it is possible to make some deductions from these data, given that one considers them in view of the outcome of comparable studies on the caudate nucleus of cats. Each section, therefore, contains an up-to-date summary of what we know about the function of neurotransmitters within the caudate nucleus of cats and, in addition, a brief survey of the present state of knowledge of these compounds in the neostriatum and nucleus accumbens in rats; in the parts dealing with rats, it is attempted to demonstrate that the feline data do offer a completely new way in which one may look for a better understanding of the mechanisms of action behind the pharmacological modulation of behavioral phenomena such as stereotyped behavior, dyskinesias, circling movements and locomotor activity.

THE INTRACAUDATE DOPAMINE "SEE-SAW"

Introduction

During the last decade, hard evidence has been presented that dopamine (DA) fulfills a crucial role as neurotransmitter in the regulation of impulse-transmission within the neostriatum. Anatomical and histochemical studies have clearly shown that DA is found within very fine, nigro-neostriatal fibres running from the substantia nigra, pars compacta, to the neostriatum, i.e., the caudate nucleus and putamen (Andèn, Dahlström, Fuxe, Olson, and Ungerstedt, 1966; Fibiger, Pudritz, McGeer, and McGeer, 1972; Fuxe, Hökfelt, and Nilsson, 1964; Ibata, Nojyo, Matsuura, and Sano, 1973; Maler, Fibiger, and McGeer, 1973; Moore, Batnagar, and Heller, 1971). Furthermore, both pharmacological and behavioral studies have revealed that neostriatal DA functions as an essential mediator in processes involved in the control and regulation of various motor activities: in animals, characteristic phenomena such as stereotyped behavioral patterns, catalepsy, choreo-athetoid movements and oro-facial-lingual dyskinesias are elicited, modified or suppressed by rather selective interference with the neostriatal DA-activity (Baker, Connor, Rossi, and Lalley, 1969; Butcher and Bryan, 1972; Connor, Rossi, and Baker, 1967; Cools, 1972; Costall and Naylor, 1972; Costall and Naylor, 1975a; Ernst and Smelik, 1966; Fog and Pakkenberg, 1971; Ungerstedt, Butcher, Butcher, Andèn, and Fuxe, 1969).

DA is also present within mesolimbic fibres running from cell bodies dorsocranial to the interpeduncular nucleus in the ventral mesencephalon to the nucleus accumbens, the nucleus interstitialis striae terminalis and the tuberculum olfactorium (Andèn et al.,

1966; Fuxe, Hökfelt, and Ungerstedt, 1969; Ungerstedt, 1971a). Since Pijnenburg and his colleagues have discovered that the dopaminergic mechanism within the nucleus accumbens is involved in the regulation of the locomotor activity (Pijnenburg and van Rossum, 1973; Pijnenburg, Woodruff, and van Rossum, 1973), many workers have focused their attention on the pharmacological and behavioral properties of this nucleus (Andèn and Jackson, 1975; Bartholini, Keller, and Pletscher, 1975; Elkhawad and Woodruff, 1975; Horn, Cuello, and Miller, 1974; Jackson, 1975; Kelly, 1975; Kelly and Miller, 1975; Kelly, Seviour, and Iversen, 1975; Miller, Horn, and Iversen, 1974; Pijnenburg, Honig, and van Rossum, 1975a-c; Pijnenburg, Honig, van der Heyden, and van Rossum, 1976; Pijnenburg, Honig, Struyker Boudier, Cools, van der Heyden, and van Rossum, in press).

Cats

Studies analysing the behavioral changes induced by injections of DA and related substances in cats have revealed that unilateral DA injections (10 μg) into the rostromedial part of the head of the caudate nucleus (CRM-area; Fig. 1) invariably result in a DA-specific "contralateral syndrome" marked by a shift from moving, walking and sitting to lying, contralateral turning of the head and eye-balls, fluttering of the ear and contractions of the facial muscles on the side contralateral to the injection, alternating ventriflexions and dorsiflexions of the contralateral paw and toes (athetoid movements) and rapid jerking, shaking-off movements of the entire contralateral forelimb (choreiform movements) (Cools and van Rossum, 1970). Similar injections into certain sites within intracaudate structures outside the CRM-area (r-CRM-area; Fig. 1) result in the display of the so-called "ipsilateral syndrome": in that case, all above-mentioned symptoms are directed to, or occur on, the side ipsilateral to the injection (Cools, Janssen, Struyker Boudier, and van Rossum, 1975a; Cools, Struyker Boudier, and van Rossum, in press). From the methodological point of view, it is of interest to note that the described syndromes only appear when the animals are tested in a well-known environment in which no changes occur during the experimental procedure (cf. Milhaud and Klein, 1974).

A more detailed behavioral analysis of effects produced by different drugs locally applied into the CRM- and r-CRM-area of the caudate nucleus has shown that this structure, indeed, contains two pharmacologically distinct types of DA-receptors: DA-receptors which are selectively activated by DA and apomorphine, selectively inhibited by haloperidol, and nearly unaffected by 1-(2-pyrimidyl)-4-piperonyl piperazine (piribedil, ET-494 or trivastal), ergometrine, 3, 4-dihydroxy-phenylamino-2-inidazoline (DPI), clonidine and noradrenaline (NA) (= DA_e-receptors); and DA-receptors which are selectively activated by DA and DPI, selectively inhibited by piribedil, ergometrine and NA, and relatively unaffected by apomorphine, haloperidol and clonidine (= DA_i-receptors) (Cools et al., 1975a; Cools et al., in press). Unilateral activation of the DA_e-receptors, which are mainly concentrated within the CRM-area, results in the contralateral syndrome, whereas unilateral activation of the DA_i-receptors, which are mainly concentrated within the anterodorsal part of the head of the caudate nucleus (r-CRM-area), results in the ipsilateral syndrome (Fig. 1). Bilateral stimulation of both types of DA-receptors within the caudate nucleus results in the appearance of athetoid and choreiform movements of the limbs, whereas only bilateral stimulation of the DA_i-sites, which are restricted to the r-CRM-area, results in the display of the so-called oro-facial-lingual dyskinesias (Cools, 1972; Cools et al., in press). Despite the fact that the number of DA_i-receptors exceeds the number of DA_e-receptors, there normally exists a well balanced see-saw between them. The fact that the DA_i-receptors are indirectly activated by 3, 4-dihydroxyphenyl-acetic acid (DOPAC) in contrast to the DA_e-receptors, which are indirectly activated by 3-methoxytyramine (Cools, 1971; Cools et al., in press), opens the question whether these distinct features reflect the presence of distinct biochemical pathways; this is especially interesting in view of the data of Olson, Seiger and Fuxe (1972), Shellenberger and Gordon (1974) and Tennyson, Barrett, Côté, Heikkila, and Mytilineou (1972), who suggested that there are different DA-systems within distinct neural systems, each of them marked by their own turnover.

A theoretical review of the concurrent research dealing with studies on the functional properties of the caudate nucleus in mammals has summarized evidence in favour of the concept that the DA_e-receptors are DA-excitation-mediating receptors presynaptically localized on GABA-ergic fibres arising from the substantia nigra in contrast to the DA_i-receptors, which are DA-inhibition-mediating receptors postsynaptically localized in synapses belonging to the well-known dopaminergic, nigro-neostriatal fibres (Cools and van Rossum, 1976; GABA section and Fig. 6). The origin of the fibres releasing DA at the DA_e-receptors is at present unknown.

Rats

In general, it is known that pharmacological manipulation with the DA-loaded neostriatum may result in turning and circling movements and/or stereotyped gnawing and biting. Furthermore, it is known that such a manipulation with the nucleus accumbens results in changes in the locomotor activity.

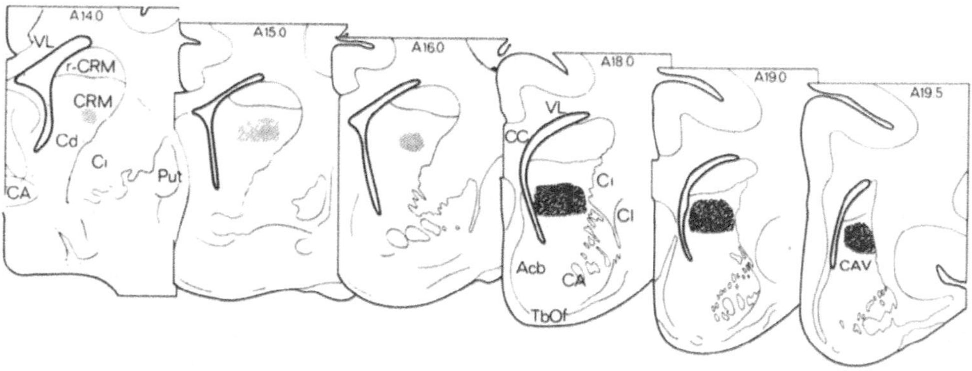

Fig. 1. Semi-diagrammatic outline of six anterior frontal planes in the caudate nucleus of cats showing the area containing DA_e-receptors (CRM-area; arced), the anterodorsal area containing DA_i-receptors (r-CRM-area) and the anteroventral area containing serotonin-sensitive sites (CAV-area; shadowed).

Acb = nucleus accumbens; CA = commissura anterior; CC = corpus callosum; Cd = nucleus caudatus; Ci = capsula interna; Cl = nucleus centrolateralis thalami; Put = putamen; TbOf = tuberculum olfactorium; VL = ventriculus lateralis.

As has been shown by Pijnenburg et al. (1973a-b; 1975a-c; 1976 and in press), Jackson (in press) and Andèn and Jackson (1975), small amounts of DA, apomorphine and dexamphetamine (1-10 μg) are able to increase the locomotor activity during a period of about 30 min following bilateral injections into the nucleus accumbens; this effect is easily blocked by 2.5 μg haloperidol, a selective antagonist of the DA_e-receptors in the cat. Ergometrine (0.5 μg), a potent antagonist of the DA_i-receptors in the cat, is able to stimulate the locomotor activity; this increase, however, appears after a latency of about 30-60 min and is long-lasting (Pijnenburg et al., 1973). Apart from the fact that this effect is attenuated by 2.5 μg haloperidol (Pijnenburg et al., 1976), this response is blocked by 5 μg DA (Fig. 2) and 5.0 μg DPI, a potent and selective agonist of the DA_i-receptors in the cat (Pijnenburg et al., in press), and potentiated by 1 μg apomorphine (Fig. 3; Cools, in press). If one considers these data in view of the mentioned feline data, it can be postulated that the nucleus accumbens of rats also contains two functionally opposing DA-systems: a DA_1-system, in which stimulation results in a short-term increase in the locomotor activity, and a DA_2-system, in which inhibition results in a long-term increase in the locomotor activity. In other words, stimulation of the DA_2-system results in "suppression" of the locomotor activity. Indeed, DPI itself produces a long-lasting suppression as shown by Pijnenburg et al. (in press). Since the short-term DA-induced increase is mimicked by apomorphine and dexamphetamine and inhibited by haloperidol in contrast to the DA-induced "suppression," which appears after a latency of about 40 min and is mimicked by DPI, attenuated by apomorphine and inhibited by ergometrine (indirectly resulting in a strong and long-lasting increase in locomotor activity), two additional deductions can be made.

First, the DA_1-system, in which stimulation results in a short-term increase, and the DA_2-system, in which inhibition results in a long-term increase, have pharmacological properties comparable to those of the feline DA_e- and DA_i-system respectively. Accordingly, the nucleus accumbens of rats might also contain a DA_e- and DA_i-system. If so, one must assume that the ability of haloperidol to attenuate the stimulating effect of ergometrine is due to its ability to restore the dysbalance between both systems caused by ergometrine rather than to its ability to block the DA_i-receptors.

Second, apomorphine, which is a potent agonist of both the DA_e-receptors in the cat and the comparable ones in the rat, has, in addition, a slight antagonistic action at the receptors in the rat, which are similar to the DA_i-receptors in the cat.

The notion that apomorphine has an antagonistic effect at the DA_i-receptors apart from its agonistic effect at the DA_e-receptors actually provides additional support for the previously reported hypothesis that the pharmacologically distinct DA-receptors within

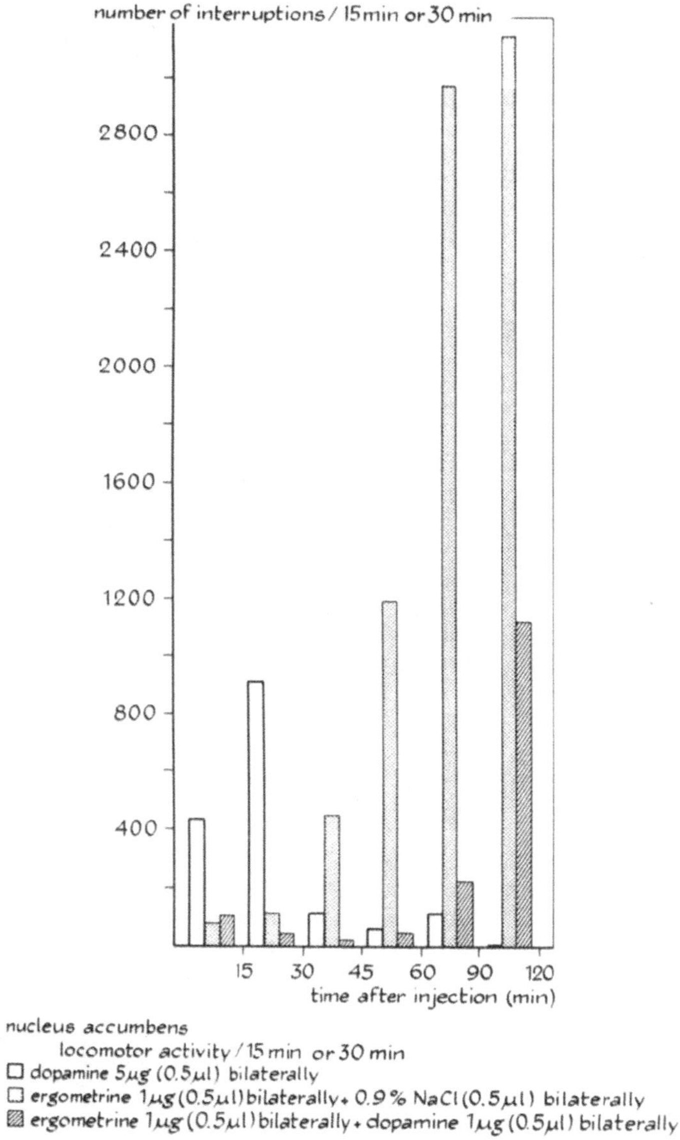

Fig. 2. Locomotor activity of rat no. 15 during successive periods (4 x 15 min + 2 x 30 min): (a) following dopamine injections into the nucleus accumbens at t = 0; (b) following ergometrine injections into the accumbens at t = -15 followed by saline injections into the accumbens at t = 0; and (c) following ergometrine injections into the accumbens at t = -15 followed by dopamine injections into the accumbens at t = 0.

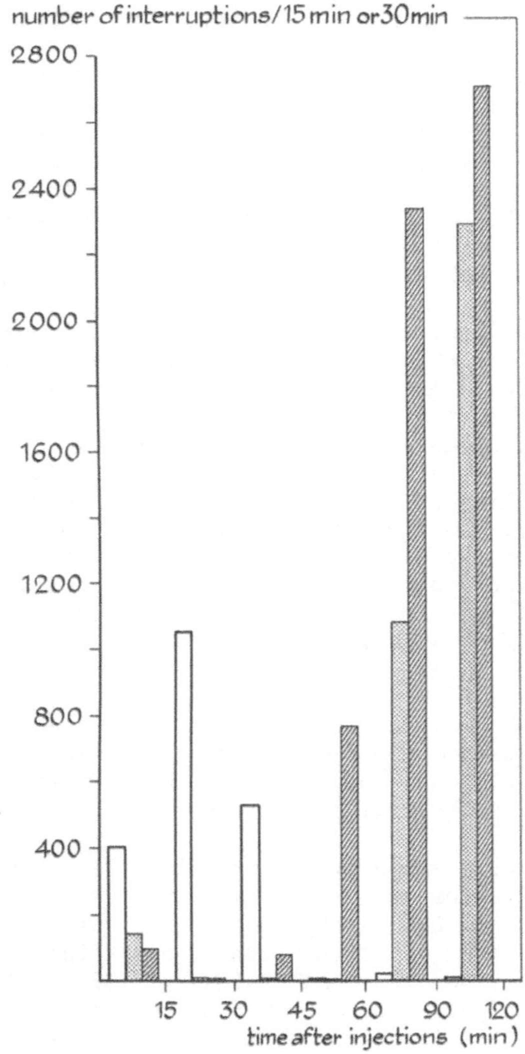

nucleus accumbens
locomotor activity/15 min or 30 min
□ apomorphine 1 μg (0.5 μl) bilaterally
▨ ergometrine 1 μg (0.5 μl) bilaterally + 0.9 % NaCl (0.5 μl) bilaterally
▨ ergometrine 1 μg (0.5 μl) bilaterally + apomorphine 1 μg (0.5 μl) bilaterally

Fig. 3. Locomotor activity of rat no. 15 during successive periods (4 x 15 min + 2 x 30 min): (a) following apomorphine injections into the nucleus accumbens at t = 0; (b) following ergometrine injections into the accumbens at t = -15 followed by saline injections into the accumbens at t = 0; and (c) following ergometrine injections into the accumbens at t = -15 followed by apomorphine injections into the accumbens at t = 0.

the mammalian brain have properties identical to those of the electrophysiologically and pharmacologically distinct DA_e- and DA_i-receptors within the snail Helix aspersa (Cools and van Rossum, 1976): as pointed out by Struyker Boudier, Gielen, Cools, and van Rossum (1974), Struyker Boudier, Teppema, Cools, and van Rossum (1975), and Struyker Boudier (1975), apomorphine exerts comparable effects at the DA_e- and DA_i-receptors within the snail Helix aspersa. On the basis of the above-mentioned data, it appears to be justified to speak about the presence of a DA_e- and DA_i-system within the nucleus accumbens of rats.

Anyhow, it is evident that an increase in the locomotor activity can be triggered either by stimulation of a DA_1-system or by inhibition of a DA_2-system. This conclusion, however, makes it rather difficult to understand that nialamide, a monoamine-oxidase inhibitor, increases the locomotor activity triggered by DA (Pijnenburg and van Rossum, 1973), since one may assume that nialamide increases the amount of DA within both systems. If one considers the data of York (1970), however, who found that nialamide inhibits the DA-induced inhibition on the one hand and potentiates the DA-induced excitation on the other hand, it becomes clear that nialamide might increase the locomotor activity because it can produce a shift in the DA_e-DA_i see-saw from a normal balance towards a predominance of the DA_e-system.

The observation that the locomotor activity can be triggered by a blockade of a certain group of DA-receptors, which are nearly insensitive to the well-known neuroleptics, has a large number of implications; two examples will be given below.

First, it is nicely shown by Maj and his colleagues that the reduction in the locomotor activity in mice induced by systemic injections of low doses of L-DOPA together with a peripheral decarboxylase inhibitor, Ro 4-4602, is significantly potentiated by a pretreatment with haloperidol (Maj and Pawlowski, 1974). Although this potentiation has been partially ascribed to the ability of L-DOPA to release serotonin, it is quite possible that it is mainly due to the fact that haloperidol, which is a selective antagonist of the DA_e-receptors, produces a shift in the DA_e-DA_i see-saw from a normal balance towards a predominance of the DA_i-system: as mentioned above, activation of the DA_i-system results in a suppression of the locomotor activity.

Second, it is known that dexamphetamine and cocaine are able to increase the locomotor activity in rats and mice: do these compounds stimulate the DA_e-receptors, or do they directly or indirectly inhibit the DA_i-receptors? As can be seen in Figs. 4 and 5, bilateral injections of the potent and selective agonist of the DA_i-receptors, DPI, into the nucleus accumbens of rats attenuate the

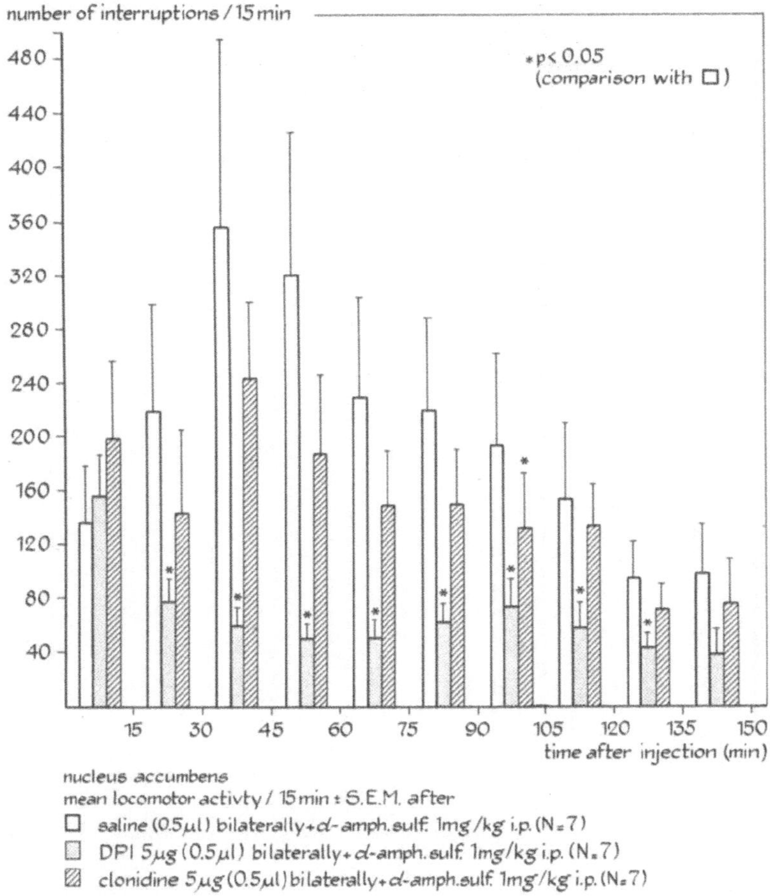

Fig. 4. Locomotor activity of rats during 10 successive 15 min periods following injections into the nucleus accumbens immediately before the d-amphetamine sulfate. Mean values ± S.E.M. are given. (Similar injections into the neostriatum do not influence the d-amphetamine-induced locomotor stimulation.) Note that clonidine, which is structurally related to DPI, remains ineffective.

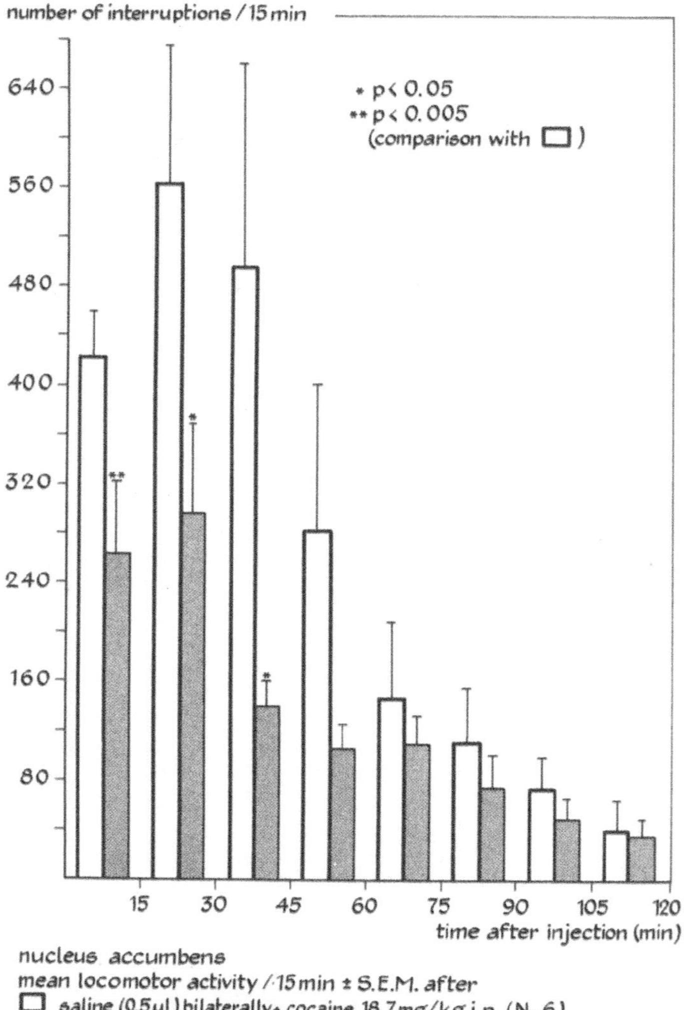

Fig. 5. Locomotor activity of rats during 10 successive 15 min periods following injections into the nucleus accumbens immediately before cocaine. Mean values ± S.E.M. are given.

increase in the locomotor activity triggered by systemic injections of these compounds. Accordingly, one must assume that both compounds produce at least an inhibition of the DA_i-receptors. Although it is at present impossible to determine which mechanism of action is involved, it is important to realize that not only ergometrine but also noradrenaline does inhibit the DA_i-receptors in the cat (Cools et al., 1975a). It is known that noradrenaline is present within the nucleus accumbens of rats (Jacobowitz, 1973; Koob, Balcon, and Meyerhoff, 1974). Since both dexamphetamine and cocaine initially increase the amount of NA and, later on, the amount of DA, it can be postulated that the locomotor stimulation produced by these compounds is due to the initial increase of NA resulting in an inhibition of the DA_i-receptors; the subsequent decrease in the locomotor activity might accordingly be due to the subsequent increase in the amount of DA within the DA_i-system. Although the available data here do not permit us to determine whether NA in this action of dexamphetamine and cocaine is acting at the level of the DA_i-receptors, it will be clear that presence of at least two pharmacologically distinct DA-systems, of which just one is modulated by NA as it has been found in the caudate nucleus of cats, opens a completely new direction in which one may look for a better understanding of the mechanism of action behind the effects of psychomotor stimulants which simultaneously interfere with DA and NA.

Finally, it is important to note that the nucleus accumbens contains a high density of dotted DA-fluorescence, which is marked by a slow turnover, and a small amount of diffuse DA-fluorescence, which is marked by a rather high turnover (Olson et al., 1972). This opens the intriguing question whether the dotted and diffuse DA-fluorescence reflect the presence of DA_i- and DA_e-system respectively; if so, the characteristic difference between the time-effect curves produced by manipulation with each single system may be due to the presence of different turnovers within the DA_e- and DA_i-system. This would fit in with the biochemical data of Shellenberger and Gordon (1974), who suggested that there are different DA-systems within distinct neural systems, each of them marked by their own turnover.

Not only the nucleus accumbens but also the neostriatum is marked by two histochemically distinct types of DA-fluorescence (Olson et al., 1972). If these types of fluorescence do reflect the presence of a DA_e- and DA_i-system respectively, one must expect that stimulation of DA-sensitive structures within the neostriatum also results in functionally distinct effects appearing at different time-intervals after the injection. Let us consider the literature.

Studies dealing with turning movements evoked from the neostriatum in rats offer the following data: (1) low doses of DA (1-5 μg) unilaterally injected into the neostriatum of non-pretreated rats produce contralateral turning movements which immediately appear after the injection and are short-lasting; this effect is mimicked by apomorphine and inhibited by chlorpromazine (Ungerstedt et al., 1969); (2) intermediate doses of DA (10-90 μg) remain ineffective during a period of 2 hr following the injection (Dill, Nickey, and Little, 1968; Bondareff, Routtenberg, Narotzky, and McLone, 1970; Costall and Naylor, 1974a; Malec and van Rossum, personal communication); (3) high doses of DA (100 μg) produce ipsilateral turning or, sometimes, bilateral turning during the first period of 25 min and contralateral turning during the following period of 120 min (Costall and Naylor, 1974a); and (4) intermediate doses of DA (50 μg) together with nialamide produce contralateral turning immediately after the injection and are long-lasting (Costall and Naylor, 1974a).

Apart from the fact that the mentioned observations are in several aspects similar to those found in studies on the caudate nucleus of cats, it is quite evident that they are not inconsistent with the possibility that the neostriatum of rats contains two functionally opposing DA-systems: one in which stimulation results in contralateral turning, and one in which stimulation results in ipsilateral turning. The finding that intermediate doses of DA together with nialamide, which might produce a shift in the DA_e-DA_i see-saw from a normal balance towards a predominance of the DA_e-system as mentioned before, immediately result in contralateral turning underlines this possibility. Since a detailed neuropharmacological analysis of these systems, however, is at present lacking, no further conclusions can be drawn.

Clearer deductions can be made by considering the studies dealing with the so-called gnawing behavior. It is known that systemically given apomorphine elicits gnawing in various species. Recently, Wolfarth, Grabowska, Lacki, Dulska, and Antkiewicz (1973) have reported that lesions in distinct parts of the neostriatum result in a potentiation of this behavior, whereas Ungerstedt (1971c) has reported that lesions in this structure just suppress this response. If it is accepted that the neostriatum does contain two functionally opposing DA-systems having pharmacological properties identical to those in the nucleus accumbens, these apparently confusing data become understandable: a lesion in the area containing DA_e-receptors, which are stimulated by apomorphine, can suppress the apomorphine-induced gnawing, whereas a lesion in the area containing DA_i-receptors, which are slightly inhibited by apomorphine, can potentiate this response. The finding that large lesions in the neostriatum do not affect the apomorphine-induced gnawing (Costall and Naylor, 1973; Divac, 1972; McKenzie, 1972) can also be explained

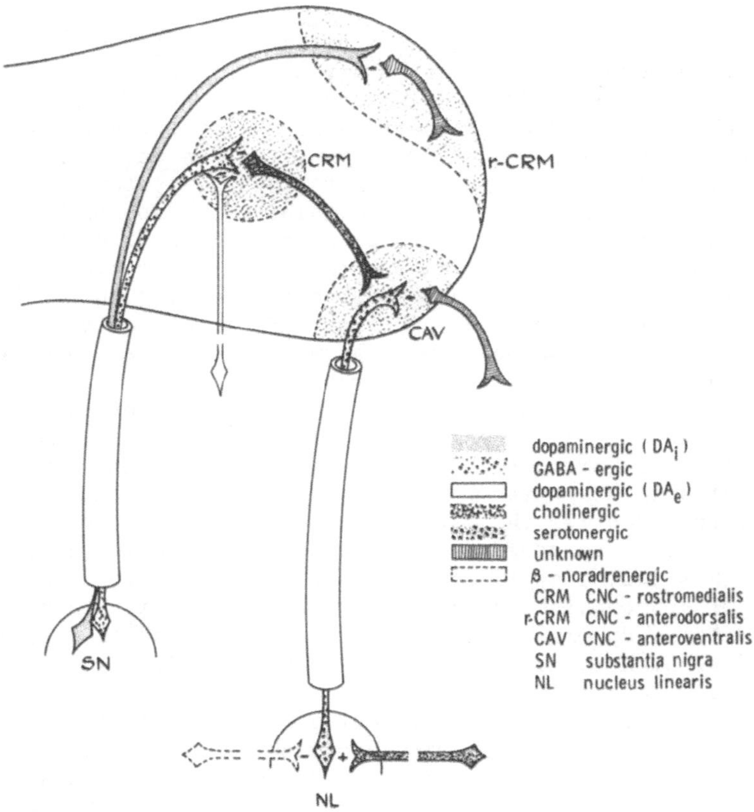

Fig. 6. Schematic diagram of the interrelationship between the excitation-mediating dopaminergic (DA$_e$-system), inhibition-mediating dopaminergic (DA$_i$-system), GABA-ergic, cholinergic and serotonergic, raphe-neostriatal system within the caudate nucleus of cats.

CNC = caput nuclei caudate.

on the basis of this concept: in that case, both areas are equally destroyed so that there still exists a balance between the DA_e- and DA_i-systems. From this point of view, it appears that the apomorphine-induced gnawing may be the result of its interaction with both types of DA-receptors: stimulation of the DA_e-receptors together with inhibition of the DA_i-receptors. This preliminary conclusion is reinforced by the data mentioned below.

Gnawing is also elicited by administering large deposits of crystalline apomorphine into the neostriatum of non-pretreated rats (Ernst and Smelik, 1966). In contrast to the turning movements, which appear immediately after the injection, gnawing appears after a latency of about 30-40 min. As has been mentioned above, pharmacological manipulation with the DA_i-system within the nucleus accumbens, which is slightly inhibited by apomorphine, results in effects appearing after a latency of about 40-60 min; such a manipulation with the DA_e-system within the nucleus accumbens, which is strongly stimulated by apomorphine, results in effects appearing immediately after the injection. From this point of view, it appears that apomorphine-induced gnawing is at least due to the inhibiting action of apomorphine at the DA_i-receptors. The finding that ergometrine, a potent inhibitor of the DA_i-receptors, does not elicit gnawing (Pijnenburg et al., 1973) shows that the mechanism of action is far more complex. Actually, the only possibility left is that both a hyperactive DA_e-system and a hypoactive DA_i-system are required for the elicitation of gnawing; recent studies in our institute have confirmed this prediction (Cools, in press). Moreover, this deduction is consistent with the finding that very low doses of apomorphine, which do not produce gnawing in non-pretreated rats, do produce gnawing when it is given to rats with a lesioned substantia nigra (Costall and Naylor, 1974b). As pointed out previously (Cools and van Rossum, 1976), the substantia nigra, pars compacta, only contains cell bodies belonging to the DA_i-system (Fig. 6): in other words, apomorphine might stimulate the unaffected DA_e-system in animals in which the DA_i-system is partially destroyed by means of the nigral lesion. An intriguing implication of this deduction is that there is no need to postulate the development of supersensitivity in such rats, as has been done by Ungerstedt (1971b): such rats might be more sensitive to apomorphine because the nigral lesion could have produced a shift in the DA_e-DA_i see-saw from a normal balance towards a predominance of the DA_e-system. The fact that apomorphine produces contralateral turning in rats with a lesioned nigra on one side, as well as the fact that the effectiveness of unilaterally, neostriatally applied dopamine in rats with a lesioned nigra at the same site remains practically unchanged (Costall, Naylor, and Pycock, 1976), can also be explained on the basis of such a shift; indeed, the failure to observe the development of supersensitivity at the biochemical level (Iversen, 1974) is not in conflict with this suggestion.

TABLE 1

Characteristic symptoms triggered by pharmacological modulation of the postulated excitation-mediating (DA_e-system) and inhibition-mediating (DA_i-system) dopaminergic systems within the neostriatum and the nucleus accumbens in rats.

Pharmacological Modulation	Drugs	Action Site/ Application	Symptoms
DA_e-system			
stimulation	apomorphine dopamine	N. accumbens	locomotor stimulation(short-term)
inhibition	haloperidol	N. accumbens	locomotor suppression
DA_i-system			
stimulation	DPI[a]	N. accumbens	locomotor suppression (long-lasting)
inhibition	ergometrine	N. accumbens	locomotor stimulation (long-lasting)
simultaneously[b]			
stimulation DA_e-system / inhibition DA_i-system	apomorphine and ergometrine	N. accumbens or neostriatum	stereotyped gnawing

[a]DPI = 3, 4-dihydroxy-phenylamino-2-imidazoline

[b]to be published (Cools, in press)

In summary, it is suggested that both the neostriatum and the nucleus accumbens of rats contain two functionally, pharmacologically, biochemically and histochemically distinct DA-systems having pharmacological properties identical to those of the DA_e- and DA_i-system within the caudate nucleus of cats. From the functional point of view it is suggested that:

1) stereotyped gnawing results from a hyperstimulation of the DA_e-system, which is accompanied by a hypostimulation of the DA_i-system;
2) contralateral turning results from unilateral stimulation of the DA_e-system or from unilateral inhibition of the DA_i-system, whereas ipsilateral turning results from unilateral stimulation of the DA_i-system or from unilateral inhibition of the DA_e-system; and
3) increase in the locomotor activity results from stimulation of the DA_e-system or from inhibition of the DA_i-system.

General

As recent studies have indicated that the presence of distinct dopaminergic systems appears to be a general principle within the brain of mammals (mice: Costentin, Protais, and Schwarz, 1975; rats: see above; guinea pigs: Costall and Naylor, 1975b; Costall, Naylor, and Pinder, 1975a; Costall, Naylor, and Neumeyer, 1975b; cats: Cools and van Rossum, 1976; Cools et al., in press; and rhesus monkeys: Cools, Hendriks, and Korten, 1975b), it becomes evident that presence of functionally distinct types of DA-receptors, each characterized by its own type of agonists and antagonists, might have a great impact upon the scientific insight into the basic mechanisms involved in the pathophysiology of psychomotor diseases in man. It is not my purpose to review these aspects of the problem, for I have done so elsewhere (schizophrenia: Cools, 1975; psychomotor diseases: Cools and van Rossum, 1976). In this context, it is just sufficient to recall the characteristic function of each DA-system. As already mentioned, bilateral stimulation of the DA_i-system, which terminates within the r-CRM-area of the caudate nucleus in cats, results in the display of the so-called oro-facial-lingual dyskinesias (Table 2); similar observations have been done in rhesus monkeys (Cools et al., 1975b). In view of these data, one may suggest that the development of such dyskinetic activities in patients treated for a long time with L-DOPA or neuroleptics is due to the development of a predominance of the DA_i-system produced by stimulation of the DA_i-system (L-DOPA) or by inhibition of the DA_e-system (neuroleptics) (cf. Costall and Naylor, 1975b; Costall et al., 1975a-b; Costall, Naylor, and Pinder, 1975c; Korczyn, 1972; cf. Fig. 6 and Table 1); if so, one might consider treating these patients with a selective inhibitor of the DA_i-receptors, i.e. piribedil, or with a potent agonist of the

TABLE 2

Characteristic symptoms triggered by pharmacological modulation of the excitation-mediating (DA_e-system) and inhibition-mediating (DA_i-system) dopaminergic, GABA-ergic, cholinergic and serotonergic systems within the rostromedial (CRM), anterodorsal (r-CRM) and anteroventral (CAV) part of the caudate nucleus in cats.

Pharmacological Modulation	Drugs	Action Site/ Application	Symptoms
DA_e-system			
stimulation	dopamine apomorphine	CRM	contralateral turning
inhibition	haloperidol	CRM	ipsilateral turning facial dyskinesias(?)
DA_i-system			
stimulation	DPI	r-CRM	ipsilateral turning facial dyskinesias
inhibition	ergometrine piribedil noradrenaline	r-CRM	contralateral turning tremor (?)
$GABA_1$-system			
stimulation	GABA	CRM	ipsilateral turning
inhibition	picrotoxin	CRM	contralateral turning
$GABA_2$-system			
stimulation	GABA	r-CRM	ipsilateral turning
inhibition	picrotoxin	r-CRM	contralateral turning
ACH_1-system			
stimulation	carbachol	CAV	contralateral turning
inhibition	scopolamine	CAV	ipsilateral turning
ACH_2-system			
stimulation	carbachol	r-CRM	contralateral turning tremor
inhibition	scopolamine	r-CRM	ipsilateral turning

TABLE 2, continued

Pharmacological Modulation	Drugs	Action Site/ Application	Symptoms
5-HT_1-system			
stimulation	serotonin	CAV	abortive grooming obstinate progression hyperkinesias contralateral turning (short-term)
inhibition	para-chloro-phenylalanine	CAV	akinesias ipsilateral turning (short-term)
simultaneous stimulation			
DA_e-system	apomorphine	CRM	choreo-athetosis
DA_i-system	DPI[a]	r-CRM	

[a]DPI = 3, 4-dihydroxy-phenylamino-2-imidazoline

DA_e-receptors, i.e. a low dose of apomorphine. With respect to the function of the DA_e-system, I have previously summarized evidence derived from our own data, as well as from neurobiological and clinical data earlier reported, that stimulation of this system results both in a break-down of previously established chains of motor responses enabling the organism to establish completely new combinations, i.e. new behavioral patterns (Cools, 1973a), and in a break-down of previously established links between different concepts and conceptual frames enabling the individual to establish completely new concepts and conceptual frames (Cools, 1975). From this point of view, it becomes clear that hyperstimulation of this system or a dysbalance between the DA_e- and DA_i-system in favour of the DA_e-system may result both in disorders in motor behavior, such as loss of the natural gracefulness of movements, and in cognitive disorders, such as impaired ability to focus and attend to relevant stimuli demanding responses, use of isolated elements and parts rather than whole concepts, inability to maintain a major set of associations, and verbal neologism, all symptoms characteristic of acute paranoid schizophrenics.

THE INTRACAUDATE DOPAMINE-GABA INTERACTION

Introduction

Apart from the fact that there is biochemical and functional evidence in favour of the presence of gamma-aminobutyric acid (GABA)-containing fibres running from the globus pallidus and/or neostriatum towards the substantia nigra (Kim, Bak, Hassler, and Okada, 1971; McGeer, McGeer, Wada, and Jung, 1971b; Sutin and McNair, 1971; Yoshida and Precht, 1971), there is some electrophysiological evidence that there are also GABA-ergic fibres running from the substantia nigra towards the neostriatum (Feltz, 1974). Indeed, a rather large amount of GABA is present in terminal nerve structures within the neostriatum and the nucleus accumbens of mammals (Fahn and Côté, 1968; Robinson and Wells, 1973). The GABA-ergic fibres terminating within the substantia nigra are believed to exert an inhibitory action at the DA-containing cell bodies within the nigra (Yoshida and Precht, 1971); since the cell bodies belonging to the DA_e-system are not localized within the substantia nigra, as has been mentioned in the previous section (cf. Fig. 6), it appears that only the DA_i-system is inhibited by these GABA-ergic fibres at the level of the substantia nigra (i.e. $GABA_3$-system: Fig. 7). The observation that inhibition of this $GABA_3$-system increases just the amount of dotted DA-fluorescence within the neostriatum (Aghajanian and Roth, 1970) underlines the earlier mentioned hypothesis concerning the relationship between the dotted DA-fluorescence and the DA_i-system (Cools and Janssen, 1976; Cools and van Rossum, 1976). Recently, some functional data have been presented that the mesolimbic, dopaminergic pathway is similarly modulated by certain GABA-ergic fibres running from the olfactory bulb towards the ventral tegmental area (Stevens, Wilson, and Foote, 1974). Despite the above-mentioned studies, histochemical evidence in favour of the existence of GABA-ergic fibres is still lacking!

Cats

At present, just one behavioral study on the effects of neostriatally applied GABA-ergic agents has been reported (Cools and Janssen, 1976). In this study, it has been found that effects triggered by unilateral injections of apomorphine and haloperidol into the CRM-area, i.e., contralateral and ipsilateral turning respectively, are completely blocked by GABA and the GABA antagonist picrotoxin respectively; on the basis of these and related data, it has been concluded that the DA_e-system within the CRM-area normally inhibits the GABA-ergic system localized within the same area (i.e. $GABA_1$-system: Fig. 7; Fig. 6). In the r-CRM-area unilaterally applied GABA mimics, apart from the so-called oro-facial-lingual

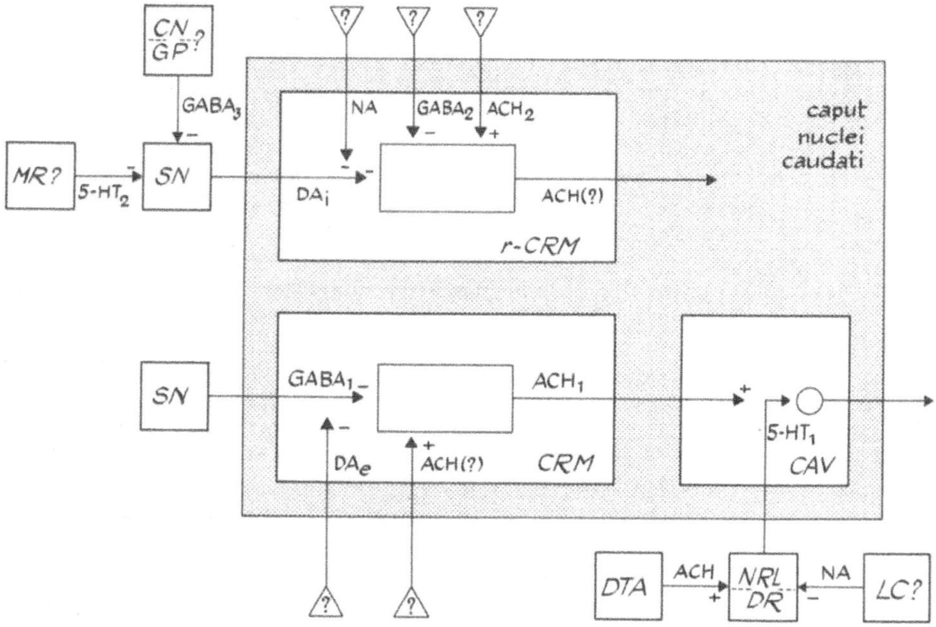

Fig. 7. Diagram of the complex interrelationship between the various neurotransmitter mechanisms within the striatum (cf. Fig. 6).

Cd = nucleus caudatus; CAV = caput nuclei caudate, anteroventral area; CRM = caput nuclei caudati, rostromedial area; r-CRM = caput nuclei caudati, anterodorsal area; DR = dorsal raphe nuclei (rats); DTA = dorsal tegmental area; LC = locus coeruleus; MR = medial raphe nuclei; NRL = nucleus linearis intermedius raphe; SN = substantia nigra; ACH = cholinergic system; DA_e = excitation-mediating dopaminergic system; DA_i = inhibition-mediating dopaminergic system; GABA = GABA-ergic system; NA = noradrenergic system; 5-HT = serotonergic system.

dyskinesias, the effects characteristic for stimulation of the DA_i-system, i.e. ipsilateral turning. From this point of view, it can be tentatively suggested that this GABA-system (i.e. $GABA_2$-system: Fig. 7) inhibits the neuronal activity within the r-CRM-area.

Rats

In 1972, McKenzie and Viik reported that unilateral injections of d-tubocurarine into the neostriatum of rats produce a syndrome marked by involuntary movements of the contralateral forelimb, contralateral rotation of the head, facial grimacing and teeth chattering (McKenzie and Viik, 1972). In a later report, they extensively describe their observations: according to that study, it appears that the GABA-antagonists, picrotoxin and bicuculline, are able to mimic these effects; they also report that both the picrotoxin-induced and the d-tubocurarine-induced effects are inhibited by GABA injections into the neostriatum (McKenzie and Viik, 1975). It is rather difficult to interpret these results because it remains unclear whether picrotoxin evokes the whole syndrome or just a part of it. This is highly important in view of the fact that hyperstimulation of the DA_e- and DA_i-system within the caudate nucleus of cats results in the appearance of athetoid-choreiform movements of the forelimbs, whereas hyperstimulation of only the DA_i-system within this structure of cats results in facial dyskinetic activities: if picrotoxin only produces involuntary movements of the contralateral forelimb and contralateral rotation of the head, we are dealing with effects similar to those evoked by picrotoxin in the cat!

Anyhow, it is intriguing to note that d-tubocurarine, which is believed to inhibit cholinergic receptors, also inhibits the DA-induced excitation (Berry and Cottrell, 1975). If this also occurs within the brain of rats, the display of the facial grimacing and teeth chattering triggered by d-tubocurarine can be ascribed to its ability to produce a shift in the DA_e-DA_i see-saw from a normal balance towards a predominance of the DA_i-system, which is known to trigger comparable effects in cats and monkeys.

General

If it is accepted that one may extrapolate the data derived from the feline studies to man, the data are highly important from the clinical point of view. The fact that stimulation of the DA_e-system normally inhibits the $GABA_1$-system within the CRM-area implies that a hyperactive DA_e-system must result in effects similar to those evoked by a hypoactive GABA-ergic system within that part of the brain (Table 1 and Figs. 6 and 7). On the other hand, it will be clear that such effects can also be elicited by an inhibition of the DA_i-system (Table 1 and Figs. 6 and 7). Since stimulation of the DA_i-system produces all effects similar to those evoked by stimulation of the $GABA_2$-system within caudate structures containing the DA_i-receptors, minus the facial dyskinesias, it is evident that a hypoactive $GABA_2$-system within that part of the brain can also produce effects similar to those elicited by a hyperactive DA_e-system (Table 1; Roberts, 1972, 1974). As has been mentioned in the final part of the foregoing section, certain psychotic disorders may be due to a predominance of the DA_e-system. In view of the above-mentioned considerations, it can be postulated that patients with such disorders can be treated with GABA-ergic agonists such as Lioresal: the advantage of such a treatment is that it bypasses the DA_i-system, in which stimulation results in the display of facial dyskinesias. Actually, this deduction is not only in agreement with earlier reported suggestions concerning the role of a defective GABA-ergic system in psychotic disorders (Roberts, 1972; Stevens, 1973), but it is also in agreement with the preliminary study of Frederiksen (1975), who has observed that Lioresal is therapeutically effective in the treatment of certain schizophrenics.

THE INTRACAUDATE DOPAMINE-ACETYLCHOLINE INTERACTION

Introduction

Apart from DA and GABA, the caudate nucleus and the nucleus accumbens contain a very high amount of acetylcholine and all of the enzymes involved in its synthesis and degradation (Hebb, 1972). Although it has been found that certain caudato-nigral, caudato-pallidal, caudato-cortical and thalamo-caudate fibres may contain ACH (McLennan, 1964; Olivier, Parent, Simard, and Poirier, 1970; Shute and Lewis, 1967), recent data have indicated that intrinsic rather than extrinsic fibres contain ACH (Butcher and Butcher, 1974; Lynch, Lucas, and Deadwyler, 1972; McGeer, McGeer, Fibiger, and Wickson, 1971a).

Today several articles, reviews and books are devoted to clinical and experimental studies dealing with the DA-ACH interaction in behavior of animals and man. The most important outcome of the clinical studies is that the parkinsonian symptoms in a great number of patients are probably due to a neostriatal DA-ACH imbalance resulting from a hyperactive cholinergic system or a hypoactive dopaminergic system (Duvoisin, 1967; Feldberg, 1945; Klawans et al., 1970). In animals too, such a "see-saw" in the brain, with DA on the one side and ACH on the other, appears to exist (Arnfred and Randrup, 1968; Connor et al., 1967; Scheel-Krüger, 1970).

Chemically selective stimulation studies, however, indicate that the relatively simple concept of the DA-ACH "see-saw" within the neostriatum needs some revision as discussed below.

Cats

Studies using chemically selective stimulation have revealed that the caudate nucleus of cats contains two functionally distinct cholinergic systems: one that is sensitive to low doses of the choline-like agent carbachol (Hull, Buchwald, and Ling, 1967; Langlois and Poussart, 1969), and one that is sensitive to high doses of carbachol (Hull et al., 1967). These studies, however, do not indicate that there is a topographical distribution of these systems.

Behavioral effects produced by stimulation of ACH-sensitive sites (carbachol: 2 μg) within the anteroventral part of the head of the caudate nucleus (CAV-area; Fig. 1) are similar to those evoked by activation of the DA_e-receptors within the CRM-area (Cools, 1974). Apart from the fact that this ACH-mechanism within the CAV-area is an indispensable link in the sequential chain of intra-caudate events triggered by activation of the DA_e-receptors, it has been found that it cooperates with this DA_e-system in the same direction (Cools, 1974). On the basis of these and related data, it has been concluded that the ACH_1-system, of which the terminal sites are concentrated within the CAV-area, is <u>in series</u> connected with the DA_e-system (Fig. 6; ACH_1-system: Fig. 7). In contrast, effects such as tremor evoked by stimulation of intracaudate ACH-mechanisms are even counteracted by intracaudate DA-mechanisms (Baker et al., 1969; Connor et al., 1967). Considering these data in view of the functional heterogeneity of DA-receptors, one might expect that the ACH-mechanism responsible for the elicitation of tremor is counteracted by the DA_i-system; indeed, we have recently found that the DA_i-system inhibits effects triggered by an increased cholinergic activity within the area containing the DA_i-receptors (Cools et al., in press). Thus, the DA_i-system, which terminates within the r-CRM-area, is able to counteract the ACH-system terminating within the same area. This might imply that cells which receive an inhibitory, dopaminergic input also receive an excitatory, cholinergic input (Fig. 6; ACH_2-system: Fig. 7). These observations are in agreement with the data of Poirier and his colleagues, who also found that distinct types of interaction between ACH and DA are involved in the elicitation of tremor and turning movements respectively (Poirier, Langelier, Bédaud, Boucher, LaRochelle, Parent, and Roberge, 1974). Studies dealing with chemically selective stimulation of the caudate nucleus of rhesus monkeys have given comparable results (Cools et al., 1975b).

Rats

Despite the fact that attention has been directed to the influence of neostriatally applied cholinergic and anticholinergic compounds upon behavior previously induced, a relatively small number of studies until now bear on the influence of these substances upon normal behavior (Costall, Naylor, and Olley, 1972; Dill et al., 1968). The main outcome of these studies is that (a) either a small amount of carbachol (1-2 μg) or a large amount of ACH (55-60 μg) produces tremor in the contralateral forepaw (Dill et al., 1968) and (b) large amounts of the choline-like compound arecoline (50 μg), or of the anticholinergic drug atropine (100 μg), produce turning towards and turning away respectively from the side injected (Costall et al., 1972).

With respect to the DA-ACH interaction, it is interesting to note that the stereotyped behavior evoked by systemic injections of amphetamine is nicely blocked by neostriatally applied atropine (Costall and Naylor, 1972). Although huge doses (100-400 μg) have been used, this inhibition can be ascribed to the interference of atropine with intracaudate structures because this effect immediately follows the injection. This observation clearly shows that there exists some cooperation between certain DA- and ACH-systems within the neostriatum of rats. Thus, the situation is far more complex than one must expect on the basis of the studies in which the effects of systemic injections have been analysed: as mentioned before, these studies have indicated that DA-systems counteract ACH-systems within the neostriatum.

General

Since the neostriatal ACH_1-system, stimulation of which does not result in tremor, is functionally in series with the DA_e-system and cooperates with this system, defects in this ACH-system may, accordingly, produce effects similar to those caused by a defective DA_e-system (Table 1; Fig. 7). Thus, certain psychomotor disorders may be due to a defective DA_e- or ACH_1-system. The same holds true for the interaction between the DA_i- and ACH_2-system. In that case, however, a hypoactive DA_i-system may result in effects similar to those produced by a hyperactive ACH_2-system (Table 1; Fig. 7). Considering the clinical studies on the DA-ACH interrelationship in patients with Parkinson's disease (see introduction of this section), it appears attractive to postulate that especially the DA_i-system is affected. In view of the fact that ACH-systems are nearly everywhere within the brain and, accordingly, also modulate systems completely different from the mentioned ones, such a postulation cannot be made. Actually, there are other, more valid arguments to postulate that a hypoactive DA_e-system is involved in this disease (Cools and van Rossum, 1976).

Anyhow, it will be clear from this section that defects in completely different neurotransmitter systems may underlie identical disorders.

THE INTRACAUDATE DOPAMINE-ACETYLCHOLINE-SEROTONIN INTERACTION

Introduction

Both fluorescent and biochemical studies in mammals have shown that certain neostriatal nerve terminals contain serotonin (5-HT) (Andèn et al., 1966; Broch and Marsden, 1972; Hökfelt and Ungerstedt, 1969). Despite the lack of histochemical evidence, anatomical, lesion, electrical and chemical stimulation studies in cats have strongly suggested that the intracaudate 5-HT containing terminal structures belong to neurons arising from the raphe nuclei, especially the nucleus linearis intermedius raphe (Askenazi, Holman, and Vogt, 1972; Bobillier, Petitjean, Salvert, Ligier, and Sequin, 1975; Brodal, Faber, and Walberg, 1960; Cools and Janssen, 1974; Holman and Vogt, 1972; Parent and Poirier, 1969). In rats too, direct and indirect evidence in favour of such an interrelationship between the neostriatum and raphe nuclei, especially the dorsal raphe nuclei, has been presented (Aghajanian, Rosecrans, and Sheard, 1967; Hökfelt and Ungerstedt, 1969; Kuhar, Roth, and Aghajanian, 1971; Lorens and Goldberg, 1974; Miller, Richardson, Fibiger, and McLennan, 1975; Nauta, Pritz, and Lach, 1974; Seiger and Olson, 1973).

The putative role of 5-HT in behavior of mammals is far from clear, although several studies have indicated that there exists a relationship between cerebral 5-HT and sleep, sexual, aggressive, and learned behavior (Aprison and Hintgen, 1972; Delorme, Froment, and Jouvet, 1966; Jouvet, 1969; Harvey, Heller, and Moore, 1963; Lints and Harvey, 1969; Tenen, 1967). Recent clinical studies have indicated that it may play a role in some psychomotor diseases (Birkmayer and Neumayer, 1972; Gumpert, Sharpe, and Curzon, 1973; Jequier and Dufresne, 1972; Stevens, 1973; Wyatt, Vaughan, Galanter, Kaplan, and Green, 1972).

With respect to the DA-5-HT interrelationship, it appears that both systems interfere with each other in at least two different ways, depending on the methods used and variables studied. Considering the locomotor activity triggered by systemically given apomorphine and amphetamine, several workers have reported that this activity is counteracted and potentiated by stimulation and inhibition of central serotonergic systems respectively (Breese, Cooper, and Müeller, 1974; Green and Harvey, 1974; Marby and Campbell, 1973). Stereotyped behavior triggered by apomorphine and amphetamine, however, is not affected by systemically given compounds, which either increase or decrease the activity within central serotonergic systems (Breese et al., 1974; Randrup and Munkvad, 1964; Rotrosen, Angrist, Wallach, and Gershon, 1972). In the final part of this section we will see that the situation is more complex than it is depicted above.

Cats

Behavioral studies on the caudate nucleus of cats have offered two sets of data: one group dealing with the elicitation of a highly complex behavioral syndrome. First, it has been found that rather large doses of 5-HT (30 μg) applied into the caudate nucleus of cats result in tremor which can be blocked by methysergide and DA. Although the tremor remains unaffected by a local pretreatment with a cholinergic blocking agent, scopolamine, it is potentiated by a local pretreatment with an inhibitor of acetylcholinesterase physostigmine (Malseed and Baker, 1973). In view of the fact that (a) 5-HT does not elicit tremor when it is applied into the neostriatum of rats (Hadzovic and Ernst, 1969), (b) large doses of 5-HT can displace DA from its stores (Ng, Chase, Colburn, and Kopin, 1970), and (c) the intracaudate DA_i-system normally inhibits the neostriatal, cholinergic system, stimulation of which results in tremor (see DA-ACH section), it is quite possible that high doses of 5-HT injected into the caudate nucleus of cats inactivate only the DA_i-system by the ability of 5-HT to displace DA from its stores and, accordingly, indirectly stimulate the cholinergic system responsible for the elicitation of tremor. The observation that DA inhibits the 5-HT elicited tremor, together with the finding that physostigmine potentiates this tremor, is consistent with this suggestion.

Second, it has been found that unilateral injections of small amounts of 5-HT (10 μg) into the CAV-area of cats (Fig. 1) result in a 5-HT-specific syndrome marked by hyperkinesias, obstinate progression, abortive and disjunctive self-directed activities, choreoathetosis, "vacuum activities," and a "conditioning effect" (Cools, 1973b). Detailed analysis of the interrelationship between the DA_e-sensitive CRM-area and the 5-HT-sensitive CAV-area has offered evidence that the DA_e-system only produces effects when the 5-HT-system within the CAV-area is unaffected. A similar analysis of the relationship between the ACH_1- and 5-HT-system within the CAV-area has indicated that the same holds true for the effects triggered by activation of the ACH_1-system (Cools, 1974). In view of earlier mentioned data concerning the close, functional relationship between the DA_e-system within the CRM-area and the ACH_1-system within the CAV-area, the above-mentioned data indicate that the DA_e-system is at least functionally in series connected with the 5-HT-system within the CAV-area by means of intracaudate, cholinergic pathways (Fig. 6; $5\text{-}HT_1$-system: Fig. 7; Cools, 1974).

Rats

According to Dill et al. (1968) no effects are elicited by injections of high doses (50 μg) of 5-HT into the neostriatum. Hadzovic and Ernst (1969), however, have reported that neostriatally applied 5-HT (25 μg) together with systemic injections of the monoamine oxidase inhibitor, ipronizid, results in the appearance of gnawing after a latency of about 60 min; the most sensitive part in this respect, the anteroventral part of the neostriatum, remains unaffected by apomorphine, suggesting a rather selective effect of 5-HT (Hadzovic and Ernst, 1969). No further studies on the effects of neostriatally applied serotonergic agents in rats are known to the author.

General

With respect to the function of the feline 5-HT-system, which is functionally in series connected with the DA_e-system, it has been found that a long-term stimulation of the DA_e-system, which gives the organism the flexibility to re-organize its ongoing behavior according to available sensory information, increases the activity within the raphe-neostriatal 5-HT pathway and, subsequently, conditions the newly acquired patterns (Cools, Janssen, and Broekkamp, 1974; Cools, in press). The implications of these data for the pathophysiology of psychomotor diseases, especially schizophrenia, have been discussed elsewhere in detail (Cools, 1975).

If it is accepted that a hyperactive DA_e-system is involved in certain psychotic disorders in man (see DA section), it will be evident from the feline data mentioned in this section that defects in the 5-HT-system, which is at least functionally in series connected, may also underlie such disorders.

Although it will be evident that our knowledge with respect to the neostriatal DA-5-HT interrelationship is limited to cats, it is important to note that studies in which the interaction between raphe nuclei, serotonergic systems, neostriatum and dopaminergic systems has been studied in rats provide some additional information. For instance, destruction of the midbrain raphe nuclei containing the majority of 5-HT-containing cell bodies within the brain does potentiate the locomotor activity triggered by systemic injections of apomorphine and amphetamine (Grabowska, 1974; Neill, Grant, and Grossman, 1972). These observations are in agreement with the data mentioned in the introduction of this section. With respect to the stereotyped behavior triggered by systemic injections of apomorphine and amphetamine, it has been reported that destruction of all 5-HT-containing cell bodies and fibres within the brain by means of intracisternal injections of 5,6-dihydroxytryptamine following systemic injections of desmethylimipramine does not affect the stereotyped behavior (Baldessarini, Amatruda, Griffith, and Gerson, 1975). This is also in agreement with the data mentioned in the introduction of this section.

Lesions restricted to medial raphe nuclei, however, inhibit the stereotyped gnawing and biting response triggered either by systemically given apomorphine (McKenzie, 1973) or by neostriatal injections of DA (100 μg) in rats pretreated with nialamide (Costall and Naylor, 1974b). Such lesions do not suppress the delicate head movements (bobbing or weaving) and involuntary movements of the forepaw triggered by the mentioned DA injections into the neostriatum of nialamide-pretreated rats (Costall and Naylor, 1974b). It is interesting to note that 5-HT locally applied into the substantia nigra, which contains 5-HT in nerve terminals (Dahlström and Fuxe, 1964; Parizek, Hassler, and Bak, 1971), also produces such head and forepaw movements (Hadzovic and Ernst, 1969).

At present, these data do not permit us to draw clear-cut conclusions. Instead, they confront us with a large number of questions. Considering the above-mentioned data together with the facts that (a) only the dorsal raphe nuclei send 5-HT fibres to the neostriatum (Miller et al., 1975); (b) the substantia nigra contains 5-HT loaded nerve terminals (see above); and (c) 5-HT applied into the nigra elicits tremor (Hadzovic and Ernst, 1969), which may result from an inhibitory action of 5-HT at cell bodies belonging to the DA_i-system which, in turn, normally inhibits the neostriatal, cholinergic system responsible for tremor, the question arises whether there are at least two distinct 5-HT-systems. One 5-HT-system running from the medial raphe nuclei towards the substantia nigra inhibits the activity in the arising DA_i-fibres and, accordingly, results in the release of the neostriatal, cholinergic system responsible for tremor and, in addition, counteracts stereotyped gnawing ($5\text{-}HT_2$-system: Fig. 7). Another system runs from the dorsal raphe nuclei towards the neostriatum. It is in series connected with the DA_e-system and mediates effects such as head bobbing and involuntary movements of the forepaws ($5\text{-}HT_1$-system: Fig. 7). The answer to these and related questions will be found only by further investigation.

CONCLUSION

At least five neurotransmitters modulate the function of the neostriatum and nucleus accumbens: dopamine, noradrenaline, serotonin, acetylcholine and GABA. Moreover, at least one neurotransmitter, i.e. dopamine, can interfere with distinct receptors within these structures. The various mechanisms involved interact in a highly complex way. A schematic diagram depicting some aspects of this complex relationship is presented in Fig. 7. Since the depicted diagram is mainly based on functional studies, it illustrates functional relationships between the various systems. That does not alter the fact that they are to a large degree consistent with our anatomical, histochemical, biochemical and electrophysiological knowledge, as has been discussed in the foregoing sections. In any case, it is clear that certain mechanisms are functionally in series connected, some of them counteracting each other and others cooperating with each other.

Considering this circuitry diagram built up from various links, each of them using its own transmitter, it becomes evident that completely different biochemical and/or structural defects may underlie more or less identical functional disorders. However, it is important to note that some systems are especially involved in the elicitation of characteristic disorders (Tables 1 and 2).

In fact the available data offer experimental support to the idea of Barbeau (1973) that: "a completely new outlook on the management of these illnesses is now permitted," (p.347) and even warranted.

REFERENCES

Aghajanian, G.K. and Roth, R.H.: γ-hydroxybutyrate-induced increase in brain dopamine: Localization by fluorescence microscopy, J. Pharmac. exp. Ther. 175, 131-138 (1970).

Aghajanian, G.K., Rosecrans, J., and Sheard, M.: Serotonin: Release in the forebrain by stimulation of midbrain raphé, Science 156, 402-403 (1967).

Andèn, N.E. and Jackson, D.N.: Locomotor activity stimulation in rats produced by dopamine in the nucleus accumbens: Potentiation by caffeine, J. Pharm. Pharmac. 27, 666-670 (1975).

Andèn, N.E., Dahlström, A., Fuxe, K., Olson, L., and Ungerstedt, U.: Ascending monoamine neurons to the telencephalon and diencephalon, Acta Physiol. Scand. 67, 313-326 (1966).

Arnfred, T. and Randrup, A.: Cholinergic mechanism in brain inhibiting amphetamine-induced stereotyped behaviour, Acta Pharmac. Tox. 26, 384-394 (1968).

Aprison, M.H. and Hintgen, J.N.: Serotonin and behavior: A brief summary, Fed. Proc. 31, 121-129 (1972).

Ashkenazi, R., Holman, R.B., and Vogt, M.: Release of transmitter on stimulation of the nucleus linearis raphe in the cat, J. Physiol. 223, 255-259 (1972).

Baker, W.W., Connor, J.D., Rossi, G.V., and Lalley, P.M.: Production of tremor by intracaudate cholinergic agents and its suppression by locally administered catecholamines. In: Progress in Neuro-Genetics. Barbeau, A. and Brunette, J.A., Eds., Vol. 1, pp. 390-403, International Congress Series No. 175. Amsterdam: Excerpta Medica, 1969.

Baldessarini, R.J., Amatruda, T.T., Griffith, F.F., and Gerson, S.: Differential effects of serotonin on turning and stereotypy induced by apomorphine, Brain Res. 93, 158-163 (1975).

Barbeau, A.: Biology of the striatum. In: Biology of Brain Dysfunction. Gaull, G.E., Ed., Vol. 2, pp. 333-350. New York: Plenum Press, 1973.

Barbeau, A., Doshey, L.J., and Spiegel, E.A., (Eds.): Parkinson's Disease: Trends in Research and Treatment. New York: Gunne and Stratton, 1965.

Barbeau, A. and McDowell, F.H.: L-DOPA and Parkinsonism. Philadelphia: F.A. Davis Company, 1969.

Barret, R.E., Yahr, M.D., and Duvoisin, R.C.: Torsion dystonia and spasmodic torticollis: Results of treatment with L-DOPA, Neurology, Minneap. 20, No. 11(2), 107-113 (1970).

Bartholini, G., Keller, H.H., and Pletscher, A.: Drug-induced changes of dopamine turnover in striatum and limbic system of the rat, J. Pharm. Pharmac. 27, 439-442 (1975).

Berry, M.S. and Cottrell, G.A.: Excitatory, inhibitory and biphasic synaptic potentials mediated by an identified dopamine containing neuron, J. Physiol. 244, 589-612 (1975).

Birkmayer, W. and Neumayer, E.: Die Behandlung der DOPA-psychosen mit L-tryptophan, Nervenarzt 43, 76-78 (1972).

Bobillier, P. Petitjean, F., Salvert, D., Ligier, M., and Sequin, S.: Differential projections of the nucleus raphe dorsalis and nucleus raphe centralis as revealed by autoradiography, Brain Res. 85, 205-210 (1975).

Bondareff, W., Routtenberg, A., Narotzky, R., and McLone, D.G.: Intra-striatal spreading of biogenic amines, Expl Neurol. 28, 213-329 (1970).

Breese, G.R., Cooper, B.R., and Mueller, R.A.: Evidence for involvement of 5-hydroxytryptamine in the actions of amphetamine, Br. J. Pharmacol. 52, 307-314 (1974).

Broch, O.J. and Marsden, C.A.: Regional distribution of monoamines in the corpus striatum of the rat, Brain Res. 38, 425-428 (1972).

Brodal, A.E., Faber, E., and Walberg, F.: The raphe nuclei of the brain stem in the cat: Efferent connections, J. comp. Neurol. 114, 239-259 (1969).

Butcher, S.G. and Butcher, L.L.: Origin and modulation of acetylcholine activity in the neostriatum, Brain Res. 71, 167 (1974).

Butcher, L.L. and Bryan, G.K.: Effects of intrastriatal dopamine application on precise motor response. In: Proceedings of the Fifth International Congress of Pharmacology, San Francisco, 1972.

Calne, D.E.: Parkinsonism: Physiology, Pharmacology and Treatment. London: Edward Arnold, 1970.

Connor, J.D., Rossi, G.V., and Baker, W.W.: Antagonism of intracaudate carbachol tremor by local injections of catecholamines, J. Pharmac. exp. Ther. 155, 545-551 (1967).

Cools, A.R.: The function of dopamine and its antagonism in the caudate nucleus of cats in relation to the stereotyped behaviour, Archs int. Pharmacodyn. Thér. 194, 259-269 (1971).

Cools, A.R.: Athetoid and choreiform hyperkinesias produced by caudate application of dopamine in cats, Psychopharmacologia 25, 229-237 (1972).

Cools, A.R.: The Caudate Nucleus and Neurochemical Control of Behaviour. Nijmegen: Brakkenstein Press, 1973a.

Cools, A.R.: Serotonin: A behaviourally active compound in the caudate nucleus of cats, Israel J. Med. Sci. 9, suppl., 5-16 (1973b).

Cools, A.R.: The transsynaptic relationship between dopamine and serotonin in the caudate nucleus of cats, Psychopharmacologia 36, 17-28 (1974).

Cools, A.R.: An integrated theory of the aetiology of schizophrenia: Impairment of the balance between certain, in series, connected dopaminergic, serotonergic and noradrenergic pathways within the brain. In: On the Origin of Schizophrenic Psychoses. van Praag, H.M., Ed., pp. 53-80. Amsterdam: De Erven Bohn, 1975.

Cools, A.R.: Two topographically, functionally and pharmacologically distinct dopamine receptors in rat and cat brain. In: Symposium on Non-striatal Dopaminergic Neurons. Gessa, G.L. and Costa, E., Eds., in press.

Cools, A.R.: Relation of dopaminergic, neostriatal and serotonergic, linear nuclei to behaviour in cats. In: Neurohumoral Correlates of Behaviour. Faridaban: Thomson Press, in press.

Cools, A.R. and van Rossum, J.M.: Caudate dopamine and stereotyped behaviour of cats, Archs int. Pharmacodyn. Thér. 197, 163-173 (1970).

Cools, A.R. and Janssen, H.J.: The nucleus linearis intermedius raphe and behaviour evoked by direct and indirect stimulation of dopamine-sensitive sites within the caudate nucleus of cats, Eur. J. Pharmacol. 28, 266-275 (1974).

Cools, A.R., Janssen, H.J., and Broekkamp, C.L.E.: The differential role of the caudate nucleus and the linear raphe nucleus in the interaction and maintenance of morphine-induced behaviour in cats, Archs int. Pharmacodyn. Thér. 210, 163-174 (1974).

Cools, A.R., Janssen, H.J., Struyker Boudier, H.A.J., and van Rossum, J.M.: Interaction between antipsychotic drugs and catecholamine receptors. In: Wenner-Gren Series, Vol. 5, pp. 73-87. Oxford: Pergamon Press, 1975a.

Cools, A.R., Hendriks, G., and Korten, J.: The acetylcholine-dopamine balance in the basal ganglia of rhesus monkeys and its role in dynamic, dystonic, dyskinetic and epileptoid motor activities, J. Neural Transm. 36, 91-105 (1975b).

Cools, A.R. and Janssen, J.H.: γ-aminobutyric acid: The essential mediator of behaviour triggered by neostriatally applied apomorphine and haloperidol, J. Pharm. Pharmac. 28, 70-74 (1976).

Cools, A.R. and van Rossum, J.M.: Excitation-mediating and inhibition-mediating dopamine-receptors: A new concept towards a better understanding of electrophysiological, biochemical, pharmacological, functional and clinical data, Psychopharmacologia 45, 243-254 (1976).

Cools, A.R., Struyker Boukier, J.A.J., and van Rossum, J.M.: Dopamine-receptors: Selective agonists and antagonists of functionally distinct types within the feline brain, Eur. J. Pharmacol., in press.

Costall, B. and Naylor, R.J.: Modification of amphetamine effects by intracerebrally administered anticholinergic agents, Life Sci. 11(1), 239-253 (1972).

Costall, B., Naylor, R.J., and Olley, J.E.: Catalepsy and circling behaviour after intracerebral injections of neuroleptic, cholinergic and anticholinergic agents into the caudate putamen, globus pallidus and substantia nigra of rat brain, Neuropharmacol. 11, 645-663 (1972).

Costall, B. and Naylor, R.J.: The role of telencephalic dopaminergic systems in the mediation of apomorphine-stereotyped behaviour, Eur. J. Pharmacol. 24, 8-24 (1973).

Costall, B. and Naylor, R.J.: Specific asymmetric behaviour induced by the direct chemical stimulation of neostriatal dopaminergic mechanisms, Naunyn-Schmiedebergs Arch. exp. Path. Pharmak. 285, 83-98 (1974a).

Costall, B. and Naylor, R.J.: Stereotyped and circling behaviour induced by dopaminergic agonists after lesions of the midbrain raphe lesions, Eur. J. Pharmacol. 29, 206-222 (1974b).

Costall, B. and Naylor, R.J.: A comparison of circling models for the detection of antiparkinson activity, Psychopharmacologia 41, 57-64 (1975a).

Costall, B. and Naylor, R.J.: Neuroleptic antagonism of dyskinetic phenomena, Eur. J. Pharmacol. 33, 301-312 (1975b).

Costall, B., Naylor, R.J., and Pinder, R.M.: Dyskinetic phenomena caused by the intrastriatal injection of phenylethylamine, phenylpiperazine, tetrahydroisoquinoline and tetrahydronaphthalene derivatives in the guinea pig, Eur. J. Pharmacol. 31, 94-109 (1975a).

Costall, B., Naylor, R.J., and Neumeyer, J.L.: Differences in the nature of the stereotyped behaviour induced by aporphine derivatives in the rat and in their actions in extrapyramidal and mesolimbic brain areas, Eur. J. Pharmacol. 31, 1-16 (1975b).

Costall, B., Naylor, R.J., and Pinder, R.M.: Design of agents for stimulation of neostriatal dopaminergic mechanisms, J. Pharm. Pharmac. 26, 753-756 (1975c).

Costall, B., Naylor, R.J., and Pycock, C.: Non-specific supersensitivity of striatal dopamine receptors after 6-hydroxydopamine lesion of the nigrostriatal pathway, Eur. J. Pharmacol. 35, 275-283 (1976).

Costentin, J., Protais, P., and Schwarz, J.C.: Rapid and dissociated changes in sensitivity of different dopamine receptors in the mouse brain, Nature 257, 405-407 (1975).

Crane, G.E.: Dyskinesia and neuroleptics, Archs gen. Psychiat. 19, 700-703 (1968a).

Crane, G.E.: Tardive dyskinesia in patients treated with major neuroleptics: A review of the literature, Am. J. Psychiat. 124, suppl. 40-48 (1968b).

Dahlström, A. and Fuxe, K.: Evidence for the existence of monoamine-containing neurons in the central nervous system, Acta Physiol. Scand. 62, Suppl. 232, 1-55 (1964).

Delorme, F., Froment, Z.L., and Jouvet, M.: Suppression du sommeil par la p-chloromethamphetamine et la p-chlorophenylalanine, C.r. Séanc. Soc. Biol. 180, 2347 (1966).

Dill, R.E., Nickey, W.M., and Little, M.D.: Dyskinesias in rats following chemical stimulation of the neostriatum, Tex. Rep. Biol. Med. 20, 101-106 (1968).

Divac, I.: Drug induced syndromes in rats with large, chronic lesions in the corpus striatum, Psychopharmacologia 27, 171-178 (1972).

Duvoisin, R.D.: Cholinergic-anticholinergic antagonism in parkinsonism, Archs Neurol., Chicago 17, 124-136 (1967).

Elkhawad, A. and Woodruff, G.N.: Studies on the behavioural pharmacology of a cyclic analogue of dopamine following its injection into the brains of conscious rats, Br. J. Pharmacol. 43, 107-114 (1975).

Ernst, A.M. and Smelik. P.G.: Site of action of dopamine and apomorphine on compulsive gnawing behaviour in rats, Experientia 22, 837-838 (1966).

Fahn, S. and Côté, L.J.: Regional distribution of γ-aminobutyric acid (GABA) in the brain of the rhesus monkey, J. Neurochem. 15, 209-213 (1968).

Feldberg, W.: Present views on the mode of action of acetylcholine in the central nervous system, Physiol. Rev. 25, 596-642 (1945).

Feltz, P.: Problems raised by the electrophysiological determination of nigro-striatal inhibitions related to a dopaminergic transmission, J. Pharmacol. 5, suppl. 1, 57 (1974).

Fibiger, H.C., Pudritz, R.E., McGeer, P.L., and McGeer, E.G.: Axonal transport in nigro-striatal neurones, Nature new Biol. 237, 177-179 (1972).

Fog, R. and Pakkenberg, H.: Combined nitoman-pimozide treatment of huntington's chorea and other hyperkinetic syndromes, Acta Neurol. Scand. 46, 249-251 (1970).

Frederiksen, P.K.: Baclophen in the treatment of schizophrenia NIH-76-145c, Lakartidningen 72(6), 456 (1975).

Fuxe, K., Hökfelt, T., and Nilsson, O.: Observations on the cellular localization of dopamine in the caudate nucleus of the rat, Histochemie 63, 701-706 (1964).

Fuxe, K., Hökfelt, T., and Ungerstedt, U.: Distribution of monoamines in the mammalian central nervous system by histochemical studies. In: Metabolism of Amines in the Brain. Hooper, C., Ed., p. 10. London: MacMillan, 1969.

Grabowska, M.: Influence of midbrain raphe lesion on some pharmacological and biochemical effects of apomorphine in rats, Psychopharmacologia 39, 315-322 (1974).

Green, T.K. and Harvey, J.A.: Enhancement of amphetamine action after interruption of ascending serotonergic pathways, J. Pharmac. exp. Ther. 190, 109-117 (1974)..

Gumpert, J., Sharpe, D., and Curzon, G.: Amine metabolites in the cerebral-spinal fluid in Parkinson's disease and the response to levodopa, J. Neurol. Sci. 19, 1-12 (1973).

Hadzovic, S. and Ernst, A.M.: The effect of 5-hydroxytryptamine and 5-hydroxytryptophan on extra-pyramidal function, Eur. J. Pharmacol. 6, 90-95 (1969).

Harvey, J.A., Heller, A., and Moore, R.Y.: The effect of unilateral and bilateral medial forebrain bundle lesions on brain serotonin, J. Pharmac. exp. Ther. 140, 103-110 (1963).

Hebb, C.: Biosynthesis of acetylcholine in nervous tissue, Pharmac. Rev. 52, 918-948 (1972).

Hökfelt, T. and Ungerstedt, U.: Electron and fluorescence microscopial studies on the N. caudato-putaminal complex of the rat after unilateral lesions of ascending nigro-neostriatal dopaminergic neurons, Acta Physiol. Scand. 76, 415-426 (1969).

Holman, R.B. and Vogt, M.: Release of 5-hydroxytryptamine from the caudate nucleus and septum, J. Physiol. 223, 243-254 (1972).

Horn, A.S., Cuello, A.C., and Miller, R.J.: Dopamine in the mesolimbic system of the rat brain: Endogeneous levels and the effects of drugs on the uptake mechanism and stimulation of adenylate cyclase activity, J. Neurochem. 22, 265-270 (1974).

Hull, C.D., Buchwald, M.A., and Ling, G.: Effects of direct cholinergic stimulation of forebrain structures, Brain Res. 6, 22-35 (1967).

Ibata, Y., Nojyo, Y., Matsuura, T., and Sano, Y.: Nigro-neostriatal projection. A correlative study with Fink-Heimer impregnation, fluorescence histochemistry and electron microscopy, Z. Zellforsch. mikrosk. Anat. 138, 333-344 (1973).

Iversen, L.L.: Summing up, Adv. Neurol. 9, 415 (1974).

Jacobowitz, D.M.: Effects of 6-hydroxydopa. In: Frontiers in Catecholamine Research. Usdin, E. and Snyder, S., Eds., p. 729. Oxford: Pergamon Press, 1973.

Jackson, D.N.: Some functional effects produced by the direct application of sympathomimetic amines to various parts of the brain and their alteration by antipsychotic agents. In: Proceedings, International Symposium on Antipsychotic Drugs, Pharmacodynamics and Pharmacokinetics. In press.

Jéquier, E. and Dufresne, J.J.: Biochemical investigations in patients with parkinson's disease treated with L-DOPA, Neurology, Minneap. 22, 15-21 (1972).

Jouvet, M.: Biogenic amines and the states of sleep, Science 163, 32-41 (1969).

Kelly, P.H.: Unilateral 6-hydroxydopamine lesions of nigrostriatal or mesolimbic dopamine-containing terminals and the drug-induced rotation of rats, Brain Res. 100, 163-169 (1975).

Kelly, P.H. and Miller, R.: The interaction of neuroleptic and muscarinic agents with central dopaminergic systems, Br. J. Pharmacol. 54, 115-121 (1974).

Kelly, P.H., Seviour, P.W., and Iversen, S.D.: Amphetamine and apomorphine responses in the rat following 6-OHDA lesions of the nucleus accumbens septi and corpus striatum, Brain Res. 74, 507-522 (1975).

Kim, J.S., Bak, I.J., Hassler, R., and Okada, Y.: Role of γ-aminobutyric acid (GABA) in the extrapyramidal motor system: Some evidence for the existence of a type of GABA-rich strio-nigral neurons, Exp. Brain Res. 14, 95-104 (1971).

Klawans, H.L.: The pharmacology of parkinsonism, Dis. nerv. Syst. 29, 805-816 (1969).

Klawans, H.L.: A pharmacological analysis of huntington's chorea, Eur. Neurol. 4, 148-163 (1970).

Klawans, H.L.: Some observations on the pharmacology of the striatum, Psychiatric Forum, 16-26 (1973).

Klawans, H.L., Ilahi, M.M., and Shenker, D.: Theoretical implications of the use of L-DOPA in parkinsonism: A review, Acta Neurol. Scand. 46, 409-441 (1970).

Koob, G.F., Balcom, G.J., and Meyerhoff, J.L.: Changes in dopamine and norepinephrine in the nucleus accumbens septi, olfactory tubercle and corpus striatum following lesions in ventral tegmental area in the rat, Fed. Proc. 33, 246 (1974).

Korczyn, A.D.: Pathophysiology of drug-induced dyskinesias, Neuropharmacol. 11, 601-607 (1972).

Kuhar, M.J., Roth, R.H., and Aghajanian, G.K.: Selective reduction of tryptophan hydroxylase activity in rat forebrain after midbrain raphe lesions, Brain Res. 35, 167-176 (1971).

Langlois, J.M. and Poussart, J.: Electrocortical activity following cholinergic stimulation of the caudate nucleus in the cat, Brain Res. 15, 581-583 (1969).

La Plante, M. and St. Laurent, J.: La recherche des bases biochimiques des syndromes schizophréniques: Une revue, Un. méd. Can. 102, 2267-2278 (1973).

Lints, C.E. and Harvey, J.A.: Altered sensitivity to footshock and decreased brain content of serotonin following brain lesions in the rat, J. comp. physiol. Psychol. 57, 23-31 (1969).

Lorens, S.A. and Guldberg, H.C.: Regional 5-hydroxytryptamine following selective midbrain raphe lesions in the rat, Brain Res. 78, 45-56 (1974).

Lynch, G.S., Lucas, P.A., and Deadwyler, S.A.: Demonstration of acetylcholinesterase containing neurones within the caudate nucleus of the rat, Brain Res. 45, 617-621 (1972).

Maj, J. and Pawlowski, L.: The effect of L-DOPA on exploratory activity after catecholamine receptors blocking agents, Pol. J. Pharmacol. Pharmac. 26, 633-638 (1974).

Maler, L., Fibiger, H.C., and McGeer, P.L.: Demonstration of the nigro-striatal projection by silver staining after nigral injection of 6-hydroxydopamine, Expl Neurol. 40, 505-515 (1973).

Malseed, R.T. and Baker, W.W.: Analysis of tremorgenic effects of intracaudate serotonin, Proc. Soc. exp. Biol. Med. 143, 1088-1093 (1973).

Marby, P.D. and Campbell, B.A.: Serotonergic inhibition of catecholamine-induced behavioral arousal, Brain Res. 49, 381-391 (1973).

McGeer, P., McGeer, E., Fibiger, H., and Wickson, V.: Neostriatal choline acetylase and cholinesterase following brain lesions, Brain Res. 35, 308-314 (1971a).

McGeer, P.L., McGeer, E.L., Wada, J.A., and Jung, E.: Effects of globus pallidus lesions and parkinson's disease on brain glutamate acid decarboxylase, Brain Res. 32, 425-431 (1971b).

McKenzie, G.M.: Role of the tuberculum olfactorium in stereotyped behaviour induced by apomorphine in the rat, Psychopharmacologia 23, 212-219 (1972).

McKenzie, G.M.: Apomorphine-induced aggression: Characteristics, pharmacological interaction, and site of action, Psychopharmac. Serv. Cent. Bull. 9(3), 19-21 (1973).

McKenzie, G.M. and Viik, K.: Chemically induced choreiform movements in the rat: Blocked by GABA and neuroleptics. Abstracts of Volunteer Papers, p. 154, from the Fifth International Congress on Pharmacology, San Francisco, 1972.

McKenzie, G.M. and Viik, K.: Chemically induced choreiform activity: Antagonism by GABA and EEG patterns, Expl Neurol. 46, 229-243 (1975).

McLennan, H.: The release of acetylcholine and of 3-hydroxytyramine from the caudate nucleus, J. Physiol. 174, 152-161 (1964).

Milhaud, C.L. and Klein, M.J.: Inhibition emotionelle de la stereotypie amphetaminique du chat, J. Pharmacol. 5, suppl. 2, 67 (1974).

Miller, R.J., Horn, A.S., and Iversen, L.L.: The action of neuroleptic drugs on dopamine stimulated adenosine-3', 5'-monophosphate production in rat neostriatum and limbic forebrain, Mol. Pharmacol. 10, 759-766 (1974).

Miller, J.J., Richardson, T.L., Fibiger, H.C., and McLennan, H.: Anatomical and electrophysiological identification of a projection from the mesencephalic raphe to the caudate-putamen in the rat, Brain Res. 97, 133-138 (1975).

Moore, R.Y., Bhatanagar, R.K., and Heller, A.: Anatomical and chemical studies of a nigro-neostriatal projection in the rat, Brain Res. 30, 119-135 (1971).

Nauta, H.J.W., Pritz, M.B., and Lasch, R.J.: Afferents to the rat caudato-putamen studied with horse radish peroxidase. An evaluation of a retrograde neuroanatomical research method, Brain Res. 67, 219-238 (1974).

Neill, D.B., Grant, L.D., and Grosman, S.P.: Selective potentiation of locomotor effects of amphetamine by midbrain raphe lesions, Physiol. & Behav. 9, 655 (1972).

Ng, K.Y., Chase, T.N., Colburn, R.W., and Kopin, I.J.: L-DOPA induced release of cerebral monoamines, Science 170, 76-77 (1970).

Olivier, A., Parent, R., Simard, H., and Poirier, L.J.: Cholinesterasic striatopallidal and striatonigral efferents in the cat and the monkey, Brain Res. 18, 273-282 (1970).

Olson, L., Seiger, A., and Fuxe, K.: Heterogeneity of striatal and limbic dopamine innervation: Highly fluorescent islands in the developing and adult rats, Brain Res. 44, 283-288 (1972).

Papeschi, R.: Dopamine, extrapyramidal system and psychomotor function, Psychiat. Neurol. Neurchir. 75, 13-48 (1972).

Parent, A. and Poirier, L.J.: The medial forebrain bundle (MFB) and ascending monoaminergic pathways in the cat, Can. J. Physiol. Pharmacol. 47, 781-785 (1969).

Parizek, J., Hassler, R., and Bak, I.J.: Light and electron microscopic autoradiography of substantia nigra of rat after intraventricular administration of tritium labelled norepinephrine, dopamine, serotonin and the precursors, Z. Zellforsch. mikrosk. Anat. 115, 137-148 (1971).

Pijnenburg, A.J.J. and van Rossum, J.M.: Stimulation of locomotor activity following injection of dopamine into the nucleus accumbens, J. Pharm. Pharmac. 25, 1003-1005 (1973).

Pijnenburg, A.J.J., Woodruff, G.N., and van Rossum, J.M.: Ergometrine induced locomotor activity following intracerebral injection into the nucleus accumbens, Brain Res. 59, 289-302 (1973).

Pijnenburg, A.J.J., Honig, W.M.M., and van Rossum, J.M.: Inhibition of d-amphetamine-induced locomotor activity by injection of haloperidol into the nucleus accumbens of the rat, Psychopharmacologia 41, 87-95 (1975a).

Pijnenburg, A.J.J., Honig, W.M.M., and van Rossum, J.M.: Antagonism of apomorphine- and d-amphetamine-induced stereotyped behaviour by injection of low doses of haloperidol into the caudate nucleus and the nucleus accumbens, Psychopharmacologia 45, 65-71 (1975b).

Pijnenburg, A.J.J., Honig, W.M.M., and van Rossum, J.M.: Effects of antagonists upon locomotor stimulation induced by injection of dopamine and noradrenaline into the nucleus accumbens of nialamide-pretreated rats, Psychopharmacologia 41, 175-180 (1975c).

Pijnenburg, A.J.J., Honig, W.M.M., van der Heyden, J.A.M., and van Rossum, J.M.: Effects of chemical stimulation of the mesolimbic dopamine system upon locomotor activity, Eur. J. Pharmacol. 35, 45-58 (1976).

Pijnenburg, A.J.J., Honig, W.M.M., Struyker Boudier, H.A.J., Cools, A.R., van der Heyden, J.A.M., and van Rossum, J.M.: Further investigation on the effects of ergometrine and other ergot derivatives following injection into the nucleus accumbens of the rat, Archs int. Pharmacodyn. Thér., in press.

Poirier, L., Langlier, P., Bédard, P., Boucher, R., LaRochelle, L., Parent, A., and Roberge, A.: Dopaminergic and cholinergic mechanisms in relation to postural tremor in the cat, Adv. Neurol. 5, 5-10 (1974).

Randrup, A. and Munkvad, I.: On the relation of tryptaminic and serotonergic mechanisms to amphetamine induced abnormal behaviour, Acta Pharmac. Tox. 21, 272-282 (1964).

Randrup, A. and Munkvad, I.: Evidence indicating an association between schizophrenia and dopaminergic hyperactivity in the brain, Orthomolec. Psychiat. 1, 2-15 (1972).

Roberts, E.: An hypothesis suggesting that there is a defect in the GABA system in schizophrenia, Neurosci. Res. Progr. Bull. 10, 468 (1972).

Roberts, E.: Disinhibition as an organizing principle in the nervous system. The role of gamma-aminobutyric acid, Adv. Neurol. 5, 127-143 (1974).

Robinson, N. and Wells, F.: Distribution and localization of sites of gamma-aminobutyric acid metabolism in the adult rat brain, J. Anat. 114, 365-378 (1973).

Rotrosen, J., Angrist, B.M., Wallach, M.B., and Gershon, S.: Absence of serotonergic influence on apomorphine stereotypy, Eur. J. Pharmacol. 20, 133-135 (1972).

Scheel-Krüger, J.: Central effects of anticholinergic drugs measured by the apomorphine gnawing test in mice, Acta Pharmac. Tox. 28, 1-16 (1970).

Seiger, A. and Olson, L.: Late prenatal ontogeny of central monoamine neurons in the rat: Fluorescence histochemical observations, Z. Anat. EntwGesch. 140, 281-318 (1973).

Shellenberger, M.K. and Gordon, J.H.: Regional differences in responses to displacement and inhibition of synthesis of catecholamines in the cat brain, Biol. Psychiat. 9(2), 131-145 (1974).

Shute, C. and Lewis, P.: The ascending cholinergic reticular system: Neocortical, olfactory and subcortical projections, Brain 90, 497-520 (1967).

Stevens, J., Wilson, K., and Foote, W.: GABA blockade, dopamine and schizophrenia: Experimental studies in the cat, Psychopharmacologia 39, 105-119 (1974).

Stevens, J.R.: An anatomy of schizophrenia, Archs gen. Psychiat. 29, 177-189 (1973).

Struyker Boudier, H.A.J.: Catecholamine Receptors in Nervous Tissue. Pp. 1-85. Nijmegen: "Stichting Studentenpers" Press, 1975.

Struyker Boudier, H.A.J., Gielen, W., Cools, A.R., and van Rossum, J.M.: Pharmacological analysis of dopamine-induced inhibition and excitation of neurones of the snail Helix aspersa, Archs int. Pharmacodyn. Thér. 209, 324-332 (1974).

Struyker Boudier, H.A.J., Teppema, L., Cools, A.R., and van Rossum, J.M.: (3, 4-dihydroxyphenylamino)-2-imidazoline (DPI): A new, potent stimulant at dopamine receptors mediating neuronal inhibition, J. Pharm. Pharmac. 27, 882-883 (1975).

Sutin, J. and McNair, J.: Suppression of cell firing in the substantia nigra by caudate stimulation, Physiologist, Wash. 14, 241 (1971).

Tenen, S.S.: The effects of p-chlorophenylalanine, a serotonin depleter on avoidance acquisition, pain sensitivity and related behavior in the rat, Psychopharmacologia 10, 204-219 (1967).

Tennyson, V.M., Barrett, R.E., Cohen, G., Côté, L., Heikkila, R., and Mytilineou, C.: The developing neostriatum of the rabbit: Correlation of fluorescence histochemistry, electron microscopy, endogeneous dopamine levels, and (H^3) dopamine uptake, Brain Res. 46, 251-285 (1972).

Ungerstedt, U.: Stereotaxic mapping of the monoamine pathways in the rat brain, Acta Physiol. Scand., Suppl. 367, 1-48 (1971a).

Ungerstedt, U.: Postsynaptic supersensitivity after 6-hydroxydopamine induced degeneration of the nigro-striatal dopamine systems, Acta Physiol. Scand., Suppl. 367, 69-93 (1971b).

Ungerstedt, U.: Adipsia and aphagia after 6-hydroxydopamine induced degeneration of the nigro-striatal dopamine system, Acta Physiol. Scand., Suppl. 367, 95-122 (1971c).

Ungerstedt, U., Butcher, L.L., Butcher, S.S., Andèn, N.E., and Fuxe, K.: Direct chemical stimulation of dopaminergic mechanisms in the neostriatum of rats, Brain Res. 14, 461-471 (1969).

Weil-Malherbe, H. and Szara, S.I.: The Biochemistry of Functional and Experimental Psychoses (American Lecture Series Publication No. 817). Springfield, Ill: Charles C. Thomas, 1971.

Wolfarth, S., Grabowska, M., Lacki, M., Dulska, E., and Antkiewicz, L.: The action of apomorphine in rats with striatal lesions, Activitas nerv. sup. 15, 132-138 (1973).

Wyatt, R.J., Fermini, B.A., and Davis, J.: Biochemical and sleep studies on schizophrenia: A review of the literature 1960-1970, Schizophrenia 4, 10-44 (1971).

Wyatt, R.J., Vaughan, T., Galanter, M., Kaplan, J., and Green, R.: Behavioural changes of schizophrenic patients given L-5-hydroxytryptophan, Science 177, 1124-1126 (1972).

York, D.H.: Possible dopaminergic pathways from substantia nigra to putamen, Brain Res. 20, 223-249 (1970).

Yoshida, M. and Precht, O.W.: Monosynaptic inhibition of neurons of the substantia nigra by caudato-nigral fibres, Brain Res. 32, 225-228 (1971).

RELEASE OF NEUROTRANSMITTERS FROM THE BRAIN *IN VIVO* BY AMPHETAMINE, METHYLPHENIDATE AND COCAINE

K. E. Moore, C. C. Chiueh and G. Zeldes

Michigan State University

East Lansing, Michigan 48824

During the past 15 years the results of indirect *in vivo* and direct *in vitro* studies suggest that a variety of central stimulant drugs exert their characteristic pharmacological effects by interacting with aminergic neuronal systems in the brain. Early behavioral and biochemical experiments indicated that amphetamines exerted central stimulant actions by releasing norepinephrine (Stein, 1964; Carr and Moore, 1969), but more recent studies suggest that the release of dopamine is more important for many of the central actions of this drug (e.g., Carlsson, 1970; Thornburg and Moore, 1937b; Hollister, Breese, and Cooper, 1974). Since the central stimulation of amphetamine is blocked by α-methyltyrosine but not by reserpine (Rech, 1964; Smith, 1965; Weissman, Koe, and Tenen, 1966), it has been postulated that amphetamine acts by preferentially releasing dopamine from a newly synthesized pool of this amine in the nerve terminals. On the other hand, the central stimulant actions of methylphenidate and cocaine are reduced by reserpine pretreatment but not by α-methyltyrosine (van Rossum, van der Schoot, and Hurkmans, 1962; Scheel-Krüger, 1971; Simon, Sultan, Chermat, and Boissier, 1972) suggesting that the actions of these two stimulants are dependent upon a storage or reserpine-sensitive pool of brain catecholamines. There has been less interest in the interactions of these central stimulants with 5-hydroxytryptamine (5HT) neuronal systems, but recent behavioral-biochemical studies (Green and Harvey, 1974; Breese, Cooper, and Mueller, 1974) suggest that tryptaminergic neurons exert an inhibitory action on amphetamine stimulation; there are few reports on the interactions of cocaine or methylphenidate with 5HT neurons.

In vitro studies employing a variety of preparations of brain tissues have demonstrated that amphetamine, methylphenidate, and cocaine release or block the specific reuptake of amines (Ferris, Tang, and Maxwell, 1972; Azzaro, Ziance, and Rutledge, 1974; Heikkila, Orlansky, and Cohen, 1975). Without minimizing the important contributions of these studies it should be pointed out that the *in vitro* situation is undoubtedly different from that *in vivo*, particularly with nervous tissue. For example, the actions of drugs on ongoing neurogenic release of putative transmitters cannot be evaluated *in vitro*.

The present report summarizes the results of some of our efforts to measure the "release" of putative neurotransmitters from nerve terminals in the brain *in vivo* by amphetamine, methylphenidate, and cocaine.

IN VIVO RELEASE FROM BRAIN OF NEUROTRANSMITTERS

The anatomical complexities and the relative inaccessibility of specific neurons in the CNS make it difficult to detect the release of putative neurotransmitters from brain *in vivo*. Furthermore, the blood brain barrier limits the transfer of most neurotransmitters from the brain into the blood. Special techniques have been developed to detect the release of neurotransmitters from brain (for review see Myers, 1972). While the polar neurotransmitter compounds do not readily transfer from brain to blood, they do diffuse from brain to CSF and vice versa. Since 1969 we have employed a modification of the cerebroventricular perfusing techniques developed by Feldberg and his co-workers (e.g., Carmichael, Feldberg, and Fleischauer, 1964) to detect the drug-induced release of catecholamines from the brain *in vivo* (see Carr and Moore, 1969).

Figure 1 is a schematic diagram of the cerebroventricular perfusion technique that we have employed. Artificial CSF is pumped into the lateral cerebral ventricle of anesthetized cats through a stereotaxically placed cannula. The effluent is collected from a catheter inserted into the cerebroaqueduct (Carr and Moore, 1970). Being unable to detect endogenous catecholamines in the effluent, we have resorted to radioactive tracer techniques. In early experiments small volumes of ^{3}H-norepinephrine or ^{3}H-dopamine were injected into the lateral ventricle before the start of the perfusion; the ^{3}H-amines are taken up by the tissues lining the ventricles and are subsequently released into the perfusing CSF by drugs or electrical stimulation of appropriate brain structures. In Fig. 1 a stimulating electrode is pictured in the lateral hypothalamus aimed at axons of the ascending dopaminergic nigrostriatal pathway. Stimulation of this electrode or of electrodes in the caudate nucleus or the substantia nigra increases

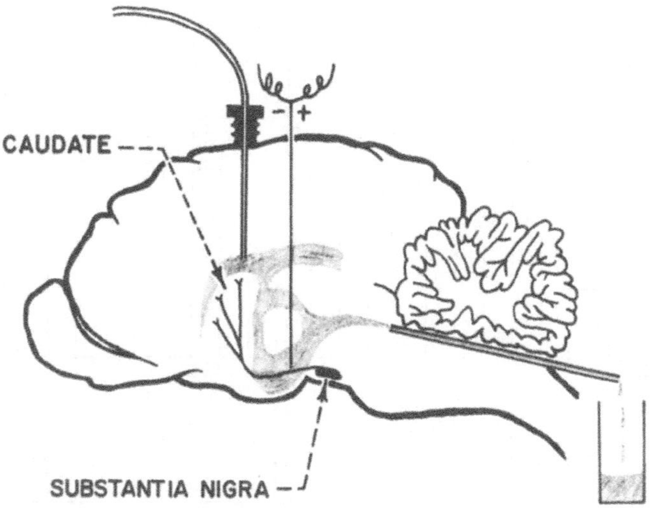

Fig. 1. Schematic diagram of the cerebroventricular perfusing technique.

the efflux of ^{3}H-dopamine (Von Voigtlander and Moore, 1971a,b). If a lesion is made in the ascending nigrostriatal bundle, the dopaminergic nerves terminating in the striatum on the side of the lesion are selectively destroyed. This is evidenced by the unilateral loss of dopamine but not 5-HT from the striatum and by the inability of the striatum to take up and retain exogenously administered ^{3}H-dopamine (Von Voigtlander and Moore, 1973a). These results suggest, therefore, that when ^{3}H-dopamine is injected into the lateral ventricle it is taken up primarily by dopaminergic nerve terminals in the striatum; the administration of certain stimulant drugs appears to release ^{3}H-dopamine from these same nerves.

DRUG-INDUCED RELEASE OF EXOGENOUSLY ADMINISTERED ^{3}H-DOPAMINE

d-Amphetamine and Tyramine

d-Amphetamine and tyramine release norepinephrine from terminals of peripheral sympathetic neurons and they also release dopamine from neurons in the brain. In the experiment illustrated in Fig. 2, an electrolytic lesion was made in the ascending

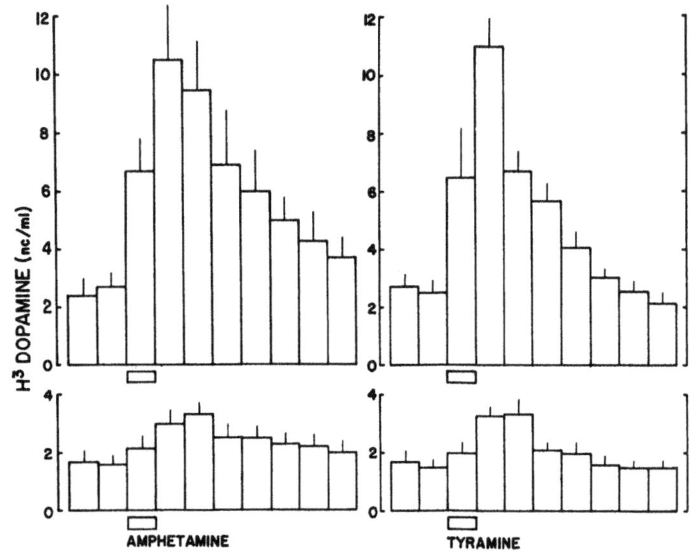

Fig. 2. Efflux of ^{3}H-dopamine evoked by an intraventricular pulse of d-amphetamine (1.6×10^{-4}M) or tyramine (3.2×10^{-4}M) in cats in which unilateral electrolytic lesions of the nigrostriatal pathway had been made 2-8 weeks prior to the experiment. The lateral ventricle contralateral to (top) and ipsilateral to (bottom) the lesions were perfused. The height of each bar represents the mean concentration of ^{3}H-dopamine in consecutive 2 min samples of perfusate (Modified from Von Voigtlander and Moore, 1973a).

nigrostriatal pathway on one side of the brains of cats some 2-8 weeks prior to the experiment. When the striatum on the non-lesioned side was perfused (top of Fig. 2), the addition of a pulse of d-amphetamine or tyramine increased the efflux of ^{3}H-dopamine. When the same procedure was repeated on the contralateral lesioned side, the drug-induced efflux of ^{3}H-dopamine was dramatically reduced. The results suggest, therefore, that the ^{3}H-dopamine released by these drugs originates primarily from dopaminergic nerve terminals lining the ventricular system.

This study indicates where the dopamine is originating but does not tell us anything about the mechanism by which the amine is released. On one hand, amphetamine and tyramine may actively replace or release dopamine; on the other hand, they may facilitate the neurogenic release or block the uptake of neurogenically released dopamine. In an attempt to determine which of these two possibilities apply, experiments were performed in which the neurogenic release of dopamine was interrupted by making acute lesions in the nigrostriatal pathway. The effects of these lesions on the abilities of amphetamine and tyramine to increase the efflux of ^{3}H-dopamine are compared in Fig. 3. The addition of a two-minute pulse of d-amphetamine or tyramine to the perfusing CSF of control cats is depicted at the top; both drugs markedly increased the efflux of ^{3}H-dopamine. The lower figures depict what happens when an electrolytic lesion is made in the ascending nigrostriatal pathway 20 minutes before the addition of the pulse of the drug solution. The lesion caused a consistent and significant decrease in the efflux of ^{3}H-dopamine, indicating that the efflux of this amine is due, in part, to ongoing activity of neurons in the nigrostriatal pathway. It is also apparent that the acute lesions reduce the ability of amphetamine but not of tyramine to evoke the release of ^{3}H-dopamine. This suggests that amphetamine-induced release of dopamine is dependent upon the activity of nerves, while the efflux caused by tyramine is independent of nerve activity. This difference could probably not be identified using *in vitro* preparations and we have concluded that amphetamine facilitates neurogenic release and/or blocks the reuptake of the released dopamine.

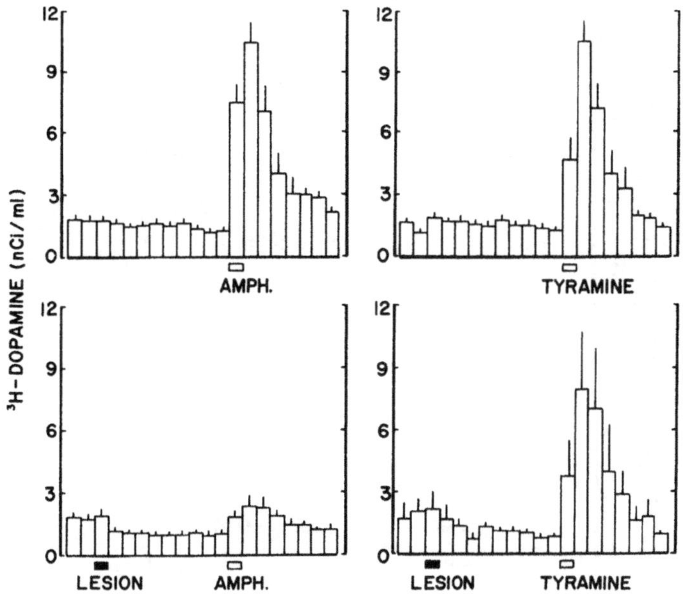

Fig. 3. Efflux of ^{3}H-dopamine evoked by ventricular infusions of d-amphetamine or tyramine contralateral to (top) and ipsilateral to (bottom) an acute unilateral lesion of the nigrostriatal pathway. See legend to Fig. 2 for additional details (Modified from Von Voigtlander and Moore, 1973a).

d-Amphetamine and 1-Amphetamine

Over the past 5 years controversy has developed over the relative abilities of d- and 1-amphetamine to influence dopaminergic and noradrenergic neuronal systems in the brain. Taylor and Snyder (1971) suggested that amphetamine-induced motor stimulation is mediated by norepinephrine, whereas stereotypy is mediated by dopamine. This hypothesis was based on a 10:1 and 2:1 potency ratio of d- and 1-amphetamine in eliciting these behaviors and in blocking the uptake of norepinephrine and dopamine, respectively. That is, these investigators reported that there was little difference in ability of the isomers of amphetamine to cause stereotypies and to block the uptake of dopamine in the striatum. In contrast, however, Ferris et al. (1972), Harris and Baldessarini (1973), and Thornburg and Moore (1973a) noted that d-amphetamine was 3-10 times more potent than 1-amphetamine in blocking ^{3}H-dopamine uptake by the preparations of the striatum. The same relative effects of these two isomers of amphetamine on the efflux of ^{3}H-dopamine was found *in vivo*

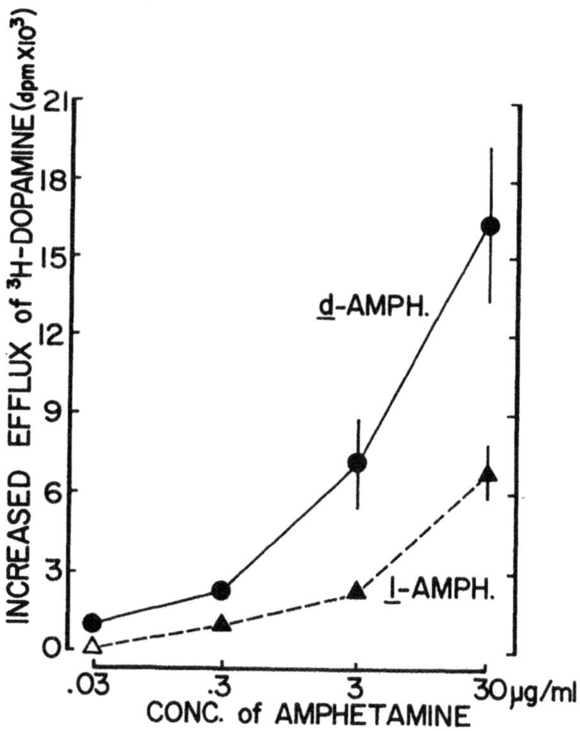

Fig. 4. The increased efflux of ^{3}H-dopamine from cat in response to 5 min intraventricular pulses of increasing concentrations of d- and 1-amphetamine (Chiueh and Moore, 1974b).

Using the cerebroventricular perfusing technique it was found that d-amphetamine was approximately 10 times more potent than l-amphetamine in increasing the efflux of ^{3}H-dopamine from the cat brain (Fig. 4).

DRUG-INDUCED RELEASE OF ENDOGENOUSLY SYNTHESIZED ^{3}H-DOPAMINE

Although intraventricularly administered ^{3}H-dopamine accumulated primarily in dopamine neurons, this amine is probably not exclusively taken up by and subsequently released from these neurons. This is evidenced in Fig. 3 by the fact that following nigrostriatal lesions the efflux of ^{3}H-dopamine does not fall to zero. Since tyrosine hydroxylase is located exclusively in catecholaminergic neurons any ^{3}H-dopamine formed from ^{3}H-tyrosine must originate exclusively from these neurons. In subsequent studies, therefore, the dopamine stores in the striatum were labelled with intraventricular perfusions of ^{3}H-tyrosine of high specific activity. The major technical problem with these experiments involved separating less than 1,000 dpm of ^{3}H-dopamine from several 100,000 dpm of ^{3}H-tyrosine; this was solved by employing a combination of ion exchange and aluminum adsorption chromatography (Chiueh and Moore, 1974a).

d-Amphetamine and Cocaine

Figure 5 illustrates the effects of intraventricular perfusion of d-amphetamine and cocaine on the efflux of endogenously synthesized ^{3}H-dopamine. The addition of 10 min pulses of increasing concentrations of d-amphetamine caused a progressive increase in the efflux of ^{3}H-dopamine, but did not alter the efflux of ^{3}H-tyrosine. In another study of identical design, increasing concentrations of cocaine also increased the efflux of ^{3}H-dopamine (Fig. 5, right). Although both drugs are equally potent, d-amphetamine appears to be more effective than cocaine in increasing the efflux of ^{3}H-dopamine. This difference may be related to the fact that cocaine may block the uptake of neurogenically released dopamine while amphetamine may facilitate neurogenic release and also block the reuptake of the released amine.

d-Amphetamine and Methylphenidate

The ability of d-amphetamine and methylphenidate to increase the efflux of endogenously synthesized ^{3}H-dopamine is compared in Fig. 6. The intraventricular and intravenous administration of both drugs increased the efflux of ^{3}H-dopamine. Although both drugs caused similar effects, the mechanism of action is quite different.

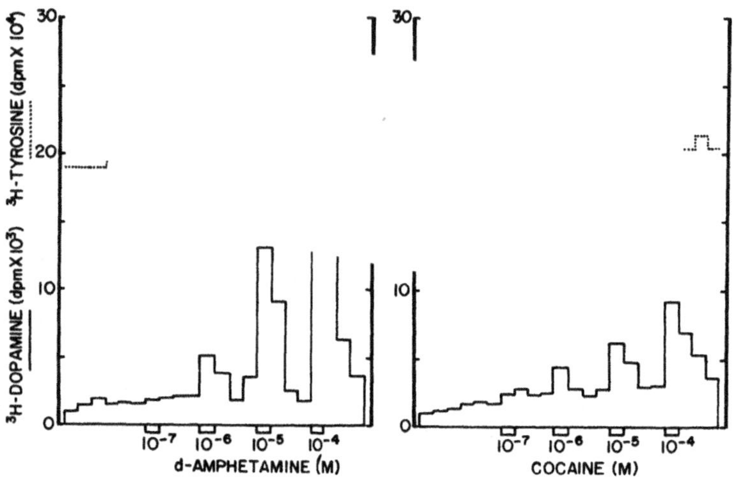

Fig. 5. Effects of adding increasing concentrations of d-amphetamine and cocaine to the perfusing CSF on the efflux of endogenously synthesized ^{3}H-dopamine. The perfusing CSF contained ^{3}H-tyrosine and each 10 min sample of perfusate was analyzed for ^{3}H-tyrosine (----) and ^{3}H-dopamine (——).

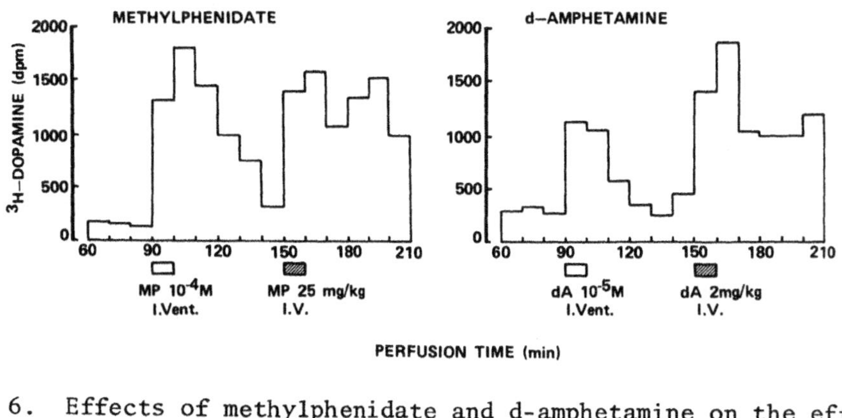

Fig. 6. Effects of methylphenidate and d-amphetamine on the efflux of endogenously synthesized ^{3}H-dopamine. CSF containing ^{3}H-tyrosine was infused into a lateral cerebroventricle for 210 min and consecutive 10 min samples of perfusate were analyzed for ^{3}H-dopamine. Methylphenidate (MP) or d-amphetamine (dA) were added to perfusing CSF for 10 min after 90 min of perfusion and injected intravenously after 150 min of perfusion.

It has been previously reported (Scheel-Krüger, 1971) that reserpine blocked the locomotor stimulation induced by methylphenidate but not by amphetamine. To determine if these behavioral differences were reflected biochemically, the effects of reserpine on the dopamine releasing abilities of d-amphetamine and methylphenidate were compared (Fig. 7). When ^{3}H-tyrosine was infused into the cerebral ventricles of control cats for 60 min, ^{3}H-dopamine appeared in the effluxing CSF in the first 10 min sample. This resting efflux increased only slightly during subsequent collection periods. CSF containing ^{3}H-tyrosine and 10^{-4}M methylphenidate was infused into the ventricles of another group of non-pretreated cats. The presence of methylphenidate caused an immediate and sustained increase in the efflux of ^{3}H-dopamine. The same experiment was then carried out in cats which had been pretreated 2 hr earlier with reserpine (0.5mg/kg i.p.). In these animals methylphenidate did not increase the efflux of ^{3}H-dopamine.

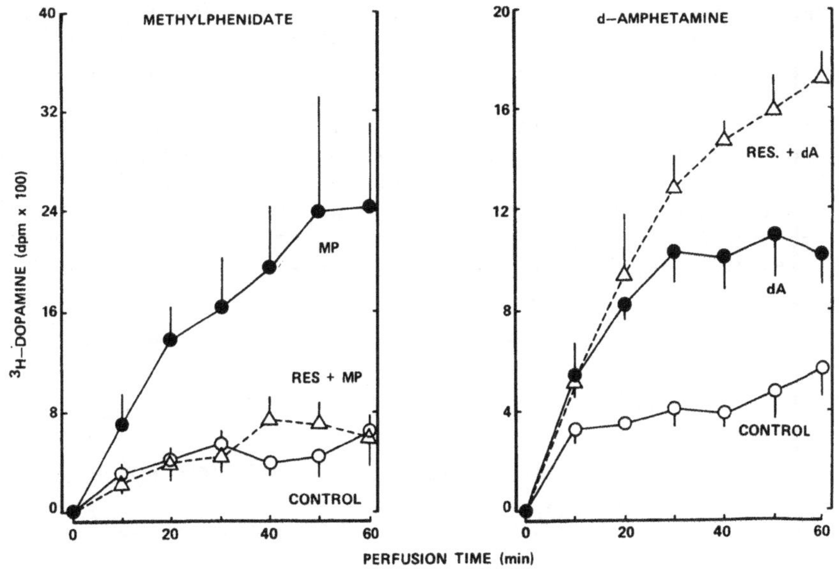

Fig. 7. Effects of methylphenidate and d-amphetamine on the efflux of endogenously synthesized ^{3}H-dopamine from the brains of control and reserpine-pretreated cats. CSF containing ^{3}H-tyrosine (○) or ^{3}H-tyrosine and drug (●) was infused into the lateral cerebral ventricles of non-pretreated cats for 60 min, and 10 min samples of perfusate were analyzed for ^{3}H-dopamine. CSF containing ^{3}H-tyrosine and drug was also infused into the lateral cerebral ventricles of cats pretreated with reserpine (0.5mg/kg, i.v.) 2 hours prior to the start of perfusion (Δ).

Quite a different pattern was seen when an experiment of identical design was carried out with perfusions of d-amphetamine (Fig. 7, right). In control non-pretreated cats, the addition of 10^{-6}M amphetamine to the perfusing CSF caused an immediate and sustained increase in the efflux of ^{3}H-dopamine. This amphetamine response was not blocked by reserpine pretreatment; rather, amphetamine-induced efflux of ^{3}H-dopamine appeared to be increased. When analyzed at the end of the experiments, the endogenous content of dopamine in the striatum of the reserpine-pretreated cats was reduced to less than 4% of that found in control cats, indicating that the reserpine had depleted the dopamine stores. In subsequent studies it has been determined that intraventricular infusions of increasing concentrations of methylphenidate (10^{-6} - 10^{-3}M) causes a progressive increase in the efflux of ^{3}H-dopamine, and this effect is completely blocked in cats pretreated with reserpine. In similar studies with amphetamine, reserpine had no effect or slightly increased the dose-related increased efflux of dopamine (Chiueh and Moore, 1975).

The results of these experiments are schematically summarized in Fig. 8. d-Amphetamine and methylphenidate both increase the efflux of dopamine from brain, but the mechanism by which they do this is different. Reserpine blocks the effects of methylphenidate but not of amphetamine. Thus, amphetamine appears to release dopamine from a newly synthesized pool, whereas methylphenidate releases dopamine from a storage or reserpine-sensitive pool. This conclusion, based on the results of direct biochemical experiments, is consistent with previous proposals made on the basis of behavioral studies by Scheel-Krüger (1971), Weissman et al., (1966), and Thornburg and Moore (1973b).

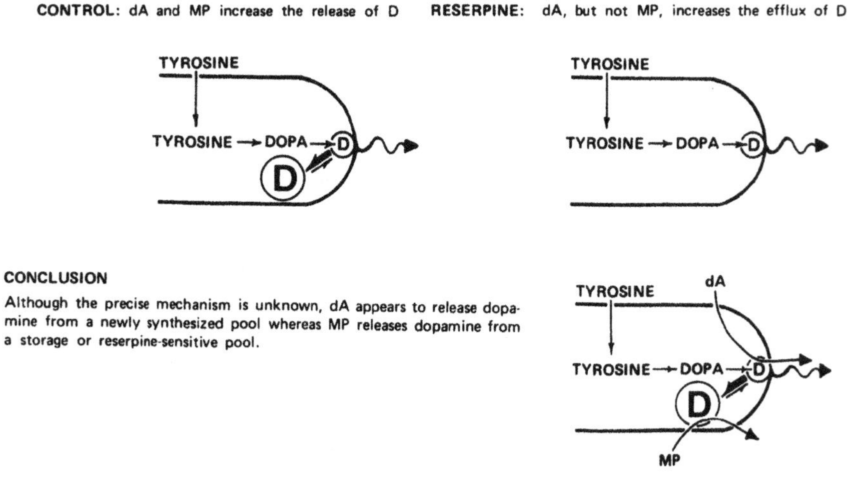

Fig. 8. Possible neuronal sites at which d-amphetamine (dA) and methylphenidate (MP) act to increase the efflux of dopamine.

RELEASE OF ENDOGENOUSLY SYNTHESIZED ^{3}H-5-HYDROXYTRYPTAMINE

Fuxe and Ungerstedt (1970) proposed that amphetamine released 5HT from granular stores, and in 1973 Azzaro and Rutledge reported that amphetamine released ^{3}H-5HT from striatal slices. Recent studies by Breese et al. (1974) and Green and Harvey (1974) suggest that 5HT neuronal systems inhibit the stimulant actions of amphetamine. That is, 5HT neuronal systems appear to inhibit the actions of catecholamine neurons responsible for amphetamine-induced motor stimulation. Accordingly, one might expect amphetamine to cause a compensatory increase in 5HT neuronal activity. To test this possibility, the ability of amphetamine to increase the efflux of ^{3}H-5HT was examined. In these experiments the same cerebroventricular perfusing technique was employed except the ventricles were perfused with ^{3}H-tryptophan and the perfusate was analyzed for effluxing ^{3}H-5HT.

The utility of the system was first tested by determining the effect of potassium on the efflux of endogenously synthesized ^{3}H-5HT. The addition of increasing concentrations of potassium to the CSF caused an increase in the ^{3}H-5HT, but did not alter the efflux of

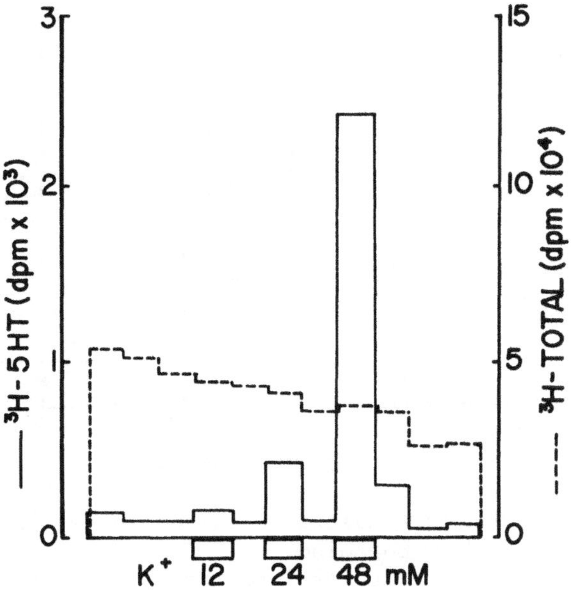

Fig. 9. Effect of potassium on the efflux of endogenously synthesized ^{3}H-5HT. Thirty min after an intraventricular injection of ^{3}H-tryptophan the cerebroventricular system was perfused with CSF and consecutive 5 min samples of perfusate were analyzed for ^{3}H-5HT. Five min pulses of increasing concentrations of potassium were added to the perfusing CSF as indicated.

^{3}H-tryptophan (Fig. 9). However, as indicated in Fig. 10, additions of amphetamine to the CSF did not markedly increase the efflux of ^{3}H-5HT. The addition of a pulse of 10^{-4}M d-amphetamine had little effect on the efflux of ^{3}H-5HT, whereas 1/10th this concentration of amphetamine (10^{-5}M) caused a marked increase in the efflux of endogenously synthesized ^{3}H-dopamine. These results indicate, therefore, that amphetamine has only a weak action on 5HT neurons when compared to its effect on dopaminergic neurons. These negative results should be tempered by the fact that the systemic administration of amphetamine could cause a compensatory release of 5HT at a site in the brain which is some distance from the cerebral ventricles, and thereby not be detected in the CSF.

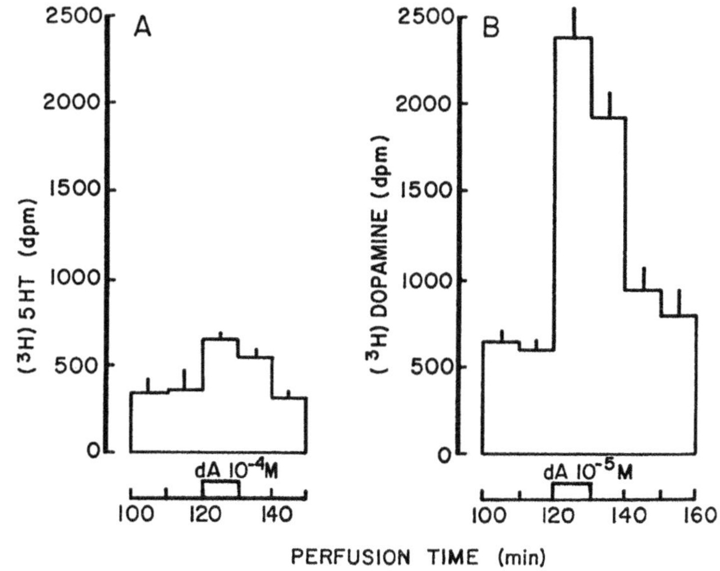

Fig. 10. Effects of d-amphetamine on the efflux of endogenously synthesized ^{3}H-5HT and ^{3}H-dopamine.

A. After an intraventricular injection of ^{3}H-tryptophan and 2 hr of perfusion a 10 min pulse of d-amphetamine was added to the perfusing CSF; 10 min samples of perfusate were analyzed for ^{3}H-5HT.

B. After 2 hr of continuous perfusion with CSF containing ^{3}H-tyrosine a 10 min pulse of d-amphetamine was added to the perfusing CSF; 10 min samples of perfusate were analyzed for ^{3}H-dopamine (Chiueh and Moore, 1976).

DISCUSSION AND SUMMARY

Evidence accumulating over the past 15 years supports the hypothesis that d-amphetamine, methylphenidate, and cocaine exert at least part of their central stimulant actions by increasing the concentrations of dopamine at specific receptors in the brain, although the mechanism by which this is accomplished may be different for each of these drugs.

Early behavioral studies implicated brain catecholamines stores in the central actions of cocaine and methylphenidate because stimulant effects of these drugs were reduced when brain catecholamines stores were depleted by reserpine pretreatment (van Rossum et al., 1962; Scheel-Krüger, 1971). Since the central stimulant actions of amphetamine were not blocked by reserpine it was proposed that this stimulant was a direct agonist on catecholamine receptors (Smith, 1965). Subsequent studies employing α-methyltyrosine, which inhibits the synthesis of both dopamine and norepinephrine, suggest that d-amphetamine acted by selectively releasing newly synthesized catecholamines (Weissman et al., 1966). When precautions were used to avoid nonspecific depressant actions of dopamine-β-hydroxylase inhibitors (Disulfiram, U-14,624, FLA-63), it was found that these compounds did not block the locomotor stimulation produced by amphetamine, prompting Thornburg and Moore (1973b) to propose that this action of amphetamine was related to its ability to release newly synthesized dopamine.

Behavioral studies in rodents with selective 6-hydroxydopamine-induced lesions of dopaminergic neuronal systems support the hypothesis that amphetamine, methylphenidate, and cocaine are indirect acting dopaminergic agonists. For example, rodents with unilateral lesions in the nigrostriatal pathway exhibit ipsilateral turning in response to these drugs, whereas direct acting dopaminergic agonists (e.g., apomorphine) caused contralateral circling (Ungerstedt, 1971; Von Voigtlander and Moore, 1973b; Wallach, 1974). Bilateral lesions of ascending dopaminergic neurons have recently been reported to block the stimulant actions of cocaine and d-amphetamine (Creese and Iversen, 1975; Kelly, Seviour, and Iversen, 1975).

Results of *in vitro* studies employing a variety of preparations of brain tissues indicate that amphetamine, methylphenidate, and cocaine influence the dynamics of catecholamines. There have been some controversies over the relative abilities of these drugs to release and/or to block the reuptake of dopamine (Ferris et al., 1972; Azzaro et al., 1974; Heikkila et al., 1975), but these controversies may not be pertinent to the *in vivo* situation. For example, behavioral and *in vivo* biochemical studies have revealed that amphetamine selectively releases newly synthesized catecholamines yet most investigators label their *in vitro* tissue preparations with exogenously administered radioactive catecholamines.

Furthermore, *in vivo* studies suggest that drugs interact with ongoing processes of neuronal activity and such interactions cannot be evaluated in slices or synaptosomal preparations. Thus, results of studies in which the actions of drugs on isolated brain tissues are evaluated may be comparable to the actions of these drugs on quiescent nerves *in vivo* (e.g., on terminals of section nerves; see Fig. 3 and Von Voigtlander and Moore, 1973a).

The experiments described in the present report indicate that d-amphetamine appears to increase the efflux of dopamine from brain tissue by facilitating neurogenic release or by blocking the reuptake of dopamine released from a newly synthesized pool; that cocaine increases the efflux of dopamine, possibly by blocking neuronal reuptake of this amine; and that methylphenidate releases dopamine from a storage or reserpine-sensitive pool. Despite the marked effect of d-amphetamine on dopamine release, this drug appears to have little effect on the efflux of 5HT.

ACKNOWLEDGMENTS

This research was supported by USPHS Grant MH 13174.

The present address of Dr. C.C. Chiueh is: Laboratory of Clinical Science, NIMH, Bethesda, Maryland.

REFERENCES

Azzaro, A.J. and Rutledge, C.O.: Selectivity of release of norepinephrine, dopamine and 5-hydroxytryptamine by amphetamine in various regions of rat brain, Biochem. Pharmacol. 22, 2801-2813 (1973).

Azzaro, A.J., Ziance, R.J., and Rutledge, C.O.: The importance of neuronal uptake of amines for amphetamine-induced release of ^{3}H-norepinephrine from isolated brain tissue, J. Pharmac. exp. Ther. 189, 110-118 (1974).

Besson, M.J., Cheramy, A., Feltz, P., and Glowinski, J.: Dopamine: Spontaneous and drug-induced release from the caudate nucleus in the cat, Brain Res. 32, 407-424 (1971).

Breese, G.R., Cooper, B.R., and Mueller, R.A.: Evidence for involvement of 5-hydroxytryptamine in the actions of amphetamine, Br. J. Pharmacol. 52, 307-314 (1974).

Carlsson, A.: Amphetamine and brain catecholamines. In: Amphetamines and Related Compounds. Costa, E. and Garattini, S., Eds., pp. 289-300. New York: Raven Press, 1970.

Carmichael, E.A., Feldberg, W., and Fleischauer, K.: Methods for perfusing different parts of the cat's cerebral ventricles with drugs, J. Physiol., Lond. 173, 354-367 (1964).

Carr, L.A. and Moore, K.E.: Norepinephrine: Release from brain by d-amphetamine *in vivo*, Science 164, 322-323 (1969).

Carr, L.A. and Moore, K.E.: Effects of amphetamine on the contents of norepinephrine and metabolites in the effluent of perfused cerebral ventricles of the cat, Biochem. Pharmacol. 19, 2361-2374 (1970).

Chiueh, C.C. and Moore, K.E.: Effects of α-methyltyrosine on d-amphetamine-induced release of endogenously synthesized and exogenously administered catecholamines from the cat brain *in vivo*, J. Pharmac. exp. Ther. 190, 100-108 (1974a).

Chiueh, C.C. and Moore, K.E.: Relative potencies of d- and l-amphetamine on the release of dopamine from cat brain *in vivo*, Res. Comm. Chem. Path. Pharmac. 7, 189-199 (1974b).

Chiueh, C.C. and Moore, K.E.: Blockade by reserpine of methylphenidate-induced release of brain dopamine, J. Pharmac. exp. Ther. 193, 559-563 (1975).

Chiueh, C.C. and Moore, K.E.: Effects of dopaminergic agonists and electrical stimulation of the midbrain raphé on the release of 5-hydroxytryptamine from the cat brain *in vivo*, J. Neurochem., in press.

Creese, I. and Iversen, S.D.: The pharmacological and anatomical substrates of the amphetamine response in the rat, Brain Res. 83, 419-436 (1975).

Ferris, R.M., Tang, F.L.M., and Maxwell, R.A.: A comparison of the capacities of isomers of amphetamine, deoxypipradrol and methylphenidate to inhibit the uptake of tritiated catecholamines into rat cerebral cortex slices, synaptosomal preparations of rat cerebral cortex, hypothalamus and striatum and into adrenergic nerves of rabbit aorta, J. Pharmac. exp. Ther. 181, 407-416 (1972).

Fuxe, K. and Ungerstedt, U.: Histochemical, biochemical and functional studies on central monoamine neurons after acute and chronic amphetamine administration. In: Amphetamines and Related Compounds. Costa, E. and Garattini, S., Eds., pp. 257-288. New York: Raven Press, 1970.

Green, T.K. and Harvey, J.A.: Enhancement of amphetamine action after interruption of ascending serotonergic pathways, J. Pharmac. exp. Ther. 190, 109-117 (1974).

Harris, J.E. and Baldessarini, R.J.: Uptake of (^{3}H)-catecholamines by homogenates of rat corpus striatum and cerebral cortex: Effects of amphetamine analogues, Neuropharmacol. 12, 669-179 (1973).

Heikkila, R.E., Orlansky, H., and Cohen, G.: Studies on the distinction between uptake inhibition and release of ^{3}H-dopamine in rat brain tissue slices, Biochem. Pharmacol. 24, 847-852 (1975).

Hollister, A.S., Breese, G.R., and Cooper, B.R.: Comparison of tyrosine hydroxylase inhibition with the effects of various 6-hydroxydopamine treatments on d-amphetamine induced motor activity, Psychopharmacologia 36, 1-16 (1974).

Kelly, P.H., Seviour, P.W., and Iversen, S.D.: Amphetamine and apomorphine responses in the rat following 6-hydroxydopamine lesions of the nucleus accumbens septi and corpus striatum, Brain Res. 94, 507-522 (1975).

McKenzie, G.M. and Szerb, J.C.: The effect of dihydroxyphenylalanine, pheniprazine and dextroamphetamine on the *in vivo* release of dopamine from the caudate nucleus, J. Pharmac. exp. Ther. 162, 302-308 (1968).

Myers, R.D.: Methods of perfusing different structures of the brain. In: Methods in Psychobiology. Myers, R.D., Ed., Vol. 2, pp. 169-211. New York: Academic Press, 1972.

Rech, R.H.: Antagonism of reserpine behavioral depression by d-amphetamine, J. Pharmac. exp. Ther. 146, 369-376 (1964).

Scheel-Krüger, J.: Comparative studies of various amphetamine analogues demonstrating different interactions with the metabolism of catecholamines in the brain, Eur. J. Pharmacol. 14, 47-59 (1971).

Simon, P. Sultan, Z., Chermat, R., and Boissier, J.R.: La cocaine, une substance amphétaminique? Un problème de psychopharmacologie expérimentale, J. Pharmacol. 3, 129-142 (1972).

Smith, C.B.: Effects of d-amphetamine upon brain amine content and locomotor activity of mice, J. Pharmac. exp. Ther. 147, 96-102 (1965).

Stein, L.: Self-stimulation of the brain and the central stimulant action of amphetamine, Fed. Proc. 23, 836-850 (1964).

Taylor, K.M. and Snyder, S.H.: Differential effects of d- and l-amphetamine on behavior and on catecholamine disposition in dopamine and norepinephrine containing neurons of rat brain, Brain Res. 28, 295-309 (1971).

Thornburg, J.E. and Moore, K.E.: Dopamine and norepinephrine uptake by rat brain synaptosomes: Relative inhibitory potencies of l- and d-amphetamine and amantadine, Res. Comm. Chem. Path. Pharmac. 5, 81-89 (1973a).

Thornburg, J.E. and Moore, K.E.: The relative importance of dopaminergic and noradrenergic neuronal systems for the stimulation of locomotor activity induced by amphetamine and other drugs, Neuropharmacol. 12, 853-866 (1973b).

Ungerstedt, U.: Striatal dopamine release after amphetamine or nerve degeneration revealed by rotational behavior, Acta Physiol. Scand., Suppl. 367, 49-68 (1971).

van Rossum, J.M., van der Schoot, J.B., and Hurkmans, J.A.T.M.: Mechanisms of action of cocaine and amphetamine in the brain, Experientia 18, 229-231 (1962).

Von Voigtlander, P.F. and Moore, K.E.: The release of ^{3}H-dopamine from cat brain following electrical stimulation of the substantia nigra and caudate nucleus, Neuropharmacol. 10, 733-841 (1971a).

Von Voigtlander, P.F. and Moore, K.E.: Nigro-striatal pathway: Stimulation-evoked release of ^{3}H-dopamine from caudate nucleus, Brain Res. 35, 580-583 (1971b).

Von Voigtlander, P.F. and Moore, K.E.: Involvement of nigro-striatal neurons in the *in vivo* release of dopamine by amphetamine, amantadine and tyramine, J. Pharmac. exp. Ther. 184, 542-552 (1973a).

Von Voigtlander, P.F. and Moore, K.E.: Turning behavior of mice with unilateral 6-hydroxydopamine lesions in the striatum: Effects of apomorphine, L-dopa, amantadine, amphetamine and other psychomotor stimulants, Neuropharmacol. 12, 451-462 (1973b).

Wallach, M.D.: Drug-induced stereotyped behavior: Similarities and differences. In: Neuropsychopharmacology of Monoamines and their Regulatory Enzymes. Usdin, E., Ed., pp. 241-260. New York: Raven Press, 1974.

Weissman, A., Koe, K.B., and Tenen, S.S.: Antiamphetamine effects following inhibition of tyrosine hydroxylase, J. Pharmac. exp. Ther. 151, 339-352 (1966).

DISTRIBUTION AND METABOLISM OF AMPHETAMINE IN TOLERANT ANIMALS

Cynthia Moreton Kuhn and Saul M. Schanberg

Duke University Medical Center

Durham, North Carolina 27710

The physiological and behavioral responses of animals to amphetamine change in a complex way when they are treated chronically with this drug. A marked tolerance develops to many of the peripheral effects of amphetamine (such as hyperthermia and increased blood pressure) and to some effects mediated by the central nervous system (Kosman and Unna, 1968; Brodie, Cho, and Gessa, 1970b). However, potentiation of other aspects of the behavioral response to amphetamine (such as stereotyped behavior and increased locomotor activity) has been observed following chronic administration (Ellinwood, 1971; Ellinwood, Sudilovsky, and Nelson, 1972; Rech, Tilson, and Marquis, 1975; Segal, 1975). The biochemical mechanisms subserving these behavioral changes are not well understood. Studies of neurotransmitter mechanisms in animals treated chronically with amphetamine suggest that compensatory reactions of many processes are involved, including increased neurotransmitter synthesis, altered receptor sensitivity, and activation of inhibitory serotonergic pathways (Koda and Gibb, 1973; Mandell and Morgan, 1970; Sparber and Tilson, 1972).

Since these biochemical findings alone still do not adequately explain the complex behavioral phenomena which have been reported, it has been suggested that alterations in the distribution and metabolism of amphetamine may also be involved in the altered responsiveness to amphetamine that develops with chronic administration. There is a large body of evidence that suggests that alteration in the metabolism of amphetamine results in profound changes in the behavioral response. For example, inhibition of amphetamine metabolism in rats causes elevation of tissue amphetamine levels and marked increases in the locomotor activity elicited by amphetamine

(Groppetti and Costa, 1969a; Lal, Missala, Sourkes, and Feldmuller, 1974; Sulser, Owens, and Dingell, 1966). Although the pattern of urinary metabolites following a single dose of amphetamine is similar in animals treated chronically and in animals not treated previously (Lewander, 1971a; Ellison, Okun, Silverman, and Siegel, 1971), there are two reports that suggest that amphetamine distribution in tissues after a single dose of amphetamine is changed by chronic treatment. In both, amphetamine content in brain after a single dose of amphetamine was higher in chronically treated animals than in controls (Magour, Coper, and Fahndrich, 1974; Ellison et al., 1971). One investigator reported that brain amphetamine content one hour after a single dose was higher in animals that had been treated chronically with amphetamine than in control animals (Magour et al., 1974). Since the doses used were very high (animals were receiving 80 mg/kg/day for 2 months), and the author observed considerable impairment of liver function in these animals, these data must be considered cautiously. In the other study, amphetamine content of lungs and cerebral cortex was higher in chronically treated cats 4 hours after administration of a single dose of amphetamine (Ellison et al., 1971).

Although these findings suggest that tissue amphetamine distribution is altered by chronic administration, several crucial factors were not evaluated. In order to compare tissue amphetamine content to critical aspects of behavioral activation, such as onset of action, intensity and duration of peak action, and decay of activity, tissue amphetamine content throughout the time of behavioral activation must be measured. Furthermore, in species that metabolize amphetamine to compounds that could contribute to the observed behavioral and physiological effects, it is vital to know the tissue content of both amphetamine and its metabolites.

In the rat, for example, the distribution of amphetamine metabolites may be a significant factor in chronic drug effects. In this species, amphetamine is converted to p-hydroxyamphetamine (POHA), which has many of the behavioral activities of amphetamine (Taylor and Sulser, 1973; Trendelenburg, 1972), and to the pseudotransmitter p-hydroxynorephedrine (POHNE) (Dring, Smith, and Williams, 1970; Goldstein and Anagnoste, 1965). It has been suggested that accumulation of POHNE in norepinephrine-containing neurons is involved in the development of tolerance to certain effects of amphetamine (Brodie, Cho, Stefano, and Gessa, 1970a). Recent evidence suggests that a complex interaction of noradrenergic, dopaminergic, and serotonergic systems determines the nature of behaviors elicited by amphetamine (Hollister, Breese, and Cooper, 1974; Creese and Iversen, 1974; Goetz and Klawans, 1974). If this is true, accumulation of POHNE in NE-containing neurons could decrease the response to effects mediated solely by NE and also enhance behaviors normally modulated by noradrenergic activity. Although both POHA and POHNE have been implicated in the behavioral effects of chronic administration, tissue content of these amphetamine metabolites during chronic administration is unknown.

In order to elucidate the role of altered amphetamine metabolism and distribution in the previously described changes in amphetamine-induced behaviors that develop during chronic administration, we are currently investigating the effect of such treatment on the distribution of amphetamine, p-hydroxyamphetamine, and p-hydroxynorephedrine in rat tissues. We have measured the tissue content of amphetamine and metabolites in brains and hearts of chronically treated rats after single or multiple doses of amphetamine as well as the effect of chronic amphetamine administration on the uptake of amphetamine into several brain regions.

METHODS

Adult male Sprague-Dawley rats were used in all studies. Because the metabolism of drugs is altered also by age of the experimental animals, stress, and time of day, these variables were controlled rigidly throughout this study. All animals were subjected to identical handling and injection procedures, and all experiments were started between 9:00 a.m. and 10:00 a.m. Two dose regimens were used in this study: animals were injected intraperitoneally for 10 days with 5 mg/kg amphetamine, or with increasing doses, starting with 10 mg/kg, increasing 1 mg/kg/injection up to 32 mg/kg/day. Both of these regimens resulted in marked tolerance to lethality and to some peripheral effects (such as hyperthermia). Potentiation of stereotyped behavior and a more rapid onset of action were also noted in these animals. Control animals were injected on the same schedule with an equivalent volume of saline. Twelve hours after the last injection, animals were injected with ^{3}H-amphetamine intraperitoneally or intracisternally as described previously (Schanberg et al., 1967), killed at various times after injection, and tissues analyzed for amphetamine, POHA, and POHNE. Amphetamine and its metabolites were analyzed by liquid scintillation spectrometry after extraction into ethyl acetate from a deproteinized tissue extract, dansylation, and separation of the dansyl derivative by thin-layer chromatography. When brain regions were assayed for amphetamine alone, regions were dissected as described by Glowinski and Iversen (1966), homogenized in 0.4 N perchloric acid, and assayed by liquid scintillation spectrometry. At the time points tested in these studies, we found that more than 98% of the total radioactivity in brain is unchanged amphetamine. Therefore, the contribution of hydroxylated metabolites to the total radioactivity was not measured. Data was analyzed with Student's t test.

RESULTS AND DISCUSSION

Effect of Chronic Amphetamine Administration on Tissue

Amphetamine and Metabolite Content. The development of tolerance to many drugs after chronic administration results from induction of microsomal drug metabolizing enzymes and a subsequent increase in the production of inactive metabolites and decrease in the half life of the parent drug in tissue (Conney, 1967). To evaluate the effect of chronic amphetamine administration on the half-life of amphetamine and its metabolites in tissues after a single dose of amphetamine, brain and heart ^{3}H-amphetamine and metabolite content was measured 1, 4, and 12 hours after administration of a single dose of ^{3}H-amphetamine (5 mg/kg) to animals injected for 10 days with saline or with amphetamine (5 mg/kg, b.i.d.). The data obtained from animals injected with this dose regimen are shown in Table 1. The concentration of ^{3}H-amphetamine in brain and heart tissue of animals treated for 10 days with amphetamine was not significantly different from that observed in control animals at 1, 4, or 12 hours. POHA and POHNE levels also were not significantly different from levels observed in control animals. Similar results were obtained when animals were treated with the high dose regimen. Also, brain and heart content of ^{3}H-amphetamine, ^{3}H p-hydroxyamphetamine, and ^{3}H p-hydroxynorephedrine after a single dose of ^{3}H-amphetamine were the same in animals treated for 10 days with either saline or increasing doses of amphetamine.

In most species, both urinary excretion of unchanged amphetamine and metabolism by the liver are rate-controlling factors in the removal of amphetamine from the body (Baggot and Davis, 1972; Beckett and Tucker, 1968). The fact that neither amphetamine nor POHA content of tissues from 1 to 12 hours after amphetamine administration was affected by repeated exposure of animals to high doses of amphetamine suggests that both processes are resistant to alteration. These findings corroborate the earlier report of Lewander (1971a), who found that the ratio of unchanged amphetamine to hydroxylated metabolites in urine was not affected significantly by chronic treatment of rats with amphetamine. It is well recognized that the hydroxylation of amphetamine by the liver is in some ways different from the well-characterized systems that hydroxylate many aromatic amines. Isolated microsomal systems that actively hydroxylate other compounds metabolize amphetamine slowly (Rommelspacher, 1974), and pretreatment of rats with known inducers of these systems, such as phenobarbital and 3-methylcholanthrene, fails to accelerate the disappearance of amphetamine *in vivo* (Groppetti and Costa, 1969b). Our results support the hypothesis that the amphetamine-hydroxylating system differs from the other drug-hydroxylating systems also in its resistance to induction following

TABLE 1

Effect of chronic amphetamine administration on tissue content of ^{3}H-amphetamine and metabolites after a single dose

	Amphetamine		p-Hydroxyamphetamine		p-Hydroxynorephedrine	
	Acute	Chronic	Acute	Chronic	Acute	Chronic
Brain						
1 hr	44.9 ± .35	40.31 ± 5.37	.29 ± .05	.33 ± .09	.09 ±.01	.09 ± .01
4 hr	7.36 ± .62	7.7 ± .82	.22 ± .04	.20 ± .04	.20 ±.04	.24 ± .03
12 hr	2.21 ± .34	2.0 ± .21	not detected		.14 ±.02	.17 ± .04
Heart						
1 hr	19.6 ± 3.23	11.0 ± 2.61	.47 ± .06	.62 ± .05	.35 ±.06	.49 ± .09
4 hr	5.10 ± 1.07	6.4 ± 0.53	.18 ± .01	.24 ± .03	.60 ±.09	.74 ± .08
12 hr	1.42 ± 0.44	1.5 ± 0.30	not detected		1.13 ±.06	1.70 ± .10

Animals received 5 mg/kg ^{3}H-amphetamine (15 μCi).
Each value represents mean ± S.E.M. N = 6.

chronic administration of substrate. However, the possibility that enzyme synthesis is increased, but balanced by some unknown inhibitory process that limits enzyme activity, cannot be eliminated on the basis of this study. There was one exception to the general finding that chronic amphetamine administration did not change the distribution of amphetamine, POHA, or POHNE in tissues after a single dose of amphetamine. Heart POHNE content 12 hours after amphetamine was significantly lower than control values in animals treated with the higher dose regimen. This finding suggests either that the systems required for the synthesis of POHNE are depressed after chronic amphetamine administration or that POHNE disappears more rapidly from tissues of chronically treated animals. There are several reports that indicate that depression of the synthesizing machinery is not involved. The amount of dopamine-beta-hydroxylase in tissue is increased by chronic administration of amphetamine (Lau and Slotkin, in press; Kuhn, unpublished data). In addition, the uptake of amines (i.e., precursor POHA) across the neuronal membrane is actually facilitated in chronically treated animals (Cook and Schanberg, 1975). Because tissue POHNE 12 hours after administration of amphetamine probably represents stored rather than newly synthesized POHNE, accelerated removal of stored POHNE may be responsible for the observed depression in metabolite content at this time point. Removal could be accelerated by several processes, including increased neuronal input, saturation of available binding sites, and displacement of POHNE by amphetamine. The failure of brain POHNE to parallel the changes in heart indicates that brain and heart differ as to the mechanisms involved in the control of POHNE formation and disappearance. It is well known that access of POHA to brain tissue is limited because this compound crosses the blood-brain barrier with difficulty (Lewander, 1971a) and changes may be masked by the limited availability of precursor POHA.

In summary, the half-life of amphetamine and its metabolites in brain and heart after a single dose of amphetamine is not affected significantly by chronic treatment with amphetamine. These findings suggest that decrease in the half-life of amphetamine in tissues does not explain the development of tolerance to amphetamine.

Effects of Chronic Amphetamine Administration on the Uptake of Amphetamine into Brain Regions After Intracisternal Administration

The peak behavioral response of amphetamine in rats occurs between 30 minutes and 1 hour after administration (Randrup and Munkvad, 1967; Creese and Iversen, 1974), and potentiation of the behavioral response to amphetamine during this time period has been observed in chronically treated animals (Rech et al., 1975; Segal, 1975; Kilbey and Ellinwood, 1976). Tissue amphetamine levels during this time period reflect the rate of absorption from the injection site, uptake into tissues, and the rate of removal. In the previous section, we demonstrated that the rate of amphetamine removal from tissues is not altered by chronic treatment. Since more rapid uptake of amphetamine into its site of action could explain the behavioral findings, we next investigated the effect of chronic amphetamine administration on the uptake of amphetamine into several brain regions. The uptake of ^{3}H-amphetamine into the pons-medulla, cerebellum, hypothalamus, midbrain, hippocampus, corpus striatum, and cerebral cortex were studied by measuring brain region content of ^{3}H-amphetamine 10 minutes after intracisternal administration of a tracer dose. At this time, brain content of drug should reflect the rate of uptake into brain tissue. The results are shown in Table 2. Tissue content of amphetamine in the pons-medulla alone of animals treated with increasing doses of amphetamine was significantly higher than control animals. These data suggest that chronic amphetamine administration causes a specific neurochemical change in the pons-medulla that does not occur elsewhere in the brain. It is interesting to note that chronic electrical stimulation of the brain or chronic administration of methamphetamine results in facilitation of ^{3}H-norepinephrine uptake into this brain region (but not other regions) after intraventricular or intracisternal administration (Thierry et al., 1968; Cook and Schanberg, 1975). Two explanations for the latter finding have been proposed (Cook and Schanberg, 1975): 1) It is possible that uptake into noradrenergic cell bodies is enhanced by these treatments. Since these cell bodies are located almost exclusively in the lower brain stem (Hillarp et al., 1966), uptake into other brain regions would not be affected, and 2) Uptake into the noradrenergic nerve terminals of the pons-medulla could be affected preferentially. If enhanced uptake resulted from increased accumulation of norepinephrine into all noradrenergic nerve terminals, uptake would be enhanced in other regions containing a high density of terminals, such as hypothalamus or midbrain. Transport of amphetamine into noradrenergic neurons by the norepinephrine uptake system which is enhanced after chronic methamphetamine administration has been demonstrated (Azarro, Ziance, and Rutledge, 1973). Therefore, the enhanced uptake of amphetamine observed in these studies could result from an increase in the uptake of amphetamine into the small, localized pool of amphetamine sequestered in the noradrenergic nerve terminals and/or cell bodies of the pons-medulla. However, intense stimulation of a group of neurons results in enhanced uptake of many compounds (such as amino acids, glucose, etc.), and the enhanced uptake of amphetamine could result also from chronic stimulation of a specific neuronal pool within the pons-medulla by amphetamine. In order to distinguish between these two possibilities, we plan to study the effect of chronic amphetamine administration on the uptake of several compounds, including amino acids and passively distributed agents such as urea. It should be mentioned that enhanced uptake into the pons-medulla cannot be attributed to the

TABLE 2

Effect of chronic amphetamine administration on the uptake of ^{3}H-amphetamine into brain regions after intracisternal administration

Brain Region	% Control	
Cerebellum	104 ± 11	N.S.
Pons-Medulla	143 ± 11	P<.02
Hypothalamus	129 ± 17	N.S.
Hippocampus	97 ± 4	N.S.
Mid-Brain	88 ± 12	N.S.
Striatum	124 ± 11	N.S.
Cortex	95 ± 11	N.S.

Animals received 5 μCi ^{3}H-amphetamine (S.A. 7.76 Ci/mm). Each value represents Mean ± S.E.M. N = 12.

high concentration of amphetamine to which this brain region is exposed after intracisternal administration. If this were the case, enhanced uptake would be observed also in the cerebellum, which contains even higher concentration of amphetamine than the pons-medulla after intracisternal administration of passively distributed agents such as urea.

Effect of Chronic Amphetamine Administration on the Uptake of Amphetamine into Brain Regions After Intraperitoneal Administration

The findings reported above seem to correlate well with the behavioral observation that the onset of amphetamine-induced stereotypies and increased locomotor activity is faster in chronically treated animals. However, these behavioral observations were made in animals that had received amphetamine intraperitoneally. Uptake into brain after this route of administration is subject to many variables that do not affect uptake after intracisternal administration. For a more relevant comparison of biochemical and behavioral data, it was necessary to study the uptake of amphetamine into brain regions after intraperitoneal administration. Rats treated chronically with increasing doses of amphetamine or saline were sacrificed 30 minutes after an intraperitoneal injection of amphetamine (5 mg/kg), and amphetamine content was assayed in various brain regions (Table 3). In contrast to the findings after intracisternal administration, uptake into all brain regions was enhanced in the chronically treated animals.

This increase could result from an increase in the amount of drug being delivered to brain. The disappearance of body fat after chronic amphetamine administration could contribute to such an effect because this tissue represents a significant reservoir for amphetamine. In addition, as a large percent of each amphetamine dose is metabolized on the first pass through the liver, a slight decrease in the rate of metabolism could increase the amount of amphetamine available for uptake into tissues. However, if either of these mechanisms were responsible for the observed changes, tissue levels would be increased at all time points, assuming amphetamine is distributed in a single pool in brain. Since amphetamine levels were not elevated from 1 to 12 hours post-administration (unpublished data), these findings suggest that tissue amphetamine distribution in chronically treated animals cannot be fitted to the simple kinetic model of first order absorption and first order elimination which describes its distribution after acute administration. An alternative explanation is that amphetamine is distributed in several pools in brain, including one with a very short half-life that is preferentially affected by chronic administration. The finding that

TABLE 3

Effect of chronic amphetamine administration on the uptake of ^{3}H-amphetamine after intraperitoneal administration

Brain Region	% Control	
Cerebellum	133 ± 9	P<.01
Pons-Medulla	146 ± 7	P<.01
Hypothalamus	131 ± 9	P<.01
Hippocampus	151 ± 7	P<.001
Mid-Brain	144 ± 6	P<.001
Striatum	161 ± 5	P<.001
Cortex	136 ± 4	P<.002

Animals received 5 mg/kg ^{3}H-amphetamine (15 μCi). Each value represents Mean ± S.E.M. N = 12.

amphetamine content of pons-medulla is enhanced in chronically treated animals 10 minutes after intracisternal administration, when tissue content reflects amphetamine concentration in a pool with a half life of 6 minutes, supports this hypothesis. However, since uptake into all brain regions after intraperitoneal administration is enhanced after chronic administration, some other mechanisms must also be involved.

Accumulation of Amphetamine and p-Hydroxynorephedrine in Tissues During Multiple Doses of Amphetamine

Because measurable amounts of both POHNE and amphetamine remain in tissue for at least 12 hours, both could accumulate with the chronic dose regimen used by most investigators (injections made twice daily at 12 hour intervals). In order to investigate this possibility, animals were injected 6 times with ^{3}H-amphetamine (5 mg/kg) at 12 hour intervals, and brain and heart amphetamine and p-hydroxynorephedrine contents were measured 12 hours after the last injection. Marked accumulation of both compounds occurred during the three day treatment (Table 4): ^{3}H-amphetamine and ^{3}H POHNE levels in brain and heart of animals treated with multiple doses were between 150-200% of those found in animals that had received a single dose of ^{3}H-amphetamine 12 hours before sacrifice. POHA still could not be detected in either tissue, suggesting that accumulation of this metabolite does not occur during chronic administration. The expected rate of accumulation calculated on the basis of the half lives reported above was greater than the amount actually observed. Similar results have been reported by other investigators, who found that the POHNE formed from a single dose of amphetamine is released by a second dose (Thoenen, Hurlimann, Gey, and Haefely, 1966; Lewander, 1971b). Although these investigators reported that heart POHNE was released more readily than brain POHNE, we found equal accumulation in both tissues. Since heart tissue synthesizes more POHNE (see above), possibly a faster rate of synthesis compensates for the greater release. The accumulation of amphetamine in brain and heart is similar to that reported by Lewander (1974). He found that the brain of animals treated with 40 mg/kg/day accumulated amphetamine up to 150% of the initial levels, and then maintained this level for the 2 weeks of chronic administration. However, the site of amphetamine accumulation cannot be detected by measuring whole tissue levels of drug, and our findings of enhanced uptake into a specific brain region indicate that further investigation of the site of amphetamine accumulation is vital to an understanding of the role of altered amphetamine distribution in chronic amphetamine effects.

TABLE 4

Accumulation of ^{3}H-amphetamine and ^{3}H p-hydroxynorephedrine in brain and heart after a single or multiple doses of ^{3}H-amphetamine

	Acute	Chronic	% Control	
Amphetamine				
Brain	1.4 ± .1	2.0 ± .1	143	P<.001
Heart	1.8 ± .4	3.2 ± .4	177	P<.02
p-Hydroxynorephedrine				
Brain	.289 ± .029	.609 ± .105	210	P<.01
Heart	.864 ± .112	1.320 ± .130	153	P<.01

Animals were injected at 12 hour intervals. Controls received 5 doses of saline followed by 1 dose of ^{3}H-amphetamine (5 mg/kg, 15 μCi). Experimental animals received 6 doses of ^{3}H-amphetamine. The last dose was given 12 hours before sacrifice. Each value represents Mean ± S.E.M. N = 6.

In summary, we have found several specific changes in the distribution of amphetamine and its metabolites that may play a significant role in the behavioral phenomena associated with chronic amphetamine intoxication. Chronic amphetamine administration is not associated with increased rate of removal from tissue or with increased production of hydroxylated metabolites. In this respect, the metabolism of amphetamine is quite unlike that of many other psychoactive drugs. In fact, the observed changes in amphetamine distribution and metabolism are correlated more with the development of supersensitivity to amphetamine than with the development of tolerance. Brain and heart levels of amphetamine at the time of peak behavioral activation actually are higher in chronically treated animals than in controls. Furthermore, amphetamine accumulates in tissues during chronic administration, forming an endogenous "pool" which could eventually disrupt cellular functions that are not affected by a single dose of amphetamine. The pseudotransmitter p-hydroxynorephedrine also accumulates during chronic amphetamine administration. However, the relationship of this accumulation to the development of tolerance to norepinephrine-mediated effects is not convincing since significant accumulation occurs before the development of measurable tolerance. These studies further emphasize the complex relationship between the distribution of amphetamine and its hydroxylated metabolites and its physiological and behavioral effects.

ACKNOWLEDGMENTS

This research was supported by a grant from the National Institute of Mental Health #MH 13688. Saul M. Schanberg is the recipient of a Research Scientist Development Award, K 5 MH 06489, from the National Institute of Mental Health.

REFERENCES

Azarro, A.J., Ziance, R.J., and Rutledge, C.O.: The importance of neuronal uptake of amines for amphetamine-induced release of ^{3}H norepinephrine from isolated brain tissue, J. Pharmac. exp. Ther. 189, 110-118 (1973).

Baggot, J.D. and Davis, L.E.: Pharmacokinetic study of amphetamine elimination in dogs and swine, Biochem. Pharm. 21, 1967-1976 (1972).

Beckett, A.H. and Tucker, G.T.: Application of the analogue computer to pharmacokinetic and biopharmaceutical studies with amphetamine-type compounds, J. Pharm. Pharmac. 20, 174-193 (1968).

Brodie, B.B., Cho, A.K., Stefano, F.J., and Gessa, G.L.: On the mechanisms of norepinephrine release by amphetamine and tyramine and tolerance to their effects. In: Advances in Biochemical Psychopharmacology. Costa, E. and Greengard, P., Eds., Vol. I, pp. 219-238. New York: Raven Press, 1970a.

Brodie, B.B., Cho, A.K., and Gessa, G.L.: Possible role of p-hydroxynorephedrine in the depletion of norepinephrine induced by d-amphetamine and in tolerance to this drug. In: Amphetamines and Related Compounds. Costa, E. and Garrattini, S., Eds., pp. 217-230. New York: Raven Press, 1970b.

Conney, A.H.: Pharmacological implications of microsomal enzyme induction, Pharm. Rev. 19, 317-366 (1967).

Cook, J. and Schanberg, S.M.: Effect of methamphetamine on norepinephrine metabolism in various regions of brain, J. Pharmac. exp. Ther. 194, 87-93 (1975).

Creese, I. and Iversen, S.D.: The role of forebrain dopamine systems in amphetamine induced stereotyped behavior in the rat, Psychopharmacologia 39, 345-357 (1974).

Dring, L.G., Smith, R.W., and Williams, R.T.: The metabolic fate of amphetamine in man and other species, Biochem. J. 116, 425-435 (1970).

Ellinwood, E.H., Sudilovsky, A., and Nelson, L.: Behavioral analysis of chronic amphetamine intoxication, Biol. Psychiat. 4, 215-230 (1972).

Ellinwood, E.H.: Effect of chronic methamphetamine intoxication in rhesus monkeys, Biol. Psychiat. 3, 25-32 (1971).

Ellison, T., Okun, R., Silverman, A., and Siegel, M.: Metabolic fate of amphetamine in the cat during development of tolerance, Arch. Int. Pharmacodyn. 190, 135-149 (1971).

Glowinski, J. and Iversen, L.L.: Regional studies of catecholamines in brain. I. Disposition of ^{3}H norepinephrine, ^{3}H dopamine and ^{3}H dopa, J. Neurochem. 13, 655-669 (1966).

Goetz, C. and Klawans, H.L.: Studies on the interaction of reserpine, d-amphetamine, apomorphine and 5-hydroxytryptophan, Acta Pharmac. Tox. 34, 119-130 (1974).

Goldstine, M. and Anagnoste, B.: The conversion *in vivo* of d-amphetamine to p-hydroxynorephedrine, Biochem. Biophys. Acta 107, 166-168 (1965).

Groppetti, A. and Costa, E.: Factors affecting the rate of disappearance of amphetamine in rats, Int. J. Neuropharm. 8, 209-215 (1969a).

Groppetti, A. and Costa, E.: Tissue concentrations of p-hydroxynorephedrine in rats injected with d-amphetamine: effect of pretreatment with desipramine, Life Sci. 8, 653-665 (1969b).

Hillarp, N., Fuxe, K., and Dahlstrom,A.: Demonstration and mapping of central neurons containing noradrenaline, 5 OH-tryptamine and their reactions to psychopharmaca, Pharmac. Rev. 18, 727-741 (1966).

Hollister, A.L., Breese, G.R., and Cooper, B.R.: Comparison of tyrosine hydroxylase and dopamine-β-hydroxylase inhibition with the effects of various 6-hydroxydopamine treatments on d-amphetamine induced motor activity, Psychopharmacologia 36, 1-16 (1974).

Kilbey, M.M. and Ellinwood, E.H.: Chronic administration of stimulant drugs: Response modification. In: Cocaine and Other Stimulants. Ellinwood, E.H. and Kilbey, M.M., Eds. New York: Plenum Press, 1976.

Koda, L.Y. and Gibb, J.W.: Adrenal and striatal tyrosine hydroxylase activity after methamphetamine, J. Pharmac. exp. Ther. 185, 42-48 (1973).

Kosman, M.E. and Unna, K.R.: Effects of chronic administration of amphetamines and other stimulants on behavior, Clin. Pharmac. Ther. 9, 240-254 (1968).

Lal, S., Missala, K., Sourkes, T.L., and Feldmuller, F.: The effect of certain drugs on amphetamine-induced stereotyped behavior and brain amphetamine levels in the rat, Biol. Psychiat. 9, 3-10 (1974).

Lau, C. and Slotkin, T.: Indirect and direct inhibition of dopamine β-hydroxylase by amphetamine in storage vesicles and synaptosomes, Br. J. Pharmac. (in press).

Lewander, T.A.: Displacement of brain and heart noradrenaline by p-hydroxynorephedrine after administration of p-hydroxyamphetamine, Acta Pharmac.Tox. 29, 20-32 (1971a).

Lewander, T.A.: A mechanism for the development of tolerance to amphetamine in rats, Psychopharmacologia 21, 17-31 (1971b).

Lewander, T.: Effect of chronic treatment with central stimulants on brain monoamines and some behavioural and physiological functions in rats, guinea pigs, and rabbits. In: Neuropsychopharmacology of Monoamines and their Regulatory Enzymes. Usdin, E., Ed., pp. 221-239. New York: Raven Press, 1974.

Magour, S., Coper, H., and Fahndrich, C.H.: Effect of chronic intoxication with amphetamine on its concentration in liver and brain and on ^{14}C leucine incorporation into microsomal and cytophasmic proteins of rat liver. J. Pharm. Pharmac. 26, 105-108 (1974).

Mandell, A.J. and Morgan, M.: Amphetamine-induced increase in tyrosine hydroxylase activity. Nature 227, 75-76 (1970).

Randrup, A. and Munkvad, I.: Stereotyped activities produced by amphetamine in several animal species and man. Psychopharmacologia 11, 300-310 (1967).

Rech, R.H., Tilson, H.A., and Marquis, W.J.: Adaptive changes in behavior after repeated administration of various psychoactive drugs. In: Advances in Biochemical Psychopharmacology. Mandell, A.J., Ed., Vol. 13, pp. 263-286. New York: Raven Press, 1975.

Rommelspacher, H.: The hydroxylation of d-amphetamine by liver microsomes of the male rat. Biochem. Pharm. 23, 1065-1071 (1974).

Schanberg, S.M., Schildkraut, J.J. and Kopin, I.J.: The effects of pentobarbital on the fate of intracisternally administered norepinephrine ^{3}H. J. Pharmac. exp. Ther. 157, 34-38 (1967).

Segal, D.S.: Behavioral and neurochemical correlates of repeated d-amphetamine administration. In: Advances in Biochemical Psychopharmacology. Mandell, A.J., Ed., Vol. 13, pp. 247-262. New York: Raven Press, 1975.

Sparber, S.B. and Tilson, H.A.: The releasability of central norepinephrine and serotonin by peripherally administered d-amphetamine before and after tolerance. Life Sci. 11, 1059-1067 (1972).

Sulser, F., Owens, M.L., and Dingell, J.V.: On the mechanism of amphetamine potentiation by desipramine. Life Sci. 5, 2005-2010 (1966).

Taylor, W.A. and Sulser, F.: Effects of amphetamine and its hydroxylated metabolites on central noradrenergic mechanisms. J. Pharmac. exp. Ther. 185, 620-632 (1973).

Thierry, A., Javoy, F., Glowinski, S., and Kety, S.: Effects of stress on the metabolism of norepinephrine, dopamine and serotonin in the central nervous system of the rat. I. Modifications of norepinephrine turnover. J. Pharmac. exp. Ther. 163, 163-171 (1968).

Thoenen, H., Hurlimann, A., Gey, K.F., and Haefely, W.: Liberation of p-hydroxynorephedrine from cat spleen by sympathetic nerve stimulation after pretreatment with amphetamine. Life Sci. 5, 1715-1722 (1966).

Trendelenburg, U.: Classification of sympathomimetic amines. In: Handbook of Experimental Pharmacology. Blaschko, H. and Muscholl, E., Eds., Berlin: Springer-Verlag 1972.

CHANGES IN BRAIN CATECHOLAMINES INDUCED BY LONG-TERM METHAMPHETAMINE ADMINISTRATION IN RHESUS MONKEYS

Lewis S. Seiden, Marian W. Fischman, and Charles R. Schuster

Department of Pharmacological and Physiological Sciences

The University of Chicago, Chicago, Illinois 60637

d-Amphetamine, methamphetamine and related psychomotor stimulants cause a decrease in food intake, increased locomotor activity and stereotypy, and disruption of behavior that is under schedule control. The dose required to produce different effects varies and depends on the nature of the behavior and the conditions under which the drug is administered. Repeated administration of amphetamine and related compounds leads to tolerance of many of its effects on behavior although the degree of tolerance depends on the frequency of administrations, the dose and the behavior examined.

Several investigators (Carlsson, 1970; Moore, Carr, and Dominic, 1970; Chieuh and Moore, 1974) have presented evidence that amphetamines increase the concentration of catecholamines at the synaptic cleft by promoting release or blocking reuptake. There is also a considerable amount of evidence to suggest that the behavioral effects of amphetamine and related drugs are mediated by their catecholamine-releasing actions (Randrup and Munkvad, 1968; Scheel-Krüger, 1971; Creese and Iverson, 1973; Rech and Stolk, 1970; Wise and Stein, 1970; Moore, 1963, 1964). Since the pharmacological action of the amphetamines is believed to be mediated by a catecholaminergic mechanism, the question arises as to what, if any, alterations occur in catecholaminergic function as a result of long term administration of amphetamines.

The overall purpose of this investigation was to determine the effect of long-term repeated intravenous administration of methamphetamine in increasing doses to rhesus monkeys. Measures were made on behavior, neuropathology and brain catecholamines. In this paper we shall report both short- and long-term changes in brain catecholamines that were caused by prolonged administration of methamphetamine. It was found that methamphetamine induced changes in regional brain catecholamines, some of which persisted even after the drug was discontinued.

Rhesus monkeys were injected intravenously 8 times daily. The dose of methamphetamine was increased until a final dose was reached which could be tolerated by the particular monkey involved. Tolerance to a particular dose was determined through observing diminished food intake and weight loss. Doses were incremented only when signs of behavioral tolerance appeared.

Two studies were carried out: in the first, monkeys were treated for 3-6 months (final dose 3.0-6.5 mg/kg/inj) eight times per day. Monkeys were either killed 24 hours or 3-6 months after the last injection. In the second study, monkeys were treated with methamphetamine for a period of two weeks (final dose 2-3 mg/kg/inj) eight times per day. These monkeys were killed either 24 hours or two weeks after the last methamphetamine injection.

On the final day of the experiment the monkeys were anesthetized with pentobarbital and killed by exsanguination after severing the ascending carotid arteries. The brain was rapidly removed (3 mins) and taken into a cold room (4° C) where it was dissected and frozen in liquid nitrogen until assay. Norepinephrine (NE) was assayed by the method of Bertler, Carlsson, and Rosengren (1958) and dopamine (DA) was assayed by the method of Carlsson and Waldeck (1958).

Monkeys killed after 3-6 months of continued daily methamphetamine administration exhibited fairly uniform depletion of NE in all brain areas 24 hours after the last methamphetamine injection. These data show the brain areas affected included the pons-medulla, the midbrain, the hypothalamus and frontal cortex. A 24 hour post injection depletion of NE is consistent with the view that methamphetamine causes blockade of reuptake and/or direct release of norepinephrine from nerve terminals. In the monkeys that were killed 3-6 months after the last methamphetamine injection, the levels of NE remained decreased in the midbrain and frontal cortex, but returned to normal in the pons-medulla and the hypothalamus. The monkeys treated with methamphetamine for a two week period showed decreased NE levels 24 hours after the last injection in each area except the hypothalamus, but there appears to be a trend to return to normal values two weeks after methamphetamine treatment (see Table 1). However, the N is not large enough for statistical testing.

The most striking change occurred in dopamine in the caudate

TABLE 1

NE - 8 INJECTIONS OF METHAMPHETAMINE DAILY FOR SEVERAL MONTHS

Treatment	Pons-Medulla	Mid-Brain	Hypothalamus	Frontal Cortex
Control N=12	0.45 ± 0.04	0.59 ± 0.03	1.8 ± 0.26	0.21 ± 0.03
Chronic meth 24 hr post meth N=5	0.23 ± 0.07 (51%) $p < 0.05$	0.40 ± 0.06 (67%) $p < 0.05$	0.76 ± 0.18 (42%) $p < 0.05$	0.08 ± 0.23 (38%) $p < 0.05$
Chronic meth 3-6 months post meth N=6	0.31 ± 0.08	0.39 ± 0.07 (66%) $p < 0.05$	1.4 ± 0.43	0.10 ± 0.01 (48%) $p < 0.05$

NE - 8 INJECTIONS OF METHAMPHETAMINE FOR A PERIOD OF TWO WEEKS

Treatment	Pons-Medulla	Mid-Brain	Hypothalamus	Frontal Cortex
Chronic meth 24 hr post meth N=3	0.21 ± 0.11 (48%)	0.41 ± 0.12 (69%)	1.77 ± 0.23 (98%)	0.12 ± 0.04 (57%)
Chronic meth 2 weeks post meth N=3	0.40 ± 0.01 (88%)	0.48 ± 0.02 (81%)	1.4 ± 0.34 (77%)	0.11 ± 0.01 (52%)

TABLE 2

DA - 8 INJECTIONS OF METHAMPHETAMINE DAILY FOR SEVERAL MONTHS

Treatment	Pons-Medulla	Mid-Brain	Hypothalamus	Caudate	Frontal Cortex
Control N=12	0.16 ± 0.01	0.51 ± 0.04	0.83 ± 0.12	10.1 ± 0.57	0.09 ± 0.01
Chronic meth 3-6 months meth N=5	0.51 ± 0.20 ns	0.61 ± 0.11 ns	1.33 ± 0.30 ns	2.0 ± 1.0 (19%) $p < 0.001$	0.19 ± 0.04 ns
Chronic meth 3-6 months post meth N=6	0.13 ± 0.03 ns	0.33 ± 0.07 ns	0.82 ± 0.17 ns	3.15 ± 0.64 (31%) $p < 0.001$	0.13 ± 0.05 ns

DA - 8 INJECTIONS OF METHAMPHETAMINE FOR A PERIOD OF TWO WEEKS

Treatment	Pons-Medulla	Mid-Brain	Hypothalamus	Caudate	Frontal Cortex
Chronic meth 24 hr post meth N=3	0.19 ± 0.01	0.43 ± 0.07	1.14 ± 0.53	3.67 ± 0.50(36%)	0.15 ± 0.02
Chronic meth 2 weeks post meth N=3	0.53 ± 0.08	0.76 ± 0.14	1.20 ± 0.45	2.3 ± 0.37 (23%)	0.30 ± 0.01

nucleus (Table 2). There was approximately 70-80% reduction of caudate dopamine, but other brain areas were unaffected. This depletion occurred in monkeys that were treated for a 3-6 month period and appeared permanent insofar as there was no difference between monkeys that were killed 24 hours after the last injection and monkeys that were killed 3-6 months after the last injection. The same changes in caudate DA were observed in monkeys treated with methamphetamine for only 2 weeks. In both the 24 hour and two week group, dopamine was depleted to a large extent.

Tonge (1974) has reported depletion of norepinephrine and serotonin in rat brain in several brain areas which appears to last for up to 36 hours after chronic oral intake of d-amphetamine. These changes observed by Tonge are consistent with some of the changes we observed in monkeys. Harris and Baldessarini (1973) have demonstrated that amphetamine inhibits tyrosine hydroxylase in the corpus striatum of rat brain but not in other areas. They propose that the inhibition of tyrosine hydroxylase is due to the activation of dopamine receptors in the corpus-striatum but not in other areas, and that the inhibition of tyrosine hydroxylase is due to the activation of dopamine receptors in the corpus striatum by accumulation of DA released by amphetamine; the increase in DA leads to feedback inhibition of DA synthesis. This mechanism can conceivably account for the effects of methamphetamine on DA seen in animals killed 24 hours after the last injection of methamphetamine. It is difficult, however, to explain the prolonged depletion of DA in these terms. One would have to assume that the feedback "tone" changes permanently as a result of prolonged administration of methamphetamine. While this appears unlikely in the absence of structural changes in the caudate, it is a possibility that must be considered.

The monkeys treated daily (8 times/day) on methamphetamine for 3-6 months exhibited tolerance to the disruptive effects of the drug on behavior maintained by a fixed ratio (FR) 10 or a differential reinforcement of low rate (DRL) schedule of food reinforcement (Fischman and Schuster, 1974, 1975). In fact, monkeys responding on the DRL schedule showed an apparently irreversible tolerance to the response suppressant effects of methamphetamine as measured by acute injection of drug 3-6 months after cessation of methamphetamine maintenance (Fischman and Schuster, in preparation). This irreversible effect is correlated with permanent changes in the catecholamine content of certain brain areas. Monkeys treated with methamphetamine for a prolonged period and killed 3-6 months after discontinuing the drug show a 70% loss of caudate DA, a 33% loss of midbrain NE, and a 52% loss of NE in the frontal cortex. The largest effect on brain catecholamines appears to occur in caudate DA with smaller effects occurring in the NE system. Which, if any, of these changes are functionally related to the apparently irreversible behavioral tolerance seen in the same monkeys can only be determined by further research.

ACKNOWLEDGMENTS

This research was supported by Grants USPHS MH-011191-10; USPHS 5-K02 MH10, 562-07; NIMH 2-R01-DA-00085-04; R01-MH-22,971.

This report has been previously published in Drug and Alcohol Dependence 1(3), 215-219 (1976).

REFERENCES

Bertler, A., Carlsson, A., and Rosengren, E.: A method for fluorimetric determination of adrenaline and noradrenaline in tissues, Acta Physiol. Scand. 44, 273-292 (1958).

Carlsson, A. and Waldeck, B.: A fluorimetric method for the determination of dopamine (3-hydroxytyramine), Acta Physiol. Scand. 44, 293-298 (1958).

Carlsson, A.: Amphetamine and brain catecholamines. In: Amphetamines and Related Compounds. Proceedings of the Mario Negri Institute for Pharmacological Research. Costa, E. and Garattini, S., Eds., pp. 289-300. New York: Raven Press, 1970.

Chiueh, C.C. and Moore, K.E.: Effects of alpha-methyltyrosine on d-amphetamine-induced release of endogenously synthesized and exogenously administered catecholamines from the cat brain *in vivo*, J. Pharmacol. exp. Ther. 190, 100-108 (1974).

Creese, I., Iversen, S.D.: Blockage of amphetamine-induced motor stimulation and stereotypy in the adult following neonatal treatment with 6-hydroxydopamine, Brain Res. 55(2), 369-382 (1973).

Fischman, M.W. and Schuster, C.R.: Tolerance development to chronic methamphetamine intoxication in the rhesus monkey, Pharm. Bio. Behav. 2, 503-508 (1974).

Fischman, M.W. and Schuster, C.R.: Behavioral, biochemical and morphological effects of methamphetamine in the rhesus monkey. In: Behavioral Toxicology. Weiss, B. and Laties, V., Eds. New York: Plenum Publishing Corporation, 1975.

Fischman, M.W. and Schuster, C.R.: Long-term behavioral changes in the rhesus monkey after chronic methamphetamine administration, (in preparation).

Harris, E. and Baldessarini, R.: Amphetamine-induced inhibition of tyrosine hydroxylation in homogenates of rat corpus striatum, J. Pharm. Pharmac. 25, 755-757 (1973).

Moore, K.E.: Toxicity and catecholamine releasing actions of d- and l-amphetamine in isolated and aggregated mice, J. Pharmacol. exp. Ther. 142, 6-12 (1963).

Moore, K.E.: The role of endogenous norepinephrine in the toxicity of d-amphetamine in aggregated mice, J. Pharmacol. exp. Ther. 144, 45-51 (1964).

Moore, K.E., Carr, L.A., and Dominic, J.A.: Functional significance of amphetamine-induced release of brain catecholamines. In: Amphetamines and Related Compounds. Proceedings of the Mario Negri Institute for Pharmacological Research. Costa, E. and Garattini, S., Eds., pp. 371-384. New York: Raven Press (1970).

Randrup, A. and Munkvad, I.: Behavioral stereotypes induced by pharmacological agents, Pharmakopsychiatrie Neuro-Psychopharmakologie 1, 18-26 (1968).

Rech, R.H. and Stolk, J.M.: Amphetamine drug interactions that relate brain catecholamines to behavior. In: Amphetamines and Related Compounds. Proceedings of the Mario Negri Institute for Pharmacological Research. Costa, E. and Garattini, S., Eds., pp. 371-384. New York: Raven Press, 1970.

Scheel-Krüger, J.: Some aspects of the mechanism of actions of various stimulant amphetamine analogues, Psychiat. Neurol. Neurochir. 75, 179-192 (1972).

Wise, C.D. and Stein, L.: Amphetamine: the facilitation of behavior by augmented release of norepinephrine from the medial forebrain bundle. In: Amphetamines and Related Compounds. Proceedings of the Mario Negri Institute for Pharmacological Research. Costa, E. and Garattini, S., Eds., pp. 463-485. New York: Raven Press (1970).

Tonge, S.R.: Noradrenaline and 5-hydroxytryptamine metabolism in six areas of rat brain during post-amphetamine depression, Psychopharmacologia (Berl.) 38, 181-186 (1974).

NEUROBIOLOGICAL ANTAGONISM OF COCAINE BY LITHIUM

Arnold J. Mandell and Suzanne Knapp

University of California at San Diego

La Jolla, California 92093

Over the past several years our group has been examining the functional characteristics of the serotonergic biosynthetic system in the brain by subjecting it to a number of challenges including various drugs (Knapp, Mandell, 1972a, 1972b, 1973, 1975, in press; Knapp, Mandell, Geyer, 1974; Knapp, 1975; Knapp, Mandell, Bullard, 1975; Rogawski, Knapp, Mandell, 1974; Geyer, Dawsey, Mandell, 1975a; Geyer, Warbritton, Menkes, Zook, Mandell, 1975b; Geyer, Puerto, Dawsey, Knapp, Bullard, Mandell, in press, a) and environmental manipulations (Segal, Knapp, Kuczenski, Mandell, 1973; Geyer, Puerto, Menkes, Segal, Mandell, in press, b). A group of biochemical measures has evolved which appears to be useful in these explorations. As depicted in Fig. 1, they include: the high affinity uptake of tryptophan into serotonergic synaptosomes; the "amount" of soluble tryptophan hydroxylase activity in cell body and nerve ending regions (median raphe and striate cortex, respectively) after hypotonic lysis of the preparations; and the overall rate of conversion of tryptophan to serotonin (5-HT) by synaptosomes. Our experimental methods have been described in detail elsewhere (Knapp et al., 1974; Knapp, Mandell, 1975). The effects on these measures of cocaine *in vitro* and *in vivo*, alone and in combination with lithium chloride, will be described in this report.

In 1972 we first reported that two narcotic drugs reduced the capacity of striate and septal synaptosomes to convert radioactive tryptophan to 5-HT (Knapp, Mandell, 1972b; Fig. 2). Morphine and cocaine achieved the same effect by different mechanisms. Morphine, in the concentrations indicated, reduced the soluble tryptophan hydroxylase activity, but did not affect synaptosomal uptake of radioactive tryptophan. Cocaine, on the other hand, did not affect the soluble enzyme activity, but did inhibit the high affinity uptake of tryptophan (K_m = 10 μM) as drug concentrations increased. Recently, Friedman, Gershon, and Rotrosen (1975), using a measure of the synthesis of 5-HT in whole rat brain, reported that cocaine reduced the rate of 5-HT turnover, thus confirming our report of the *in vitro* effects of cocaine on striate synaptosomal conversion.

As a concomitant of the cocaine-induced reductions in the uptake of tryptophan and its conversion to 5-HT, the soluble tryptophan hydroxylase activity from cell body regions was augmented, which is consistent with our model of adaptive regulation in the synthesis of biogenic amines in brain (Mandell, 1975).

We have begun to re-examine these phenomena with *in vivo* studies. Figure 3 shows that, one hour after the administration of a large dose of cocaine hydrochloride (100 mg/kg), there was a reduction in the conversion of tryptophan to 5-HT by striate synaptosomes and a compensatory increase in nerve ending soluble tryptophan hydroxylase activity. Note that, at least as far as these *in vivo* experiments were concerned, cocaine administration had no effect on 5-HT reuptake. Thus, cocaine inhibits the high affinity uptake of radioactive tryptophan, reduces the conversion of radioactive tryptophan to 5-HT, and leads to a compensatory increase in intraneuronal soluble

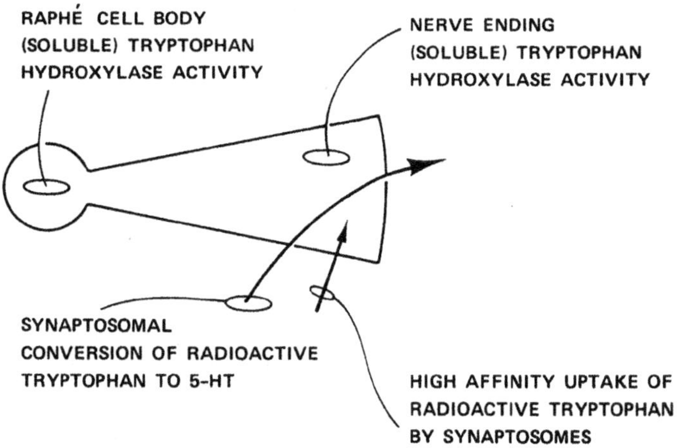

Fig. 1. Four measures used to assess the activity of the 5-HT neuronal system. Soluble tryptophan hydroxylase measures require the addition of an artificial pteridine cofactor, dithiothreitol, and exogenous aromatic-L-amino acid decarboxylase, while the measurement of synaptosomal conversion of tryptophan to 5-HT does not (Ichiyama, Nakamura, Nishizuka, Hayaishi, 1968, 1970; Knapp, Mandell, 1975).

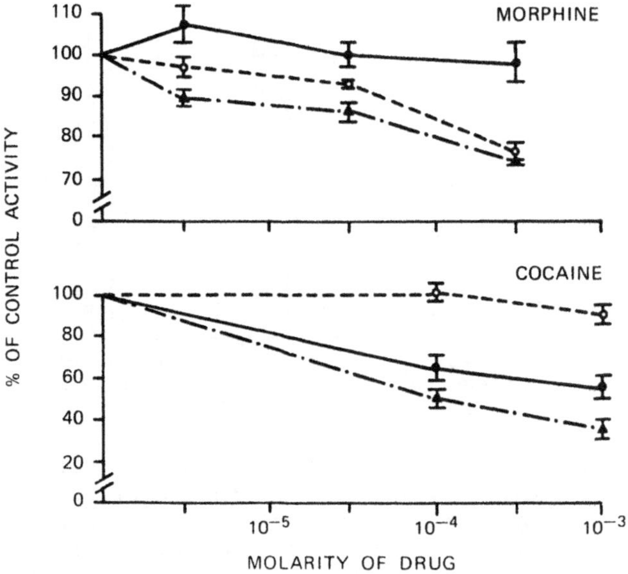

Fig. 2. *In vitro* effects of morphine and cocaine on uptake of tryptophan by septal synaptosomes (—•—), midbrain soluble tryptophan hydroxylase (—o—), and synaptosomal conversion of tryptophan to 5-HT (·—▲·—). Control velocities: uptake, 450-500 pmol/mg/10 min; soluble enzyme, 100 pmol/mg/hr; conversion, 125 pmol/mg/45 min. Enzyme and conversion activities were reduced by morphine; substrate uptake and conversion were reduced by cocaine ($p < 0.05$).

tryptophan hydroxylase. This sequence of effects has two other interesting features: brief duration and anatomical specificity in the raphe system.

Figure 4 demonstrates the anatomical specificity. The area we call medial midbrain contained the dorsal and median nuclei of the median raphe, which are also known as the B7 and B8 nuclear groups (Dahlstrom, Fuxe, 1964). The area we call lateral midbrain contained the cells of the B9 nuclear groups. Enzyme activity was determined in both regions using an homogenization medium that leaves the synaptosomes intact (0.32 M sucrose) and one that lyses them (1.0 mM Tris buffer). Note that the compensatory increase in tryptophan hydroxylase activity in these serotonergic cell body regions was seen only in the area encompassing B9. This specificity is identical to that we reported earlier with amphetamine treatment (Knapp et al., 1974). Others have reported the same specificity with parachloroamphetamine (Harvey, McMaster, Yunger, 1975). The specificity could not be due

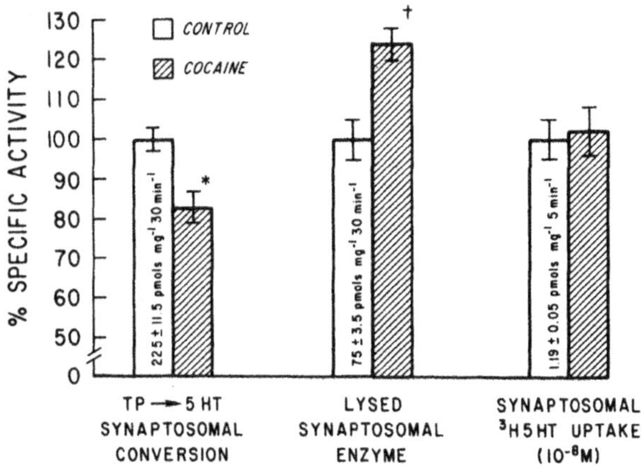

Fig. 3. Effects of cocaine administered one hour before sacrifice on striate synaptosomal tryptophan-to-5-HT conversion, intrasynaptosomal tryptophan hydroxylase activity, and synaptosomal uptake of ^{3}H-5-HT, graphed as percentages of the control specific activities shown in the white bars. Substrate concentration was 10 μM for enzyme assays; 0.08 μM for uptake determination. Cocaine significantly reduced conversion activity and significantly increased soluble enzyme activity (*$p < 0.001$; †$p < 0.032$).

simply to the drug's acting on short-axoned nerve endings because the anatomical differentiation was seen with both intact and lysed nerve endings. Thus, the B9 region appears uniquely implicated in the changes we have seen in the striate. Fuxe and Jonsson (1967) have demonstrated, using histofluorescence staining techniques, that the B9 cells project to the striate cortex in the rat.

Figure 5 demonstrates again this interesting anatomical specificity for the lateral midbrain of the compensatory increase in tryptophan hydroxylase activity. In addition, it shows the remarkable speed of the effect, which reached a peak in one hour and returned to control levels by two hours. The amphetamine-induced effects that we reported (Knapp et al., 1974) occurred with like rapidity, but took several hours more to subside. Of all the drugs studied with our multiple measures of the serotonergic biosynthetic system, cocaine produced the quickest and briefest effect. Before presenting our data on the effects of the interaction between lithium and cocaine on this system, we shall reiterate briefly the effects of lithium alone.

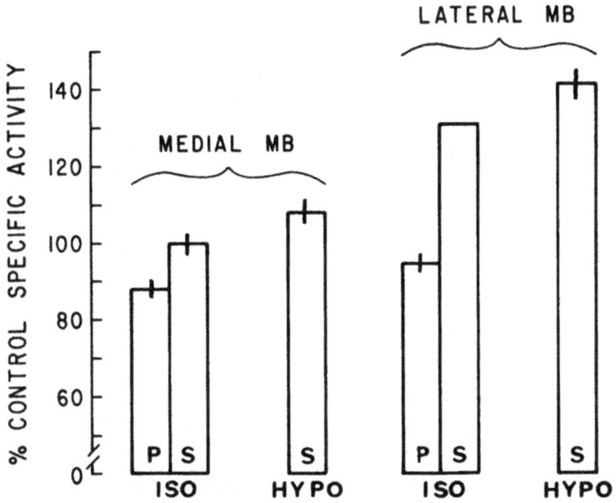

Fig. 4. Cocaine-induced effects one-half hour after injection on medial and lateral midbrain (MB) tryptophan hydroxylase prepared by isotonic homogenization in 0.32 M sucrose and centrifugation at 12,000 _g_ (which keeps synaptosomes intact) and by hypotonic homogenization in 1.0 mM Tris buffer (pH 7.4) and centrifugation at 35,000 _g_ (which destroys synaptosomal integrity). Data are presented as mean (N=6) percentages of corresponding control activities from saline-treated animals. Of the isotonic preparations from medial MB, control activity in pellet (P) was 139 ± 5 pmol/mg/30 min; in supernate (S), 750 ± 25.2. Of the isotonic preparations from lateral MB, control activity in pellet (P) was 51.5 ± 3.0 pmol/mg/30 min; in supernate (S), 90.6 ± 4.0. Of the hypotonic preparations, control activity was 770 ± 20 pmol/mg/45 min in medial MB and 103.6 ± 4 pmol/mg/30 min in lateral MB. There was a mean decrease in synaptosomal conversion in pellets from both midbrain areas. The activity in neither supernate from medial MB changed significantly after cocaine; both soluble enzyme measures from lateral MB rose significantly after cocaine ($p < 0.005$ for isotonic preparation; $p < 0.013$ for hypotonic preparation).

Figure 6 summarizes the changes in serotonergic pathways from the midbrain to the striate cortex induced by short-term, repeated administration of lithium chloride (10 meq/kg/day). Rats, weighing 125 to 150 g each, were sacrificed 24 hours after the last dose, and blood levels of lithium at that time ranged from 0.9 to 1.4 meq/liter. Lithium ion, when compared with equimolar sodium, stimulated the high affinity uptake of radioactive tryptophan into the

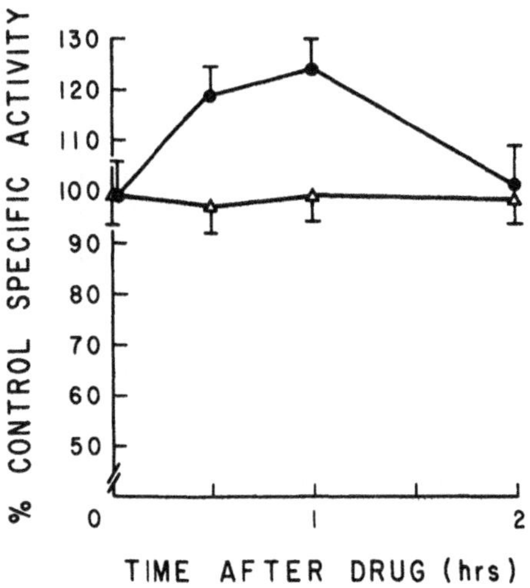

Fig. 5. Time course of the selective effects of cocaine (100 mg/kg) on medial midbrain (—Δ—), B7 and B8 serotonergic cell bodies, and on lateral midbrain (—●—), B9 cell bodies. Whereas there was no detectable cocaine-induced change in tryptophan hydroxylase prepared from medial MB (control = 750 ± 25.8 pmol/mg/30 min), enzyme from lateral MB (control = 125 ± 5 pmol/mg/30 min) was increased 30 min and 60 min after drug treatment ($p < 0.005$).

synaptosomes, and there was an associated increase in synaptosomal conversion of radioactive tryptophan to radioactive 5-HT. These two changes are represented by the upper two lines of Fig. 6. Mediated by neuronal feedback, or by some other mechanism indigenous to the serotonergic neuron, was a slightly delayed (one day in this instance) decrease in the specific activity of soluble tryptophan hydroxylase in both cell body (raphe nuclei) and nerve ending (striate cortex) regions. After three weeks of lithium treatment (5 meq/kg/day), the stimulation of the high affinity uptake and the decrease in the activity of soluble tryptophan hydroxylase in both midbrain and striate remained (Fig. 7). However, there was a return to control levels of the capacity of the serotonergic synaptosomes to convert radioactive tryptophan to 5-HT (second of the three bar graphs): conversion was made possible by the joint functions of an increased uptake of substrate and a reduced level of intrasynaptosomal tryptophan hydroxylase activity.

Because both these parameters of brain serotonergic biosynthetic activity are capable of adaptive change in response to a variety of

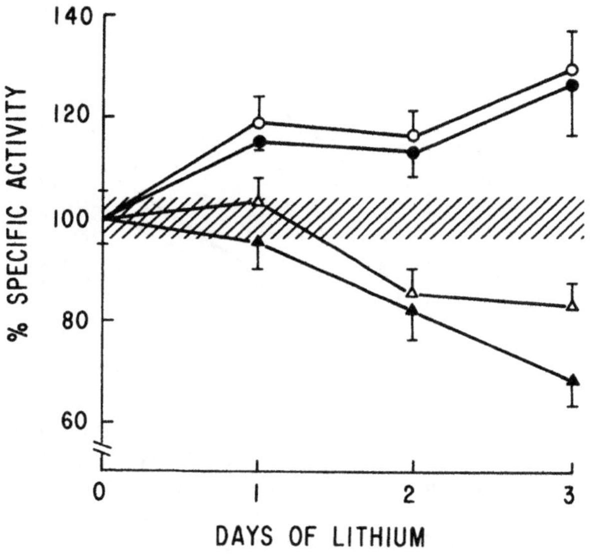

Fig. 6. Simultaneous short-term effects of three daily lithium injections (10 meq/kg) on four measures relevant to 5-HT synthesis, expressed as percentages of the following control specific activities: {^{14}C}tryptophan uptake (o), 1200 ± 50 pmol/mg/4 min; synaptosomal conversion of tryptophan to 5-HT (●), 250 ± 20 pmol/mg/45 min; midbrain soluble tryptophan hydroxylase (Δ), 525 ±20 pmol/mg/45 min; intrasynaptosomal enzyme (▲), 150 ± 5 pmol/mg/45 min. Uptake and conversion were significantly elevated each day ($p < 0.05$). Soluble enzyme activities were significantly reduced at Day 2 (midbrain, $p < 0.05$) and Day 3 (striate, $p < 0.02$). Substrate concentration was invariably 10 μM.

pharmacological and environmental manipulations (Knapp, Mandell, 1972a, 1972b, 1975; Knapp et al., 1974; Knapp, 1975; Rogawaski et al., 1974; Segal et al., 1973), we interpret our data as showing that lithium-induced changes "use up" two potential adaptive mechanisms without changing the normal range of overall synaptosomal biosynthetic capacity. Substrate uptake is maximized, and soluble enzyme activity is minimized. Figure 8 is a diagram showing this lithium-induced sequence of changes. An obvious assumption in this model is that cell body soluble enzyme is somehow related to the experience of the postsynaptic receptors.

Recent clinical studies have suggested that lithium pretreatment eliminates or significantly alters the euphoric experience usually

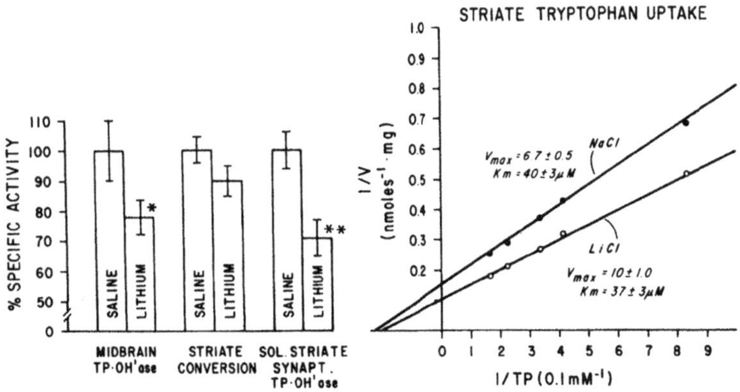

Fig. 7. Simultaneous long-term effects of 21 daily lithium injections (5 meq/kg) on four measures relevant to 5-HT synthesis. Control velocities: midbrain soluble tryptophan hydroxylase, 475 ± 20 pmol/mg/45 min (*p < 0.05); striate synaptosomal conversion, 200 ± 10 pmol/mg/45 min; striate solubilized (intrasynaptosomal) enzyme, 160 ± 5 pmol/mg/45 min (**p < 0.001). High affinity uptake (12 μM to 53 μM substrate) is plotted as nmol L-{3-^{14}C}-tryptophan retained/mg/4 min, and V_{max} and K_m ± S.E. were estimated according to the method of Wilkinson (1961).

induced by a number of drugs, including amphetamine and cocaine (Flemenbaum, 1974; Bunney, W., 1975). This is interesting in light of lithium's antimanic action. Schou has suggested that lithium administered on a chronic basis is equally prophylactic against depression and mania. His challenge to those attending a recent Neurosciences Research Program workshop on lithium (Schou, in press) was that any explanation of the action of lithium based on a single neurotransmitter system would have to show how the drug can inhibit both extremes of behavior and yet maintain a normal range of function under control conditions. As seen in Figs. 7 and 8, such a circumstance is possible during treatment with lithium. Although the role of the brain's serotonergic system in affective disorder is far from clear, the fixation of adaptive mechanisms so that they resist further change in either direction and the gradual resulting stability in the system so achieved suggest an interesting model for further exploration of the mechanisms by which lithium might achieve such symmetrical prophylaxis of manic-depressive disease (Mandell, Knapp, 1975).

After examining the effects of cocaine and lithium separately, we studied the effects of their interaction on the serotonergic

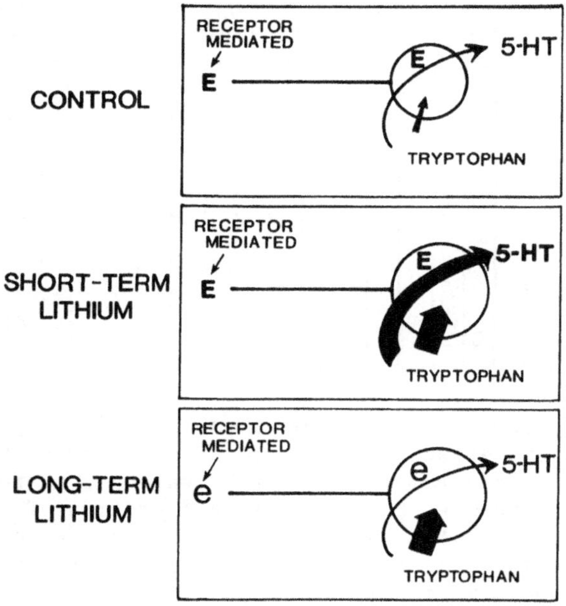

Fig. 8. Hypothetical presynaptic mechanisms in the action of lithium. In the control neuron, tryptophan hydroxylase (E) is optimal in cell body and nerve ending. Tryptophan (substrate) is taken up through the neuronal membrane and converted by E to 5-HT, which is released from the nerve ending. After short-term lithium treatment, tryptophan uptake is augmented and, consequently, synthesis and release of 5-HT are increased because E is not saturated with regard to substrate. After long-term lithium treatment, "amount" of enzyme has been reduced (E → e) to compensate for the initial 5-HT bombardment of the receptor. Tryptophan uptake is still elevated, but 5-HT synthesis and release at the nerve ending have returned to control levels because of the enzyme deficit (e instead of E).

system. Sprague-Dawley rats (150 to 200 g each) were treated with lithium chloride or sodium chloride (10 meq/kg) for three days before cocaine injection (100 mg/kg s.c.) and sacrificed one hour later. Figure 9 summarizes the individual effects of cocaine and lithium as well as the effect of the interaction of the drugs on the four parameters related to 5-HT biosynthesis. Note (bars to the far right) that cocaine alone reduced the high affinity uptake of radioactive tryptophan, lithium alone stimulated the same system, and their interaction led to values approximating 100% of control. Similar changes were seen in the capacity of striate synaptosomes to convert radioactive tryptophan to 5-HT (bars second from left):

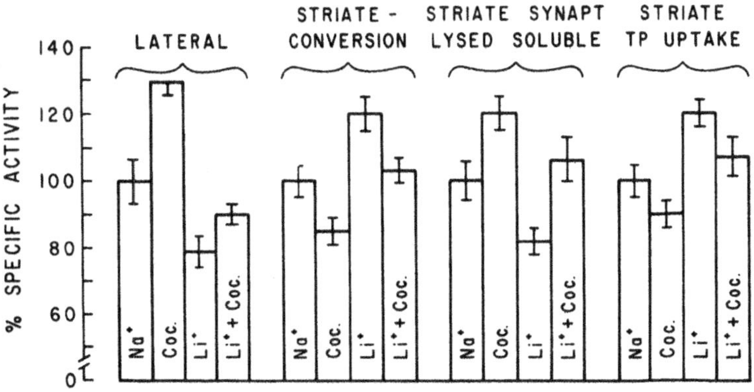

Fig. 9. The independent effects of cocaine (100 mg/kg) and lithium (10 meq/kg) and the effects of cocaine after three days of lithium pretreatment on four parameters of 5-HT synthesis in rat brain. On each graph Na+ represents control (animals pretreated with NaCl), and the data are presented as percentages of the following control specific activities: lateral midbrain soluble tryptophan hydroxylase activity, 200 ± 5 pmol/mg/30 min; striate conversion, 180 ± 7 pmol/mg/30 min; striate synaptosomal lysed soluble enzyme, 111 ± 4.5 pmol/mg/30 min; striate uptake of L-{3-^{14}C}-tryptophan, 1150 ± 60 pmol/mg/5 min. Independently, cocaine and lithium altered lateral midbrain and striate enzyme activities ($p < 0.028$) as well as striate conversion of tryptophan to 5-HT ($p < 0.05$). Lithium increased radioactive tryptophan uptake whereas cocaine decreased it. Pretreatment with lithium chloride prevented the cocaine-induced changes in 5-HT biosynthesis reflected in all four parameters.

cocaine reduced it; lithium increased it; and the result of their combined presence approached control value. The bars at the far left and those second from the right reflect the compensatory changes in intraneuronal soluble tryptophan hydroxylase activity from the lateral midbrain raphe and the striate cortex, respectively. Cocaine produced an increase in tryptophan hydroxylase activity in the lateral midbrain and the striate cortex. Lithium produced a decrease in tryptophan hydroxylase activity in both midbrain and striate. When lithium and cocaine treatments were combined, the values for the soluble enzyme activities approached control values. Thus, in all four parameters of 5-HT biosynthesis examined in this study, the cocaine-induced changes were antagonized by those induced by lithium.

A question arises concerning the behavioral significance of the apparent neurobiological antagonism between these two drugs in the brain's serotonergic system. Not a great deal of work relevant to the question can be cited. Although, to our knowledge, there has been no animal behavioral study of a cocaine and lithium antagonism, lithium has been shown to antagonize the behavioral effects of two drugs that, like cocaine, reduce the biosynthesis of 5-HT. Furukawa (1975) demonstrated that lithium pretreatment antagonized the motoric effects of amphetamine. Cassens and Mills (1973) showed that amphetamine and lithium have opposite effects on the threshold for maintaining intracranial self-stimulation. We demonstrated that amphetamine, like cocaine, acutely reduced the biosynthesis of 5-HT (Knapp et al., 1974). Carroll and Sharp (1971) showed that lithium antagonized the behavioral activation induced by morphine in mice. We showed that morphine reduced the synaptosomal conversion of tryptophan to 5-HT (Knapp, Mandell, 1972b).

Although the relationship between 5-HT synthesis and behavioral inhibition is not established definitively, it is generally believed that the indoleamine neurotransmitter has the capacity to inhibit such behaviors as spontaneous motor movement, startle, and self-stimulation (Brodie, Shore, 1957; Sheard, Aghajanian, 1968; Appel, Sheard, Freedman, 1970; Connor, Stolk, Barchas, Levine, 1970; Swonger, Rech, 1972; Geyer et al., 1975a, 1975b, in press a, b). Cocaine tends to have the opposite effects (Crow, 1970; Fog, 1969; van Rossum, 1968).

Perhaps the antagonism observed in the measures of serotonergic function used in our studies have similar behavioral correlates. Recently two manic-depressive patients in treatment with lithium whom we have seen reported that illicitly obtained cocaine failed to affect them when used in the presence of others who experienced the expected effects. Whether lithium has a place in the treatment of compulsive stimulant users awaits appropriate clinical research.

ACKNOWLEDGMENT

This work is supported by USPHS Grant DA-00265-04.

REFERENCES

Appel, M.B., Sheard, M.H., and Freedman, D.X.: Alterations in the behavioral effects of LSD by midbrain raphe lesions, Comm. behav. Biol. 5, 237-241 (1970).

Brodie, B.B. and Shore, P.A.: A concept for a role of serotonin and norepinephrine as chemical mediators in the brain, Ann. N.Y. Acad. Sci. 66, 631-642 (1957).

Carroll, B.J. and Sharp, B.P.: Rubidium and lithium: Opposite effect on amine-mediated excitement, Science 172, 1355-1357 (1971).

Cassens, G.P. and Mills, A.W.: Lithium and amphetamine: Opposite effects on threshold of intracranial reinforcement, Psychopharmacologia 30, 283-290 (1973).

Connor, R.L., Stolk, J.M., Barchas, J.D., and Levine, S.: Parachlorophenylalanine and habituation to repetitive auditory startle stimuli in rats, Physiol. Behav. 5, 1215-1219 (1970).

Crow, T.J.: Enhancement by cocaine of intracranial self-stimulation in the rat, Life Sci. 9, 375-381 (1970).

Dahlström, A. and Fuxe, K.: Evidence for the existence of monoamine-containing neurons in the central nervous system, Acta Physiol. Scand. 62, Suppl. 232, 1-55 (1964).

Flemenbaum, A.: Does lithium block the effects of amphetamine? A report of three cases, Am. J. Psychiat. 131, 820-821 (1974).

Fog, R.: Stereotyped and non-stereotyped behavior in rats induced by various stimulant drugs, Psychopharmacologia 14, 299-304 (1969).

Friedman, E., Gershon, S., and Rotrosen, J.: Effects of acute cocaine treatment on the turnover of 5-hydroxytryptamine in the rat brain, Br. J. Pharmacol. 54, 61-64 (1975).

Furukawa, T.: Modification by lithium of behavioral responses to methamphetamine and tetrabenazine, Psychopharmacologia 42, 243-248 (1975).

Fuxe, K. and Jonsson, G.: A modification of the histochemical fluorescence method for the improved localization of 5-hydroxytryptamine, Histochemie 11, 161-166 (1967).

Geyer, M.A., Dawsey, W.J., and Mandell, A.J.: Differential effects of caffeine, d-amphetamine, and methylphenidate on individual raphe cell fluorescence: A microspectrofluorometric demonstration, Brain Res. 85, 135-139 (1975a).

Geyer, M.A., Warbritton, J.D., Menkes, D.B., Zook, J.A., and Mandell, A.J.: Opposite effects of intraventricular serotonin and bufotenine on rat startle responses, Pharmacol. Biochem. Behav. 3, 687-691 (1975b).

Geyer, M.A., Puerto, A., Dawsey, W.J., Knapp, S., Bullard, W.P., and Mandell, A.J.: Histologic and enzymatic studies of the mesolimbic and mesostriatal serotonergic pathways, Brain Res. (in press, a).

Geyer, M.A., Puerto, A., Menkes, D.B., Segal, D.S., and Mandell, A.J.: Behavioral studies following lesions of the mesolimbic and mesostriatal serotonergic pathways, Brain Res. (in press, b).

Harvey, J.A., McMaster, S.E., and Yunger, L.M.: p-Chloroamphetamine: Selective neurotoxic action in brain, Science 187, 841-843 (1975).

Ichiyama, A., Nakamura, S., Nishizuka, Y., and Hayaishi, O.: Tryptophan hydroxylase in mammalian brain, Adv. Pharmacol. 6A, 5-17 (1968).

Ichiyama, A., Nakamura, S., Nishizuka, Y., and Hayaishi, O.: Enzymic studies on the biosynthesis of serotonin in mammalian brain, J. biol. Chem. 245, 1699-1709 (1970).

Knapp, S.: Differential drug effects on brain serotonergic systems. In: Neurobiological Mechanisms of Adaptation and Behavior. Mandell, A.J., Ed., pp. 155-168. New York: Raven Press, 1975

Knapp, S. and Mandell, A.J.: Parachlorophenylalanine: Its three phase sequence of interactions with the two forms of brain tryptophan hydroxylase, Life Sci. 11, 761-771 (1972a).

Knapp, S. and Mandell, A.J.: Narcotic drugs: Effects on serotonin biosynthetic systems of the brain, Science 177, 1209-1211 (1972b).

Knapp, S. and Mandell, A.J.: Short- and long-term lithium administration: Effects on the brain's serotonergic systems, Science 180, 645-647 (1973).

Knapp, S. and Mandell, A.J.: Effects of lithium chloride on parameters of biosynthetic capacity for 5-hydroxytryptamine in rat brain, J. Pharmac. exp. Ther. 193, 812-823 (1975).

Knapp, S. and Mandell, A.J.: Coincidence of blockade of synaptosomal 5-hydroxytryptamine uptake and decrease in tryptophan hydroxylase activity: Effects of fenfluramine, J. Pharmac. exp. Ther. (in press).

Knapp, S., Mandell, A.J., and Bullard, W.: Calcium activation of brain tryptophan hydroxylase, Life Sci. 16, 1583-1594 (1975).

Knapp, S., Mandell, A.J., and Geyer, M.A.: Effects of amphetamines on regional tryptophan hydroxylase activity and synaptosomal conversion of tryptophan to 5-HT in rat brain, J. Pharmac. exp. Ther. 189, 676-689 (1974).

Mandell, A.J.: Neurobiological mechanisms of presynaptic metabolic adaptation and their organization: Implications for a pathophysiology of the affective disorders. In: Neurobiological Mechanisms of Adaptation and Behavior. Mandell, A.J., Ed., pp. 1-32, New York: Raven Press, 1975.

Mandell, A.J. and Knapp, S.: A model for the neurobiological mechanisms of action involved in lithium prophylaxis of bipolar affective disorder. In: Aminergic Hypotheses of Behavior: Reality or Cliche? Bernard, B.K., Ed., pp. 97-107. Washington: DHEW (NIDA Research Monograph Series 3), 1975.

Rogawski, M.A., Knapp, S., and Mandell, A.J.: Effects of ethanol on tryptophan hydroxylase activity from striate synaptosomes, Biochem. Pharmacol. 23, 1955-1962 (1974).

Schou, M.: Clinical prophylactic effects and clinical pharmacology of lithium. In: The Neurobiology of Lithium. Bunney, W.E., Jr. and Murphy, D.L., Eds. Cambridge: MIT Press (Neurosciences Research Program Bull. 13), in press.

Segal, D.S., Knapp, S., Kuczenski, R.T., and Mandell, A.J.: The effects of environmental isolation on behavior and regional rat brain tyrosine hydroxylase and tryptophan hydroxylase activities, Behav. Biol. 8, 47-53 (1973).

Sheard, M.H. and Aghajanian, G.K.: Stimulation of midbrain raphe neurons: Behavioral effects of serotonin release, Life Sci. 7, 19-25 (1968).

Swonger, A.K. and Rech, R.H.: Serotonergic and cholinergic involvement in habituation of activity and spontaneous alternation of rats in a Y maze, J. comp. Physiol. Psychol. 81, 509-522 (1972).

van Rossum, J.M.: Mode of action of psychomotor stimulant drugs, Int. Rev. Neurobiol. 12, 307-383 (1968).

Wilkinson, G.N.: Statistical estimation in enzyme kinetics, Biochem. J. 80, 324-332 (1961).

ON FOOD DEPRIVATION IN RELATION TO AMPHETAMINE TOLERANCE

Tommy Lewander

Psychiatric Research Center, Ulleråker Hospital

University of Uppsala, S-750 17 UPPSALA, Sweden

INTRODUCTION

Previous studies on amphetamine tolerance in rats have shown that tolerance develops to some effects of the drug; e.g., hyperthermia, anorexia, increase in brain tryptophan concentrations (Lewander, 1971, 1974, unpublished observations), while not to others; e.g., motor hyperactivity, sterotyped behaviour (Lewander, 1971). In fact, reverse tolerance, *viz.* a progressive augmentation of stereotypies on chronic administration of low to medium doses of amphetamine, has been reported (Segal and Mandell, 1974).

Tolerance to the hyperthermic action of d-amphetamine was initially shown to be related to the accumulation of p-hydroxynorephedrine, a metabolite of d-amphetamine, as a false transmitter in noradrenergic neurons in rats (Brodie, Cho, Stefano, and Gessa, 1969; Brodie, Cho, and Gessa, 1970; Costa and Groppetti, 1970; Lewander, 1970, 1971). However, this mechanism of tolerance was later found to apply to male but not to female rats (Sever, Caldwell, and Williams, 1974). Further, the rate of development and disappearance of tolerance to the hyperthermic effect of amphetamine did not parallel the displacement and replacement of brain and heart noradrenaline during chronic administration and after withdrawal of amphetamine (Lewander, Moliis, and Brus, 1975). In addition, tolerance to the amphetamine-induced hyperthermia developed also after chronic administration of l-amphetamine, an isomer that is not converted to the false transmitter (Lewander et al., 1975), and on chronic administration of d-amphetamine in the guinea pig, a species that does not metabolize amphetamine by *para*-hydroxylation and, therefore, cannot accumulate p-hydroxynorephedrine (Sever and Caldwell, 1974). The conclusion seems to be that, although p-hydroxynorephedrine accumulation might contribute to amphetamine tolerance in some cases, other mechanisms of tolerance explaining all presently known facts must be sought.

In the study of mechanisms of tolerance to the hyperthermic effect of amphetamine by Lewander et al. (1975), it was accidentally found that the feeding conditions markedly influenced the pattern of tolerance development in rats. Tolerance developed to a maximal degree; i.e., there was no increase in body temperature at one hour after amphetamine injection in rats that had received chronic administration of amphetamine twice daily for 8-10 days and had been fed during the 16 hours before each morning injection of amphetamine. In another group of rats, however, food was not available during the 16 hours before each morning injection, but only for 7 hours after the morning injections; in this group a hypothermic response to amphetamine began to appear after 6-8 days of chronic administration of the drug. These findings led to the question of whether or not a reduction of the food intake might affect the temperature response to a single dose of amphetamine in drug naive animals.

It is reported in the present communication in a preliminary form that the hyperthermic response to amphetamine is gradually abolished in rats subjected to starvation for 1-4 days and that the response reappears after refeeding. In addition, the effect of amphetamine on food intake and some biochemical parameters in fed rats and in rats starved for 4 days were investigated.

METHODS

Male Sprague-Dawley (Anticimex, Uplands Väsby, Sweden) rats, 250-300 g body weight, were used in all experiments. The animals were kept in individual Macrolon^{R} cages. Food (Anticimex rat pellets No. 214) was available according to various feeding schedules described under Results. Water was given *ad libitum*. The animals were kept in a temperature-constant room (21°C) at 70 per cent humidity for at least one week before the start of, and during, all experiments. Light was present between 6 a.m. and 6 p.m.

Body temperature was measured with electric thermometer (El-lab, Copenhagen) and the thermocouple was inserted into the colon 4 cm from the anal orifice. The animals were habituated to the handling procedures and body temperature was measured several times daily for one week before starting the experiment.

Food intake was measured by weighing in- and out-going portions of pellets to the nearest 0.05 g. Spillage into the bottoms of the cages was always eaten by the rats, and therefore no corrections were necessary.

Brain and plasma concentrations of amphetamine were measured by gas chromatography (Änggård, Gunne, and Niklasson, 1970). Catecholamines, trytophan, and 5-hydroxyindoles were determined by standard fluorimetric procedures as described elsewhere (Lewander, 1974). Free tryptophan in plasma was assayed after centrifugation of 2 ml of heparinized plasma through Centriflo ultrafilters (Amicon Corp.) at 2500 rpm for 30 min. at +4°C. A rigid time schedule was followed for the treatment of the plasma samples. Plasmas from control animals were always run simultaneously with samples from treated rats in order to avoid differences between groups due to possible temperature and pH changes during the procedures (McMenamy and Oncley, 1958). Student's t-test was used for the statistical evaluation of the results.

RESULTS

Body Temperature

The time response curves for the hyperthermic effect of 20 mg/kg d-amphetamine in groups of rats starved for 1, 2, and 4 days, respectively, and in a group of fed rats are shown in Fig. 1. The body temperature was measured 30 min. before and at hourly intervals for 7 hours after injection of amphetamine at 9 a.m. The temperature response at 1 and 2 hour intervals after injection was successively decreased depending on the duration of starvation; after 4 days of starvation, the 1 hour response was totally absent. The late temperature response, 3-7 hours after the injection, was less affected in the starved rats. One day of re-feeding for rats that had been subjected to 4 days of starvation did not restore the hyperthermic response to amphetamine while 2 (and 4) days of re-feeding restored, although incompletely, the temperature response (Fig. 2).

Food Intake

Rats tested for the anorexigenic effect of amphetamine were trained for 12 days before the experiment to eat between 9 a.m. and 4 p.m. only. Twelve rats were starved for 4 days before the test while 12 other rats continued to be fed *ad libitum*. The animals were further sub-divided at the day of the test into 4 groups of 6 rats each. One starved group and one fed group received amphetamine immediately before food was made available while the remaining rats were given saline. Food consumption was measured at hourly intervals for 7 hours after the injection and the food intake was plotted cumulatively for each group (Fig. 3). The results showed that the starved rats given saline ate less than the fed controls

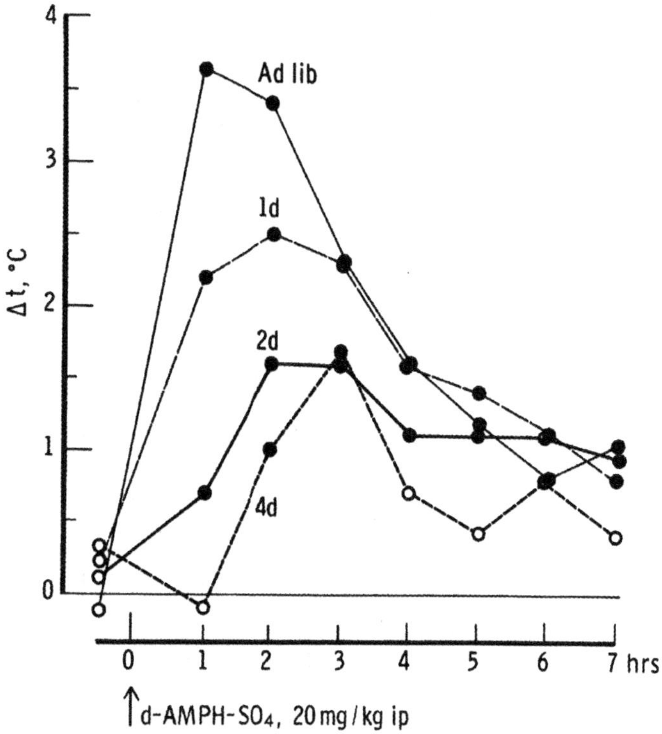

Fig. 1. Effect of d-amphetamine sulphate (d-AMPH. SO_4; 20 mg/kg i.p.) on body temperature in rats fed *ad libitum* (ad lib) daily between 4 p.m. and 9 p.m. and in rats starved for 1, 2 and 4 days (1d, 2d, 4d), respectively, before the injection of amphetamine or saline. Body (colonic) temperature was measured 30 min before and at hourly intervals after the drug administration. Values are given as the mean difference in body temperature (Δt°C) between amphetamine-treated rats and saline-injected controls. Filled circles represent statistically significant differences ($p < 0.02$) from saline-injected control rats, whereas open circles represent non-significant differences. N = 5 in each group.

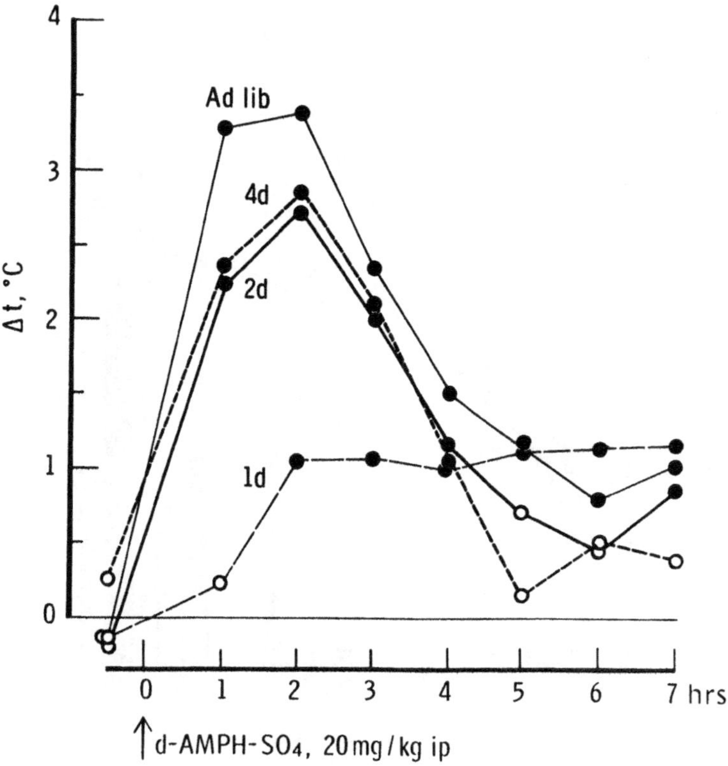

Figure 2. Effect of re-feeding (25 g pellets/day between 4 p.m. and 9 a.m.) for 1, 2 and 4 days (1d, 2d, 4d), respectively, on the amphetamine-elicited hyperthermic response in rats previously starved for 96 hours. A group of rats given access to food daily between 4 p.m. and 9 a.m. (ad lib.) were injected also with amphetamine sulphate (AMPH. SO_4; 20 mg/kg i.p.) and served as fed amphetamine-treated controls. For further information see text to Fig. 1.

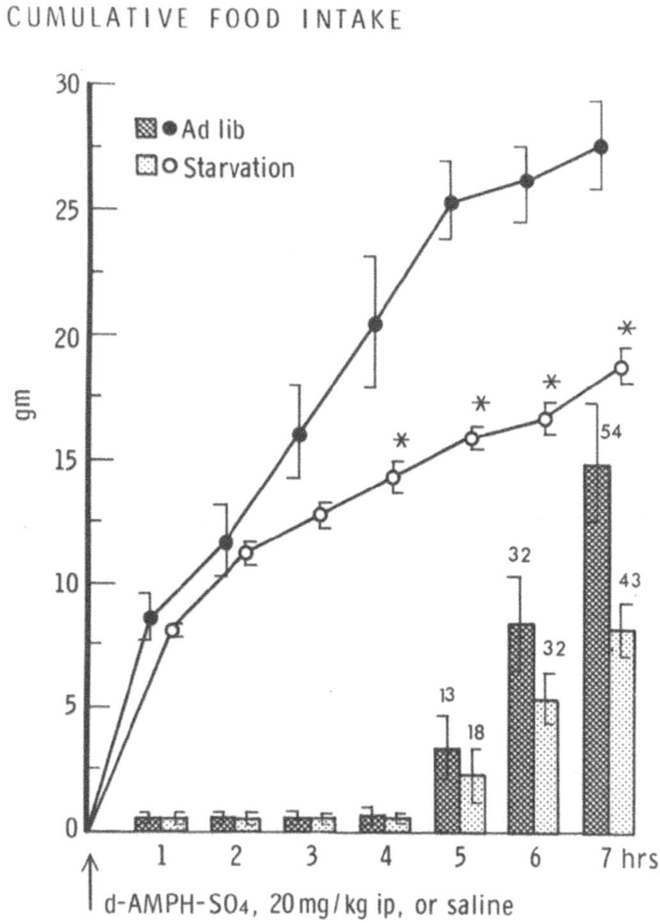

Fig. 3. Cumulative food intake for 7 hours after 20 mg/kg d-amphetamine sulphate i.p. in rats fed *ad libitum* and rats starved for 96 hours before the experiments. Dots (mean ± SEM) and bars connected with lines represents the food intake (cumulated hourly) for saline-injected rats. Columns (and bars) represent the food intake in fed and starved rats after amphetamine. Figures above columns represent the food intake in percentages of the respective control groups. There were six rats in each group.

throughout the experiment. Amphetamine administration caused a decrease in the food intake to a similar degree in both starved and fed rats as shown by the percentage figures in Fig. 3. The duration of complete anorexia after the amphetamine injection was the same for both groups.

Body Weight

Four days of starvation was followed by a reduction in the mean body weight of approximately 50 g (Table 1).

Biochemical Findings

A series of endogenous substances in brain and plasma, including tryptophan, 5-HT, 5-HIAA, DA and NA, as well as the amphetamine concentrations were measured at 2 hours after administration of amphetamine to fed rats and rats starved for 4 days (Table 1). In spite of the differences in body weight between the starved and the fed rats (above), the concentrations of amphetamine in brain and plasma did not differ significantly between the groups.

Brain tryptophan was increased about three-fold after amphetamine in fed rats while there was no significant change after starvation. The plasma concentrations of tryptophan (total and free) in the fed rats were increased after amphetamine although not as much as brain tryptophan. Again, there was no change in these measures in the starved rats.

Brain 5-HT decreased by 23 per cent after amphetamine in the fed control rats while there was an increase by 29 per cent in the starved animals. Similarly, brain 5-HIAA was higher in starved than in fed rats after amphetamine. However, the tendencies to a decrease in 5-HIAA in fed rats and an increase in the starved rats were not statistically significant, which makes this comparison uncertain.

Brain and heart NA concentrations were decreased by amphetamine both in fed and starved rats. However, the degrees of depletion were less after starvation, being 29 per cent in starved rats versus 47 per cent in fed rats for the brain and 9 per cent versus 33 per cent, respectively, for the heart.

Brain DA was not affected by amphetamine in either group of rats.

TABLE 1

Effects of d-Amphetamine in Fed and Starved Rats

Measure	Feeding Schedule	Amphetamine 2 hrs	Saline	AMPH vs. saline $p <$
Body Weight, g	fed	300 ± 5 (5)	301 ± 2 (5)	NS
	starved	251 ± 5^{xxx}(5)	255 ± 4^{xxx}(5)	NS
Amphetamine, brain, μg/g	fed	7.22 ± 0.68 (5)	-	
	starved	6.02 ± 0.75 (5)	-	
Amphetamine, plasma, μg/ml	fed	1.02 ± 0.10 (5)	-	
	starved	0.82 ± 0.25 (5)	-	
Tryptophan, brain μg/g	fed	11.81 ± 1.47 (4)	3.61 ± 0.21 (5)	0.001
	starved	5.34 ± 0.28^{xxx}(4)	4.30 ± 0.38 (4)	NS
Tryptophan, plasma, total μg/ml	fed	25.87 ± 2.12 (5)	18.83 ± 1.29 (5)	0.05
	starved	15.26 ± 1.16^{xx}(5)	18.17 ± 1.11 (5)	NS
Tryptophan, plasma, free μg/ml	fed	3.61 ± 0.51 (5)	1.65 ± 0.28 (5)	0.01
	starved	1.77 ± 0.17^{xx}(5)	1.38 ± 0.20 (5)	NS
5-HT, brain, μg/g	fed	0.24 ± 0.01 (4)	0.31 ± 0.01 (5)	0.01
	starved	0.44 ± 0.04^{xx}(4)	0.34 ± 0.01 (4)	0.05
5-HIAA, brain, μg/g	fed	0.27 ± 0.02 (4)	0.25 ± 0.01 (5)	NS
	starved	0.41 ± 0.05^{x}(4)	0.29 ± 0.04 (5)	NS

TABLE 1 (continued)

Measure	Feeding Schedule	Amphetamine 2 hrs	Saline	AMPH vs. saline p <
DA, brain, μg/g	fed	0.93 ± 0.12 (5)	0.73 ± 0.07 (5)	NS
	starved	0.65 ± 0.04 (4)	0.74 ± 0.06 (5)	NS
NA, brain, μg/g	fed	0.18 ± 0.01 (5)	0.34 ± 0.02 (5)	0.001
	starved	0.24 ± 0.01^{xxx}(5)	0.34 ± 0.01 (5)	0.001
NA, heart, μg/g	fed	0.38 ± 0.01 (5)	0.57 ± 0.03 (5)	0.05
	starved	0.66 ± 0.06^{xx}(4)	0.72 ± 0.03^{xx}(5)	NS

Effects of d-amphetamine (AMPH) in rats fed daily between 4 p.m. and 9 a.m. (fed) or totally deprived of food for 96 hours before the injection (starved) on the following measures: body weight, tryptophan in brain, tryptophan in plasma (total plus free), brain 5-hydroxytryptamine (5-HT), brain 5-hydroxyindole acetic acid (5-HIAA), brain dopamine (DA), brain and heart noradrenaline (NA). Brain and plasma concentrations of amphetamine were also determined. The animals were killed 2 hours after the i.p. injection of 20 mg/kg of d-amphetamine sulphate.

Values are means ± S.E.M.; number of observations within brackets.

NS = not significant

Starved versus *ad libitum* feeding (fed): x = $p < 0.05$, xx = $p < 0.01$, xxx = $p < 0.001$, according to Student's t-test.

DISCUSSION

The present experiments show that food deprivation markedly influences several pharmacological effects of amphetamine in rats.

The reduction of amphetamine-elicited hyperthermia was directly correlated to the duration of starvation, showing that the nutritional status of the animals is of considerable importance for this effect of the drug. This finding confirms the conclusions drawn from a previous experiment on tolerance to the hyperthermic effect of amphetamine during chronic amphetamine administration under various feeding schedules (Lewander et al., 1975, see Introduction). Interestingly, the pattern of the time response curve for hyperthermia in starved rats; i.e., a complete abolishment of the initial (1 hour) response, is strikingly similar to the time response curve in amphetamine-tolerant rats (of Fig. 2 in Lewander et al., 1975). Re-feeding for more than 2 days restored the temperature response to amphetamine. The present results, thus, lend support to the hypothesis (Lewander et al., 1975) that depletion of pool(s) of calorigenic substances might constitute an important mechanism of amphetamine tolerance in addition to the false transmitter mechanism which seems to be valid only under certain conditions (see Introduction). It still remains to be demonstrated, however, which calorigenic substances are involved.

Tolerance also develops to the amphetamine-induced increase in brain tryptophan concentrations on chronic administration of the drug (Lewander, 1974; Lewander et al., 1975; Lewander, unpublished observations). Therefore, it is an interesting finding that this effect of amphetamine was also completely abolished after 4 days of starvation. There does not seem to be a causal relationship, however, between changes in brain tryptophan and hyperthermia since tolerance development and disappearance to these two effects are not parallel (cf Lewander, 1974).

The changes in plasma total and free tryptophan concentrations paralleled the changes in brain tryptophan concentration. It is not yet clear, however, whether or not it is the pool of free tryptophan (Tagliamonte, Biggio, Vargiu, and Gessa, 1973a,b: Curzon, Friedel, and Knott, 1973) or the bound form (Fernström and Wurtman, 1974) that is in equilibrium with the brain compartment of tryptophan. Anyhow, tolerance to the amphetamine-induced increase in free tryptophan occurs during chronic administration; the mechanism, though, is obscure (Lewander, unpublished observations).

Tolerance develops to the anorexigenic effect of amphetamine (Shapiro and Freedman, 1957; Tormey and Lasagna, 1960; Lewander, 1971, 1974). There is no explanation for the tolerance to this effect of amphetamine; the false transmitter hypothesis has previously been refuted (Lewander, 1971). Some authors (Panksepp and Booth, 1973) have claimed that food restriction during chronic amphetamine treatment might build up a hunger state that eventually overcomes the anorexigenic effect of the drug. The present results are against this view since 4 days of complete starvation, which is certainly a drastic treatment, changed neither the duration nor the degree of amphetamine-induced anorexia. Thus, starvation and the hypothetical depletion of some calorigenic substances are of no consequence for the tolerance development to the anorexigenic effect of amphetamine.

The mitigation of the amphetamine-elicited depletion of brain and heart NA caused by starvation is not easily explained at present. Should this finding mean that less NA is released by amphetamine, it is certainly of interest in relation to amphetamine tolerance since many effects, peripheral at least, are mediated through release of this transmitter. Among other possibilities, amphetamine might be less efficiently *para*- and/or β-hydroxylated in starved rats so that less p-hydroxynorephedrine (see Introduction) is accumulating in NA neurons. Direct experiments are required for elucidation of these matters.

In summary, starvation of rats for up to 4 days markedly changes a number of pharmacological effects of amphetamine. Earlier studies (Campbell and Fibiger, 1971; Fibiger, 1973) have shown a potentiation of amphetamine-induced hyperactivity in rats. The present study demonstrates that the amphetamine-induced increase in body temperature and in brain and plasma concentrations of tryptophan are almost completely abolished and that the depletion of NA in central and peripheral NA neurons is mitigated after administration of amphetamine in starved rats. In contrast, the anorexigenic effect of amphetamine is not affected by starvation. The present observations confirm and extend previous findings on the importance of the nutritional status for amphetamine-induced changes of body temperature, and provide an explanation, in addition to suggesting a possible mechanism, for the development of tolerance of some effects of amphetamine in chronically treated rats. A more detailed account of the present observations and subsequent findings along these lines is in progress.

ACKNOWLEDGMENTS

The investigations were supported by the Swedish Medical Research Council, Grant Nos. B75-25X-1017-11 and B76-04P-4288-03C. Ms. Sonja Ahlén is gratefully acknowledged for skillful technical assistance.

REFERENCES

Änggård, E., Gunn, L-M., and Niklasson, F.: Gas chromatographic determination of amphetamine in blood, tissue and urine, Scand. J. clin. lab. Investig. 26, 137-144 (1970).

Brodie, B.B., Cho, A.K., and Gessa, G.L.: Possible role of p-hydroxynorephedrine in the depletion of norepinephrine induced by d-amphetamine and in tolerance to this drug. In: International Symposium on Amphetamines and Related Compounds. Costa, E. and Garattini, S., Eds., pp. 217-230. New York: Raven Press, 1970.

Brodie, B.B., Cho, A.K., Stefano, F.J.E., and Gessa, G.L.: On mechanisms of norepinephrine release by amphetamine and tyramine and tolerance to their effects, Adv. biochem. Pharmac. 1, 219-238 (1969).

Campbell, B.A. and Fibiger, H.C.: Potentiation of amphetamine-induced arousal by starvation, Nature (Lond.) 233, 424-425 (1971).

Costa, E. and Gropetti, A.: Biosynthesis and storage of catecholamines in tissues of rats injected with various doses of d-amphetamine. In: International Symposium on Amphetamines and Related Compounds. Costa, E. and Garattini, S., Eds., pp. 231-255. New York: Raven Press, 1970.

Curzon, G., Friedel, J., and Knott, P.J.: The effect of fatty acids on the binding of tryptophan to plasma protein, Nature (Lond.) 242, 198-200 (1973).

Fernström, J.D. and Wirtman, R.J.: Control of brain serotonin levels by the diet, Adv. biochem. Pharmac. 11, 133-142 (1974).

Fibiger, H.C.: Behavioural pharmacology of d-amphetamine: Some metabolic and pharmacological considerations. In: Frontiers in Catecholamine Research. Usdin, E. and Snyder, S., Eds., pp. 933-937. New York: Pergamon Press, 1973.

Lewander, T.: Catecholamines turn-over studies on chronic amphetamine intoxication. In: International Symposium on Amphetamines and Related Compounds. Costa, E. and Garattini, S., Eds., pp. 317-329. New York: Raven Press, 1970.

Lewander, T.: A mechanism for the development of tolerance to amphetamine in rats, Psychopharmacologia (Berl.) 21, 17-31 (1971).

Lewander, T.: Effect of chronic treatment with central stimulants on brain monoamines and some behavioural and physiological functions in rats, guinea pigs and rabbits. In: Neuropsychopharmacology of Monoamines and Their Regulatory Enzymes. Usdin, E., Ed., pp. 221-239. New York: Raven Press, 1974.

Lewander, T., Moliis, G., and Brus, I.: Mechanisms of tolerance to the hyperthermic effect of d- and l-amphetamine in rats. In: Neuropsychopharmacology. Boissier, J.R., Hippius, H., and Pichot, P., Eds., pp. 323-334. Amsterdam: Excerpta Medica Press, 1975.

McMenamy, R.H. and Oncley, J.L.: The specific binding of L-tryptophan to serum albumin, J. biol. Chem. 233, 1436-1447 (1958).

Panksepp, J. and Booth, D.A.: Tolerance to the depression of intake when amphetamine is added to the rat's food, Psychopharmacologia (Berl.) 29, 45-54 (1973).

Segal, D.S. and Mandell, A.J.: Long-term administration of d-amphetamine--progressive augmentation of motor activity and stereotypy, Pharmacol. Biochem. Behav. 2, 249-255 (1974).

Sever, P.S. and Caldwell, J.: Species differences in amphetamine tolerance, J. Pharmacologie (Paris) 5 (supplementum 2), 91 (1974).

Sever, P.S., Caldwell, J., and Williams, R.T.: Evidence against the involvement of the false neurotransmitters in tolerance to amphetamine-induced hyperthermia in the rat, J. Pharm. Pharmac. 26, 823-826 (1974).

Shapiro, S.L. and Freedman, L.: Effects of dosage level of amphetamine tartronate on weights of castrate rats, Arches int. Pharmacodyn. Thér. 112, 419-426 (1957).

Tagliamonte, A., Biggio, G., Vargiu, L., and Gessa, G.L.: Free tryptophan in serum controls brain tryptophan level and serotonin synthesis, Life Sci. 12, 277-287 (1973a).

Tagliamonte, A., Biggio, G., Vargiu, L., and Gessa, G.L.: Increase in brain tryptophan and stimulation of serotonin synthesis by salicylate, J. Neurochem. 20, 909-912 (1973b).

Tormey, J. and Lasagna, L.: Relation of thyroid function to acute and chronic effects of amphetamine in the rat, J. Pharmacol. exp. Ther. 128, 201-209 (1960).

COCAINE: DISTRIBUTION AND METABOLISM IN ANIMALS

Salvatore J. Mulé and Anand L. Misra

New York State ODAS Testing and Research Laboratory

Brooklyn, New York 11217

The abuse potential of cocaine primarily initiated through the intense euphoric effect of the drug with subsequent inducement of psychic dependence (Deneau, Yanagita, and Seevers, 1969) has prompted us to study the physiological disposition and metabolism of this drug in acutely- and chronically-treated animals. Although several reports have appeared in the literature (Woods, McMahon, and Seevers, 1951; Ortiz, 1966; Montesinos, 1965; Fish and Wilson, 1969), there is a paucity of data on the general pharmacodynamics of cocaine, especially in regards to disposition, metabolism, psychic dependence, tolerance, and the central mechanisms of action of this drug.

Earlier studies lacked adequate sensitivity (nanogram-picogram) to determine the levels of cocaine, especially in brain after days or weeks following drug usage. Also, there was little, if any, reliable data on the metabolism of cocaine in the acutely- and chronically-treated animal. In this report we present the data obtained through the use of highly sensitive radiochemical techniques on the disposition and metabolism of [^{3}H] cocaine in the rat and dog.

METHODS

The method for the preparation of [^{3}H] cocaine has been described (Nayak, Misra, Patel, and Mulé, 1974). Other essential details concerning radiochemical purity, sp. activity, method of estimation of [^{3}H] cocaine in biological materials, recoveries, specificity of the extraction, details on the acute and chronic animal experimental design, techniques for the identification of both brain and urinary metabolites of cocaine have previously been described (Nayak et al., 1974; Nayak, Misra, and Mulé, in press; Misra, Patel, Alluri, Mulé, and Nayak, submitted for publication; Misra, Pontani, and Mulé, 1973; Misra, Nayak, Patel, Vadlamani, and Mulé, 1974).

RESULTS

1. Rat

a. Tissue and plasma studies. The data obtained on the distribution of [^{3}H] cocaine in acutely- and chronically-treated rats appear in Tables 1 and 2. In acute animals peak levels of drug were observed at 4 hr, except for the heart which peaked at 0.5 hr. An abrupt fall in drug occurred between 4-6 hrs, resulting in very low levels in brain, testes, and plasma and the absence of cocaine in these tissues and plasma at 24 hr. The T 1/2 of cocaine in brain and plasma was 4.8 and 5.0 hrs, respectively.

In chronically-treated rats peak levels of drug were observed between 1 and 2 hours. The levels of cocaine were lower in the chronically-treated animals as compared to the acute group or there was a faster disappearance of cocaine from the tissues and plasma. Significant detectable levels of cocaine were observed through 48 hrs, except for plasma. Thus, even 4 weeks after [^{3}H] cocaine, levels of this drug were observed in brain and especially fat tissue. The T 1/2 for cocaine in brain and plasma of chronically-treated rats was 3.8 and 2.9 hrs, respectively.

b. Urinary and fecal excretion. The results obtained on the percentage of free cocaine and total radioactivity in urine and feces observed over a period of 7 days in acutely- and chronically-treated rats appears in Table 3. Less than 1% of free cocaine was excreted in either urine or feces of the acutely- or chronically-treated rat. Similar levels of total radioactivity (free cocaine plus metabolites) were observed in the urine of both acute and chronic animals (49-52%). However, significantly higher levels of total radioactivity were observed in the feces of the chronic animals as compared to the acute. Cumulative total radioactivity excreted in urine and feces was higher in the chronically-treated rats (87.5%) as compared to the acute group (71.4%).

c. Urinary metabolites. Column and thin layer chromatographic techniques and methods provided a comparative profile of known and probable metabolites of cocaine. Benzoylecgonine (11.6% in acute and 14.6% in chronic animals); benzoylnorecgonine (0.7% acute and 0.4% chronic); ecgonine (2.0% acute and 1.4% chronic); ecgonine methyl ester (0.6% acute and 8.7% chronic). Norcocaine and norecgonine were not found in urine; neither were glucuronide sulfate or amino acid conjugates. Suggestive evidence for the presence of a phenolic metabolite and other hydroxylated polar non-phenolic metabolites was obtained.

TABLE 1

DISTRIBUTION OF [^{3}H] COCAINE AFTER A SINGLE SUBCUTANEOUS INJECTION OF 20 mg/kg (FREE BASE) IN RATS

Tissue or Fluid	ACUTE (ng/g or ml)				
	1 h	2 h	4 h	6 h	24 h
Brain	2320 ± 205	2963 ± 195	3439 ± 362	485 ± 194	0
Kidney	4330 ± 252	5204 ± 476	6456 ± 384	765 ± 347	45 ± 11
Lung	4526 ± 383	4318 ± 268	6348 ± 827	1147 ± 436	41 ± 2
Spleen	2720 ± 241	3881 ± 435	4319 ± 373	718 ± 274	46 ± 1
Fat	1624 ± 226	3232 ± 637	2528 ± 194	428 ± 103	32 ± 9
Testes	1976 ± 252	2987 ± 209	3849 ± 333	1170 ± 275	0
Intestine	2247 ± 515	2865 ± 387	3401 ± 379	556 ± 188	10 ± 2
Muscle	978 ± 61	1340 ± 175	1475 ± 185	255 ± 78	2 ± 1
Liver	727 ± 86	927 ± 187	1352 ± 221	272 ± 66	61 ± 2
Heart	1465 ± 184	1246 ± 101	1059 ± 119	281 ± 105	8 ± 1
Plasma	378 ± 31	448 ± 74	494 ± 59	78 ± 35	0

TABLE 2

DISTRIBUTION OF [^{3}H] COCAINE IN CHRONICALLY-TREATED RATS AFTER SUBCUTANEOUS INJECTIONS OF 20 mg/kg (FREE BASE) IN RATS[1]

Tissue or Fluid	CHRONIC (ng/g or ml)						
	1 h	2 h	4 h	12 h	24 h	96 h	4 w
Brain	2408 ± 271	3046 ± 136	1788 ± 221	76 ± 32	26 ± 1	22 ± 3	16 ± 1
Kidney	4718 ± 659	5592 ± 402	3323 ± 416	481 ± 26	415 ± 11	80 ± 11	16 ± 2
Lung	6852 ± 1802	5838 ± 684	3287 ± 412	430 ± 115	220 ± 13	141 ± 52	6 ± 1
Spleen	5223 ± 492	5363 ± 372	4017 ± 542	555 ± 56	404 ± 18	133 ± 23	0
Fat	3494 ± 497	6102 ± 2244	3601 ± 297	2388 ± 131	1243 ± 212	655 ± 79	180 ± 32
Testes	1869 ± 100	2573 ± 184	1951 ± 321	39 ± 6	29 ± 3	23 ± 4	7 ± 1
Intestine	2375 ± 346	2957 ± 295	1174 ± 323	115 ± 13	55 ± 4	41 ± 12	9 ± 7
Muscle	876 ± 74	1279 ± 100	790 ± 76	223 ± 70	65 ± 15	41 ± 5	0
Liver	1045 ± 178	1250 ± 120	1196 ± 172	428 ± 28	283 ± 20	65 ± 3	0
Heart	1563 ± 370	1801 ± 137	1037 ± 93	84 ± 3	44 ± 2	8 ± 4	0
Plasma	502 ± 100	377 ± 81	208 ± 24	10 ± 1	6 ± 0	0	-

1. The rats were given 20 mg/kg s.c. injections twice daily for 21 days, then the same dose of ^{3}H-cocaine by the same schedule for five consecutive injections.

TABLE 3

URINARY AND FECAL EXCRETION OF FREE ^{3}H-COCAINE AND TOTAL RADIOACTIVITY AFTER SUBCUTANEOUS INJECTION OF 20 mg/kg (FREE BASE) IN ACUTELY- AND CHRONICALLY-TREATED MALE RATS

	Mean Percentage of Excreted Drug	
	0-24 h	Total
ACUTE		
Free cocaine (urine)	0.8	0.9
Free cocaine (feces)	0.1	0.3
Total radioactivity (urine)	41.6	49.3
Total radioactivity (feces)	14.7	22.1
CHRONIC[1]		
Free cocaine (urine)	0.5	0.6
Free cocaine (feces)	0.5	0.9
Total radioactivity (urine)	41.3	51.6
Total radioactivity (feces)	26.2	35.9

1. Treated as in Table 2. Biological material was collected over a period of seven days.

2. Dog

a. Tissue and plasma studies. The distribution of free cocaine in tissues and plasma of the acutely- and chronically-treated dogs is given in Tables 4 and 5. In general, the values of cocaine in the tissues and plasma were higher in the chronic animals as compared to the acute. Cocaine disappearance from bile was faster from the chronically-treated dogs 4 hours after the dose in comparison to the acute. Cocaine was not present in plasma by 12 hrs in either the acutely- or chronically-treated dogs. By 24 hrs, there were extremely low levels of the drug in all tissues except for the liver and bile and cocaine was still detectable 7 days later (19-83 ng/g or ml) in both the acute and chronic animals. Significant high levels of total radioactivity were present in all tissues and plasma 7 days after drug administration in both groups. The half-lives for cocaine in plasma and liver in the acute and chronic groups were 1.2 and 1.0 and 2.2 and 1.8, respectively.

b. CNS distribution of cocaine. In Tables 6 and 7 appear the data obtained on the distribution of cocaine. The concentration of cocaine in general was higher in the chronic animals as compared to the acute in all CNS areas. Essentially, complete disappearance of free cocaine from the CNS occurred by 24 hrs after drug administration. Significant levels of total radioactivity were observed in the CNS 7 days after drug administration in both groups. The half-lives of free cocaine in selected areas of CNS for acute dogs ranged between 1.5-1.6 hrs and in the chronic group were 1.2-1.5 hrs.

c. Urinary and fecal excretion. The results obtained on the urinary and fecal excretion of free cocaine and total radioactivity in urine and feces appear in Table 8. The quantity of free cocaine excreted in the urine over a period of 7 days in the acute dogs was 0.9-5.0% and in the chronic dogs, 2.2-3.3%. In the feces 1.1-1.6% and 0.2-0.3% were excreted in the acute and chronic dog, respectively. The excretion of total radioactivity occurred primarily in urine during the 0-24 hr period and continued for several days. The values of urine for 7 days of the acute dog (48.3-49.1%) were somewhat less than that observed for the chronic (59.1-60.0%). In feces the total radioactivity during a 7 day period ranged from 13.0-20.4% in the acute and 5.4-5.7% in the chronic dog.

d. Cocaine metabolites in brain and urine. (a) Brain--Norcocaine, benzoylecgonine, benzoylnorecgonine, and ecgonine were found as metabolites of cocaine in the acutely- and chronically-treated dogs. The quantity of norcocaine in brain at various intervals in the chronic dogs was considerably higher than in the acute group

TABLE 4

DISTRIBUTION OF [^{3}H] COCAINE IN VARIOUS TISSUES AND FLUIDS OF THE DOG AFTER A SINGLE 5 mg/kg^{-1} (FREE BASE) INTRAVENOUS INJECTION OF THE DRUG[1]

Tissues and Fluids	(ng/g or ml) 1 h	2 h	4 h	12 h	24 h
Bile	15438	17855	21206	15339	9979
Liver	8598	3300	871	254	232
Kidney	4210	1408	679	62	35
Lungs	3482	1462	492	80	43
Spleen	4318	1496	499	91	41
Small Intestine	1631	654	252	83	14
Duodenum	1982	871	627	36	8
Fat	2061	1540	396	29	8
Heart	1569	534	182	32	18
Muscle	1460	483	146	7	0
Plasma	460	124	38	0	0

1. Two dogs were sacrificed at each time interval. The data represent mean values.

TABLE 5

DISTRIBUTION OF [^{3}H] COCAINE IN VARIOUS TISSUES AND FLUIDS OF CHRONICALLY-TREATED DOGS AFTER A 5 mg/kg (FREE BASE) INTRAVENOUS INJECTION OF THE DRUG[1]

Tissues and Fluids	(ng/g or ml) 1 h	2 h	4 h	6 h	24 h
Bile	8669	39113	38244	10963	5780
Liver	6171	2059	1458	872	316
Kidney	5200	2224	1138	307	87
Lungs	4887	1419	1143	316	126
Spleen	6901	2603	1220	451	187
Small Intestine	2155	1008	739	139	19
Duodenum	2056	1399	749	168	19
Fat	2202	1812	687	220	43
Heart	2745	839	351	163	58
Muscle	1644	742	271	78	9
Plasma	563	310	92	24	0

1. Beagle dogs were subcutaneously injected with a 5 mg/kg dose of nonradioactive cocaine twice daily for 6 weeks, then with a 5 mg/kg s.c. dose of randomly labeled [^{3}H] cocaine twice daily for two days followed by a terminal injection of the same dose by i.v. route. Two dogs were sacrificed at each time interval, except 6 and 24 hrs., at which time one animal each was used.

TABLE 6

DISTRIBUTION OF [^{3}H] COCAINE IN SELECTED TISSUES OF THE CNS OF THE DOG AFTER A SINGLE 5 mg/kg^{-1} (FREE BASE) INTRAVENOUS INJECTION OF THE DRUG[1]

Selected tissues of the CNS	(ng/g or ml ± SEM) 0.5 h	1 h	2 h	4 h	12 h	24 h
Temporal Cortex (gray)	4505 ± 660	2705	1027	308	18	2
Temporal Cortex (white)	4918 ± 639	2688	1147	296	17	2
Cerebellum	3522 ± 639	2184	808	238	15	2
Spinal Cord	4164 ± 628	2442	1229	390	17	4
Hypothalamus	3800 ± 571	2098	832	276	14	6
Thalamus	4208 ± 559	2457	912	279	17	2
Medulla	3751 ± 495	2203	899	267	15	4
Pons	3993 ± 507	2258	949	266	15	1
Mesencephalon	3671 ± 667	2107	833	273	15	2
Caudate Nucleus	4285 ± 551	2442	1184	355	22	4
Cerebrospinal Fluid	1069	570	244	30	0	0

1. Two dogs were sacrificed at each time interval. Data represent mean values.

TABLE 7

DISTRIBUTION OF [^{3}H] COCAINE IN SELECTED TISSUES OF THE CNS OF CHRONICALLY-TREATED DOGS AFTER A 5 mg/kg (FREE BASE) INTRAVENOUS INJECTION OF THE DRUG[1]

Selected tissues of the CNS	(ng/g or ml)					
	0.5 h	1 h	2 h	4 h	6 h	24 h
Temporal Cortex (gray)	5935	3172	1260	480	205	11
Temporal Cortex (white)	5696	3060	1351	490	200	6
Cerebellum	4916	2448	1037	417	162	6
Spinal Cord	4335	2741	1538	611	314	8
Hypothalamus	4652	2646	1040	431	162	11
Thalamus	5359	2947	1216	462	189	8
Medulla	4547	2590	1151	426	209	7
Pons	4727	2563	1353	478	188	7
Mesencephalon	4491	2549	1090	428	185	8
Caudate Nucleus	5110	3473	1368	517	245	13
Cerebrospinal Fluid	925	425	228	76	24	0

1. As in Table 5.

TABLE 8

URINARY AND FECAL EXCRETION[1] OF FREE COCAINE AND TOTAL RADIOACTIVITY AFTER INTRAVENOUS INJECTION OF 5 mg/kg (FREE BASE) [^{3}H] COCAINE IN ACUTELY- AND CHRONICALLY-TREATED DOGS[2]

		Mean percentage of dose excreted				
		0-24 hr	24-28 hr	48-72 hr	3-7 days	Total
ACUTE						
Free cocaine in urine	(A)	0.9	0	0	---	0.9
	(B)	5.0	0	0	---	5.0
Free cocaine in feces	(A)	1.1	0.3	0.1	0.1	1.6
	(B)	0	0.8	0.1	0.2	1.1
Total radio-activity in urine	(A)	44.2	2.2	1.1	1.6	49.1
	(B)	41.6	4.4	1.3	1.0	48.3
Total radio-activity in feces	(A)	13.7	2.4	1.6	2.7	20.4
	(B)	0	10.5	0.8	1.7	13.0
CHRONIC						
Free cocaine in urine	(A)	2.2	0	0	---	2.2
	(B)	3.3	0	0	---	3.3
Free cocaine in feces	(A)	0.2	0	0	---	0.2
	(B)	0.3	0	0	---	0.3
Total radio-activity in urine	(A)	55.8	1.6	0.7	1.0	59.1
	(B)	55.9	2.5	0.8	0.8	60.0
Total radio-activity in feces	(A)	4.8	0.5	0.2	0.2	5.7
	(B)	3.5	1.3	0.2	0.4	5.4

1. Data represent mean values obtained from two female beagle dogs A and B.

2. Beagle dogs were subcutaneously injected with a 5 mg/kg dose of nonradioactive cocaine twice daily for six weeks, then with 5 mg/kg i.v. dose of ring-labeled [^{3}H] cocaine.

although the rate of disappearance of norcocaine was similar. Neither cocaine nor norcocaine persisted in the CNS of acute or chronic dogs. Benzoylecgonine and benzoylnorecgonine were present in the CNS of chronic dogs one week after a 5 mg/kg i.v. injection. (b) Urine--The metabolites of cocaine identified in urine of both acutely- and chronically-treated dogs were: norcocaine, benzoylecgonine, benzoylnorecgonine, norecgonine, ecgonine methyl ester, and ecgonine. Benzoylnorecgonine and ecgonine were excreted in higher amounts in the acute (9.1 and 37.1%) as compared to the chronic (6.9 and 33%). Benzoylecgonine and norecgonine were lower in the acute (2.5, 0.9%) in comparison to the chronic (3.8, 2.2%). No differences were observed in the excretion of norcocaine (0.8%) and the methyl ester of ecgonine (0.1%) between the two groups.

DISCUSSION

Due to the extremely low levels of cocaine in biological materials, a very sensitive method was developed that allowed the detection of 1 ng of [^{3}H] cocaine.

After a 10 mg/kg i.v. convulsive dose of cocaine, the concentration of free cocaine in rat brain and plasma within 1-2 min of the convulsions was 35 μg and 5 μg/ml, respectively. Norcocaine was observed as a metabolite during the convulsions (Misra et al., 1974). The metabolites norcocaine, benzoylecgonine, and benzoylnorecgonine were shown to have pharmacological activity (Misra, Nayak, and Mulé, 1975) after intracisternal injection in the rat. Following systemic injection (200 ng/kg), benzoylecgonine and benzoylnorecgonine were not active. Lipid solubility and permeability through the blood-brain barrier play an important role in the pharmacological action of cocaine and metabolites.

The chronically-treated rats were given consecutive, labeled cocaine injections after non-labeled cocaine in order to label free drug or metabolites in tissues. A single, labeled injection of cocaine in the chronic animals would not furnish the total value of drug in the biological material. A significant reduction in the half-lives of chronically-treated rats occurred in brain and plasma as compared to the acute. This suggests a faster rate of metabolism of cocaine in the chronic group.

The presence of drug in the brains of chronic rats several weeks after administration of labeled cocaine may not be due solely to free cocaine. It is possible that such polar metabolites as benzoylecgonine, benzoylnorecgonine, ecgonine, and norcocaine may be present in brain at later time intervals. This may be due to the relatively slow clearance of these metabolites from tissues.

The metabolites identified in the rat study were benzoylecgonine, benzoylnorecgonine, ecgonine methyl ester, and ecgonine. Norcocaine was detected in rat brain but not in urine, probably due to further metabolism to benzoylnorecgonine. In the rat a higher excretion of benzoylecgonine and ecgonine methyl ester was observed in the chronic group as compared to the acute. In addition to these metabolites, suggestive evidence for the presence of phenolic and hydroxylated metabolites was obtained. No evidence for the presence of glucuronide conjugates of the hydroxylated metabolites was obtained. Comparatively higher levels of total radioactivity, which includes free cocaine and metabolites, were present in the bile and tissues of dogs; and, although this persisted for at least 1 week in acute and chronic dogs, no accumulation occurred in the tissues of the chronic dogs. Cocaine did not persist in plasma or selected areas of the CNS of acutely and chronically-treated dogs. The level of cocaine in the CNS of dogs in two groups coincided with the changes in plasma, suggesting fairly rapid and easily reversible binding to the cell structure.

Norcocaine was observed in the brains of dogs at higher levels 6 hrs after injection in the chronic dogs as compared to the acute. Benzoylecgonine, benzoylnorecgonine, and ecgonine were also observed in the brains of acutely- and chronically-treated dogs. At 1 week post injection, only benzoylecgonine and benzoylnorecgonine were detectable.

Cocaine is rapidly metabolized in dog and only a small fraction of the dose is excreted free in urine and feces. Higher total radioactivity values in the urine of chronic dogs indicated rapid elimination of cocaine metabolites. The polar nature of the unidentified metabolites was indicated in partition characteristic studies.

Hypothetically, cocaine may act partially through a displacement of neuronal membrane-bound Ca^{++} which may conceivably cause a conformational change in membrane proteins leading to alterations in Na^{+} and K^{+} permeability and depolarization of the membrane. Simultaneously, a reduction in Ca^{++} binding sites on membrane protein could also affect the release of neurotransmitters.

ACKNOWLEDGMENTS

The authors are grateful for the excellent technical assistance of Drs. Nayak and Giri and Messrs. Patel and Alluri. The research was supported in part by USAMRDC Contract DADA-17-73-C-3080.

REFERENCES

Deneau, G.A., Yanagita, Y., and Seevers, M.H.: Self-administration of psychoactive substances by the monkey--a measure of psychological dependence, Psychopharmacologia 16:30-48 (1969).

Fish, F. and Wilson, W.D.C.: Excretion of cocaine and its metabolites in man, J. Pharm. Pharmacol. 21:135S-138S (1969).

Misra, A.L., Pontani, R.B., and Mulé, S.J.: Separation of cocaine, some of its metabolites and congeners on glass-fibre sheets, J. Chromat. 81:167-169 (1973).

Misra, A.L., Nayak, P.K., Patel, M.N., Vadlamani, N.L., and Mulé, S.J.: Identification of norcocaine as a metabolite of [^{3}H] cocaine in rat brain, Experientia 30:1312-1314 (1974)

Misra, A.L., Nayak, P.K., Bloch, R., and Mulé, S.J.: Estimation and disposition of [^{3}H] benzoylecgonine and pharmacological activity of some cocaine metabolites, J. Pharm. Pharmacol. 27: 784-786 (1975).

Misra, A.L., Patel, M.A., Alluri, V.R., Mulé, S.J., and Nayak, P.K.: Disposition, metabolism and regional brain distribution of [^{3}H] cocaine in acute and chronically-treated dogs, Xenobiotica (submitted for publication).

Montesinos, F.: Metabolism of cocaine, Bull. Narc. (U.N.) 17:11-17 (1965).

Nayak, P.K., Misra, A.L., Patel, M.N., and Mulé, S.J.: Preparation of radiochemically pure randomly-labeled and ring-labeled [^{3}H] cocaine, Radiochem. Radioanal. Letters 16:167-171 (1974).

Nayak, P.K., Misra, A.L., and Mulé, S.J.: Physiological disposition and biotransformation of [^{3}H] cocaine in acute and chronically-treated rats, J. Pharmacol. exp. Ther. (in press, 1976).

Ortiz, R.V.: Distribution and metabolism of cocaine in the rat, An. Fac. Quim. Farm. (U. of Chile) 18:15-19 (1966).

Woods, L.A., McMahon, F.G., and Seevers, M.H.: Disposition and metabolism of cocaine in the dog and rabbit, J. Pharmacol. exp. Ther. 101:200-204 (1951).

BEHAVIORAL EFFECTS OF COCAINE--METABOLIC AND NEUROCHEMICAL APPROACH

Beng T. Ho, Dorothy L. Taylor, Vicente S. Estevez,

Leo F. Englert and Mary L. McKenna

Texas Research Institute of Mental Sciences

Houston, Texas

Cocaine is known to be a local anesthetic and a potent CNS stimulant. Several reports indicate an increase in locomotor activity with low acute doses of the drug, and involvement of brain amines in this psychomotor stimulation has been proposed (Van Zwieten, Widhalm, and Hertting, 1965; Groppetti, 1974).

Although it is generally accepted that brain catecholamines are implicated in the central action of stimulant drugs, reports are conflicting as to whether norepinephrine (NE) or dopamine (DA) or both are involved in specific behavioral changes. It also has been suggested that stereotyped behavior as shown by d-amphetamine is related to the dopaminergic system, whereas locomotor activity involves the noradrenergic system (Randrup and Scheel-Krüger, 1966; Coyle and Snyder, 1969). Other reports indicate that cocaine, and possibly amphetamine, decreases the rate of synthesis and turnover of serotonin (5-HT) (Schubert, Fyrö, Nybäck and Sedvall, 1970). It appears, therefore, that stimulant drugs affect not only brain catecholamines but also the neurotransmitter 5-HT.

There are conflicting reports as to whether tolerance is developed to cocaine (Caldwell and Sever, 1974; Kosman and Unna, 1968). Some evidence of a pronounced increase in the intensity of toxic reactions with repeated daily administration has been reported (Downs and Eddy, 1932; Gutierrez-Noriega, 1944; Post, 1975). Studies on tolerance to cocaine currently in progress in our laboratory also revealed an initial excitation period resulting from daily administration of cocaine.

The purpose of the present studies was to correlate neurochemical and metabolic changes associated with the behavioral effects of cocaine during this excitation period.

METHOD

Spontaneous Locomotor Activity Measurement

Spontaneous locomotor activity was measured using a Motron electronic motility cage. Movement of animals across the floor of the cage interrupted light paths from overhead infrared lamps to photo cells located under the floor and was registered as number of counts. Sixteen male Sprague-Dawley rats, weighing 200-250 g, were injected for the first three days with saline to assure stabilization of locomotor activity. Thereafter, eight of the animals were injected with cocaine hydrochloride (10 mg/kg, i.p.) in saline, while the eight control animals received daily administration of saline. Every other day, motor activity was measured immediately following injection for 30 min.

Discrimination Studies

Five two-lever sound-insulated operant chambers (Scientific Prototype Model PLS-100) programmed with solid state equipment (Grason-Stadler 1200 series) were used for behavioral training and testing. Male Sprague-Dawley rats (350-450 g) were trained to perform a differential reinforcement of low response rate (DRL), 15 sec schedule for a food reward. Reward was contingent upon correct lever choices to the induced differential cue conditions of cocaine hydrochloride (10 mg/kg, i.p.) or saline. Upon acquisition of discriminative response control all animals responded more than 80% on the correct lever during a 15-min extinction test in which the reinforcement was terminated. Details of the procedure have been previously published (Huang and Ho, 1974; Browne, Harris and Ho, 1974).

Having attained a stabilized percentage correct response, a group of six animals were pretreated with pimozide (1 mg/kg, i.p.) in 30% propylene glycol 4 hr prior to the administration of 5 mg/kg of cocaine. Animals receiving pimozide plus cocaine were compared in performance with one group of four animals receiving 5 mg/kg of cocaine alone and one group of seven animals receiving first pimozide then saline.

Metabolic Studies

Sixteen rats were injected daily for six days with cocaine hydrochloride (10 mg/kg, i.p.), while a group of the same number of rats received only saline. On the seventh day all animals received a final injection of 10 mg/kg of N-^{14}C-labeled cocaine hydrochloride (8.7 μCi/mg) and were sacrificed at 5, 15, 45, and 60 min intervals. Brain was homogenized in nine volumes of water; aliquots of the homogenate were assayed in Insta Gel (Packard Co.) for radioactivity by liquid scintillation spectrometry. Blood was first decolorized with ten per cent hydrogen peroxide in methanol, then digested in 1N sodium hydroxide at 70°C for 2 hr. After neutralization with 2-ethyl-hexanoic acid and the addition of Insta Gel, the radioactivity was determined. For chromatography, blood and the brain homogenates were extracted four times with methanol. The methanol extracts were evaporated to dryness and the residue was redissolved in a very small amount of the solvent. After centrifugation, the supernatant was applied on precoated TLC sheets (E. Merck Co.) containing Silica Gel F-254 and chromatographed in ethyl acetate/methanol/25% ammonium hydroxide (20:1.5:1) against reference compounds; Rf of cocaine was 0.91. Sections of 1x1 cm^2 of the chromatogram were then assayed for radioactivity.

Neurochemical Studies

Male Sprague-Dawley rats, weighing 150-175 g, were injected daily with a dose of 10 mg/kg cocaine hydrochloride and sacrificed by decapitation 24 hr after the last injection; the specific brain areas were pooled from three rats and homogenized in 0.4N perchloric acid. The isolation procedure of Anton and Sayre (1962) was followed. NE was oxidized by the method of Laverty and Taylor (1968) and DA was oxidized according to Schellenberger and Gordon (1971). 5-HT in both brainstem and septum/caudate was measured by pooling tissues from two rats and following the procedure of Curzon and Green (1970). Tyrosine hydroxylase activity was determined in the striatum and hypothalamus/thalamus by a coupled reaction of hydroxylase and decarboxylase using L-tyrosine-^{14}C (U) as substrate (Waymire, Bjur, and Weiner, 1971); the product was ^{14}C-DA/mg tissue/hr. For the measurement of tryptophan hydroxylase activity, the cerebellum, medulla, and cortex were dissected from the whole brain, and the remaining subcortical area was homogenized in five volumes of 0.32M sucrose. After centrifuging for 20 min, the supernatant was separated and the particulate fraction resuspended in three ml of 0.05M phosphate buffer, pH 7.4. The enzyme was assayed by hydroxylation of the substrate, L-tryptophan-3-^{14}C, using the procedure of Lovenberg, Jequier and Sjoerdsma (1967), then coupled with decarboxylation as described by Waymire et al. (1971). ^{14}C-5-HT was separated by the method of McCaman, McCaman, and Lees (1972) and the enzyme activity calculated as n mole ^{14}C-5-HT/mg protein/hr.

RESULTS AND DISCUSSION

In the course of studying the change in spontaneous locomotor activity of rats with daily administration of cocaine (10 mg/kg, i.p.), a continuous increase in the motor activity was observed for about 7 days, after which time this increase was no longer seen following the administration of the drug through 45 days (Fig. 1). The initial excitation period was examined to determine the levels of unchanged labeled cocaine by TLC in animals receiving daily injection of cocaine for 6 days followed by a final injection of N-$^{14}CH_3$-cocaine. Corresponding with the peak of motor activity, which occurs 5 to 10 min post-injection, there were increases of 127 and 40% in unchanged cocaine in the blood and brain, respectively, at 5 min compared to control animals injected daily with saline (Table 1).

Preliminary data showed that the half-life of unchanged cocaine in the brain of animals receiving repeated injections of cocaine was shorter than that of the saline animals following an acute injection of the drug (Fig. 2). It is suggested that, although cocaine is metabolized faster in animals injected repeatedly with cocaine compared to an acute injection, the continuous accumulation of the unchanged drug in tissues and fluids may account for the linear increase of motor activity observed in the period of 7 days (Fig. 1).

TABLE 1

Levels of unchanged ^{14}C-cocaine in the brain and blood of rats receiving repeated administration of unlabeled cocaine (repeated) or saline (acute)

TIME (MIN)		UNCHANGED COCAINE	
		Blood (n mole/ml)	Brain (n mole/g)
5	Acute:	1.40 ± 0.04	6.15 ± 0.13
	Repeated:	3.55 ± 0.06 $p < 0.001$	8.75 ± 0.26 $p < 0.001$
15	Acute:	0.78 ± 0.03	5.17 ± 0.07
	Repeated:	0.83 ± 0.03 N.S.	6.08 ± 0.19 $p < 0.01$

Each value represents the mean (± S.E.M.) of 4 rats.

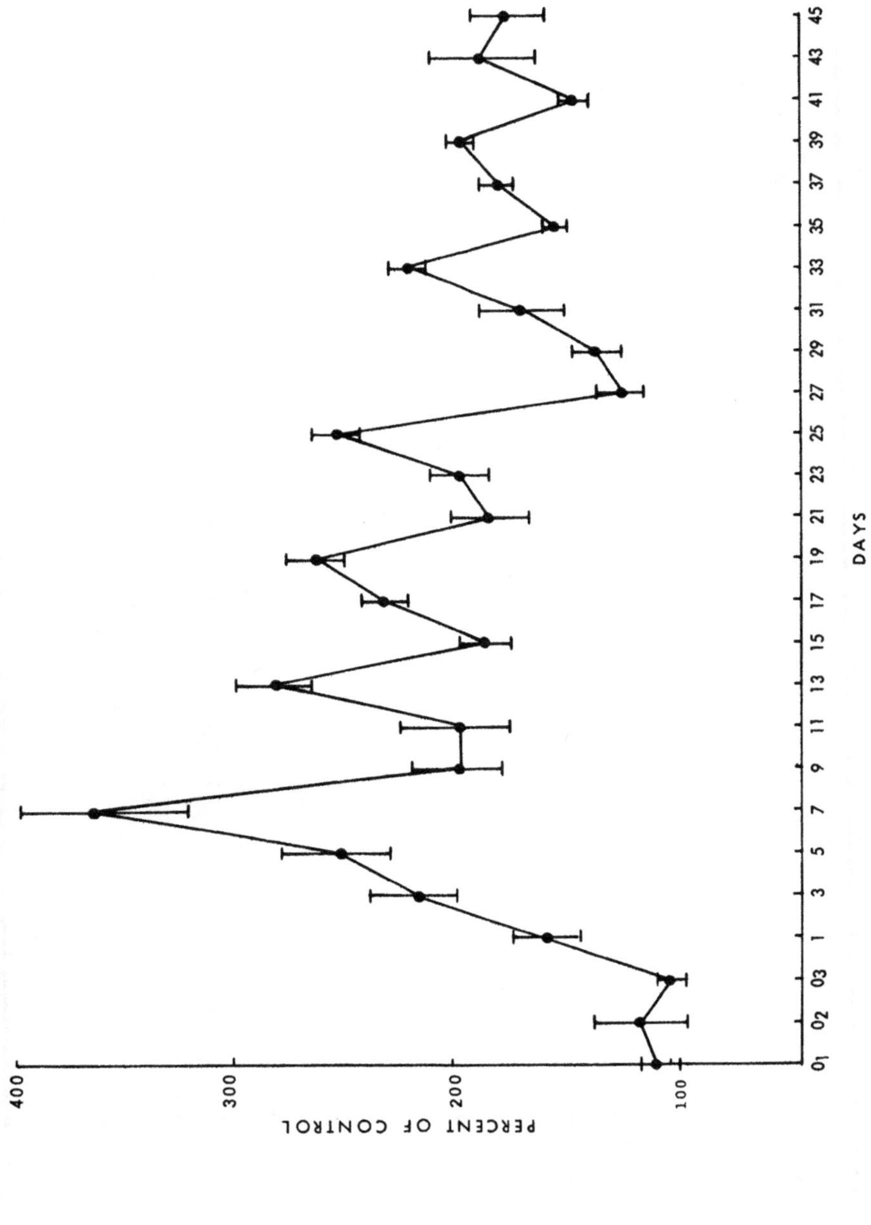

Fig. 1. Spontaneous locomotor activity of rats receiving daily injections (10 mg/kg, i.p.) of cocaine hydrochloride.

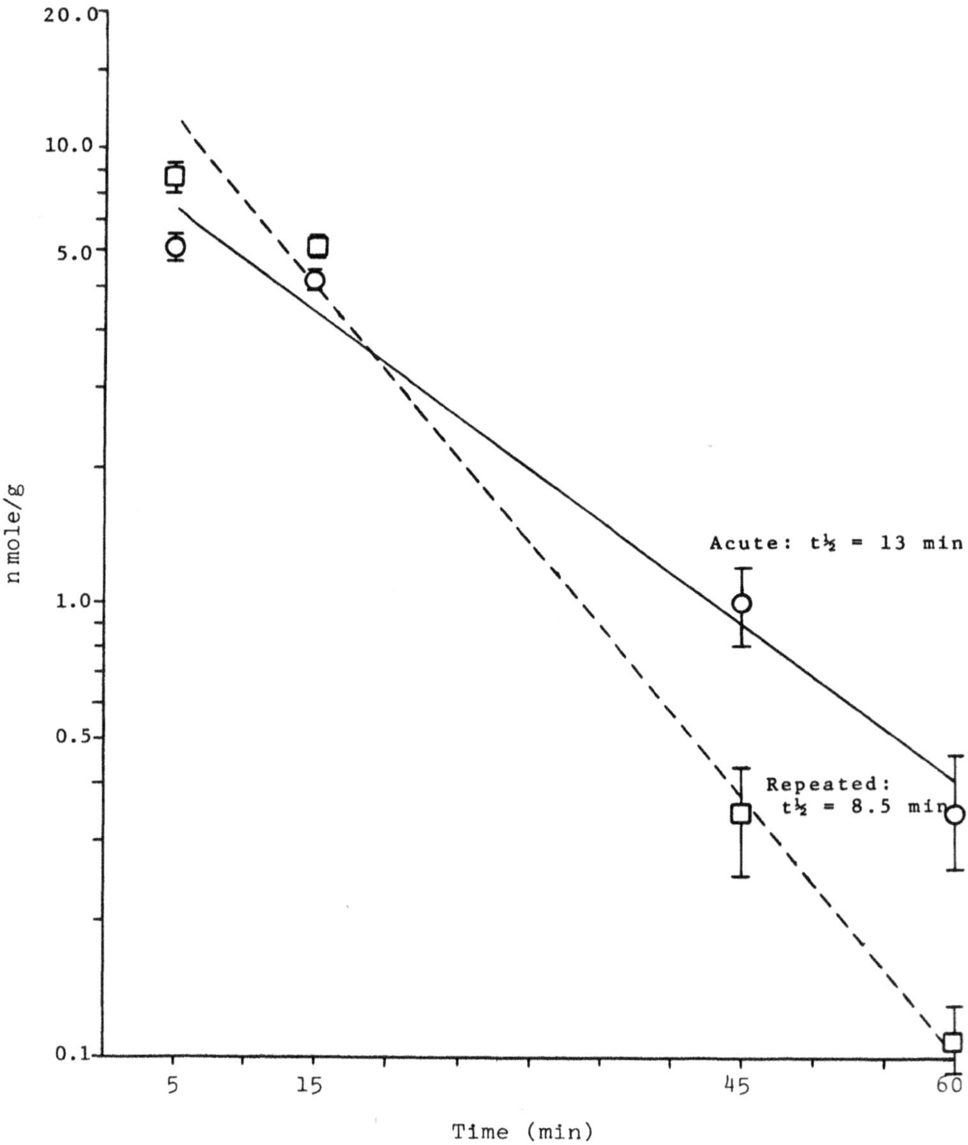

Fig. 2. Determination of half-life of unchanged ^{14}C-cocaine in the brain of rats receiving repeated doses of unlabeled cocaine. (□- - - -□) or saline (○——○).

Repeated administration of cocaine significantly reduced (36%) the concentration of norepinephrine (NE) in the hypothalamus/thalamus area (Table 2). A concomitant increase (25%) in normetanephrine (NM), although not statistically significant, would indicate an increase in the turnover of NE (a decrease in NE/NM ratio) caused by the drug. A similar change was observed for striatal dopamine (DA) in the same animals (Table 3). The increase of tyrosine hydroxylase activity in both the striatal and hypothalamic areas (Table 4) may be due to a decrease in concentrations of catecholamines; it is believed that the biosynthesis of intraneuronal catecholamines is regulated by "product-feedback" inhibition. Following repeated administration of cocaine, concentrations of 5-hydroxytryptamine (5-HT) in both brainstem and septum/caudate areas significantly diminished by 14 and 18%, respectively (Table 5). In addition, the activity of soluble tryptophan hydroxylase from the subcortical structures was substantially reduced in cocaine-treated animals (Table 6). It is conceivable that the behavioral effects of cocaine following repeated injections are partly due to a direct stimulation of central 5-HT receptors, which, through a neuronal feedback mechanism, reduces the activity of the biosynthetic enzyme in the presynaptic cells and, consequently, decreases the concentration of 5-HT.

TABLE 2

Effects of repeated administration of cocaine on the levels of rat brain norepinephrine (NE) and normetanephrine (NM)

TREATMENT	HYPOTHALAMUS/THALAMUS		RATIO
	NE (μg/g)	NM (μg/g)	NE/NM
Controls	1.75 ± 0.14	0.61 ± 0.04	2.9
Cocaine (10 mg/kg, 7 days)	1.12 ± 0.05*	0.76 ± 0.10	1.5

Each value represents the mean (±S.E.M.) of 6 samples (3 rats per sample)

*$p < 0.01$

TABLE 3

Effects of repeated administration of cocaine on the levels of rat brain dopamine (DA) and homovanillic acid (HVA)

TREATMENT	STRIATUM DA (μg/g)	STRIATUM HVA (μg/g)	RATIO DA/HVA
Controls	6.12 ± 0.36	2.10 ± 0.15	2.9
Cocaine (10 mg/kg, 7 days)	5.09 ± 0.40	2.50 ± 0.14	2.0

Each value represents the mean (± S.E.M.) of 6 samples (3 rats per sample)

TABLE 4

Effects of repeated administration of cocaine on tyrosine hydroxylase activity

	TYROSINE HYDROXYLASE (n mole/mg tissue/hr)	
	STRIATUM	HYPOTHALAMUS-THALAMUS
Controls	0.828 ± 0.048	0.676 ± 0.059
Cocaine (10 mg/kg, 5 days)	1.19 ± 0.088*	1.39 ± 0.078**

Each value represents the mean (±S.E.M.) of duplicate determination from 3 samples (2 rats per sample)

*$p < 0.01$
**$p < 0.001$

TABLE 5

Effects of repeated administration of cocaine on the levels of rat brain 5-hydroxytryptamine (5-HT) and 5-hydroxyindoleacetic acid (5-HIAA)

TREATMENT	SEPTUM/CAUDATE 5-HT (μg/g)	SEPTUM/CAUDATE 5-HIAA (μg/g)	RATIO 5-HT/5-HIAA
Controls	1.40 ± 0.04	0.58 ± 0.03	2.4
Cocaine (10 mg/kg, 7 days)	1.21 ± 0.04*	0.50 ± 0.02†	2.4
	BRAINSTEM		
Controls	1.28 ± 0.04	0.75 ± 0.04	1.7
Cocaine (10 mg/kg, 7 days)	1.05 ± 0.04*	0.75 ± 0.01	1.4

Each value from septum/caudate area represents the mean (±S.E.M.) of 10 samples (2 rats per sample) and that from brainstem 10 samples (one rat per sample)

*$p < 0.01$
†$p < 0.05$

TABLE 6

Effects of repeated administration of cocaine on subcortical tryptophan hydroxylase activity

TREATMENT	TRYPTOPHAN HYDROXYLASE PARTICULATE (n mole/mg protein/hr)	TRYPTOPHAN HYDROXYLASE SOLUBLE (n mole/ml/hr)
Controls	0.165 ± 0.037	0.621 ± 0.077
Cocaine (10 mg/kg, 5 days)	0.156 ± 0.029	0.332 ± 0.053*

Each value represents the mean (±S.E.M.) of duplicate determinations from each of 6 rats

*p < 0.02

In discrimination studies, rats were trained to discriminate 10 mg/kg of cocaine vs. saline. A lower dose (5 mg/kg) of cocaine was shown to produce generalization (over 96%) to the cue produced by the training dose (Table 7). Pretreatment with pimozide, a dopamine receptor blocker, blocked the ability of animals to perform cocaine lever responding. These results thus indicate dopamine is involved in the cocaine-induced discriminative behavior.

TABLE 7

Effects of pimozide on the discriminative stimulus property of cocaine

	DOSE (mg/kg)	% COCAINE LEVER CHOICE 5 min	% COCAINE LEVER CHOICE 10 min
Pimozide + cocaine	1 + 5	39.7 ± 1.6*	47.8 ± 1.2*
cocaine	5	96.5 ± 1.3	98.5 ± 0.9
Pimozide + saline	1	15.7 ± 6.8	19.6 ± 9.0

*p < 0.001 compared to cocaine control

ACKNOWLEDGMENTS

This work was supported in part by U.S. Public Health Service grant DA-00795 from the National Institute on Drug Abuse. The authors wish to thank Mrs. Mary B. O'Brien for performing the motor activity study and Mr. David P. Barnes, Miss Mary Beth Hughes and Mrs. Ann Rougeaux for technical assistance.

REFERENCES

Anton, A.H. and Sayre, D.F.: A study of the factors affecting the aluminum oxide-trihydroxyindole procedure for the analysis of catecholamines, J. Pharmac. exp. Ther. 138, 360-375 (1962).

Browne, R.G., Harris, R.T., and Ho, B.T.: Stimulus properties of mescaline and n-methylated derivatives: Difference in peripheral and direct central administration, Psychopharmacologia 39, 43-56 (1974).

Caldwell, J. and Sever, P.: The biochemical pharmacology of abused drugs. I. Amphetamines, cocaine and LSD, Clin. Pharmacol. Therap. 16, 625-638 (1974).

Coyle, J.T. and Snyder, S.H.: Catecholamine uptake by synaptosomes in homogenates of rat brain: Stereospecificity in different areas, J. Pharmac. exp. Ther. 170, 221-231 (1969).

Curzon, G. and Green, A.R.: Rapid method for the determination of 5-hydroxytryptamine and 5-hydroxyindoleacetic acid in small regions of rat brain, Br. J. Pharmacol. 39, 653-655 (1970).

Downs, A.W. and Eddy, N.B.: The effects of repeated doses of cocaine on the rat, J. Pharmac. exp. Ther. 46, 199-200 (1932).

Groppetti, A., Zambotti, F., Biazzi, A., and Mantegazza, P.: Amphetamine and cocaine on amine turnover. In: Frontiers in Catecholamine Research. Usdin, E. and Snyder, S., Eds., pp. 917-925. New York: Pergamon, 1974.

Gutierrez-Noriega, C. and Zapata-Ortiz, V.: Cocainismo experimental. I. Toxicologia general, acostumbramiento y sensibilizacion, Revta Med. exp. 3, 280-306 (1944).

Huang, J.T. and Ho, B.T.: Discriminative stimulus properties of d-amphetamine and related compounds in rats, Pharmac. Biochem. Behav. 2, 669-673 (1974).

Kosman, M.E. and Unna, K.R.: Effects of chronic administration of the amphetamines and other stimulants on behavior, Clin. Pharmacol. Therap. 9, 240-254 (1968).

Laverty, R. and Taylor, K.M.: The fluorometric assay of catecholamines and related compounds, Anal. Biochem. 22, 269-279 (1968).

Lovenberg, W., Jequier, E., and Sjoerdsma, A.: Tryptophan hydroxylation: Measurement in pineal gland, brainstem and carcinoid tumor, Science 155, 217-219 (1967).

McCaman, M.W., McCaman, R.E., and Lees, G.J.: Liquid cation exchange - a basis for sensitive radiometric assays for aromatic amino acid decarboxylases, Anal. Biochem. 45, 242-252 (1972).

Post, R.M. and Kopanda, R.T.: Cocaine, kindling and reverse tolerance, Lancet i, 409-410 (1975).

Randrup, A. and Scheel-Krüger, J.: Diethyldithio carbamate and amphetamine stereotype behavior, J. Pharm. Pharmac. 18, 752 (1966).

Schellenberger, M.K. and Gordon, J.H.: A rapid, simplified procedure for simultaneous assay of norepinephrine, dopamine and 5-hydroxytryptamine from discrete brain areas, Anal. Biochem. 39, 356-371 (1971).

Schubert, J., Fyrö, B., Nybäck, H., and Sedvall, G.: Effects of cocaine and amphetamine on the metabolism of tryptophan and 5-hydroxytryptamine in mouse brain *in vivo*, J. Pharm. Pharmac. 22, 860-862 (1970).

Van Zwieten, P.A., Widhalm, S., and Hertting, G.J.: Influence of cocaine and of pretreatment with reserpine on the pressor effect and the tissue uptake of injected *dl*-catecholamines-2-^{3}H, J. Pharmac. exp. Ther. 149, 50-56 (1965).

Waymire, J.C., Bjur, R., and Weiner, N.: Assay of tyrosine hydroxylase by coupled decarboxylation of dopa formed from 1-^{14}C-L-tyrosine, Anal. Biochem. 43, 588-600 (1971).

SMALL VESSEL CEREBRAL VASCULAR CHANGES FOLLOWING CHRONIC AMPHETAMINE INTOXICATION

Calvin L. Rumbaugh

Departments of Neurology and Radiology, LAC-USC

Medical Center, Los Angeles, California

Over the past seven years the authors have observed an increasing number of young and middle-aged patients, presenting for cerebral angiography for a variety of neurological problems, including stroke, in whom eventually a history of drug abuse is obtained. Such a history is only rarely volunteered; in fact, usually considerable questioning of the patient, the patient's family, relatives, and friends is required before such a history is brought to light. In many of these patients cerebral angiography demonstrates vascular changes thought to be related to drug abuse (Rumbaugh, Bergeron, Fang, and McCormick, 1971a). These patients present a diagnostic problem, however, in that their histories often are unreliable or not available regarding the specific drugs or combination of drugs, dosages, impurities, etc. Neither the pathologic nature of the cerebral vascular changes nor the mechanism whereby drug abuse results in these vascular changes is well-understood. It is not known whether one or two specific drugs are responsible for most of the changes or whether many of the misused drugs are capable of producing cerebral damage.

The problem is exemplified by the following clinical case. A 28-year-old male, confused and lethargic, was admitted to the hospital. The cerebral spinal fluid was xanthochromic and, clinically, a subarachnoid bleed was suspected. Cerebral angiography demonstrated no aneurysm or vascular malformation; however, extensive small vessel occlusive disease, characteristic of the findings observed in drug abuse patients (Fig.1), was present, bilaterally. On the initial questioning of the patient, there was no drug history. Later, however, the patient did admit to the fact that he occasionally took "Contac" tablets for colds and it eventually developed that he was taking up to 60 "Contac" tablets a day for severe colds. The patient did not have a very good memory and was confused. There is no reason to think that he was not trying to cooperate; but it is quite possible and, in fact, probable that he was taking other things besides "Contac" tablets in excessive amounts. (Incidentally, each "Contac" capsule contains 50 mg of phenylpropanolamine hydrochloride which is a sympathomimetic drug like methamphetamine). This patient admitted only to taking "Contac" tablets; others have admitted taking some type of tranquilizer and nothing else; others report some specific barbiturate and, in all sincerity, state that they never have had any other drug. Yet, the same general abnormal vascular pattern is seen with these different drug histories. It has been practically impossible to do any type of controlled investigative study with the drug abuse population seen at the L.A. County USC Medical Center because of the difficulty in obtaining a reliable history and because most of these patients are incapable of cooperating in such a study. Therefore, in an effort to gain more insight into the nature of this hazard, an experimental drug abuse research project was designed using the Rhesus monkey and the Simonson-Albino rat in which an effort is made to approximate the clinical drug abuse situation and yet control the variables as much as possible. This is a summary of the findings thus far with i.v. administration of amphetamines. This continues an earlier pilot study (Rumbaugh, Bergeron, Scanlan, Teal, Segall, Fang, and McCormick, 1971b).

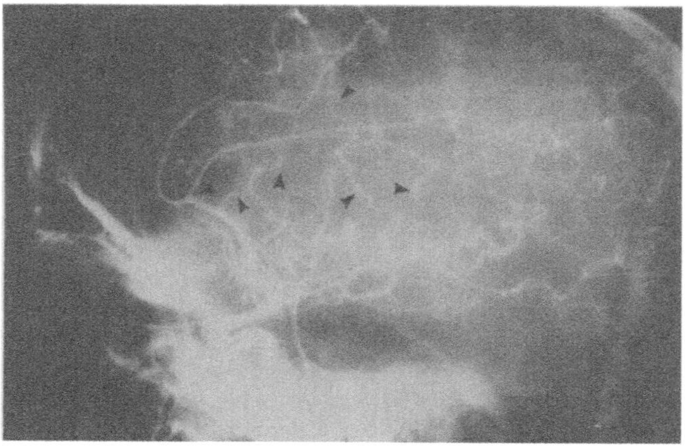

Fig. 1. Lateral view, left common carotid arteriogram in 28-year old male who gave a history of ingesting up to 60 "Contac" tablets a day. Note the numerous small arteries which are blocked or deformed. These changes can be appreciated even better when the serial sequential films are viewed together and compared.

Fifteen monkeys, each weighing between 4 and 6 kgs., were used in this i.v. amphetamine study.

In the long-term one-year group, five monkeys received methamphetamine, 1.5 mg/kg body weight, i.v. twice a week. Desoxyn 5 mg. tablets were crushed and dissolved in saline about 20 minutes before injection. Two additional animals served as controls. These received intravenous saline injections twice a week for the one-year period. All animals had preliminary cerebral arteriograms, EKGs, and blood pressure recordings. Rectal temperatures were monitored continuously. These studies were repeated again just before sacrifice. Serial cerebral angiography demonstrated occlusions and slow blood flow in small arteries in three of the drug animals (Figs. 2a, 2b). One drug animal showed only questionable minimal vascular changes and another appeared normal. The two control animals were negative. Benzadine stains of the histologic sections showed rather extensive changes involving the small arterioles and capillary beds in all of the drug animals (Figs. 3a, 3b). These changes were characterized by patchy areas of vascular filling or nonfilling, attenuation, and fragmentation of vessels. Stagnant, dilated venules were common in many of these areas. The changes were most prominent in the cortex of the frontal, temporal, and occipital lobes. H and E (Hematoxylin and Eosin), C/V (Cresyl Echt Violet), and LF/B (Luxol-Fast Blue Hematoxylin) stains demonstrated primarily chronic changes characterized by pyknotic nuclei, some loss of neurons with increased glial cells, satellitosis, and chromatolysis (Fig. 4). In one animal there were areas of microhemorrhage in the cerebellum and thalamus; a few microaneurysms in the putamen also were identified. Occasionally talc crystals were noted in some surface vessels; more commonly talc granules were seen in vessel walls, but there was no granuloma formation.

An intermediate term one-month study group consisted of three drug animals and one control animal. The general format was similar to the one-year group. Cerebral angiography in two drug animals demonstrated decreased caliber or nonfilling of a moderate number of small arteries, particularly in the region of the insula, at the end of one month. In the other drug animal, only questionable changes were seen. The control animal was negative. Benzadine stains demonstrated patchy areas of cortical avascularity in two animals, primarily in the frontal lobes. The conventional histologic stains showed subacute neuronal cell damage in all three drug animals. A few arterioles were thrombosed; an occasional capillary was partially blocked, and a few areas of aneurysmal dilatation of small arterioles surrounded by these small round cell focal infiltrates were found. Scattered talc crystals in the lumina of the capillaries were noted. The control animal was not remarkable.

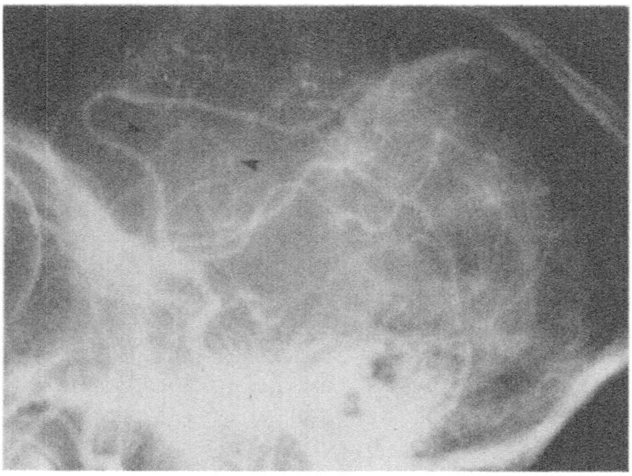

Fig. 2a. Preliminary arteriogram, a normal study, in a one-year amphetamine monkey before the animal had received any drug. Note the normal small opercular vessels.

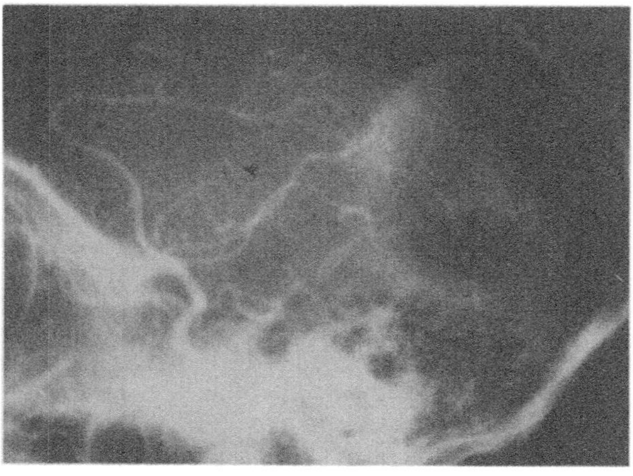

Fig. 2b. Same animal as Fig. 2a, repeat arteriogram one year later. The animal had been receiving i.v. amphetamine for one year. Note that a number of the small opercular vessels are not filling and others are considerably decreased in caliber.

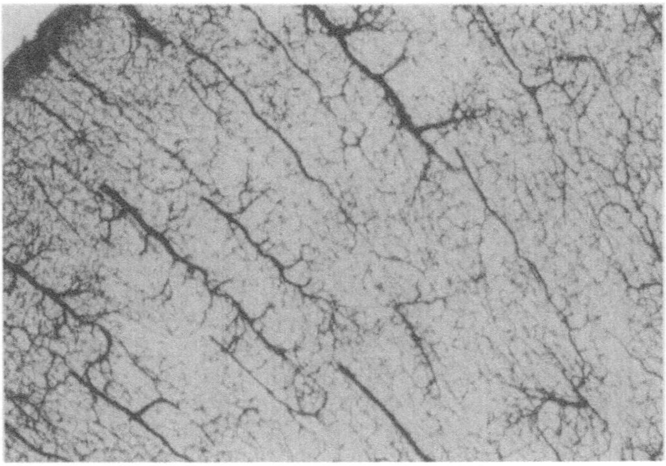

Fig. 3a. Normal benzadine stain in a one-year control methamphetamine monkey. This is the normal microvascular cerebral architecture in the cortex of the frontal lobe in the monkey.

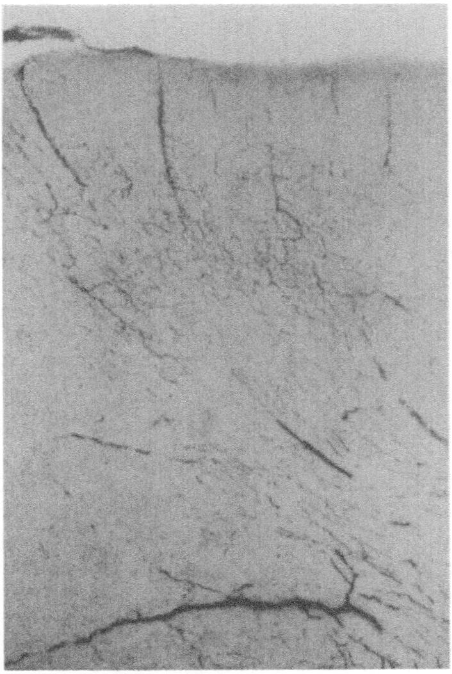

Fig. 3b. Benzadine stain cerebral cortex frontal lobe in a one-year amphetamine monkey. This animal had been on i.v. amphetamine for one year. Note the paucity of vessels; there is substantial disruption of the normal microvascular architecture.

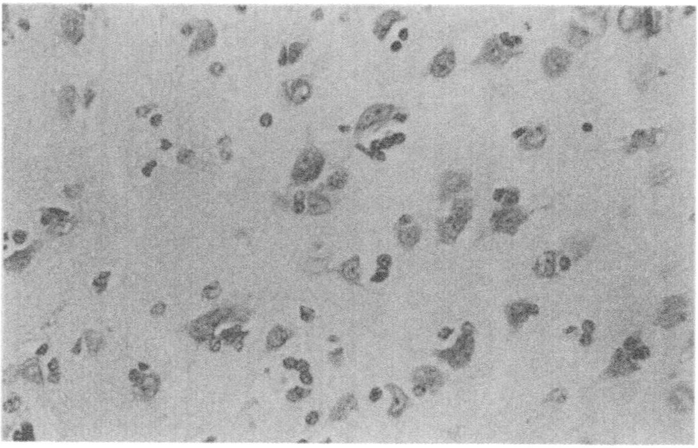

Fig. 4. C/V stain (Cresyl Violet stain) of a one-year amphetamine monkey. The section is from the frontal cortex; chronic degenerative changes characterized by neuronophagia and reactive astrocytes are evident. Clusters of small round cells are about degenerating neurons.

The short-term one-week study group consisted of three drug animals and one control animal (Figs. 5a, 5b). The animals received 1.5 mg/kg body weight of methamphetamine i.v. every other day for one week. In two of the drug animals cerebral angiography at the end of one week demonstrated a diffuse decrease in caliber of most cortical arteries in the 100-200 μ size range. One drug animal showed no changes and the control animal showed no changes. Histologically, two of the drug animals had acute changes; in one, there was disruption of the connecting channels and perforators in the frontal cortex. A recent thrombus in a small arteriole was identified in this animal also. In the other animal, engorged vessels with red cells leaking from the walls were identified. The final drug animal and the control animal were not remarkable.

Finally, there was a one-month placebo study group identical to the one-month Desoxyn study, but the placebo of Desoxyn was used. Everything was the same, same filler, binder, etc., but there was no active drug in the placebo. In this study neither the angiographic nor the histologic findings were very impressive.

In conjunction with the monkey studies, some parallel short-term i.v. drug studies were carried out in the rat (Figs. 6a, 6b, 7).

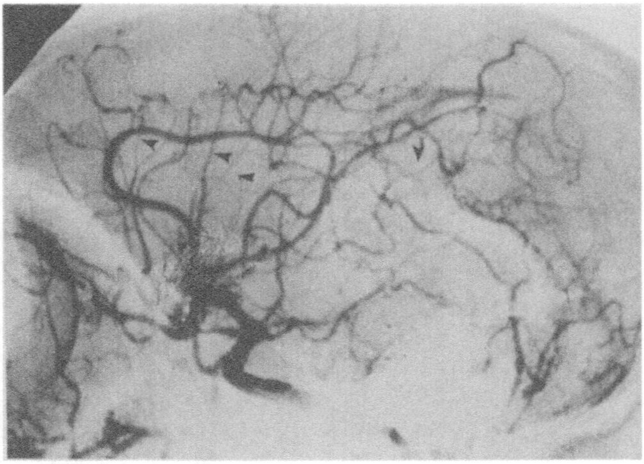

Fig. 5a. Lateral arteriogram in one-week amphetamine monkey before the monkey had received any drug. This is a normal arteriogram. Note the small arteries in the frontal-parietal opercular region.

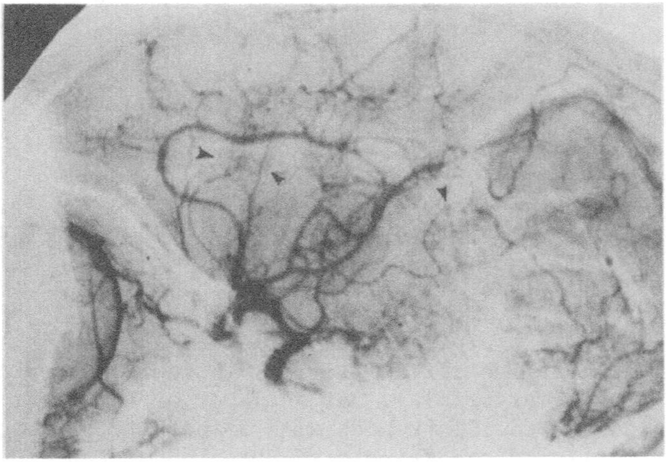

Fig. 5b. Repeat lateral cerebral arteriogram in the same animal as Fig. 5a, but 15 minutes following the administration of i.v. methamphetamine. Note that already at the end of 15 minutes in this particular animal some of the small opercular vessels have decreased in caliber considerably and some are not filling at all.

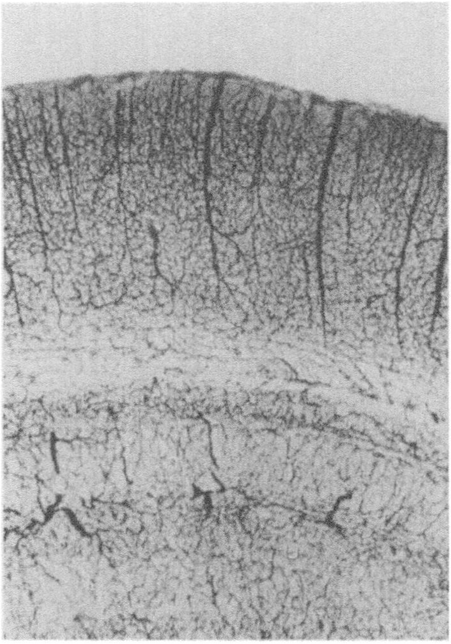

Fig. 6a

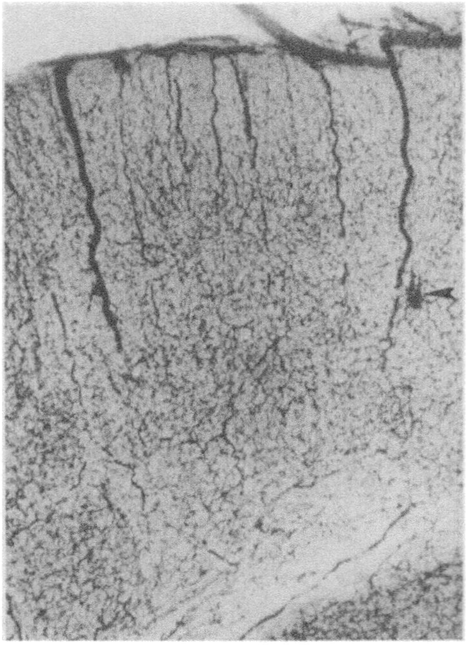

Fig. 6b

Fig 6a. Benzadine stain-parietal cortex of a control rat. This demonstrates the normal microvascular architecture of the cerebral cortex in the rat.

Fig. 6b. Benzadine stain-parietal cortex of a rat which had received i.v. amphetamine for two weeks. There is marked disruption of the perforating arterioles, particularly of the inner connecting arterioles and capillary beds with a sparsity of vascular filling, primarily of the arterioles but also of the venules. Note the area of petechial hemorrhage deep in the cortex near the edge of the figure.

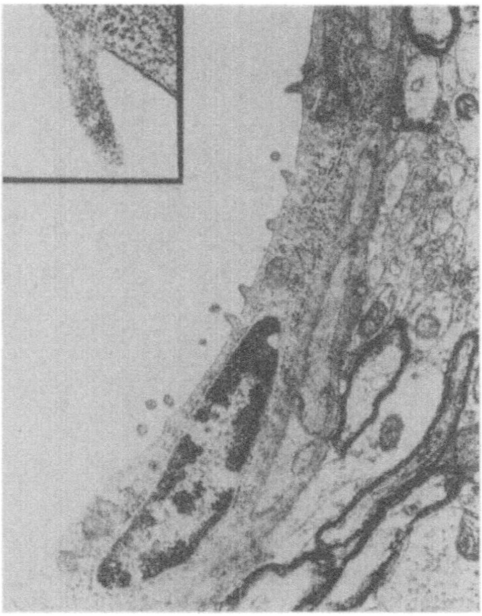

Fig. 7. Electron microscopic print of the capillary wall in a section from the cerebral cortex of a rat. This rat had been on i.v. amphetamine for two weeks. The dose was 6 mg/kg body weight five times a week. There is extensive budding and vacuolation of the endothelial luminal cytoplasmic membrane. Occasionally, similar budding was seen in the vessels of the control animals but never to the degree observed in these animals which received methamphetamine.

Figures 8a, 8b, and 8c demonstrate some of the preliminary findings in the current series of Rhesus monkey studies in which the animals are started at the same i.v. amphetamine dose as the other Rhesus monkey studies discussed earlier (1.5 mg/kg body weight amphetamine three times a week). However, in the present series the dose is being progressively increased. Each animal receives 1.5 mg/kg body weight three times a week the first week, then 3 mg/kg body weight the next week, then 4.5 mg., etc. However, there may be some delay in increment increase; if the animal shows respiratory depression, episodes of unconsciousness, and/or unsteadiness of gait, etc., that might result in secondary head injury.

Oral methamphetamine studies both in rats and monkeys recently have been initiated. Preliminary findings indicate that the oral route of administration probably results in cerebral vascular

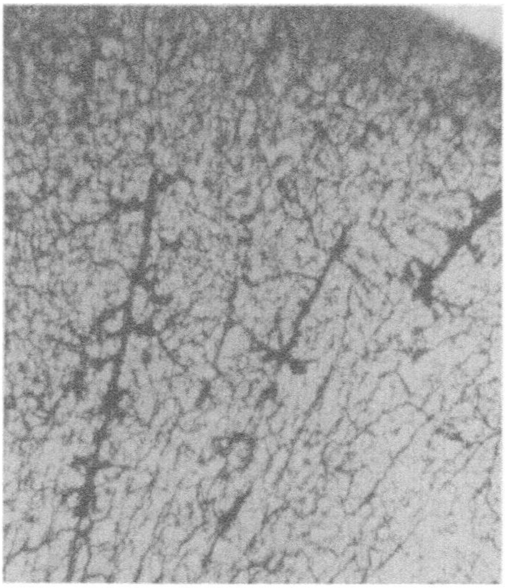

Fig. 8a. Benzadine stain of frontal cortex section in a Rhesus monkey that had been on i.v. methamphetamine approximately three months. The animal was started on a dose of 1.5 mg/kg body weight that had been progressively increased up to the time of death. At the time of death the animal was receiving 10.5 mg/kg body weight three times a week. There is marked disruption of the normal microvascular architecture. Arterioles and venules show severe injury with numerous areas of petechial hemorrhage.

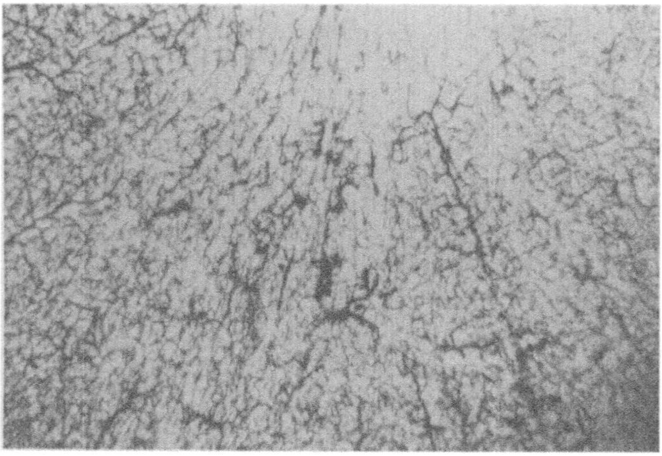

Fig. 8b. Benzadine stain of frontal cortex, same animal as Fig. 8a. Again petechial hemorrhages are numerous with prominent beading of the venules. Arterioles show constriction and extravasation along axis of penetrating vessels. There is extensive disarrangement of the microvasculature.

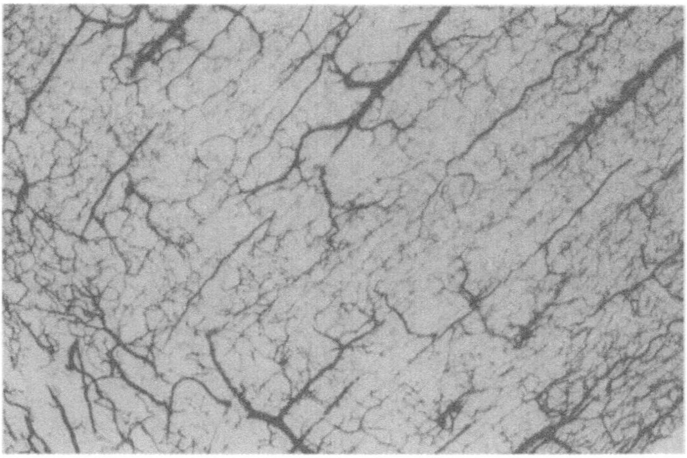

Fig. 8c. Benzadine stain-frontal cortex, normal control monkey. This demonstrates the normal microvascular pattern in the white matter for comparison purposes with Figs. 8a and 8b.

changes as severe as the intravenous route. Also, there is a suggestion that the cerebral vascular changes may develop earlier in the oral animals than in the intravenous animals.

In conclusion, on the basis of animal studies which have been completed thus far, it appears that methamphetamine, when taken in large doses, either orally or intravenously, is an extremely dangerous drug and is capable of producing severe brain damage. At least part of the damage is a result of direct vascular injury, arterial and venous.

REFERENCES

Rumbaugh, C.L., Bergeron, R.T., Fang, H.C.H., McCormick, R.: Cerebral angiographic changes in the drug abuse patient, Radiology 101, 335-344 (1971).

Rumbaugh, C.L., Bergeron, R.T., Scanlan, R.L., Teal, J.S., Segall, H.D., Fang, H.C.H., McCormick, R.: Cerebral vascular changes secondary to amphetamine abuse in the experimental animal (Preliminary report), Radiology 101, 345-351 (1971b).

ENHANCEMENT OF COCAINE-INDUCED LETHALITY BY PHENOBARBITAL

M. A. Evans, C. Dwivedi, and R. D. Harbison

Department of Pharmacology and Center in Toxicology

Vanderbilt Medical Center, Nashville, Tennessee 37232

Cocaine is a powerful central nervous system stimulant that produces intense excitation, euphoria, and restlessness in man. In laboratory animals the cortical action of cocaine is first manifested by an increase in well coordinated motor activity. As dosage is increased, the lower centers of the brain are progressively affected--producing tremors, convulsions, and, eventually, clonic-tonic convulsions. This central stimulation is followed by a progressive wave of depression beginning at the cortex and spreading downwards to the cerebrospinal axis (Ritchie and Chen, 1975). Lethality related to direct cardiac depression from cocaine overdose has been demonstrated within 2-3 minutes of intravenous administration; in 2-3 hours death due to respiratory paralysis associated with CNS depression has been observed (Casarett, 1975).

Although rapidly distributed following absorption, the vasoconstrictive action of cocaine acts to limit its release from subcutaneous injection sites and mucosal membranes. Woods, McMahon, and Seevers (1951) demonstrated that, in dog, the half-life of cocaine following intravenous administration was approximately 1.5 hours. Subcutaneous administration prolonged the duration of cocaine activity to approximately seven hours. Early investigators demonstrated that, following absorption, cocaine is rapidly hydrolyzed by blood serum esterases to produce benzoylecgonine, ecgonine methyl ester, and ecgonine (Kalow, 1952; Montesinos, 1965). A study by Misra, Nayak, Bloch, and Mulé (1975) showed that, in the rat, intravenous doses up to 200 mg/kg of these metabolites had no demonstrable pharmacological effect. Thus, due to its relatively rapid inactivation by the serum esterases and lack of activity of the metabolites, no prolonged toxicity, physical dependence or tolerance have been reported with cocaine. Recent studies by Misra, Nayak, Patel, Vadlamani, and Mulé (1974) have suggested that cocaine can also undergo microsomal oxidation similar to lidocaine. Biotransformation may produce N-dealkylated products of norcocaine and benzoylnorecgonine that are active pharmacologically. However, the relatively slow release of cocaine from injection sites and the large capacity of the serum esterases would seem to suggest that the hepatic microsomes would have a very small part in the bioactivation of cocaine.

Drug oxidations, including C-hydroxylations and N-dealkylations, are known to be catalyzed by liver microsomal enzymes and to be dependent on oxygen and reduced nicotinamide adenine dinucleotide phosphate (NADPH) for activity. However, while the classical drug-oxidative reactions and the N-oxygenation of primary amines are dependent on the NADPH-linked monooxygenase system, which includes cytochrome-P-450, several studies indicate that the enzymic N-oxygenation of secondary and tertiary amines is independent of cytochrome P-450 (Masters and Ziegler, 1971; Ziegler and Mitchell, 1972).

Recent reports by Miller (1970) and Uehleke (1965) have indicated that the N-oxidation of secondary and tertiary amines can involve formation of an active N-oxide intermediate that is capable of undergoing biological reaction resulting in tissue binding.

The purpose of this investigation was to examine the influence of sex on cocaine distribution and lethality and the possible effect of alteration in microsomal metabolism on the systemic toxicity of cocaine.

METHODS

Animals

Male and virgin female Swiss Webster mice (Harlan Industries, Cumberland, Indiana) weighing 20-25 g were randomized 10 per cage according to sex and allowed food (Purina Laboratory Chow) and tap water *ad libitum*.

Treatment

All drugs were made in a vehicle to deliver the appropriate dosage in a volume of 0.1 ml/10 g of body weight. Control animals were treated with the appropriate vehicle solution. Total number of dead animals was recorded at 3 hours and on day 3 following administration of cocaine. Each treatment group consisted of 10-15 animals and was replicated at least once.

Cocaine, phenobarbital sodium (PB), and SKF 525A (β-diethylaminoethyldiphenylpropylacetate hydrochloride) were dissolved in 0.9% NaCl and administered intraperitoneally. Phenobarbital sodium at a dose of 60 mg/kg was administered once daily for 4 days, and cocaine was administered 24 hr after the last injection of phenobarbital. SKF 525A was administered, 40 mg/kg, 1 hr before cocaine.

Analytical Methods

Baker-analyzed silica gel, 60-160 mesh, was used for column chromatography, and Baker-flex silica gel 1B plates were used for thin layer chromatography. Radioscans of chromatograms were prepared by sectioning 1 cm strips of the plates, transferring them to counting vials, adding toluene counting solution, 15 ml, and determining the radioactivity in a Packard tri-carb model 3320 liquid scintillation counter.

Cocaine base (50 mg, 1.7 x 10^{-4} mol) was tritiated (New England Nuclear Laboratory, Boston, Massachusetts) in solutions of glacial acetic acid in the presence of a platinum catalyst, 25 mg and ^3H_2O, 10 curies, by stirring the reaction mixture overnight at 50°C. After filtration of the catalyst, labile tritium was removed *in vacuo* and the crude ^{3}H-cocaine residue taken up in methanol.

The methanol solution of ^{3}H-cocaine was mixed with nonlabeled cocaine, 150 mg, 5.1 x 10^{-4} mol and the solution evaporated to dryness in a stream of nitrogen. The residue, dissolved in 3 ml of chloroform, was chromatographed on a silica gel column, 15 x 1 cm, and cocaine was eluted with 200 ml of chloroform. The residue from the chloroform eluate was dissolved in 3 ml of 1N HCl, basified to pH 9.5 with 1N Nh_4OH, and extracted with benzene. The benzene extract was dried over anhydrous sodium sulfate. Residue obtained on evaporation of benzene extract had a specific activity of 53 μCi/mg and a yield of 164 mg. The chemical and isotopic purity (95%) of ^{3}H-cocaine were checked by TLC using two separate solvent systems (Nayak, Misra, Patel, and Mulé, 1974).

Tissue and plasma samples for liquid scintillation counting were prepared and counted by a previously described method (Harbison and Mantilla-Plata, 1972). The dosage of ^{3}H-cocaine was 32 μCi/50 mg/kg of body weight.

In Vitro Metabolism

N-dealkylation of cocaine *in vitro* was estimated by product formation of formaldehyde. Fasted male mice were sacrificed and livers immediately removed and homogenized in 5 volumes of cold 1.15%

KCL. The homogenate was centrifuged at 10,000 g for 20 min and the supernatant decanted. Incubation media, at a final volume of 3 ml, contained phosphate buffer, pH 7.4, 0.1 M; $MgCl_2 \cdot 6H_2O$, 15 μmoles; nicotinamide, 20 μmoles; glucose-6-phosphate, 10 μmoles; nicotinamide adenine dinucleotide phosphate, 0.48 μmoles; semicarbazide, 40 μmoles; and 1 ml of microsomal suspension. The media was preincubated for 10 min in an oxygen atmosphere at 37°C before addition of cocaine, 20 μmoles, 0.2 ml. After 20 min, the reaction was stopped with 4ml of Nash reagent and heated in boiling water for 10 min. The developed color was read at 415 nm using an Hitachi Spectrophotometer Model 100-20. Microsomal protein was isolated and protein estimated by the Biuret method (Gornall, Bardowill, and David, 1949). Liver homogenates from six untreated and six phenobarbital treated mice in duplicate were used.

RESULTS

Cocaine, 75 mg/kg, i.p., produced 53% mortality in males and 74% mortality in females (Fig. 1). All deaths in both groups occurred during the first three hours following treatment and were the result of respiratory failure. The female is more sensitive to acute cocaine-induced toxicity than the male.

The effects of phenobarbital and SKF 525A on cocaine-induced lethality in male mice is shown in Fig. 2. The incidence of mortality in untreated animals was 55%; no deaths were observed after the first three hours. Pretreatment with phenobarbital reduced the three hour acute toxicity of cocaine to 14% but produced a delayed toxicity resulting in 62% lethality of the animals surviving the first three hours. Deaths in this group occurred up to the 3rd day following cocaine administration and appeared to be due to organ damage rather than acute respiratory failure. Phenobarbital pretreatment reduces the acute central nervous system toxicity of cocaine but promotes a delayed toxicity related to organ damage in greater than 60% of the surviving animals. Pretreatment with SKF 525A had no significant effect on cocaine-induced toxicity. The incidence of cocaine-induced mortality during the first 3 hr was 50%; no deaths beyond that time were observed.

^{3}H-labeled cocaine dissolved in saline was used to measure total plasma and tissue concentrations of cocaine plus metabolites. No attempts were made to quantitatively separate cocaine and metabolites in these tissues, and results reported as disintegrations per minute/100 mg tissue are considered to be cocaine plus metabolites (CM). Plasma concentrations of CM at selected time intervals for both male and female mice are shown in Fig. 3. Peak plasma concentrations for CM in both male and female mice were reached within the first 30 min following administration and declined rapidly during the next 3½ hr. Concentrations in the female were slightly higher

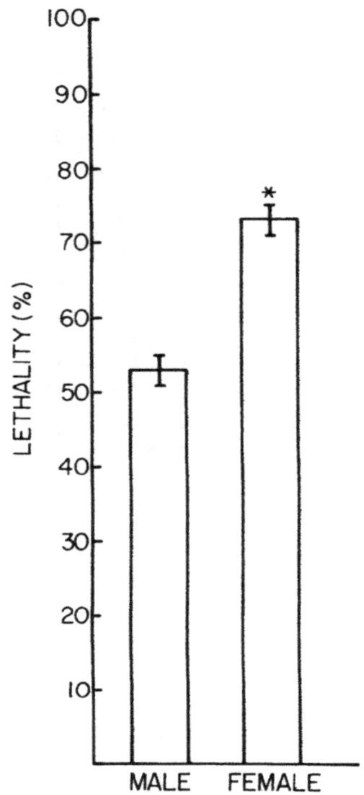

Fig. 1. Effect of sex on cocaine-induced lethality. Cocaine was administered intraperitoneally at a dosage of 75 mg/kg.

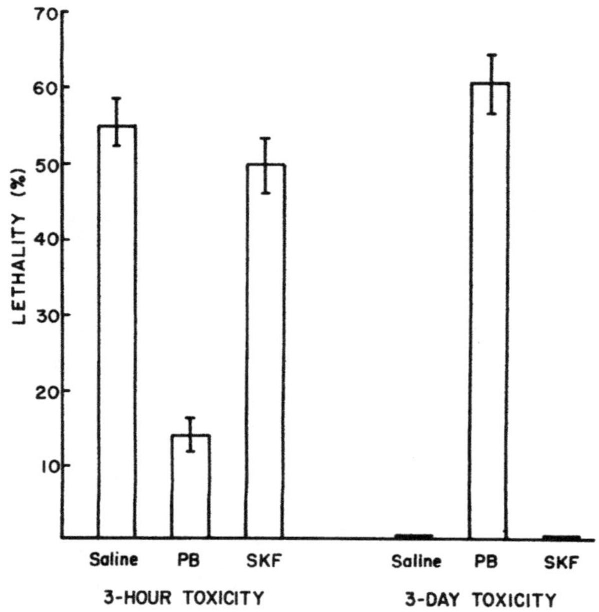

Fig. 2. Effect of phenobarbital, 60 mg/kg i.p., and SKF 525A, 40 mg/kg i.p., on cocaine toxicity in male mice. Mortality was recorded at 3 hr and again at 3 days following treatment with cocaine.

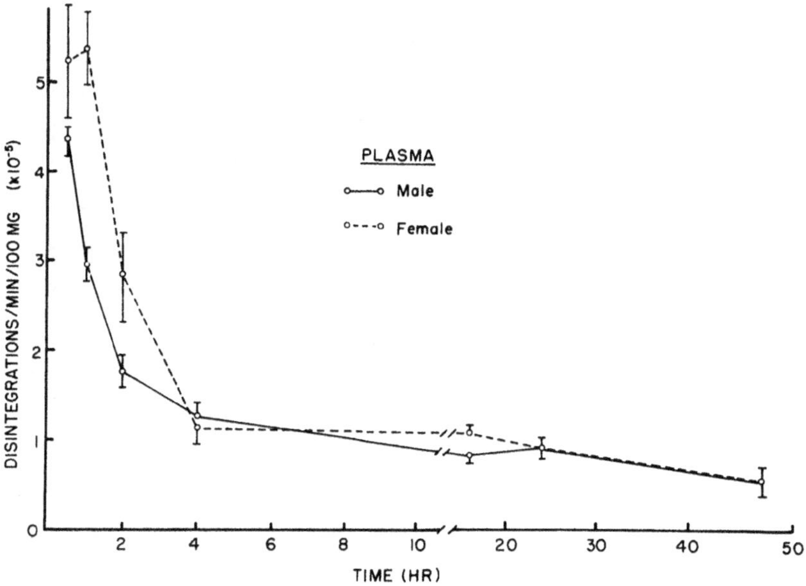

Fig. 3. Effect of sex on plasma concentrations of cocaine plus metabolites.

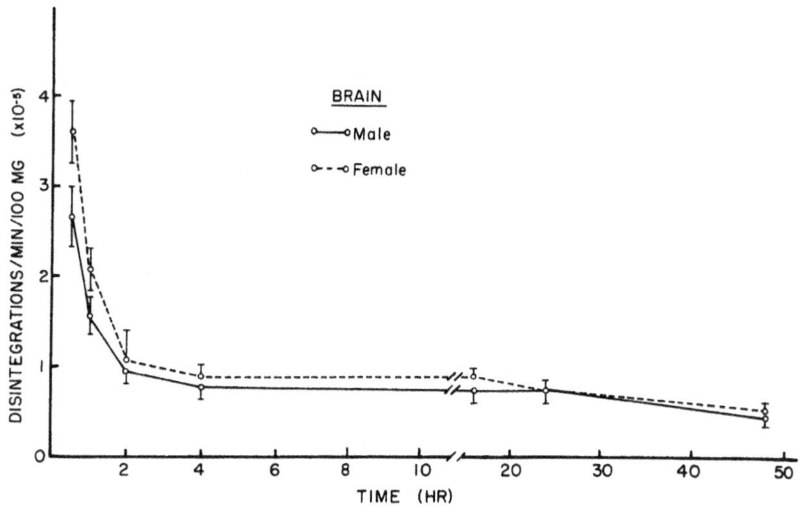

Fig. 4. Effect of sex on brain concentration of cocaine plus metabolites.

than in males during the initial 2 hr following administration, but after the second hour no significant difference between the two groups was observed. Figure 4 illustrates CM concentration in the brain tissue for both male and female mice. The concentration of total radioactivity in brain for both groups paralleled plasma concentrations, demonstrating slightly higher levels of CM in the female than in males during the first hour following administration. Mean concentration of radioactivity in the brain of females 30 min following ^{3}H-cocaine was approximately 30% higher than in the brain of males. However, tissue to plasma ratios for both groups were similar. At 30 min following administration, the brain/plasma ratio was 0.68 for female and 0.65 for male.

The effect of phenobarbital pretreatment on concentration of total radioactivity in plasma is shown in Fig. 5. Peak concentrations in both groups were reached within 30 min of treatment with ^{3}H-cocaine. Pretreatment with phenobarbital slightly reduced the total CM plasma concentration during the first hour. However, no differences in plasma concentrations could be demonstrated beyond this time period. Concentration of CM in brain paralleled plasma concentrations for both groups, demonstrating a slightly reduced level of radioactivity in the phenobarbital-pretreated group during the first two hours. Figure 6 illustrates the tissue plasma ratio of CM in brain for untreated and phenobarbital-treated animals during

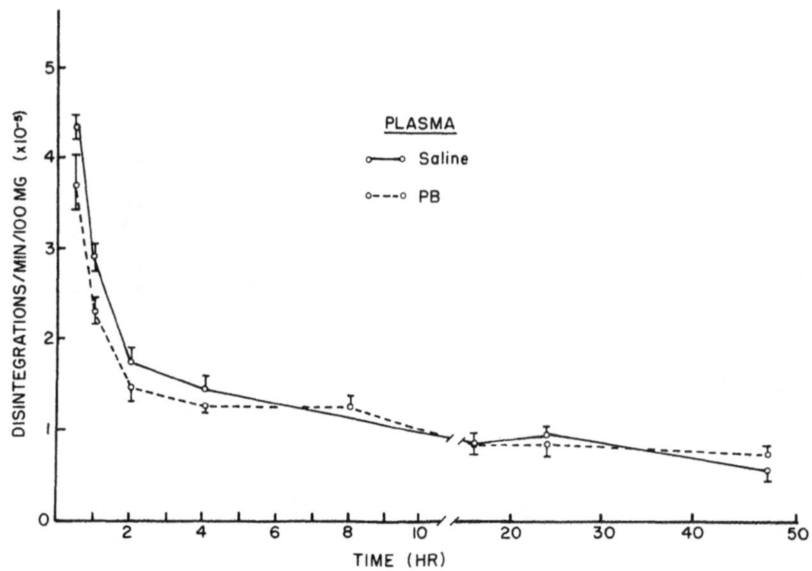

Fig. 5. Effect of phenobarbital, 60 mg/kg i.p., on plasma concentrations of cocaine plus metabolites in male mice.

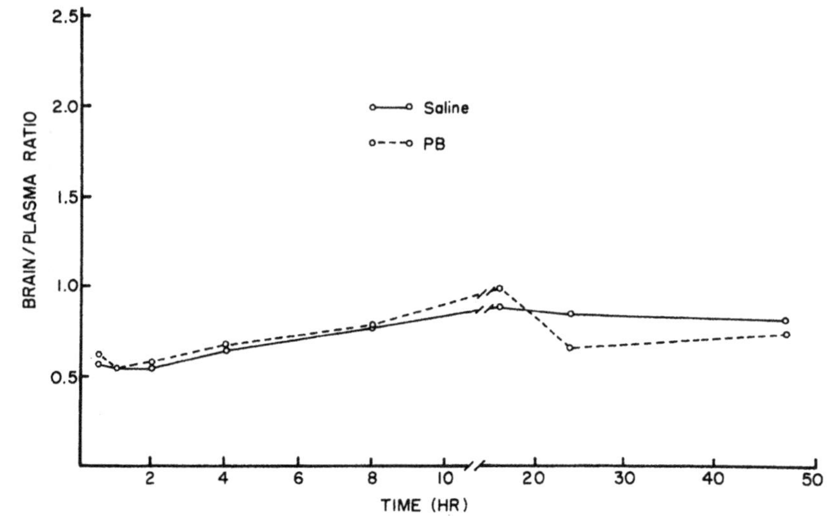

Fig. 6. Effect of phenobarbital, 60 mg/kg i.p., on the brain tissue to plasma ratio of cocaine plus metabolites in male mice.

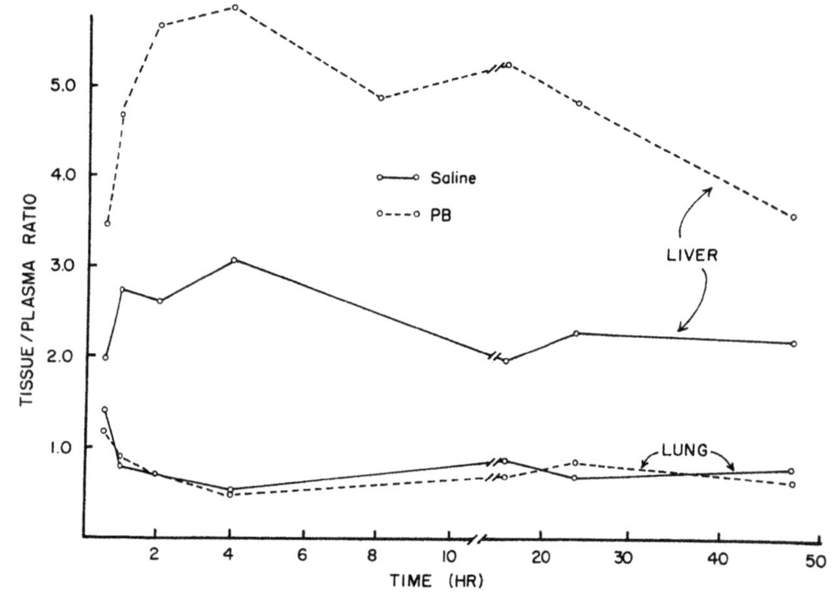

Fig. 7. Effect of phenobarbital, 60 mg/kg i.p., on the lung and liver tissue/plasma ratio of cocaine plus metabolites in male mice.

the initial 48 hr following ^{3}H-cocaine administration. During the first 4 hr the tissue/plasma ratio was significantly less than one, indicating some diffusion impairment across the blood-brain barrier. No difference in the brain tissue/plasma ratio between the two groups was observed at any time period. The ratio of tissue/plasma of CM for both lung and liver tissue are shown in Fig. 7. The ratio in lung approximated unity, indicating complete equilibration of drug and metabolite between the plasma and tissues. No difference in lung tissue/plasma ratio was demonstrable between phenobarbital-pretreated animals and untreated animals.

The liver tissue/plasma ratio of total radioactivity in untreated animals, as shown in Fig. 7, ranged between 2 and 3 during the first 48 hr following ^{3}H-cocaine, suggesting hepatic uptake and retention of radioactive material from the plasma. Pretreatment with phenobarbital significantly enhanced the liver concentration of cocaine plus metabolites; and tissue/plasma ratio of CM, as shown

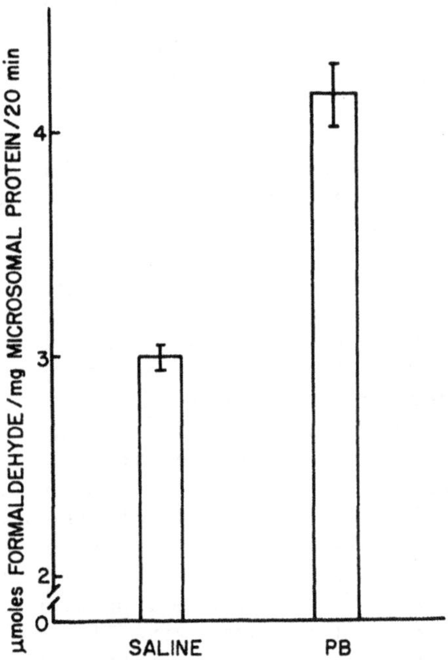

Fig. 8. Effect of phenobarbital, 60 mg/kg i.p., on *in vitro* N-dealkylation of cocaine by liver microsomes.

in Fig. 7, was increased 100% over that of untreated animals. Peak ratio of liver/plasma CM for both groups was reached within 4 hr of ^{3}H-cocaine administration.

N-dealkylation of cocaine as measured by product formation of formaldehyde is shown in Fig. 8. Liver homogenates from untreated animals produced a final formaldehyde concentration of 3.0 μmoles per mg microsomal protein for 20 min incubation. Pretreatment with phenobarbital significantly increased *in vitro* N-dealkylation of cocaine by 40% with a final formaldehyde concentration of 4.2 μmoles per mg microsomal protein. Total microsomal protein per gram of liver was also increased in the phenobarbital-treated animal. In comparison to untreated males, the concentration of microsomal protein was elevated 20% in phenobarbital-treated animals.

DISCUSSION

Females are more susceptible to acute cocaine-induced lethality. Brain tissue and plasma of females contained more cocaine at early time periods when compared to males. This suggests that distribution of cocaine and/or metabolism of cocaine is different in the female and consequently produces higher brain levels of cocaine in the female. The increase in cocaine toxicity among females, therefore, corresponds to the increased levels of cocaine in the brain. Brain tissue/plasma ratios of total radioactivity in both sexes were equal, indicating that relative distribution of the drug to brain is not altered.

Phenobarbital has two clearly distinguishable pharmacological actions. It is a central nervous system depressant and anticonvulsant as well as a stimulator of hepatic mixed function of oxidase activity. The drug produces a sharp rise in liver Δ-aminolevulinic acid synthetase, the initial and rate limiting enzyme in heme biosynthesis (Marver, 1969). Pretreatment of animals for several days with phenobarbital can promote increases in liver NADPH-cytochrome C and cytochrome P-450, the essential components of microsomal drug oxidizing systems, and correspondingly stimulate microsomal drug metabolism (Orrenius and Ernster, 1964). Metabolism of cocaine, like procaine and other esters, is non-microsomal, being metabolized primarily by the hydrolytic enzymes of blood serum and other tissue esterases (La Du and Snody, 1971). Recent studies by Misra et al. (1974), however, have demonstrated the presence of norcocaine and benzoylnorecgonine following administration of radiolabeled cocaine to rats. This indicates that at least a portion of administered cocaine is metabolized by microsomal mixed function oxidases. Pretreatment of Swiss Webster mice with phenobarbital to stimulate microsomal metabolism significantly antagonized the acute 3 hr cocaine-induced lethality. However, observation during the next 3 days revealed that over 60% of the surviving animals died from systemic organ damage. Since no cocaine-associated deaths were recorded in untreated male or female mice after the third hour, it seems likely that phenobarbital pretreatment may alter the mechanism of cocaine-induced lethality by shifting metabolism from the esterase path to the microsomal pathway. Plasma and brain levels of total radioactive material were slightly lower in the phenobarbital-treated animals during the first 2 hr following treatment with ^{3}H-cocaine, which may account for the initial protective action of phenobarbital. Beyond the second hour no differences in total levels of cocaine plus metabolites were observed in either brain tissue or plasma, indicating that the delayed toxicity is not related to altered distribution of total CM to the brain.

Recent reports have demonstrated that, during N-dealkylation of secondary and tertiary amines by the mixed function oxidase, an N-oxide is formed as an intermediate metabolite (Pettit and Ziegler, 1963). The ability of a compound to undergo N-dealkylation may be of toxicological importance since certain nitrogen-containing compounds, following incubation with liver microsomes, can produce methemoglobinemia (Rane and Ackermann, 1972). Various secondary and tertiary amines are also known to have carcinogenic and other adverse effects that are ascribed to their N-oxygenated metabolites (Radomski and Bidl, 1970; Uehleke, 1965). Distribution of total radioactivity in the liver following treatment with ^{3}H-cocaine revealed a 100% increase in the tissue/plasma CM ratio for phenobarbital-treated animals when compared to untreated controls. Other tissues, including brain and lung, showed no differences in distribution with phenobarbital pretreatment. *In vitro* studies revealed that cocaine does undergo N-dealkylation in the presence of liver microsomes, and pretreatment with phenobarbital can significantly enhance norcocaine formation.

Figure 9 illustrates a proposed pathway for the biochemical transformation of cocaine. With pharmacologically active doses, serum esterase activity (E) is sufficient to account for the disposition of most of the administered drug. The major metabolites from this pathway would include benzoylecgonine, ecgonine methyl ester, and ecgonine. Stimulation of microsomal enzymes to enhance the activity of the mixed function oxidase (MFO) would increase the. N-dealkylation of available cocaine in the liver to produce norcocaine and benzoylnorecgonine. However, due to cocaine's rapid plasma distribution and enzymatic hydrolysis, the availability of free cocaine in the liver would be restricted, limiting the formation of norcocaine and benzoylnorecgonine. Systemic organ damage from the formation of an N-oxide intermediate would be limited and restricted to discrete focal lesions. Administration of high doses of cocaine, on the other hand, would act to make available a large pool of free cocaine in the liver capable of undergoing MFO metabolism and N-oxide formation. Overall metabolism of cocaine during

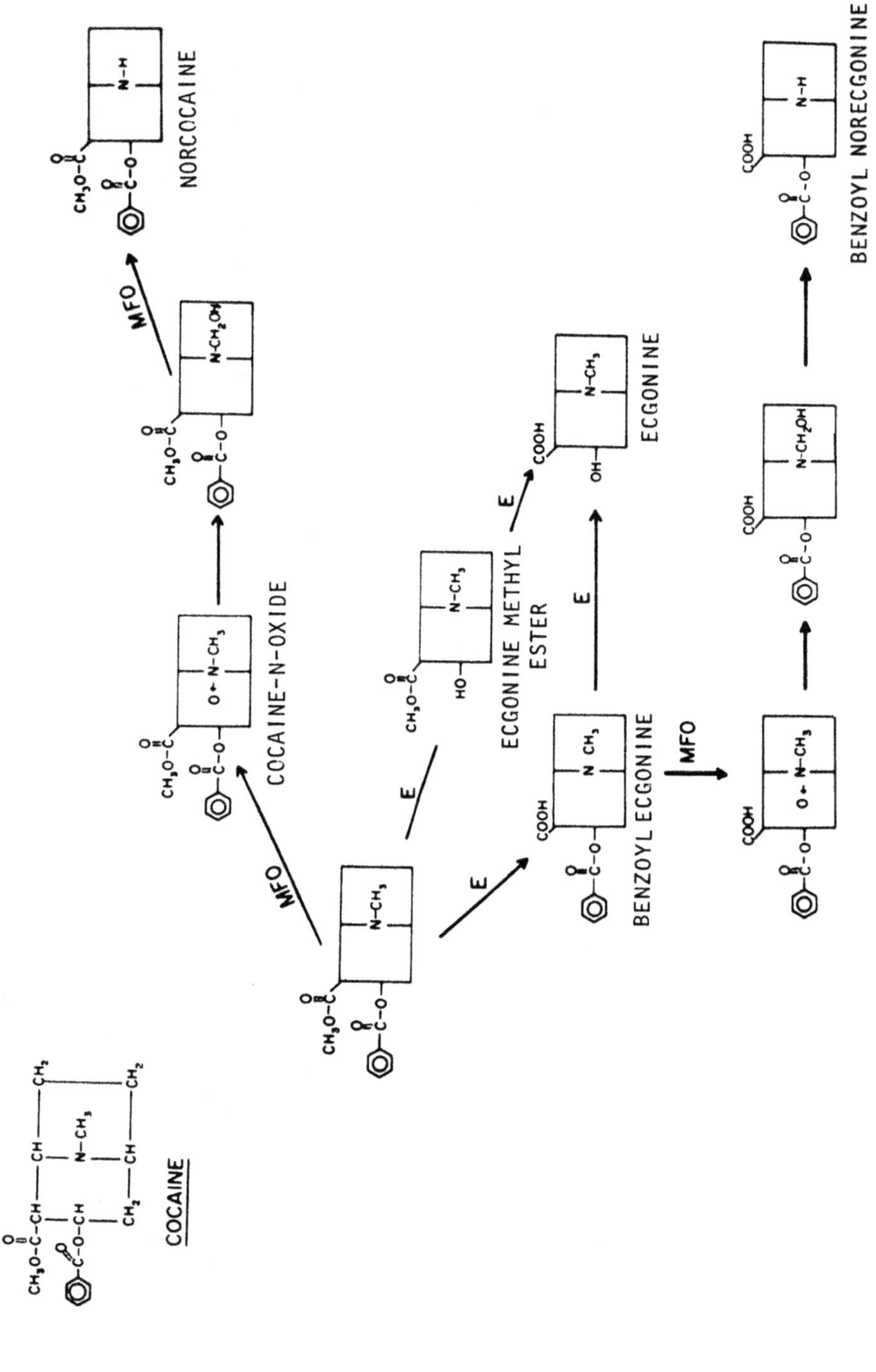

Fig. 9. Biological transformation of cocaine.

phenobarbital treatment would be increased due to activity of both the esterase and MFO, resulting in an initial decreased plasma level of free cocaine and, consequently, a decrease in acute cocaine lethality. With the increased formation of an MFO active metabolite, systemic organ damage with a delayed toxicity would be observed in the surviving animals.

The implications of this hypothesis are that habituated use of cocaine, particularly in high doses, by multiple drug users could possibly result in organ tissue damage unrelated to the CNS pharmacological action of cocaine. Thus, stimulation of the MFO system may shift the metabolism of cocaine to a more toxic metabolite.

In conclusion, stimulation of microsomal metabolism can produce delayed cocaine lethality probably related to organ tissue damage. Distribution and *in vitro* metabolism studies suggest that the delayed toxicity may be associated with the formation of an N-oxide intermediate during the microsomal N-dealkylation of cocaine to norcocaine.

REFERENCES

Casarett, M.G.: Social poisons. In: Toxicology, the Basic Science of Poisons. Casarett, L.J. and Doull, J., Eds., pp. 627-654. New York: MacMillan, 1975.

Gornall, A.G., Bardowill, C.S., and David, M.M.: A rapid method of protein estimation, J. biol. Chem. 177, 751-756 (1949).

Harbison, R.D. and Mantilla-Plata, B.: Prenatal toxicity, maternal distribution, and placental transfer of tetrahydrocannabinol, J. Pharmac. exp. Ther. 180, 446-453 (1972).

Kalow, W.: Hydrolysis of local anesthetics by human serum cholinesterase, J. Pharmac. exp. Ther. 104, 122-127 (1952).

La Du, B.N. and Snody, H.: Esterases of human tissues. In: Concepts of Biochemical Pharmacology. Brodie, B.B. and Gillette, J.R., Eds., Vol. 28, Part 2, pp. 474-482. New York: Springer-Verlag, 1971.

Marver, H.S.: The role of heme in the synthesis and repression of microsomal protein. In: Microsomes and Drug Oxidation. Gillette, J.R., Conney, A.H., Cosmides, G.J., Estrabrooks, R.W., Fouts, J.R., and Mannering, G.J., Eds., pp. 126-137. New York: Academic Press, 1969.

Masters, B.S.S. and Ziegler, D.M.: The distinct nature and function of NADPH-cytochrome c reductase and the NADPH-dependent mixed-function amine oxidase of porcine liver microsomes, Archs. Biochem. Biophys. 145, 358-364 (1971).

Miller, J.A.: Carcinogenesis by chemicals: An overview. G.H.A. Clowers Memorial Lecture, Cancer Res. 30, 559-576 (1970).

Misra, A.L., Nayak, P.K., Patel, M.N., Vadlamani, N.L., and Mulé, S.J.: Identification of norcocaine as a metabolite of ^{3}H-cocaine in rat brain, Experientia 69, 1312-1314 (1974).

Misra, A.L., Nayak, P.K., Bloch, R., and Mulé, S.J.: Estimation and disposition of ^{3}H-benzoylecgonine and pharmacological activity of some cocaine metabolites, J. Pharm. Pharmac. 27, 784-787 (1975).

Montesinos, F.: The metabolism of cocaine, Bull. Narcot. 17, 11-26 (1965).

Nayak, P.K., Misra, A.L., Patel, M.N., and Mulé, S.J.: Preparation of radiochemically pure randomly labeled and ring labeled ^{3}H-cocaine, Radiochem. Radioanal. Letters 16, 167-171 (1974).

Orrenius, S. and Ernster, L.: Phenobarbital-induced synthesis of the oxidative demethylating enzymes of rat liver microsomes, Biochem. Biophys. Res. Commun. 16, 60-67 (1964).

Pettit, F.H. and Ziegler, D.M.: The catalytic demethylation of N, N-dimethylaniline-N-oxide by liver microsomes, Biochem. Biophys. Res. Commun. 13, 193-197 (1963).

Radomski, J.L. and Brill, E.: Bladder cancer induction by aromatic amines: Role of N-hydroxy metabolites, Science 167, 992-993 (1970).

Rane, A. and Ackermann, E.: Evidence for drug metabolism in the human fetal liver. Studies in different cell fractions, Acta Pharmac. Tox., Suppl. 29, 84 (1971).

Ritchie, J.M. and Chen, P.J.: Local anesthetics. In: The Pharmacological Basis of Therapeutics. Goodman, L.S. and Gilman, A., Eds., pp. 379-403. New York: MacMillan, 1975.

Uehleke, H.: Biologische Oxydation und Reduktion am Stickstoff aromatischer Aminound Nitroderivate und ihre Folgen für den organismus, Progr. Drug Res. 8, 195-260 (1965).

Woods, L.A., McMahon, F.G., and Seevers, M.H.: Distribution and metabolism of cocaine in the dog and rabbit, J. Pharmac. exp. Ther. 101, 200-204 (1951).

Ziegler, D.M. and Mitchell, C.H.: Microsomal oxidases. IV. Properties of a mixed-function amine oxidase isolated from pig liver microsomes, Arch. Biochem. Biophys. 150, 116-125 (1972).

CHANGES IN NEURONAL ACTIVITY IN THE NEOSTRIATUM AND RETICULAR FORMATION FOLLOWING ACUTE OR LONG-TERM AMPHETAMINE ADMINISTRATION

Philip M. Groves and George V. Rebec*

University of Colorado, Boulder, Colorado 80302

*University of California, San Diego, School of Medicine

La Jolla, California 92093

There is now considerable evidence to suggest that the sequential patterns of hyperkinesia and behavioral stereotypes observed in a wide variety of species following an injection of amphetamines are due, in large measure, to a facilitation of catecholaminergic transmission in the central nervous system (e.g., as recently reviewed by Groves and Rebec, 1976). Additional recent work (e.g., Roberts, Zis, and Fibiger, 1975; Kelly, Seviour, and Iversen, 1975) further implicates the caudate-putamen, or neostriatum, and its dopaminergic input from the substantia nigra, pars compacta, and associated dopaminergic cell groups in the brainstem, in the expression of the psychomotor stimulant effects of amphetamine. The reticular formation of the brainstem is supplied, in part, by noradrenergic terminals and, as suggested by Bradley and associates (e.g., Bradley and Elkes, 1957; Bradley and Key, 1958), this area may contribute to the expression of amphetamine-induced electroencephalographic arousal. This view is consistent with the wide variety of evidence suggesting that the reticular formation of the brainstem mediates electroencephalographic and behavioral arousal (e.g., Moruzzi and Magoun, 1949; Lindsley, Bowden, and Magoun, 1949; Lindsley, Schriener, Knowles and Magoun, 1950; Segal and Mandell, 1970) and the elementary forms of plasticity that these phenomena exhibit (e.g., Sharpless and Hasper, 1956; Groves and Lynch, 1972; Groves, Wilson, and Miller, in press).

In order to further characterize the effects of amphetamine on central catecholaminergic transmission and neuronal activity, we have studied amphetamine-induced changes in neuronal firing rates in the caudate-putamen and reticular formation of the brainstem under experimental conditions in which alterations in neuronal firing are monitored over the time-course of the known behavioral and biochemical effects of amphetamine administration in experimental animals.

Male Sprague-Dawley rats were prepared with ether anesthesia and the points of surgical and stereotaxic contact were thoroughly infiltrated with local anesthetic, supplemented regularly. The animals were immobilized with d-tubocurarine chloride and artificially respired as we have described in detail elsewhere (e.g., Groves, Miller, Parker, and Rebec, 1973; Rebec and Groves, 1975a). Heartbeat, body temperature and, in later experiments, expired carbon dioxide were monitored continuously throughout the experiments. Glass-coated tungsten microelectrodes were used to record single unit discharges which were amplified and displayed by conventional means. Neuronal firing rates were recorded on-line by means of a Schmidt-trigger circuit and high speed printer-counter on a minute-by-minute basis. Unit activity also was stored on magnetic tape and in some cases photographic film for later analysis.

NEURONAL CORRELATES OF ACUTE AMPHETAMINE ADMINISTRATION

Figure 1 illustrates the effects of four acute doses of d-amphetamine sulfate on the spontaneous firing rates of neurons in the caudate-putamen with each graph representing the mean activity for five neurons, recorded in each case from five different locally anesthetized, paralyzed subjects (Groves, Rebec, and Segal, 1974). These graphic representations are constructed to illustrate deviations from pre-drug firing rates, defined for each neuron by the mean firing rate for 10 minutes prior to drug administration, and represented for each neuron as 100%. Subsequent deviations from this baseline firing rate are also represented as a percent of this mean, pre-drug control rate. This procedure allows group data to be averaged and displayed despite individual variability with respect to absolute pre-injection firing rates for individual neurons. Since there is also variability from unit to unit with respect to the duration of these amphetamine-induced alterations in firing rate, and since additional alterations in firing may continue beyond these initial effects (e.g., Rebec and Groves, 1975a), slashes are used to indicate the times at which each neuron returned to a recovery criterion (50% of control firing rate in Fig. 1) following these drug-induced changes and to indicate the points at which subsequent data collected for each neuron are deleted from the averaged, group curves. Unit activity that did not return to this recovery criterion was excluded from our samples, since in such cases the alterations in neuronal firing could be attributed to spontaneous variations in the preparation, cell loss, or other sources of variability unrelated to drug administration.

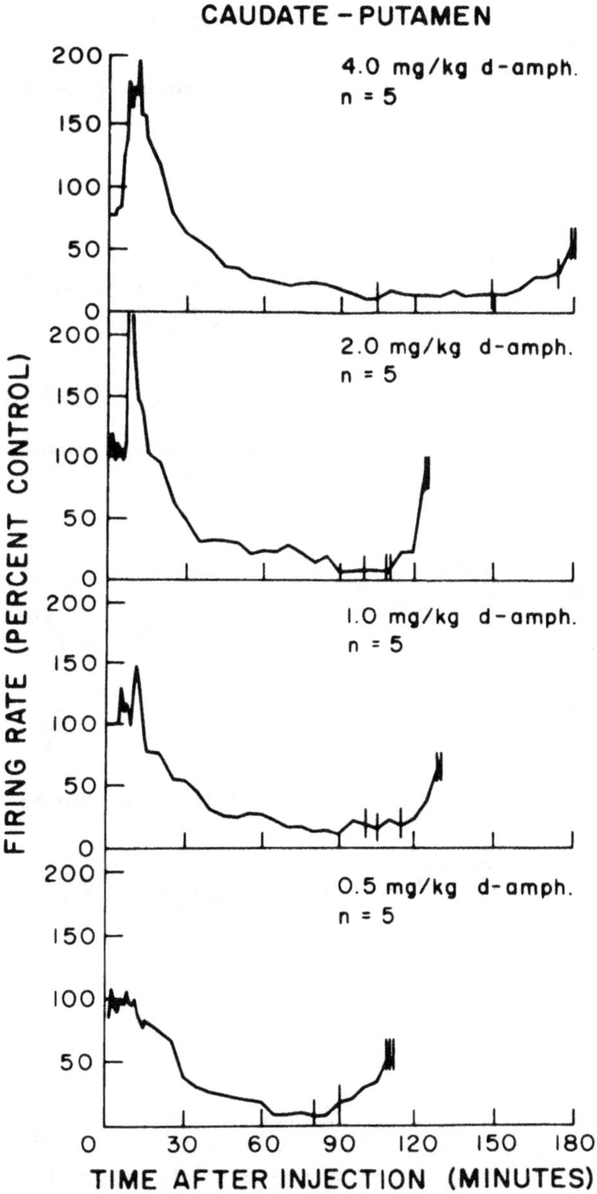

Fig. 1. Changes in spontaneous activity in the caudate-putamen following intraperitoneal injection of d-amphetamine sulfate. Each graph represents alterations in the mean firing rate of five single neurons recorded from five different animals, for doses of 0.5, 1.0, 2.0, and 4.0 mg/kg from bottom to top, respectively. In this and all subsequent figures, amphetamine was injected at time zero. (From: Groves, Rebec, and Segal, 1974.)

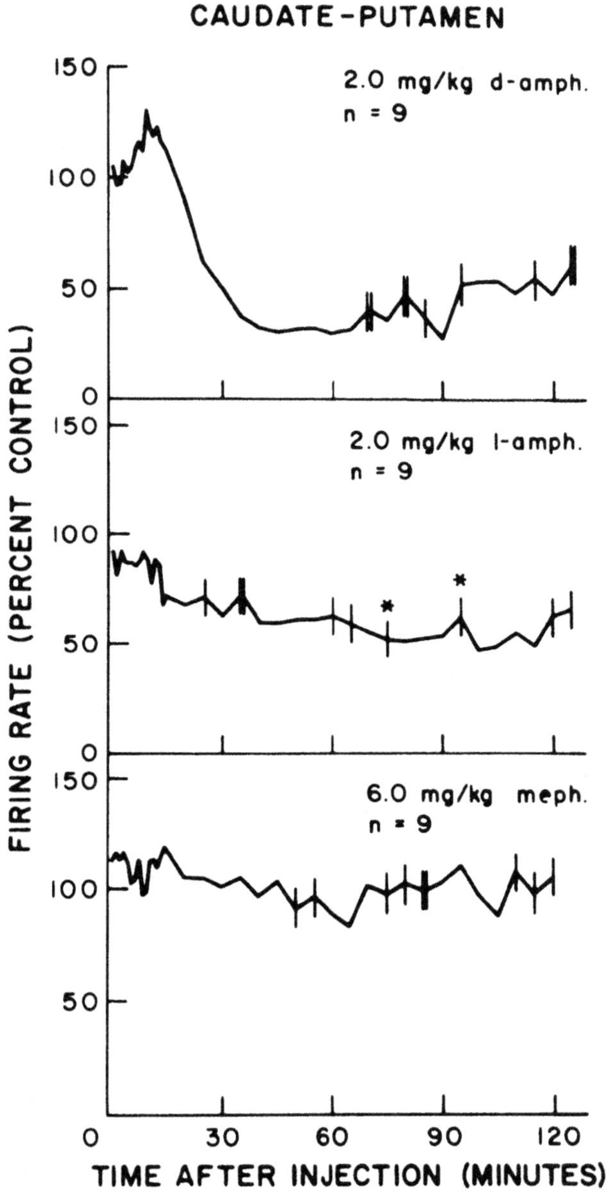

Fig. 2. Changes in caudate-putamen neuronal activity following intraperitoneal injection of 2.0 mg/kg d-amphetamine sulfate (top graph), 2.0 mg/kg l-amphetamine sulfate (middle graph), or 6.0 mg/kg mephentermine sulfate (bottom graph). The asterisks mark the duration that two neurons in the l-amphetamine group that did not depress to below 60% of pre-drug, control firing rate were held for observation. (From: Rebec and Groves, 1975a.)

As shown in Fig. 1, intraperitoneal administration of d-amphetamine sulfate to naive subjects typically produces a biphasic alteration in neuronal firing consisting of an initial, brief potentiation of neuronal activity which emerges within 10 minutes after injection, and a subsequent, prolonged depression of neuronal activity typically lasting from one to several hours. Both of these effects are dose-dependent as depicted sequentially from bottom to top in Fig. 1 for doses of 0.5, 1.0, 2.0, and 4.0 mg/kg, respectively.

Figure 2 reiterates this typical response pattern of caudate-putamen neurons to an injection of 2.0 mg/kg d-amphetamine sulfate in the top graph as it occurred in another sample of nine neostriatal neurons, and offers an interesting comparison with the alterations in neostriatal firing rates elicited by an injection of the same dose of l-amphetamine in nine additional neurons in the middle graph and by an injection of 6.0 mg/kg mephentermine sulfate, a presumed peripheral sympathomimetic with only weak central nervous system action, in the bottom graph (Rebec and Groves, 1975a).

Considering the view that the effects of amphetamine on dopaminergic transmission and stereotyped behavior were not stereospecific whereas its effects on noradrenergic transmission and locomotor behavior were stereospecific (e.g., Coyle and Snyder, 1969; Taylor and Snyder, 1970), and considering our previously published dose-response data shown in Fig. 1, we anticipated that the effects of d-amphetamine and l-amphetamine on neuronal firing rates in the neostriatum would be strikingly similar. In contrast to this result, we anticipated that the effects of these optical isomers of amphetamine on neuronal activity in the reticular formation of the brainstem would be quite markedly different. These data are presented later (see Fig. 5). In any event, our expectations were not borne out, as illustrated in Fig. 2. d-Amphetamine sulfate produced the typical initial increase in neuronal firing followed by a prolonged depression of neuronal activity in neostriatal neurons whereas l-amphetamine at the same dose produced no initial potentiation of firing rate and only minimal depressions of neuronal activity in the caudate-putamen, suggesting a difference in potency between these two isomers of considerably greater magnitude than the potency ratio of two-to-one or less that we expected. Nevertheless, our data are consistent with the general view that amphetamine-induced stereotyped behavior and locomotor behavior are mediated, in part, by dopaminergic nigro-neostriatal and noradrenergic reticular formation influences, respectively, as stated previously (e.g., Rebec and Groves, 1975a). A final point with regard to the data shown in Fig. 2 is that mephentermine sulfate did not produce any substantial alteration in caudate-putamen neuronal activity when it was administered to a sample of nine animals, suggesting that the amphetamine-induced-alterations in neostriatal firing rates that we have observed are not due to the peripheral sympathomimetic effects of amphetamine. The slashes in this graph indicate how long each neuron was held for observation.

In a recent, careful, and quantitative analysis of the behavioral effects of the optical isomers of amphetamine, Segal (1975) has shown that both the magnitude and pattern of locomotor and stereotyped behaviors produced by a dose of 2.5 mg/kg d-amphetamine can be virtually duplicated by 11.5 mg/kg l-amphetamine, with the exception that the time-response curve for the behavioral effects of l-amphetamine is shifted to the right, thus exhibiting a slightly longer latency. Data for d-amphetamine are illustrated in Fig. 3. The curious similarity of this curve to the effects of amphetamine on single neuron activity in the caudate-putamen at comparable doses is particularly interesting and is the subject of continuing analysis.

Figure 4 provides examples of single neuron activity photographed directly from data film and illustrates sequentially, in the upper four traces, the activity of a single caudate neuron prior to d-amphetamine administration, the potentiation of activity 10 minutes after the injection, the subsequent depression of neuronal firing 50 minutes after injection, and recovery to pre-injection rate at 120 minutes after d-amphetamine. The bottom four traces, representing a similar sequence, illustrate the activity of another caudate neuron in response to l-amphetamine administration. Essentially similar effects occur in response to amphetamine when recording from small populations of neurons (e.g., Groves, Wilson, Young, and Rebec, 1975), suggesting that such changes are widespread and not restricted to occasional, isolated single neostriatal neurons.

In the reticular formation, an acute intraperitoneal injection of d-amphetamine sulfate elicits a quite different response alteration than in the neostriatum (e.g., Groves, et al., 1974); Rebec and Groves, 1975a) and this is illustrated in Fig. 5. A prolonged increase in neuronal firing in the reticular formation following 2.0 mg/kg d-amphetamine sulfate is illustrated for a sample of eight neurons recorded from eight different subjects in the top graph of Fig. 5, where the slashes indicate a return to within 135% of control firing rate following this acceleration of activity. In the middle graph, the same dose of l-amphetamine elicited in eight additional reticular formation neurons an increase in activity that was considerably less pronounced and less prolonged than that produced by the d-isomer of the drug. Interestingly, the response to 6.0 mg/kg mephentermine sulfate in seven additional reticular formation neurons, as shown in the bottom graph, was not different from that produced by 2.0 mg/kg l-amphetamine sulfate. The slashes in the lowest graph illustrate how long each neuron was held for observation.

The depression of neuronal activity in the neostriatum may be presumed to result from the ability of amphetamine to promote the release and block the reuptake of dopamine from terminals of the

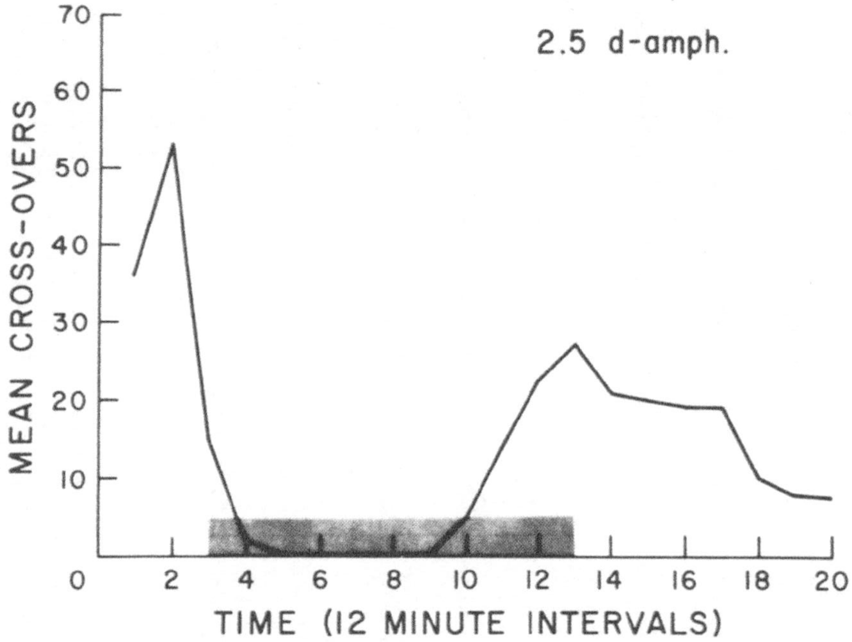

Fig. 3. The time course of locomotor and stereotyped behavior produced by 2.5 mg/kg d-amphetamine in the albino rat. The ordinate (cross-overs) is a measure of locomotor behavior. The shaded portion of the figure indicates stereotyped behavior in the absence of normal, forward locomotion. (From: Segal, 1975. Used by permission of the author.)

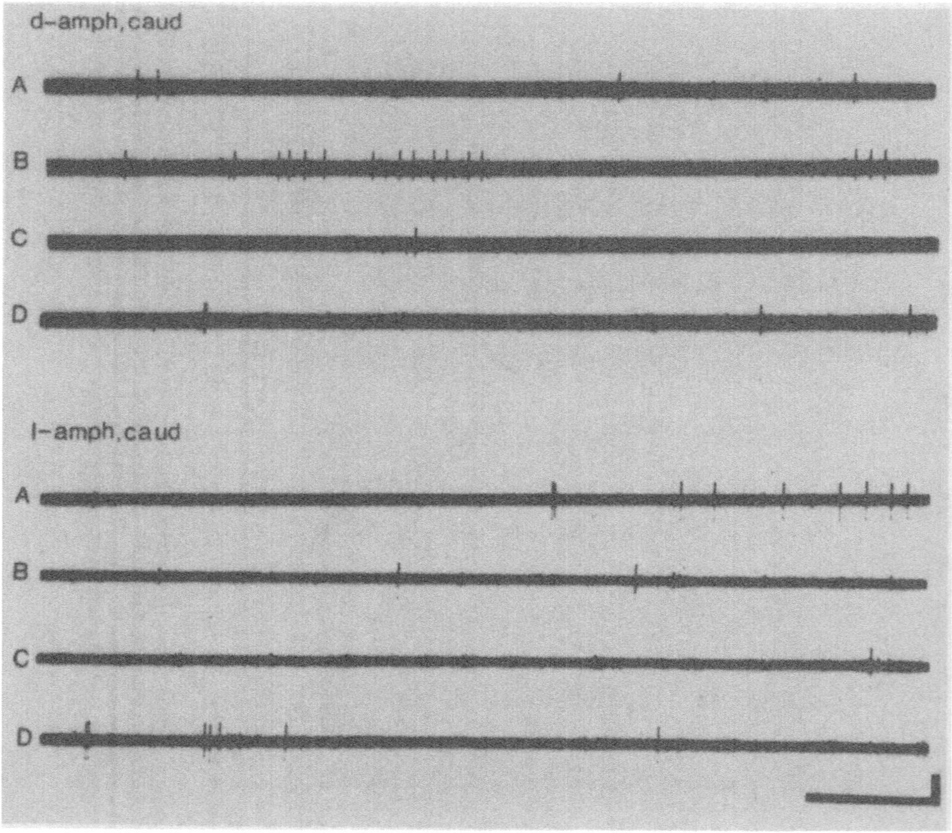

Fig. 4. Illustrative examples of single neuron activity in the caudate-putamen prior to (A in each set of traces), and 10 min (B), 50 min (C), and 120 (D, top) or 80 (D, bottom) min following administration of 2.0 mg/kg d-amphetamine sulfate (upper four traces) or l-amphetamine sulfate (lower four traces). Calibration mark is 1 sec (horizontal) and 100 μv (vertical). (From: Rebec and Groves, (1975a.)

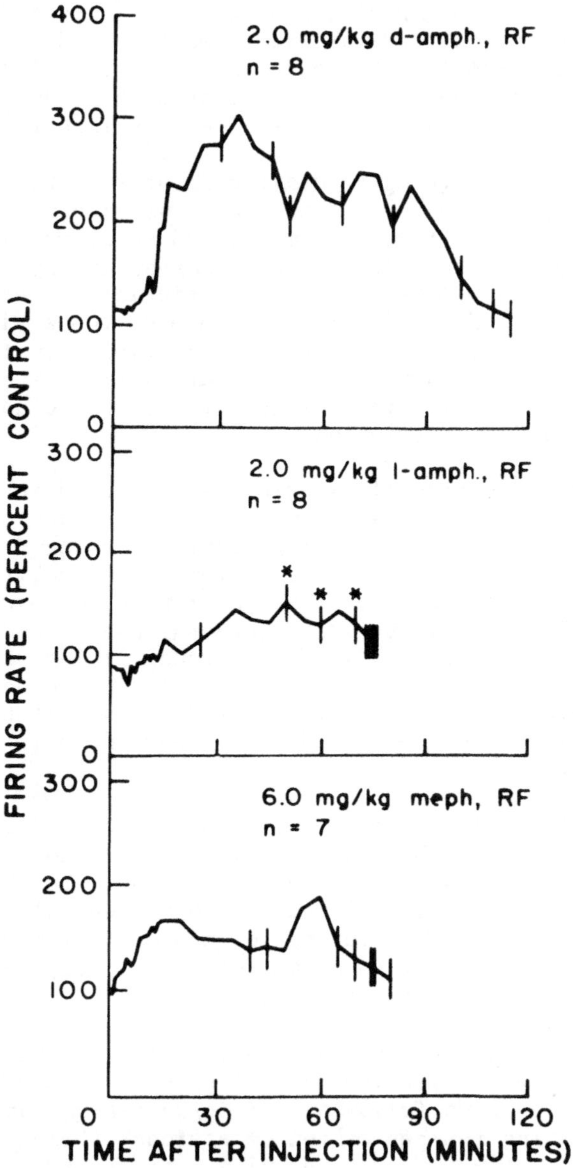

Fig. 5. Changes in reticular formation neuronal activity following intraperitoneal administration of 2.0 mg/kg d-amphetamine sulfate (top graph), l-amphetamine sulfate (middle graph), and 6.0 mg/kg mephentermine sulfate (bottom graph). The asterisks indicate three neurons in the l-amphetamine sample that did not increase firing rate to above 140% of pre-drug baseline firing rate. (From: Rebec and Groves, 1975a.)

nigro-neostriatal dopaminergic projection (Groves and Rebec, 1976). We have also performed several experiments in order to confirm this view. For example, the depression of neuronal firing can be blocked by intra-peritoneal administration of haloperidol, a dopaminergic blocking agent. This effect is illustrated in Fig. 6.

An injection of 1.0 mg/kg d-amphetamine sulfate produced a marked slowing of firing rate in this sample of five neostriatal neurons recorded from five different animals, and in every case the slowing of firing rate could be blocked by a subsequent injection of 2.0 mg/kg haloperidol 50 minutes after amphetamine administration. An injection of 2.0 mg/kg haloperidol also produces a significant, although not dramatic, increase in neuronal firing in the neostriatum as illustrated for a sample of five neurons from five different animals in Fig. 7, in which the slashes also indicate how long each neuron was held for observation.

In a separate series of experiments performed in collaboration with John Harvey of the University of Iowa, we examined alterations in caudate-putamen neuronal firing rates following d-amphetamine administration in animals with ipsilateral electrolytic lesions of the ascending nigro-neostriatal projection which resulted in a depletion of telencephalic dopamine (Groves, Rebec, and Harvey, 1975). Alterations in neostriatal neuronal firing rates in animals with unilateral nigro-neostriatal bundle lesions produced by 2.0 mg/kg d-amphetamine sulfate administered intraperitoneally are compared to alterations elicited by the same dose in intact control animals in Fig. 8.

Although the initial potentiation of neuronal firing remains unaffected in animals with unilateral lesions of the nigro-neostriatal projection, the depression of neuronal firing rate is markedly reduced or abolished. This evidence is consistent with the view that the amphetamine-induced depression of neuronal firing is due to an indirect mechanism of action of amphetamine; i.e., release of dopamine from nigro-neostriatal terminals.

Recently, Groves, Wilson, and Juraska (unpublished observations) have been able to abolish the initial potentiation of firing rate in neostriatal neurons following 2.5 mg/kg d-amphetamine administration while leaving the depression of neuronal firing relatively unaffected. This effect occurs in animals pretreated 15 minutes prior to amphetamine administration by intraperitoneal administration of 1.0 mg/kg scopolamine. Similar pretreatment with 1.0 mg/kg methscopolamine does not block the initial potentiation of firing rate despite the markedly greater peripheral effects of this peripheral cholinergic blocking agent at this dose. Indeed, both methscopolamine and, to a lesser extent, scopolamine potentiated the increased heart rate typically seen following d-amphetamine administration (e.g., Groves, et al., 1974).

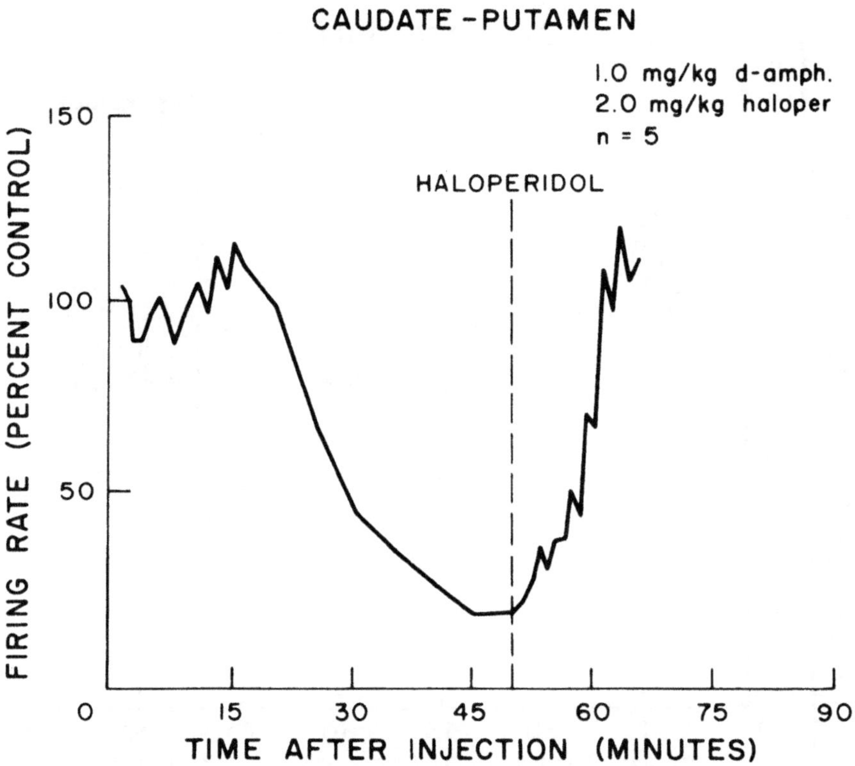

Fig. 6. Reversal of the d-amphetamine depression of spontaneous neuronal firing in the caudate-putamen by 2.0 mg/kg Haloperidol injected intraperitoneally. (From: Groves, Rebec, and Segal, 1974.)

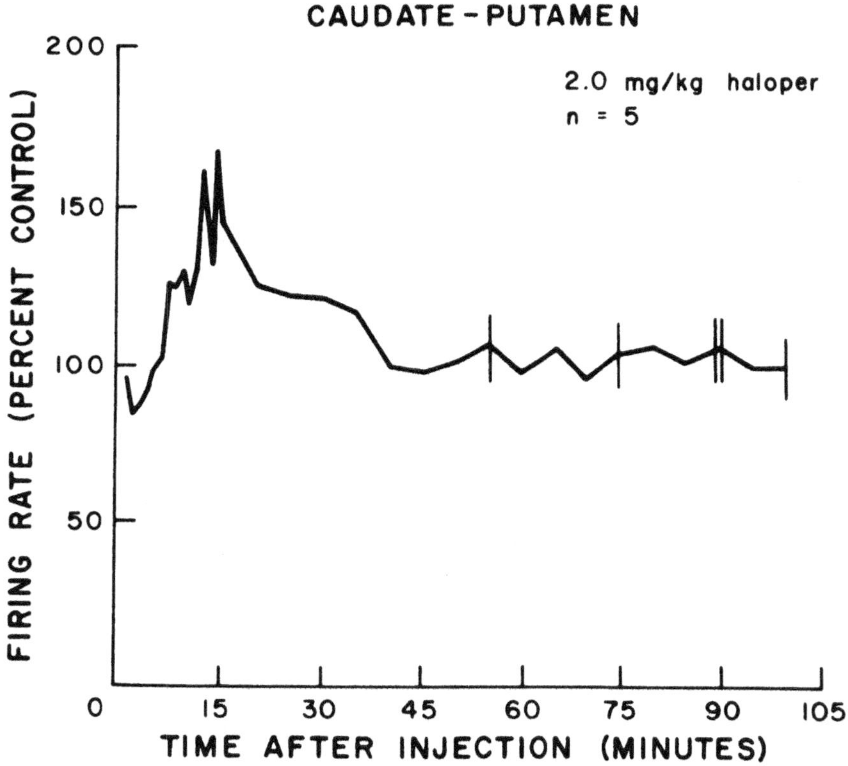

Fig. 7. Changes in spontaneous neuronal activity in the caudate-putamen following 2.0 mg/kg Haloperidol injected intraperitoneally at time zero. (From: Groves, Rebec, and Segal, 1974.)

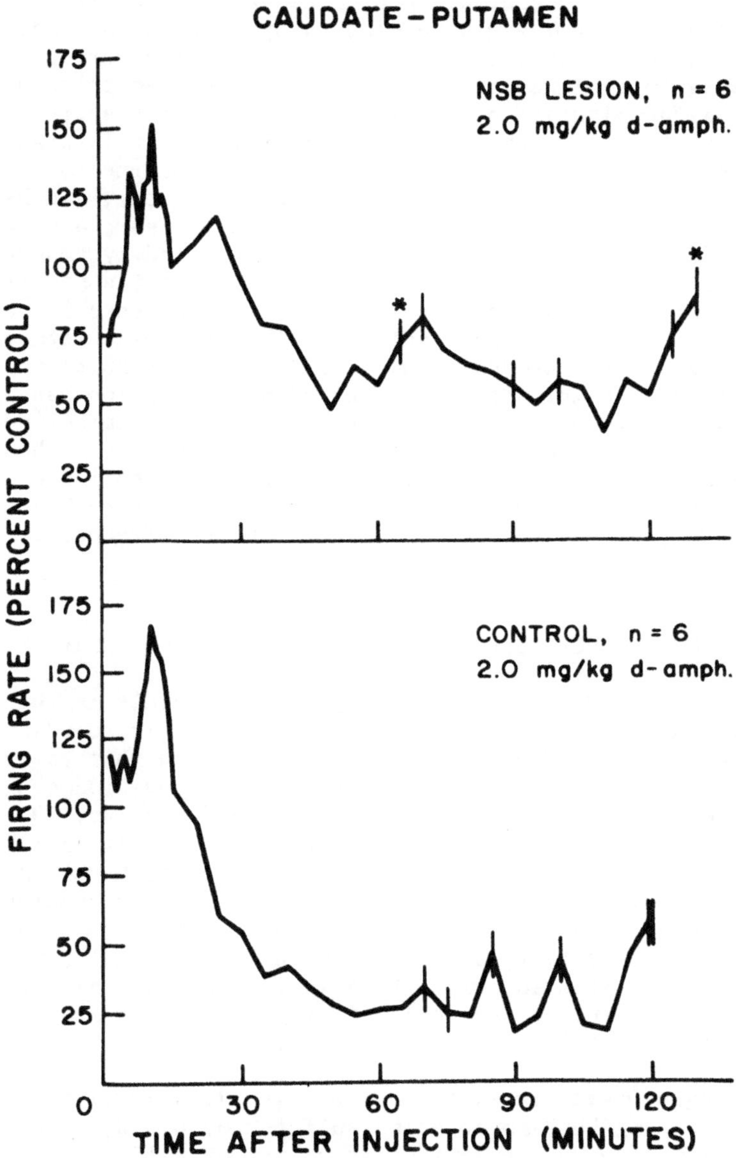

Fig. 8. Alterations in caudate-putamen neuronal firing rates following 2.0 mg/kg d-amphetamine sulfate at time zero, for animals with unilateral lesions of the nigro-neostriatal bundle (top graph, n = 6) or intact control animals (bottom graph, n = 6). Asterisks mark two neurons in the animals with unilateral lesions for which neuronal firing never fell below 60% of control firing rate. (From: Groves, Rebec, and Harvey, 1975.)

Since the initial potentiation produced by intraperitoneally administered d-amphetamine can be blocked by scopolamine pretreatment, it would appear that this initial increase may reflect a transient increase in cholinergic transmission in the neostriatum, perhaps due to a facilitation of cholinergic interneuron activity. It is tempting to speculate that amphetamine promotes an initial, transient release of acetylcholine from cholinergic interneurons that are intrinsic to the basal ganglia (e.g., Lynch, Lucas, and Deadwyler, 1972; Butcher and Butcher, 1974; McGeer, McGeer, Grewaal, and Singh, 1975) before these elements are inhibited by amphetamine's facilitation of dopaminergic transmission in the neostriatum. In addition, since a similar initial, transient increase in neuronal firing can be produced by local infusion of amphetamine into the caudate-putamen (e.g., Groves et al., 1975), these results appear to be well-accounted for without invoking an explanation based upon increased excitatory drive originating from an amphetamine-induced increase in excitatory afferents to the caudate-putamen. These results are also consistent with the view that the cholinergic interneurons of the neostriatum are mutually excitatory (e.g. Trabucchi, Cheney, Racagni, and Costa, 1975; Racagni, Cheney, Trabucchi, and Costa, in press).

ALTERATIONS PRODUCED BY LONG-TERM AMPHETAMINE PRETREATMENT

Although repeated injections of amphetamine result in the development of tolerance to amphetamine-induced anorexigenic, cardiovascular, and hyperthermic effects, it has been observed that tolerance does not develop to the hyperactivity and stereotypy produced by the drug (Lewander, 1971, 1974; Kalant, LeBlanc, and Gibbins, 1971). In the first systematic study of this phenomenon involving rats continuously exposed to their experimental chambers, Segal and Mandell (1974) reported that repeated injections of d-amphetamine for 36 consecutive days caused a progressive augmentation of locomotor activity and/or stereotypy, depending on the dose. In light of such evidence, we have extended our work to include an examination of the effects of amphetamine on neuronal activity in animals pretreated with the drug for extended periods of time.

Male Sprague-Dawley rats, housed individually, received an i.p. injection of 2.5 mg/kg d-amphetamine sulfate for 6, 18, or 36 days. Control animals received an equivalent volume of saline for 36 days. On the day immediately following the appropriate pretreatment period, the subjects were prepared for the recording session as previously described.

Figure 9 illustrates what happens to the initial amphetamine-induced potentiation and subsequent depression of neuronal activity in the neostriatum following long-term saline or amphetamine pretreatment (Rebec and Groves, unpublished observations). The top

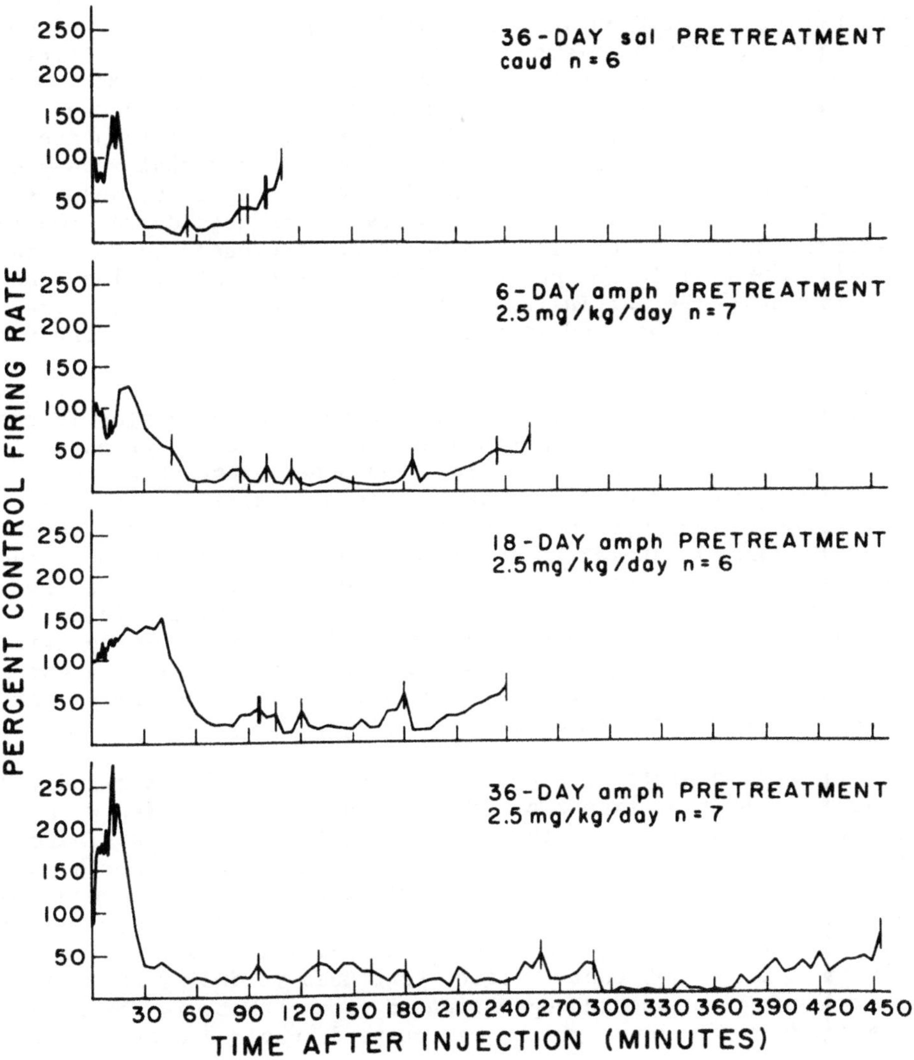

Fig. 9. Changes in neuronal firing rates in the caudate-putamen following an intraperitoneal injection of 2.5 mg/kg d-amphetamine sulfate at time zero, in animals pretreated with 36 daily saline injections, or 6, 18, or 36 days of d-amphetamine sulfate, from top to bottom, respectively. The slashes indicate recovery to 65% of control firing rate for each neuron and points at which data from each neuron are deleted from subsequent averaged values. (From: Rebec and Groves, unpublished observations.)

graph represents the mean responses over time of six neostriatal neurons in animals that were pretreated with saline for 36 days and subsequently received an injection of 2.5 mg/kg d-amphetamine. Note that the two prominent d-amphetamine effects (the initial potentiation and subsequent depression of activity) are, for the most part, identical to the effects of amphetamine reported in our acute studies. The lower three graphs depict, in order, the response to an injection of 2.5 mg/kg d-amphetamine for animals that were pretreated with the drug for 6, 18, or 36 days. Note that, despite some individual variability, the amphetamine-induced depression in neostriatal neuronal activity progressively increased in duration following these prolonged periods of exposure to amphetamine. An augmentation of the initial amphetamine-induced potentiation of activity was also observed in animals pretreated with the drug for 36 days.

Two individual examples of amphetamine-induced changes in the activity of single caudate-putamen neurons in saline pretreated animals are illustrated in Fig. 10. The upper graph shows that amphetamine produced a brief potentiation of activity which was followed by a pronounced depression of firing rate that returned to 65% of control rate at approximately 90 minutes after the injection. When unit activity was monitored beyond this point, a prolonged secondary increase in activity of substantial magnitude emerged before a second return to control firing rate became evident. A qualitatively similar but less dramatic series of events in response to amphetamine are illustrated in the lower graph for another saline pretreated animal.

Figure 11 depicts some changes in the activity of two individual neurons obtained from two different animals pretreated with amphetamine for 36 days. In these examples, the amphetamine-induced potentiation of firing rate is quite pronounced and, although quantitative differences exist with respect to the degree of depression produced by amphetamine, the slowing of activity persists, in both cases, for several hours. Following the initial recovery of unit activity to above 65% control rate, continued recording revealed the existence of a second depression of firing that, in the case of the example in the lower graph, was quite dramatic and of significant duration.

As in our acute experiments, we attempted to block the amphetamine-induced depression of caudate activity in chronically treated animals by a subsequent injection of 2.0 mg/kg haloperidol. In all cases, this dopamine antagonist was capable of reversing the amphetamine effect in animals pretreated with the drug for 36 days. Figure 12 depicts this rapid, albeit transient, reversal as it occurred in one caudate neuron. Following the initial amphetamine-induced potentiation of activity, which in this case was quite pronounced, neuronal activity rapidly decreased to well below baseline firing

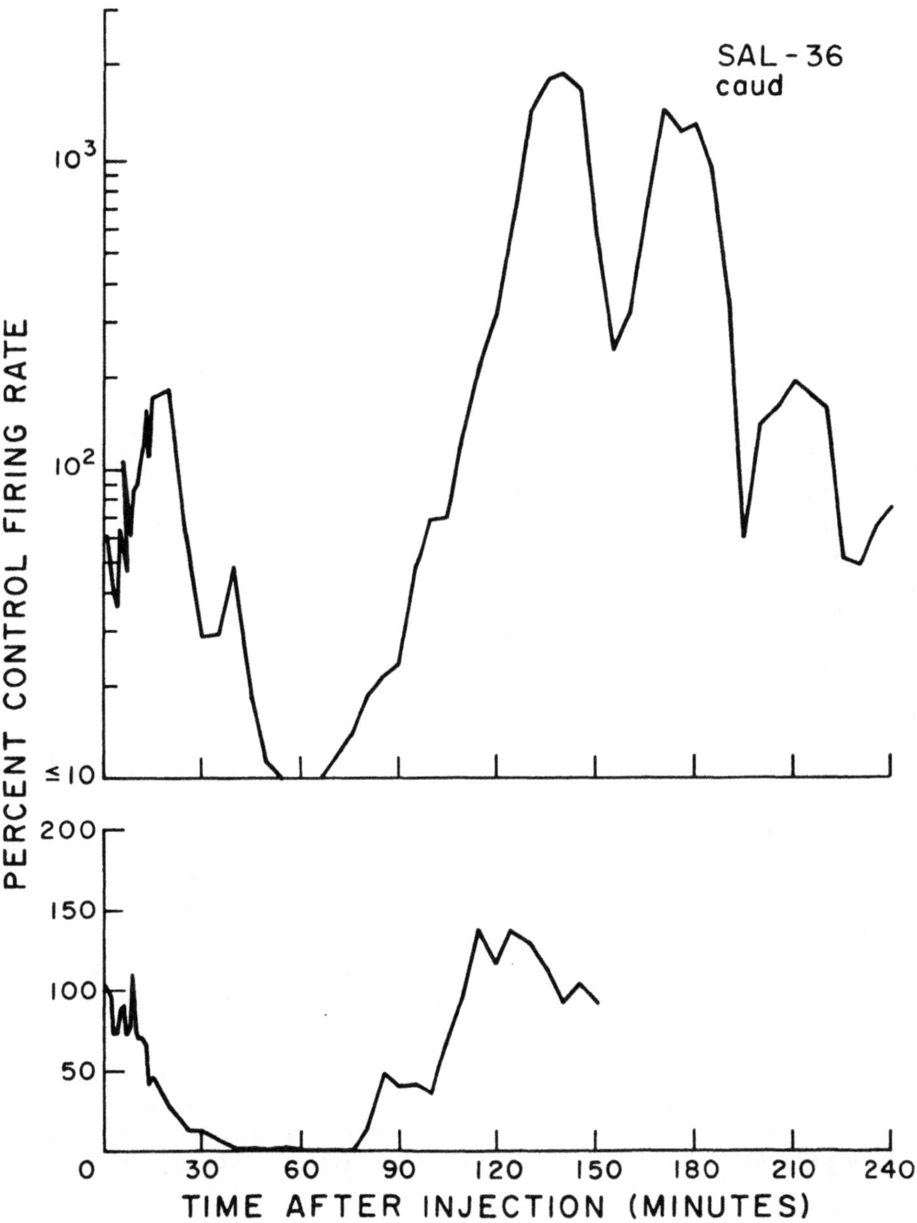

Fig. 10. Changes in the spontaneous firing rates of two neurons recorded from two different animals pretreated with saline for 36 consecutive days. Amphetamine was injected intraperitoneally (2.5 mg/kg) at time zero in both cases. (From: Rebec, 1975.)

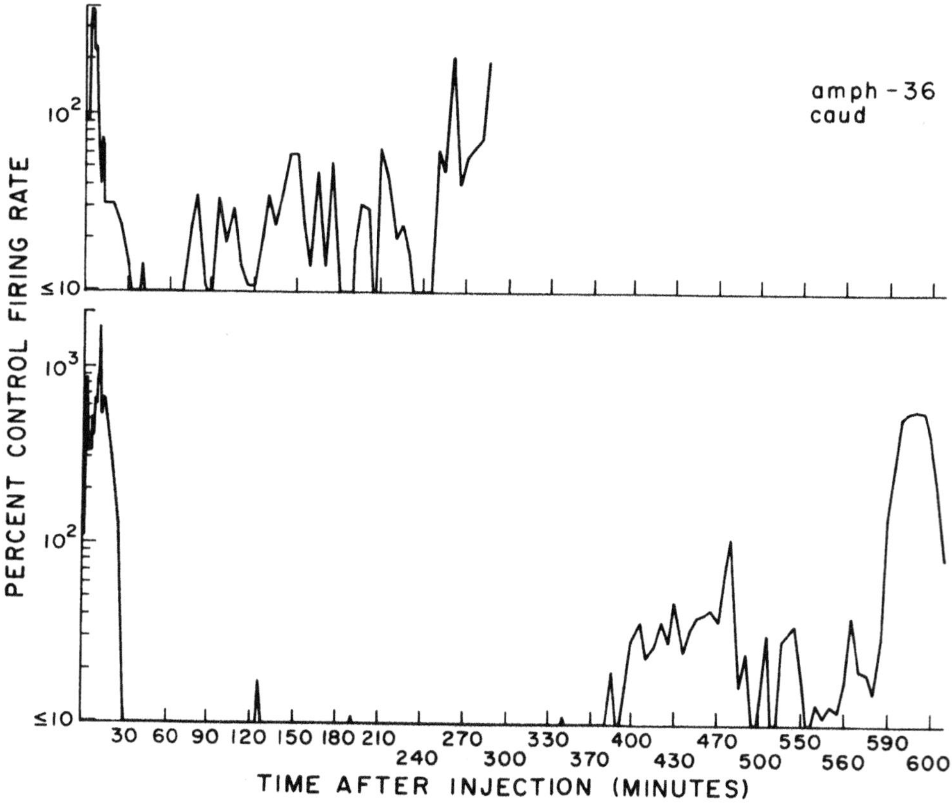

Fig. 11. Changes in the spontaneous firing rates of two neurons recorded from two different animals pretreated with amphetamine for 36 consecutive days. Amphetamine was injected intraperitoneally (2.5 mg/kg) at time zero in both cases. (From: Rebec, 1975.)

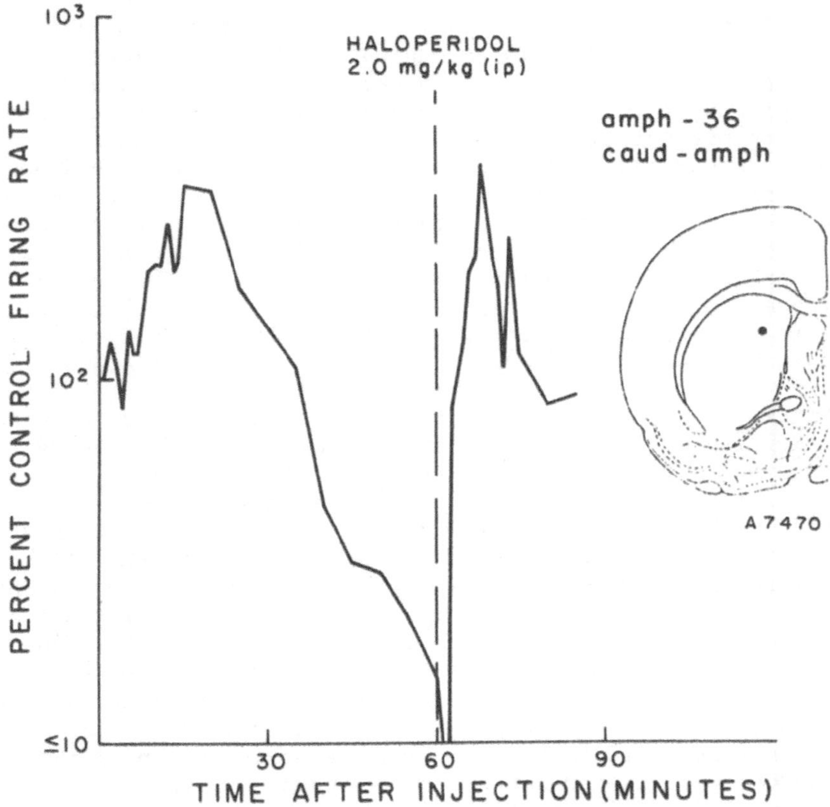

Fig. 12. Changes in the firing rate of a single neuron in the caudate-putamen recorded from a subject pretreated with d-amphetamine for 36 days. An intraperitoneal injection of haloperidol 60 minutes after d-amphetamine reversed the depression of firing rate. (From: Rebec, 1975.)

rate. The administration of haloperidol at 60 minutes after amphetamine produced a reversal of the amphetamine depression. In one additional case, shown in Fig. 13, we encountered a caudate neuron in an animal pretreated with amphetamine for 36 days that demonstrated a prolonged increase in responsiveness to a subsequent injection of amphetamine and this atypical response was also rapidly reversed following haloperidol administration. We have seen similar, atypical prolonged increases in neostriatal neuronal activity following amphetamine administration in a variety of experimental paradigms (e.g., Rebec and Groves, 1975a, unpublished observations; Groves, Wilson, and Juraska, unpublished observations). Thus, these less typical prolonged increases in neuronal activity in the caudate-putamen are not restricted to chronically pretreated animals and may form another class of responses in the neostriatum to amphetamine administration. Interestingly, infrequent excitatory effects of dopamine applied iontophoretically to neurons in the caudate-putamen have also been reported (e.g., York, 1967; Connor, 1970), and it has been suggested that, on some neurons of the neostriatum, dopamine may act as an excitatory transmitter, although in our experiments an indirect effect of amphetamine by way of intrastriatal connections or other pathways cannot be ruled out.

Figure 14 illustrates the effects of reticular formation neuronal activity of 2.5 mg/kg d-amphetamine administered to animals pretreated with saline for 36 days or with amphetamine for varying periods of time. The slashes indicate, in these graphs, the total time that each reticular formation neuron was held for observation. The top graph depicts the effects of saline pretreatment on the neuronal response to amphetamine. Not surprisingly, the response closely resembles that produced by amphetamine in other acute experiments. The lower three graphs illustrate, in order, the effects of 2.5 mg/kg d-amphetamine in subjects pretreated with the drug for 6, 18, or 36 consecutive days. One prominent feature of the amphetamine-induced changes in reticular formation activity in chronically treated rats appeared to be a progressive prolongation of the initial drug-induced increase in activity. The mean durations of the initial, amphetamine-induced increases in firing rate of reticular formation neurons are depicted for these different pretreatment groups in Fig. 15. The duration of increased firing for each neuron was defined as the time after injection that each unit remained above 135% control firing rate before falling below this criterion level for 10 minutes or more. The electrode tip placements where neuronal activity in the reticular formation was recorded are illustrated in Fig. 16. The increase in reticular formation unit responsiveness produced by amphetamine has been attributed, in part, to the drug-induced release of norepinephrine (e.g., Groves, et al., 1974; Rebec and Groves, 1975a, b) which, when applied iontophoretically, mimics the action of iontophoretically applied amphetamine among brainstem neurons (Boakes, Bradley, and Candy, 1972).

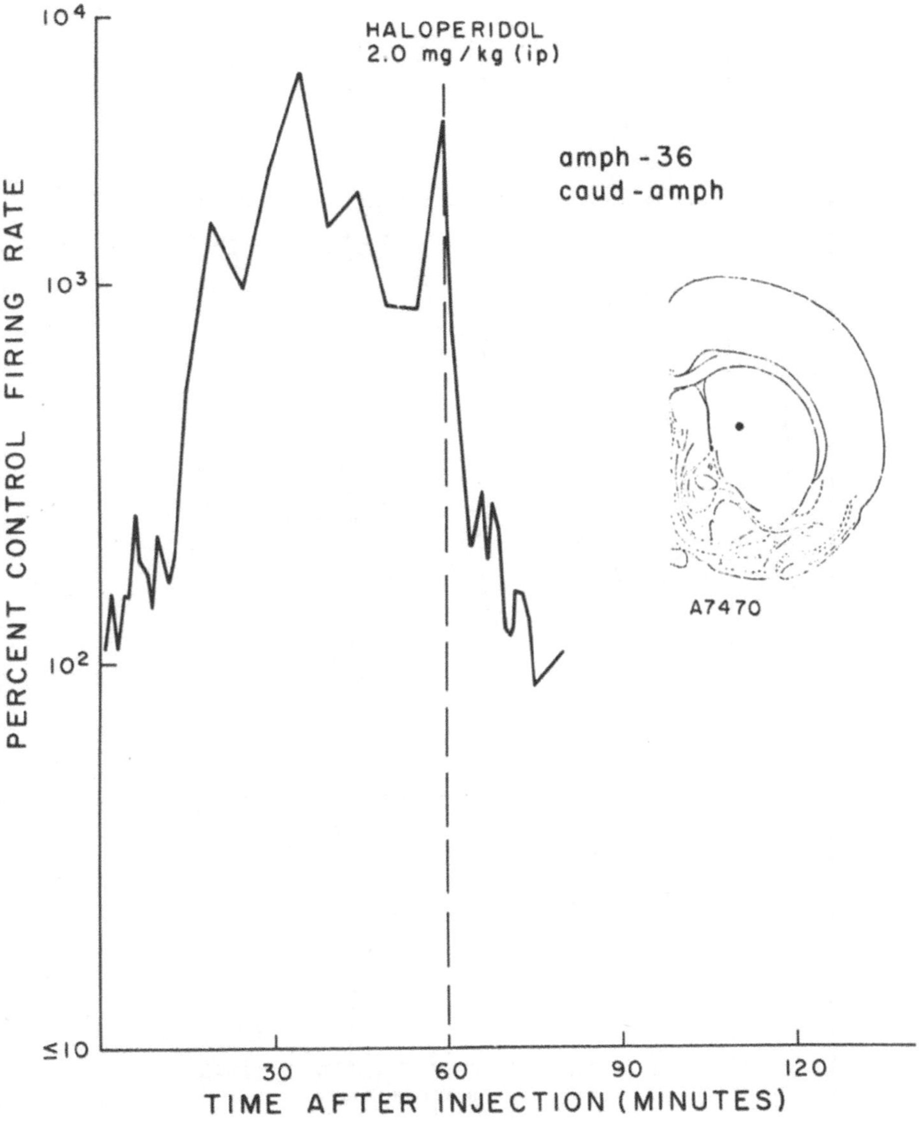

Fig. 13. An atypical increase in neuronal firing rate of a caudate-putamen neuron recorded in a subject pretreated with d-amphetamine for 36 days. The increase in firing rate was blocked by a subsequent injection of 2.0 mg/kg haloperidol. (From: Rebec, 1975.)

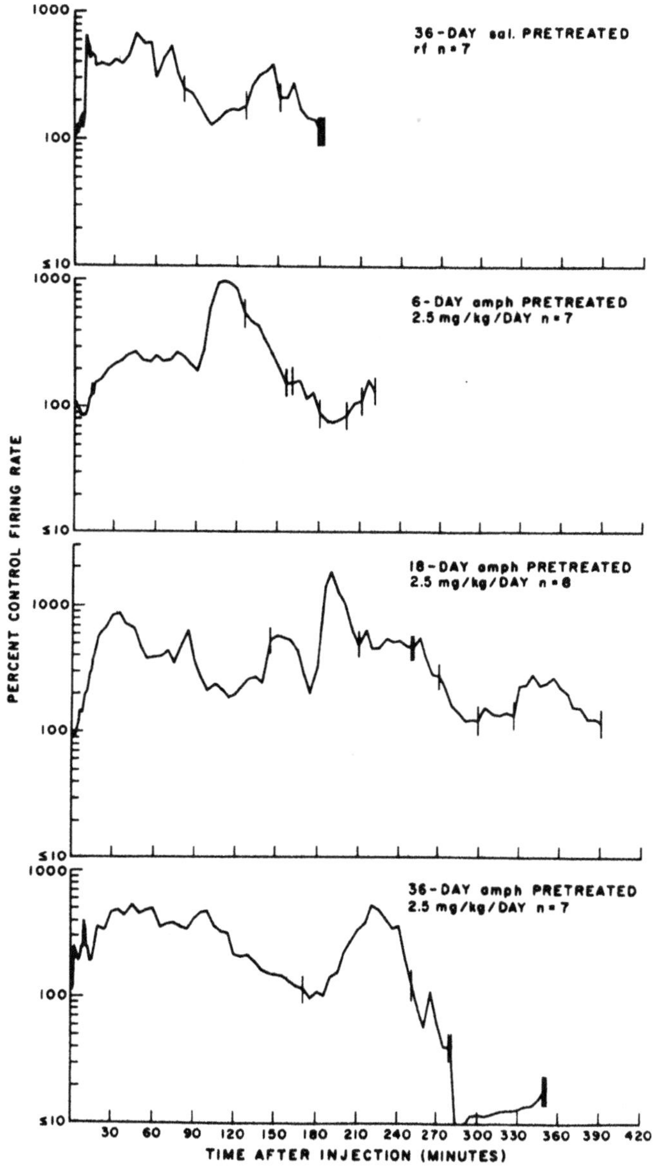

Fig. 14. Changes in neuronal firing rates in the reticular formation following an intraperitoneal injection of 2.5 mg/kg d-amphetamine sulfate at time zero, in animals pretreated with 36 daily saline injections, or 6, 18, or 36 days of d-amphetamine sulfate, from top to bottom, respectively. The slashes indicate the time that each neuron was held for observation and the points at which data from each neuron no longer contribute to subsequent averaged values. (From: Rebec, 1975.)

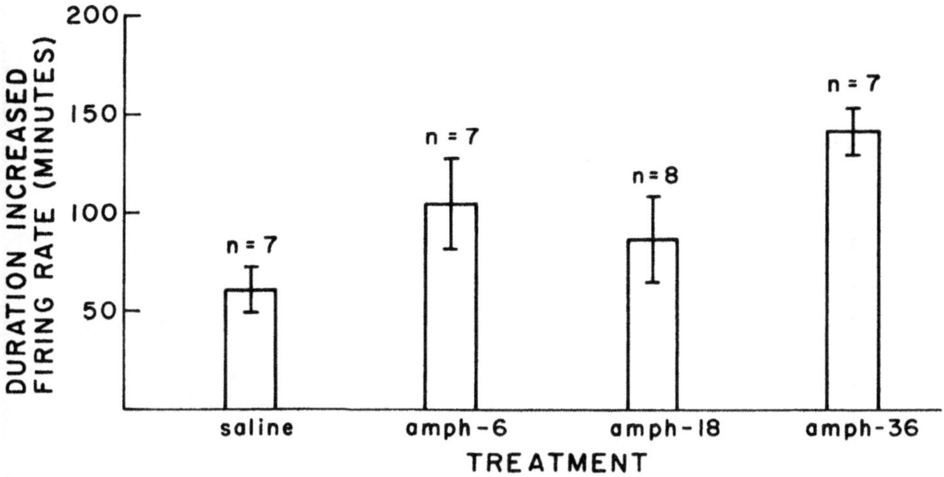

Fig. 15. The mean duration of increased neuronal activity in the reticular formation produced by amphetamine administration, in animals pretreated with saline or d-amphetamine for varying periods of time. The brackets indicate one standard error above and below the mean values. (From: Rebec, 1975.)

In several cases, activity in the reticular formation was monitored beyond recovery from the initial, amphetamine-induced increase in firing rate. In many cases, a marked depression of firing became evident and was followed by a second, prolonged increase in activity. These effects are illustrated for two individual neurons in Fig. 17. The upper traces illustrate the activity of one reticular formation neuron recorded from an animal pretreated with saline for 36 consecutive days, while the lower traces illustrate the response of a single neuron in a subject pretreated with amphetamine for 36 days. In both examples activity increases dramatically after amphetamine administration (B), compared to neuronal firing prior to administration of the drug (A). Also in both cases, a marked depression of firing rate follows the initial acceleration (C), a secondary increase in neuronal activity occurs (D), and a second recovery to predrug firing rate follows this (E).

Although we have observed an enhancement of caudate-putamen and reticular formation neuronal responses to amphetamine following long-term pretreatment, we have also observed, in agreement with previous reports, the development of tolerance to the weight loss effect of amphetamine. Figure 18 illustrates that, for a sample of 25 animals receiving single daily injections of 2.5 mg/kg d-amphetamine, a decline in body weight occurred during the first week of treatment but tolerance to this effect developed rapidly. An additional 25

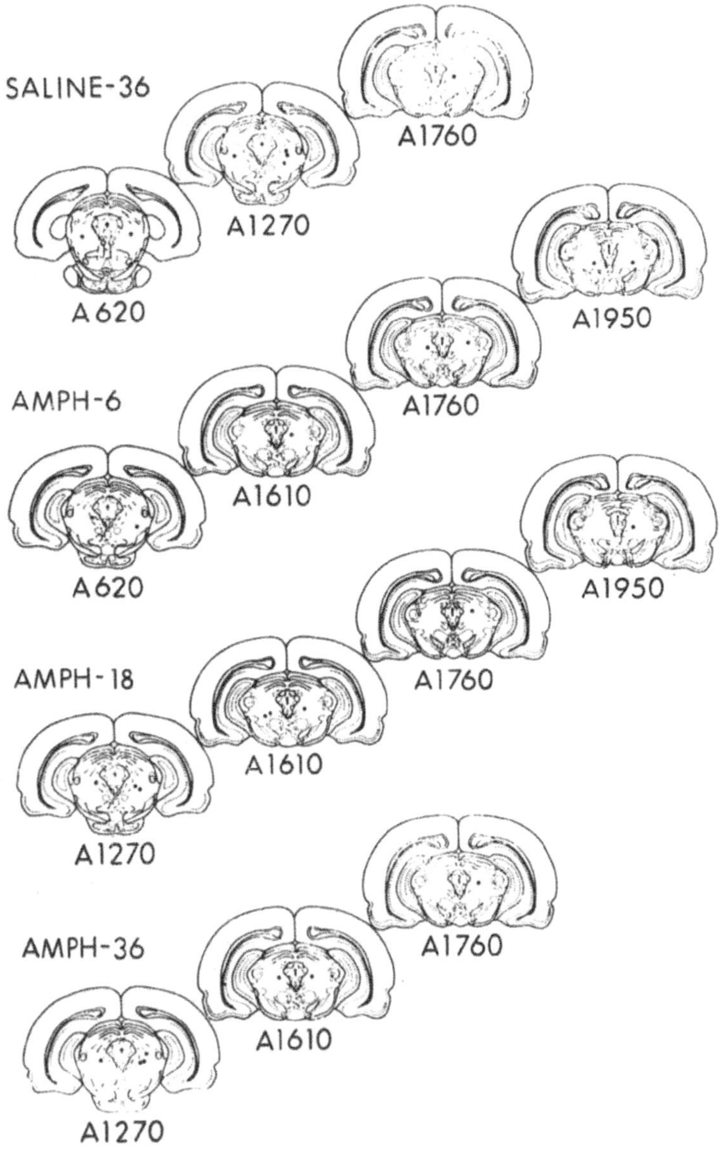

Fig. 16. Electrode tip placements in the reticular formation where neuronal activity was recorded in various pretreatment groups are illustrated by small black dots. Histological sections are after Koenig and Klippel (1963). (From: Rebec, 1975.)

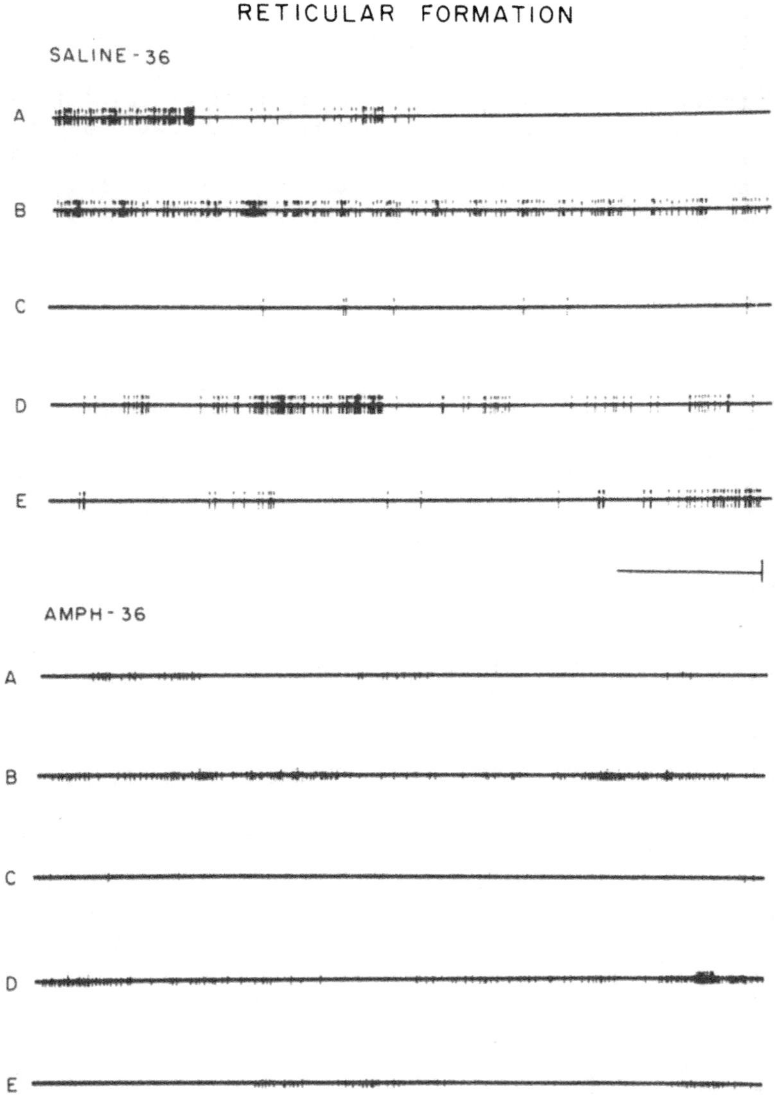

Fig. 17. Examples of extracellular unit activity in the reticular formation of one subject pretreated with saline for 36 consecutive days (upper traces) and one subject pretreated with amphetamine for 36 days (lower traces). The upper traces illustrate spontaneous firing prior to amphetamine administration (A), increased firing rate 30 minutes after the drug was injected (B), a slowing of firing rate 70 minutes after injection (C), a second increase in neuronal firing 120 minutes after injection (D), and recovery to control rate 150 minutes after injection (E). In the lower traces, control activity is illustrated prior to injection (A), the initial increase

(Fig. 17 continued)
in activity still evident 80 minutes after drug administration (B), a marked depression of activity 140 minutes following injection (C), a secondary increase in activity 160 minutes after injection (D), and a return to baseline firing rate 220 minutes following amphetamine administration (E). The calibration marks represent 2 seconds (horizontal) and 15 μv (upper traces) or 200 μv (lower traces, vertical). (From: Rebec, 1975.)

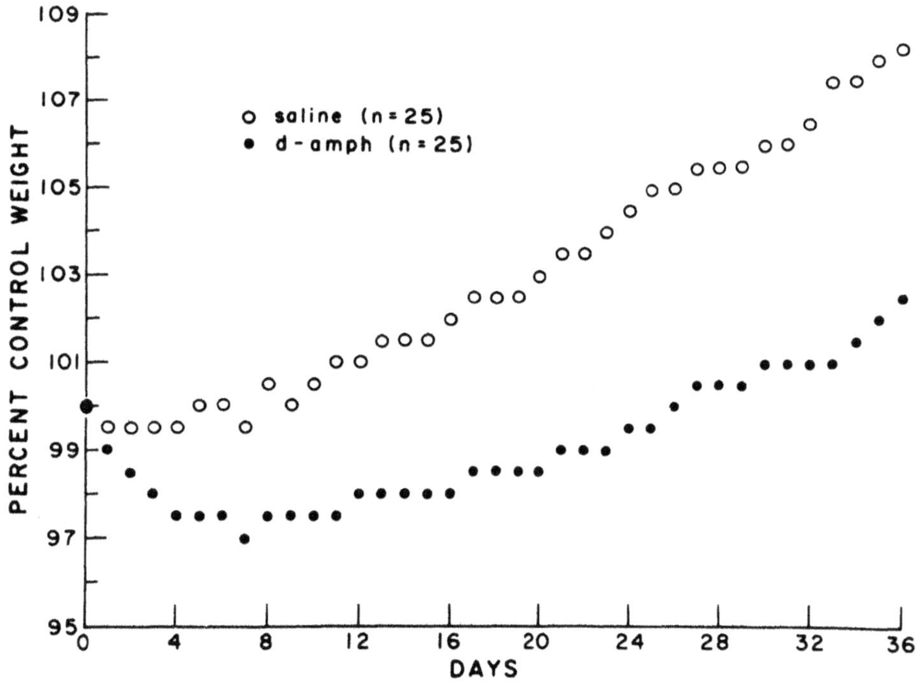

Fig. 18. Mean body weight, plotted as percent of control weight as measured on the day prior to treatment, for 25 rats given 2.5 mg/kg d-amphetamine sulfate intraperitoneally (solid circles) or 25 rats given an equivalent volume of saline (open circles) once each day for 36 consecutive days. (From: Rebec, 1975.)

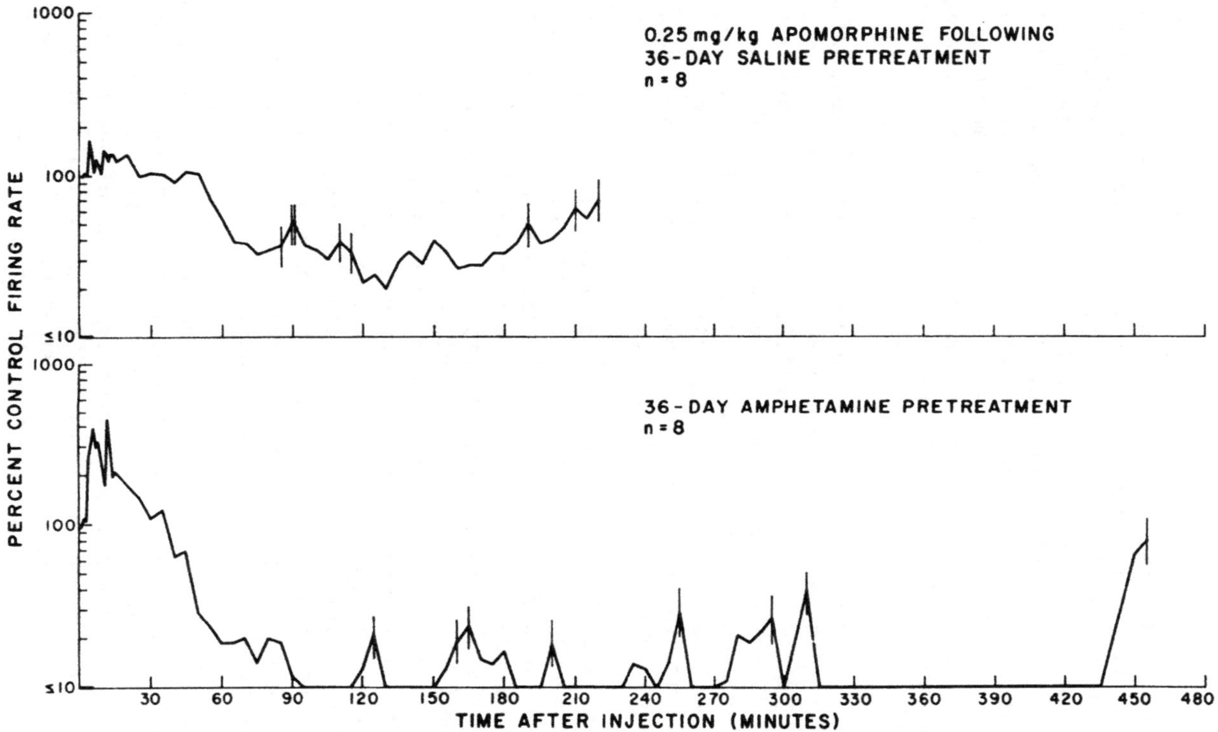

Fig. 19. Alterations in spontaneous neuronal firing rates in the caudate-putamen produced by intraperitoneally administered apomorphine (0.25 mg/kg), in animals pretreated with 36 daily saline injections (upper graph) or 36 daily injections of 2.5 mg/kg d-amphetamine sulfate. (Rebec and Groves, unpublished observations.)

saline animals continued to gain weight on a regular basis. Body weights are shown as percent of the pre-injection weight which was given a value of 100 percent.

It has been suggested that the depletion of brain catecholamines that accompanies long-term amphetamine treatment results in such heightened sensitivity of central catecholamine receptors, perhaps analogous to functional disuse or denervation (e.g., Sharpless, 1964, 1975), that repeated injections of the drug elicit enhanced psychomotor stimulant effects (Ellinwood, Sudilovsky, and Nelson, 1973). In support of this notion, Klawans and associates (Klawans, Crossett, and Dana, 1975) reported that the administration of apomorphine, a dopamine receptor stimulant, to animals maintained on amphetamine for two to five weeks elicited full-blown stereotyped behaviors at a dose that had no effect in naive animals.

In order to determine whether chronic exposure to amphetamine alters the sensitivity of central dopamine receptors, we recorded the alterations in neostriatal unit activity produced in animals administered 0.25 mg/kg d-amphetamine once daily for 36 days and in animals that had received an equivalent volume of saline for an identical period (Rebec and Groves, unpublished observations). In accord with the hypothesis of a chronic amphetamine-induced heightened sensitivity of central catecholamine receptors, we found that apomorphine elicited considerably more pronounced effects on caudate-putamen neuronal activity in amphetamine-pretreated rats than in saline-pretreated controls. This is illustrated in Fig. 19. The top graph shows the effects of 0.25 mg/kg apomorphine on the activity of eight single neurons in the neostriatum recorded from saline-pretreated animals. In this case, apomorphine elicited an initial transient potentiation of firing rate followed by a gradual slowing of activity. As illustrated in the lower graph for eight additional neurons recorded from chronically intoxicated animals, the apomorphine-induced effects appeared to be significantly enhanced by long-term amphetamine treatment. Note especially that the apomorphine-induced depression of neuronal firing is not only increased in duration following chronic amphetamine treatment but is also more pronounced than in saline-pretreated controls.

The origin of the initial potentiation of neuronal firing in the caudate nucleus following apomorphine administration is unknown and could reflect an action of this drug on striatal afferents or inter-neurons. The apomorphine-induced depression of neostriatal activity appears to be the result of a direct action of this drug on postsynaptic dopamine receptors (e.g., Ungerstedt, Ljungberg, Hoffer, and Siggins, 1975). The enhancement of this apomorphine-induced response following long-term amphetamine treatment is consistent with the hypothesis (Ellinwood, 1974) that chronic amphetamine intoxication produces a heightened sensitivity of postsynaptic catecholamine receptors which may be secondary to the chronic amphetamine-induced depletion of brain catecholamines. This interpretation is compatible with data showing that the inhibition of caudate neuronal activity produced by iontophoretically applied apomorphine is enhanced following depletion of striatal dopamine (e.g., Ungerstedt et al., 1975). Similarly, the stereotyped behaviors produced by apomorphine are enhanced following long-term amphetamine treatment and after functional denervation of dopaminoceptive neurons in the neostriatum (Klawans et al., 1975; Iversen and Creese, 1975).

The enhancement of amphetamine- and apomorphine-induced effects on neuronal activity following long-term amphetamine pretreatment provides additional support for the view that catecholaminergic transmission in the central nervous system is enhanced following chronic amphetamine administration which may reflect an increase in postsynaptic receptor sensitivity. However, while our results are consistent with other evidence and speculation suggesting that long-term amphetamine administration produces increased efficacy of catecholaminergic transmission in the central nervous system, the changes in neuronal activity produced by acute as well as long-term amphetamine administration are complex and widespread, and surely reflect a variety of as yet unknown influences. The enhanced behavioral effects of amphetamine following long-term administration may be regarded as an experimental model for understanding the mechanisms by which chronic stimulant intoxication produces the psychotic disorder, amphetamine psychosis (e.g., Angrist and Gershon, 1974; Wallace, 1974; Snyder, Benerjee, Yamamura, and Greenberg, 1974). Our results are consistent with the view that significant alterations in dopaminergic transmission occur following long-term amphetamine treatment in experimental animals. Changes in reticular formation function in human thought disorders also have been regarded as significant (e.g., Mirsky, 1969), and our results provide additional evidence for the role of the reticular formation in such disorders.

ACKNOWLEDGMENTS

Portions of this chapter were presented by George V. Rebec at the conference on Contemporary Issues in Stimulant Research, Duke University School of Medicine, Durham, North Carolina, November 10-12, 1975.

Supported in part by Grant MH 19515 and Research Scientist Development Award K02 MH 70706 (to Philip M. Groves) from the National Institute of Mental Health.

REFERENCES

Angrist, B. and Gershon, S.: Dopamine and psychotic states: Preliminary remarks. In: Neuropsychopharmacology of Monoamines and Their Regulatory Enzymes. Usdin, E., Ed., pp. 211-219. New York: Raven Press, 1974.

Boakes, R.J., Bradley, P.B., and Candy, J.M.: A neuronal basis for the altering action of (+)-amphetamine, Br. J. Pharmacol. 45, 391-403 (1972).

Bradley, P.B. and Elkes, J.: The effects of some drugs on the electrical activity of the brain, Brain 80, 77-117 (1957).

Bradley, P.B. and Key, B.J.: The effect of drugs on arousal responses produced by electrical stimulation of the reticular formation of the brain, Electroenceph. clin. Neurophysiol. 10, 97-110 (1958).

Butcher, S.G. and Butcher, L.L.: Origin and modulation of acetylcholine activity in the neostriatum, Brain Res. 71, 167-171 (1974).

Connor, J.D.: Caudate nucleus neurones: Correlation of the effects of substantia nigra stimulation with iontophoretic dopamine, J. Physiol. 208, 691-703 (1970).

Coyle, J.T. and Snyder, S.H.: Catecholamine uptake by synaptosomes in homogenates of rat brain: Stereospecificity in different areas, J. Pharmac. exp. Ther. 170, 221-231 (1969).

Ellinwood E.H.: Behavioral and EEG changes in the amphetamine model of psychosis. In: Neuropsychopharmacology of Monoamines and Their Regulatory Enzymes. Usdin, E., Ed., pp. 281-297. New York: Raven Press, 1974.

Ellinwood, E.H., Sudilovsky, A., and Nelson, L.M.: Evolving behavior in the clinical and experimental amphetamine (model) psychosis, Am. J. Psychiat. 130, 1088-1093 (1973).

Groves, P.M. and Lynch, G.S.: Mechanisms of habituation in the brainstem, Psychol. Rev. 79, 237-244 (1972).

Groves, P.M., Miller, S.W., Parker, M.V., and Rebec, G.V.: Organization by sensory modality in the reticular formation of the rat, Brain Res. 64, 167-187 (1973).

Groves, P.M. and Rebec, G.V.: Biochemistry and behavior: Some central actions of amphetamine and antipsychotic drugs, A. Rev. Psychol. 27, 91-127 (1976).

Groves, P.M., Rebec, G.V., and Harvey, J.A.: Alteration of the effects of (+)-amphetamine on neuronal activity in the striatum following lesions of the nigrostriatal bundle, Neuropharmacol. 14, 369-376 (1974).

Groves, P.M., Rebec, G.V., and Segal, D.S.: The action of d-amphetamine on spontaneous activity in the caudate nucleus and reticular formation of the rat, Behav. Biol. 11, 33-47 (1974).

Groves, P.M., Wilson, C.J., and Miller, S.W.: Habituation of the acoustic startle response: A neural systems analysis of habituation in the intact animal. In: Advances in Psychobiology. Riesen, A. and Thompson, R.F., Eds., Vol. 3. New York: Wiley, in press.

Groves, P.M., Wilson, C.J., Young, S.J., and Rebec, G.V.: Self-inhibition by dopaminergic neurons, Science 190, 522-529 (1975).

Iversen, S.D. and Creese, I.: Behavioral correlates of dopaminergic supersensitivity, Adv. Neurol. 9, 81-92 (1975).

Kalant, H., LeBlanc, A.E., and Gibbins, R.J.: Tolerance to and dependence on some non-opiate psychotropic drugs, Pharmac. Rev. 23, 135-191 (1971).

Kelly, P.H., Seviour, P.W., and Iversen, S.D.: Amphetamine and apomorphine responses in the rat following 6-OHDA lesions of the nucleus accumbens septi and corpus striatum, Brain Res. 94, 507-522 (1975).

Klawans, H.L., Crossett, P., and Dana, N.: Effect of chronic amphetamine exposure on stereotyped behavior: Implications for pathogenesis of L-dopa induced dyskinesias, Adv. Neurol. 9, 105-112 (1975).

Koenig, J.F.R. and Klippel, R.A. The Rat Brain: A Stereotaxic Atlas of the Forebrain and Lower Parts of the Brain Stem. Baltimore: Williams and Wilkins, 1963.

Lewander, T.: Effect of chronic treatment with central stimulants on brain monoamines and some behavioral and physiological functions in rats, guinea pigs, and rabbits. In: Neuropsychopharmacology of Monoamines and Their Regulatory Enzymes. Usdin, E., Ed., pp. 221-240. New York: Raven Press, 1974.

Lewander, T.: A mechanism for the development of tolerance to amphetamine in rats, Psychopharmacologia 13, 17-31 (1971).

Lindsley, D.B., Bowden, J., Magoun, H.W.: Effect upon EEG of acute injury to the brain stem activating system, Electroenceph. clin. Neurophysiol. 1, 475-486 (1949).

Lindsley, D.B., Schriener, L.H., Knowles, W.B., Magoun, H.W.: Behavioral and EEG changes following chronic brain stem lesions in the cat, Electroenceph. clin. Neurophysiol. 2, 483-498 (1950).

Lynch, G.S., Lucas, P.A., Deadwyler, S.A.: The demonstration of acetylcholinesterase containing neurons within the caudate nucleus of the rat, Brain Res. 45, 617-621 (1972).

McGeer, E.G., McGeer, P.L., Grewaal, D.S., and Singh, V.K.: Striatal cholinergic interneurons and their relation to dopaminergic nerve endings, J. Pharmacol. 6, 143-152 (1975).

Mirsky, A.F.: Neuropsychological bases of schizophrenia, A. Rev. Psychol. 20, 321-348 (1969).

Moruzzi, G. and Magoun, H.W.: Brain stem reticular formation and activation of the EEG, Electroenceph. clin. Neurophysiol. 1, 455-473 (1949).

Racagni, G., Cheney, D.L., Trabucchi, M., and Costa, E.: *In vivo* actions of clozapine and haloperidol on the turnover rate of acetylcholine in rat striatum, J. Pharmac. exp. Ther., in press.

Rebec, G.V. and Groves, P.M.: Differential effects of the optical isomers of amphetamine on neuronal activity in the reticular formation and caudate nucleus of the rat, Brain Res. 83, 301-318 (1975a).

Rebec, G.V. and Groves, P.M.: Apparent feedback from the caudate nucleus to the substantia nigra following amphetamine administration, Neuropharmacol. 14, 275-282 (1975b).

Rebec, G.V.: Neurophysiological correlates of long-term amphetamine treatment in rats. Unpublished Ph.D. dissertation, University of Colorado, 1975.

Roberts, D.C.S., Zis, A.P., and Fibiger, H.C.: Ascending catecholamine pathways and amphetamine-induced locomotor activity: Importance of dopamine and apparent non-involvement of norepinephrine, Brain Res. 93, 441-454 (1975).

Segal, D.S.: Behavioral characterization of d- and l-amphetamine: Neurochemical implications, Science 190, 475-477 (1975).

Segal, D.S. and Mandell, A.J.: Long-term administration of d-amphetamine: Progressive augmentation of motor activity and stereotypy, Pharmacol. Biochem. Behav. 2, 249-255 (1974).

Sharpless, S.: Reorganization of function in the nervous system--use and disuse, A. Rev. Physiol. 26, 357-388 (1964).

Sharpless, S.: Supersensitivity-like phenomena in the central nervous system, Fed. Proc. 34, 1990-1997 (1975).

Sharpless, S. and Jasper, H.H.: Habituation of the arousal reaction, Brain 79, 6550-680 (1956).

Snyder, S.H., Banerjee, S.P., Yamamura, H.I., and Greenberg, D.: Drugs, neurotransmitters and schizophrenia, Science 184, 1243-1253 (1974).

Taylor, K.M. and Snyder, S.H.: Amphetamine: Differentiation by d- and l-isomers of behavior involving brain norepinephrine or dopamine, Science 168, 1487-1489 (1970).

Trabucchi, M., Cheney, D.L., Racagni, G., and Costa, E.: In vivo inhibition of striatal acetylcholine turnover by L-DOPA, apomorphine and (+)-amphetamine, Brain Res. 85, 130-134 (1975).

Ungerstedt, U., Ljundberg, T., Hoffer, B., and Siggins, G.: Dopaminergic supersensitivity in the neostriatum, Adv. Neurol. 9, 57-66 (1975).

Wallach, M.B.: Drug-induced stereotyped behavior: Similarities and differences. In: Neuropsychopharmacology of Monoamines and Their Regulatory Enzymes. Usdin, E., Ed., pp. 241-260. New York: Raven Press, 1974.

York, D.H.: The inhibitory action of dopamine on neurones of the caudate nucleus, Brain Res. 5, 263-266 (1967).

AMYGDALA HYPERSPINDLING AND SEIZURES INDUCED BY COCAINE

E.H. Ellinwood, Jr., M.M. Kilbey, S. Castellani, C. Khoury

Behavioral Neuropharmacology Section, Department of Psychiatry, Duke University Medical Center

Durham, North Carolina 27710

INTRODUCTION

The temporal-lobe-like seizures produced by local anesthetics (deJong and Walts, 1966) have at least two possibly important contributions to human pathological conditions: 1) they may help explain the mechanisms underlying temporal lobe epilepsy and/or psychosis occasionally associated with this condition; 2) they may help elucidate the intervening links between the association of the overactivity of the limbic spindle and limbic discharges, with hyperarousal and hyperactive behaviors noted in animal models of chronic stimulant psychosis (see Ellinwood, 1974a for review). Chronic high-dose amphetamine (25-35 mg/kg) administration, or self-administration, in the cat results in bizarre hyperreactive behavior and associated high voltage limbic spindles that may precede tonic-clonic seizures. Furthermore, in chronic high dose amphetamine-intoxicated animals, specific hyperreactive behaviors (at times the animal appears to be reacting to non-existent stimuli) are often immediately preceded by a high voltage spindle and/or discharge in the amygdala, accumbens, and olfactory tubercle (Ellinwood, 1974a; Ellinwood, Sudilovsky, and Nelson, 1974). Much lower doses of amphetamine (10 mg/kg) when administered concomitantly with disulfiram (a dopamine beta hydroxylase inhibitor blocking norepinephrine [NE] synthesis) for only two to three days produces bizarre hyperreactive behavior with hyperspindling leading to tonic-clonic seizures (Ellinwood, Sudilovsky, and Grabowy, 1973).

Cocaine, or any local anesthetic, produces a similar hyperspindling with subsequent seizure when administered in moderately large doses systemically, but the behaviors are characterized by postural collapse in a muscularly rigid or tonic state. Still higher doses produce tonic-clonic seizures (Eidelberg, Lesse, and Gault, 1963; Tuttle and Elliott, 1969; Wagman, deJong, and Prince, 1968; Wagman, deJong, and Prince, 1967; Riblett and Tuttle, 1970; deJong, 1969; Ellinwood, Khoury, Kilbey, and Benignus, unpublished observations). Subsequently the hyperspindling and/or seizures give way to normal but high voltage levels of spindling with hyperarousal stereotypy and relatively fixed postures. This occurs within 10 to 15 min after a moderately high dose of cocaine (e.g., 5-9 mg/kg i.v.). Lidocaine and other synthetic local anesthetics do not, of course produce the stereotypy phase.

The observation that disulfiram markedly lowered the amphetamine dose necessary to produce amygdala hyperspindling and seizures indicated that NE might have an inhibitory action on the hyperspindling mechanism. In one of the original studies on the effects of pretreatments on cocaine seizures in rats, Eidelberg et al. (1963) demonstrated that such diverse compounds as hydroxylamine, pyridoxine chlorpromazine, dibenamine, and reserpine significantly reduced the behavioral seizure produced by cocaine. Subsequently, Sanders (1967) confirmed that chlorpromazine protected against cocaine seizures, but found dibenamine and reserpine were ineffective. Eidelberg et al. (1963) also noted that isopropyl phenylhyrazine (IPH), a monoamine oxydase inhibitor (MAOI), lowered the threshold to the cocaine seizures, but pyrogallol, a catecholamine O-methyl-transferase inhibitor, had no effect. They reasoned that serotonin might be involved in the potentiation since only the former drug potentiated both serotonin and catecholamines. More recently, deOliveira and Bretas (1974) reported that pretreatment with high doses of 5-hydroxytryptophan (100 mg/kg) decreased the threshold for lidocaine-induced seizures. This dose of 5-hydroxytryptophan is a rather overwhelming one. deOliveira and Bretas (1974) subsequently reported that p-chlorolphenylalanine in serotonin-depleting doses elevated the threshold for lidocaine-induced seizures. They also demonstrated an additive effect in reducing seizure threshold to lidocaine when the MAOI iproniazide (which lowered the threshold to seizures alone) was given prior to the 5-hydroxytryptophan. The discrepant results of different investigators for the effects of dibenamine and reserpine on cocaine-induced seizures suggested that systematic investigation of the catecholamine effects, and perhaps acetylcholine effects as well, was warranted.

Another major concern in our laboratory is the potential relationship between chronic pre-seizure and seizure activity induced by chronic intoxication with cocaine and amphetamine and the induction of reverse tolerance for seizures. The mechanisms involved may be similar to the "kindling" phenomena (Goddard, 1967). Goddard demonstrated that daily unilateral low-level electrical stimulation of certain areas of the brain, especially the amygdala and limbic system, initially had no behavioral effects but produced progressive increments in pre-seizure behavior until finally behavioral convulsions were induced by the originally sub-seizure electrical stimulation. Previously we had postulated (Ellinwood, 1974b) that the high voltage synchronous activity induced by cocaine and local anesthetics may produce neuronal alterations in the limbic system qualitatively similar to those produced by low-level electrical stimulation. Chronic daily administration of these drugs may produce a gradual augmentation in the propagation of the drug-induced amygdaloid activity to other areas of the limbic system correlated with increases and/or qualitative changes in the behavioral effects of the drug similar to kindling. Post (1976) has a similar formulation. Furthermore, depletion of catecholamines by either 6-hydroxydopamine or reserpine has been found to increase the rate at which kindling occurs (Corcoran, Fibiger, McCaughran, and Wada, 1974; Arnold, Racine, and Wise, 1973). In addition, rats which have not been gentled (and for which the kindling procedure is presumably more stressful, causing a greater turnover of NE) kindle at a slower rate than gentled rats (Arnold et al., 1973). Finally, Pinel, Phillips, and MacNeil (1973) demonstrated that foot shock, administered just prior to stimulation of the amygdala, blocks the expression of previously kindled seizure. We have already discussed the effect of disulfiram on amphetamine-induced seizures. We also have preliminary data indicating that small doses of amphetamine (0.5 mg/kg) sufficient to enhance the NE effect markedly reduce cocaine spindle effects. These data suggest that there may be a NE inhibitory effect on both cocaine-induced spindling and the reverse tolerance to seizure induction induced by long-term cocaine stimulation.

Although our primary interest is in the chronically-induced, more permanent CNS changes (Stripling and Ellinwood, 1976), we reasoned that investigation of the effects of neurochemical manipulation of acutely-induced cocaine hyperspindling and seizure might provide information as to the neurotransmitters underlying these phenomena. In this study, we were concerned with 1) administering cocaine and various agents which alter the availability of neurotransmitters; 2) examining the onset and spread of hyperspindling and seizure activity, including measurement of spindle parameters and degree of synchrony between unilateral and/or contralateral limbic sites; 3) measuring the limbic spindle pre-seizure activity. The measurement of the limbic spindle provides a specific and quantifiable phenomenon, emphasizing the early electrophysiological changes preceding the behavioral seizure state rather than the behavioral seizure end point itself. The measurement of the spindle instead of the convulsive end point (as used, for example, by

Eidelberg et al. in 1963) eliminates confounding by variables intrinsic to the major motor seizure. For our own interest, the mesolimbic spindle and discharge provide information concerning the electrophysiological events preceding limbic seizures or during non-drug periods that may relate more intimately to the psychotic phenomena associated with temporal lobe epilepsy and stimulant psychosis than to the final seizure episode, since the psychosis associated with temporal lobe epilepsy is not correlated with greater frequency of the seizure itself but is related to long interictal periods (Flor-Henry, 1968).

METHODS

Sixteen cats weighing 2.5 to 3 kg were implanted with electrodes in sites including the olfactory bulb, amygdala, the olfactory tubercle, accumbens, the mesencephalic reticular formation, hippocampus, and cortex. An indifferent electrode was placed on the occiput. A catheter was introduced into the jugular vein, run underneath the skin to the dorsal surface of the skull, and attached to a 20-gauge needle (Balster, Kilbey, and Ellinwood, 1976). The needle and an Amphenol connecting plug for the electrodes were imbedded in an acrylic base attached to the skull. The animals rested for three weeks prior to recording or administration of drugs. Subsequently, electrophysiological activity was recorded. The electrophysiological output from a Grass Model 78 Polygraph was recorded on a Hewlett Packard analog tape deck. Behavior was videotaped. One-sec synch signals were placed on the voice channel of the TV tape and a channel of the analog tape. For one study of behavior and EEG (Group I), FLA-63 (a dopamine beta hydroxylase inhibitor) was administered i.p. 24 hr prior to the cocaine injections. Cocaine alone (5 mg/kg given intravenously at 0.25 mg/kg/sec) and cocaine plus FLA-63 sessions were counterbalanced between cats and within the same cat. One week between administrations was allowed for recovery from previous drug effects. In another study (Group II) pretreatments of acetylcholine and dopamine agonists and antagonists were run in a counterbalanced order preceding weekly cocaine injections (described more fully in text).

Spindles were recognized and subsequently digitized using a computer program (Grabowy and Ellinwood, 1971). In this study, 4 cycles of the spindle were recognized and the small laboratory PDP-8 computer digitized the preceding 288 msec. These programs have the capability of analyzing voltage, frequency, and number of spindles. Additional analyses included cross-correlation between various electrodes.

RESULTS

Cocaine Electrophysiological Changes

The initial effect of cocaine in animals from both groups is an increased regularization of hippocampal theta and/or hyperspindling in the amygdala. During this initial phase the olfactory bulb activity usually is suppressed (Fig. 1). Within 30 sec after injection the olfactory tubercle and later the olfactory bulb usually join in the hyperspindling response. High voltage spindling may also be induced in the opposite amygdala, but in some subjects the spindling response is notably unilateral. In animals demonstrating tonic behavioral collapse without the subsequent clonic seizure stage, hyperspindling may be the only major electrographic change. The intensity of the tonic phase appears to be related to the degree of hyperspindling. The sequence leading to tonic seizure collapse often occurs in the absence of electrographic manifestations at the cortex. Spikes and spike-spindle complexes are noted preceding the tonic-clonic seizure stage and are usually the only electrographic manifestation leading to hypersynchronous discharge bursts if the seizure onset is extremely rapid. When the clonic stage ensues, pervasive (including the cortex) hypersynchronous discharge bursts are interspersed with electrical suppression.

A dramatic decrease in the frequency of the amygdala spindle from 40 hz to an average of approximately 30 hz, not infrequently to 15-20 hz, occurs within 12 sec of the end of an i.v. injection of 5 mg/kg of cocaine (Fig. 2). The frequency remains at this low level for approximately 1 min and then begins a steady increase, usually reaching 35 to 40 cycles/sec within 4 min. The frequency continues to increase slightly after this period for approximately 10 to 15 min, when it has usually recovered to its original level. The response in the olfactory tubercle and the olfactory bulb lags somewhat behind the amygdala.

The increased amygdala spindle amplitude following cocaine reaches a plateau in approximately ½ min, then begins dropping rapidly after 2 min (Fig. 3). The average maximum voltage increase is approximately 30% for the 5 mg/kg dose; however, individual cats may have a greater increase in amplitude. The number of amygdala spindles (Fig. 4) also increases to a plateau at about 1 min post-injection, then gradually decreases over the next ½ hr. Cocaine suppresses the olfactory bulb spindle amplitude during the initial 20-30 sec phase. The amplitude gradually increases over the next 2-4 min. During the phase of increasing amygdala and decreasing bulb amplitude, the amygdala spindle often is initiated earlier than the bulb spindle. The time effect post-cocaine for the amplitude and frequency spindle parameters in the amygdala and olfactory bulb were statistically significant (Table 1). The number of spindles was significantly greater in the amygdala sites following cocaine.

TABLE 1

F Values and Associated Probability Level*
for Three Parameters of Electrophysiological Brain Activity:
Number of Spindles, Amplitude, and Frequency; for Three Electrode Sites:
Right and Left Amygdala and Left Olfactory Bulb

Site	Number of Spindles			Amplitude			Frequency		
	F	df	p	F	df	p	F	df	p
Right Amygdala	15.1	1,7	≤ 0.001	76.8	1,7	≤ 0.001	244.6	1,7	≤ 0.001
Left Amygdala	6.7	1,7	≤ 0.05	76.8	1,7	≤ 0.001	70.8	1,7	≤ 0.001
Left Olfactory Bulb	7.7	4,1	≤ 0.26	743.9	4,1	≤ 0.02	822.8	4,1	≤ 0.02

*Determined by a multivariable analysis of intervals 0-19 over Days 1 through 4.

(McCall and Appelbaum, 1973; Appelbaum, 1974.)

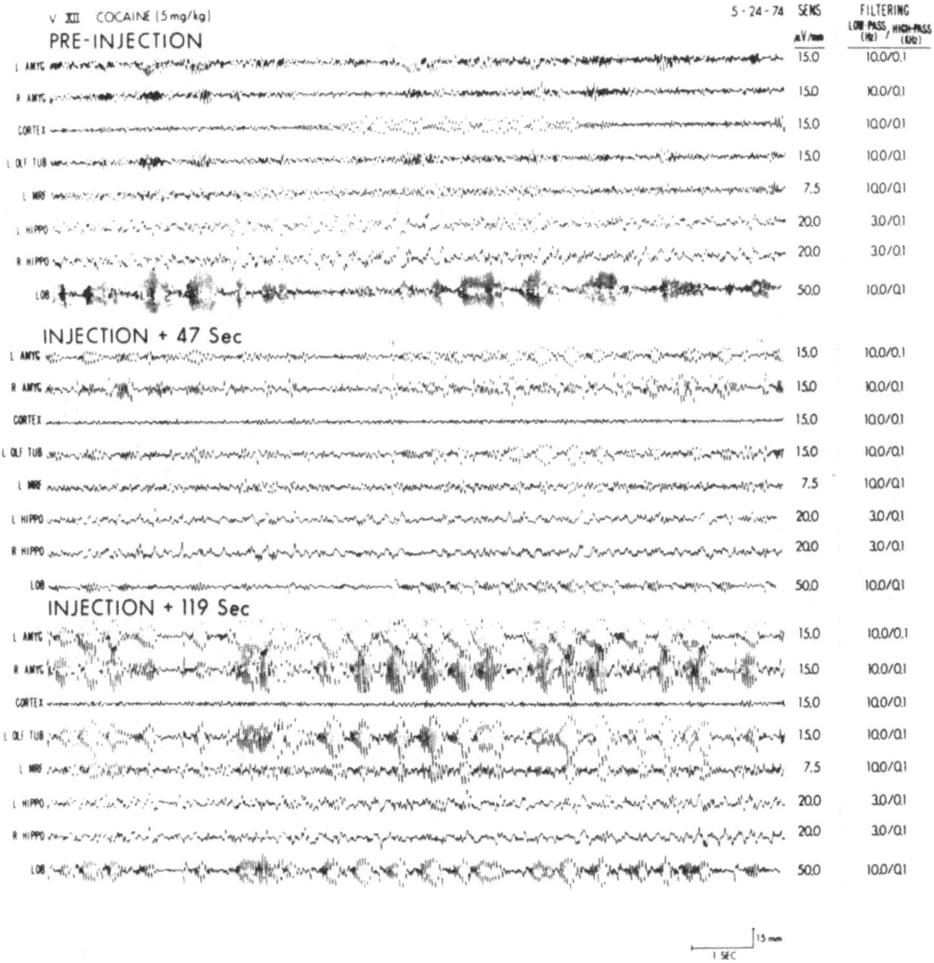

Fig. 1. Electrographic response to i.v. cocaine. AMYG = amygdala; OLF TUB = olfactory tubercle; MRF = mesencephalic reticular formation; HIPPO = hippocampus; OB = olfactory bulb.

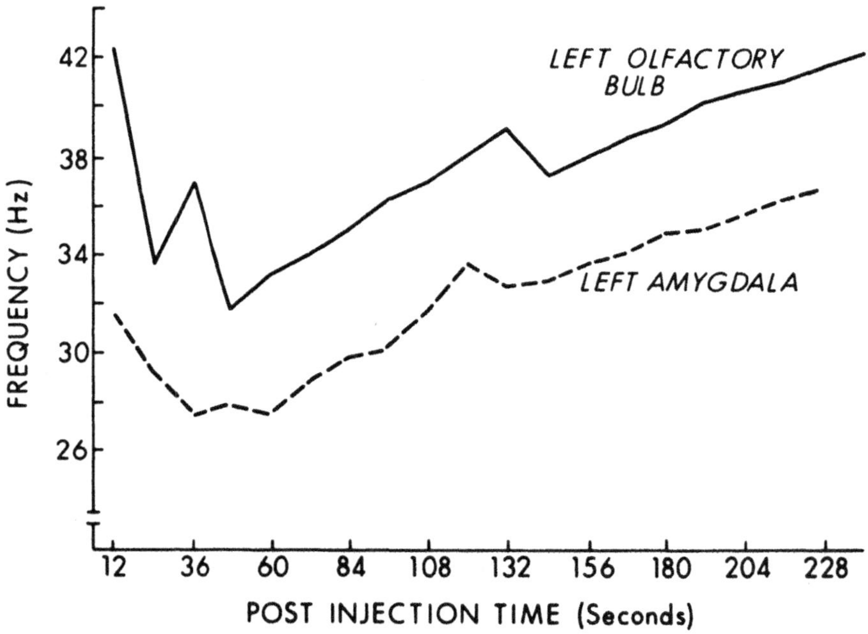

Fig. 2. Average spindle frequency for cocaine injections.

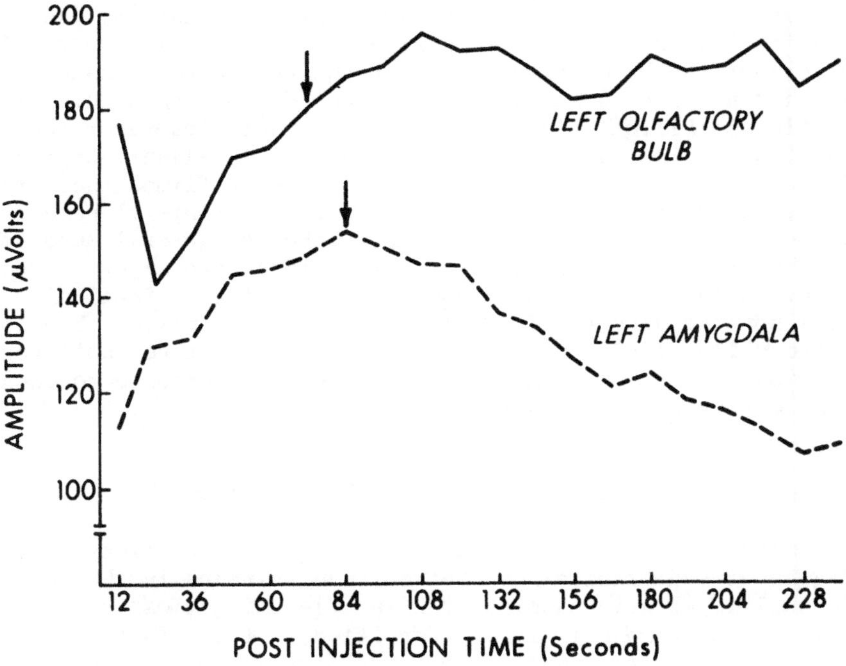

Fig. 3. Average spindle amplitude for cocaine injections. Amygdala arrow indicates peak effect, which is approximately the same time as the olfactory bulb amplitude recovery.

Although our experiments are run on a weekly basis, at the same 5 mg/kg dose, it is important to ascertain whether tolerance or reverse tolerance occurs in this paradigm. Analysis of the various electrodes and parameters in the Group I experiment over a 4-week period indicated that there is no Day effect over that time period. In the Group II experiment, carried out over 12 weeks, there was a significant decrease in spindle amplitude from the 1st to the 12th injection; change in the other parameters was nonsignificant.

The greater responsiveness of the amygdala also raises the question whether the origin of the activity for the cocaine spindle is primarily emanating from the amygdala or from what is, under normal conditions, the "usual pacing site," i.e., the olfactory bulb. The origin of the high-voltage, slow-frequency cocaine-induced spindle has not been conclusively delineated. Wagman et al. (1967) and Tuttle and Elliott (1969) demonstrated that closure of the nares blocked the cocaine-induced limbic spindle. Castellani, Kilbey, and Ellinwood (unpublished observations) have confirmed these findings and, in addition, have demonstrated that unilateral nare occlusion blocks the spindle response in the ipsilateral mesolimbic nuclei, but the contralateral side may in fact have an even greater response. Bilateral occlusion does not block the tonic-clonic seizures nor the associated hypersynchronous polyspikes. Eidelberg, Neer, and Miller (1965) reported that bilateral but not unilateral destruction of the amygdala blocked the seizure response to cocaine, thus indicating a primary site in the amygdala.

Synchronization Between Limbic Sites

In order to examine the phase and frequency relationship (i.e., the degree of synchronization) between the spindles in the various limbic nuclei, we have examined the spindle using cross-correlation programs. The spindle is first identified in the olfactory bulb using our computer programs. The first 4 cycles of the spindle are recognized and act as a trigger to store 288 msec of the digital sample. Figure 5 demonstrates an average of 93 spindle cross-correlations between the left olfactory bulb, amygdala, and tubercle (same animal as used in Fig. 1). The peak negative correlations near "0" indicate that the amygdala is approximately 180° out of phase with the other two sites. The relationship of the highest positive peak between the olfactory bulb/amygdala and amygdala/tubercle correlation indicates that there is a major leading component in the olfactory bulb. The olfactory tubercle and the olfactory bulb are remarkably in phase with the positive peak, indicating that the olfactory bulb is leading by a 4 to 5 msec phase difference.

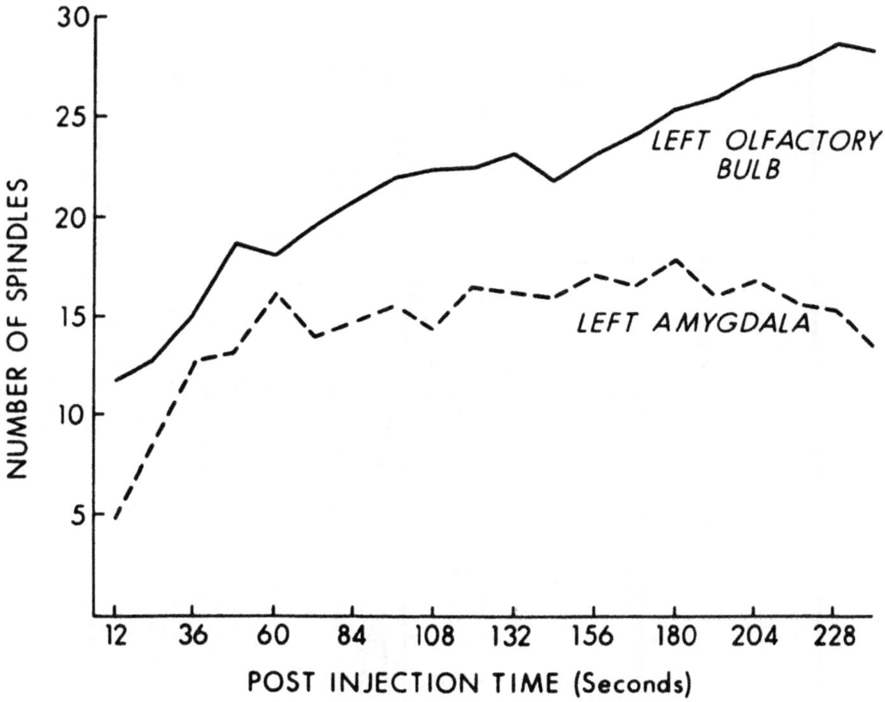

Fig. 4. Average number of spindles for cocaine injections.

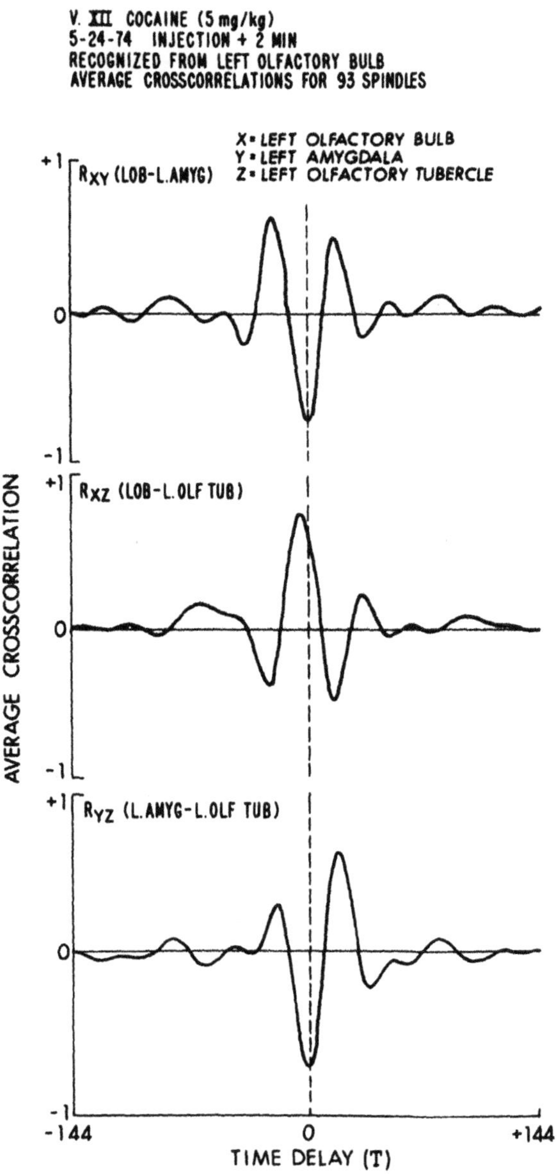

Fig. 5. Average 2 min of post-injection spindle cross-correlations.

In order to assess the overall as well as differential spindle correlation between the limbic nuclei induced by cocaine, we calculated the degree of correlation between the nuclei, either positive or negative correlations, and derived what we have called the maximum squared average correlation (MSAC). An average cross-correlogram is computed from the cross-correlograms corresponding to each spindle in a 1-min interval. This average cross-correlogram is then squared and its maximum point denoted as the MSAC. The highest degree of maximum squared average correlation induced by cocaine is between the amygdala and the ipsilateral olfactory tubercle (Fig. 6). Examination of the records shows that these two nuclei also have the greatest spindling response to cocaine. Although the right and left amygdala not infrequently have a simultaneous hyperspindling response to cocaine, the level of correlation for phase and frequency does not increase (and may in fact decrease), indicating an independent pacing mechanism for cocaine spindling for the two sides. A similar lack of correlation between the olfactory bulb and the contralateral amygdala has been found.

Although the maximum squared average correlation is a derived estimate of spindle correlation between olfactory nuclei, it has proven to be the most stable, least variable, and one of the more sensitive measures of the cocaine CNS response, especially the correlation between the tubercle and ipsilateral amygdala. Figure 7 demonstrates the stability of the maximum squared average correlation of the amygdala and tubercle for 5 cats in the pre-injection period across the 4 weeks of one experiment. Using such a measure, one can note that there is a significant difference between pre-injection and 1 min post-injection on Day One and Day Two. This response decreases over the 4-week period (4 test days) to a point where there is no discernible drug effect; thus this derived estimate of correlation may provide a sensitive indicator of tolerance in the early stages of weekly injections.

Influence of Neurotransmitter Manipulation on Cocaine Spindles and Seizures

Considerable effort has been directed toward quantifying the pre-seizure electrographic events in order to provide a stable measure that is sensitive to manipulation of the cocaine-induced syndrome prior to the final stage of behavioral seizures. The behavioral seizure stage is, of course, a final common pathway but is subject to a great variety of metabolic influences; changes in behavioral seizure threshold or duration following experimental manipulation may only partially elucidate the pre-seizure triggering mechanisms. We have focused on the cocaine-induced hyperspindling as one such pre-seizure mechanism. Obviously, the amygdala spikes are another important pre-seizure event that needs assessment.

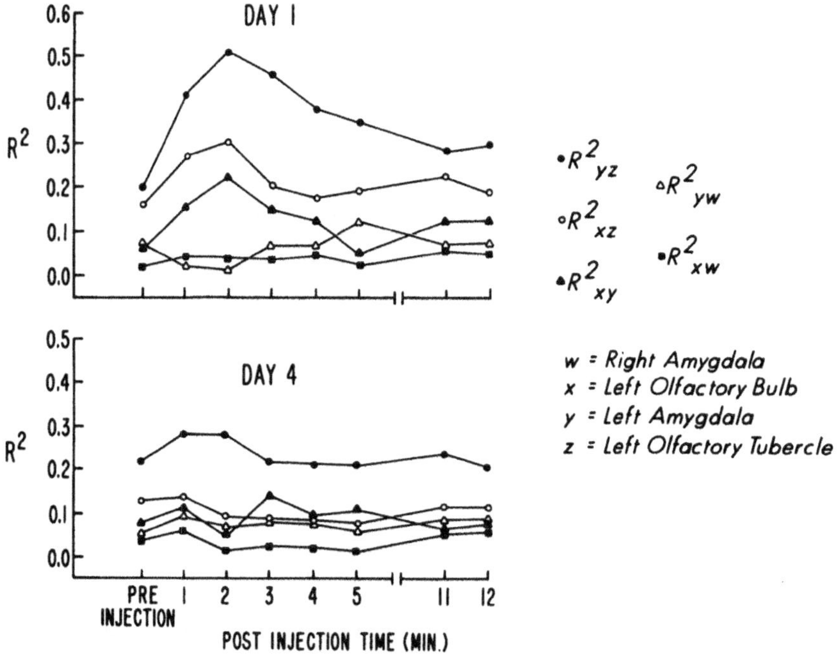

Fig. 6. Maximum squared average cross-correlation (R^2).

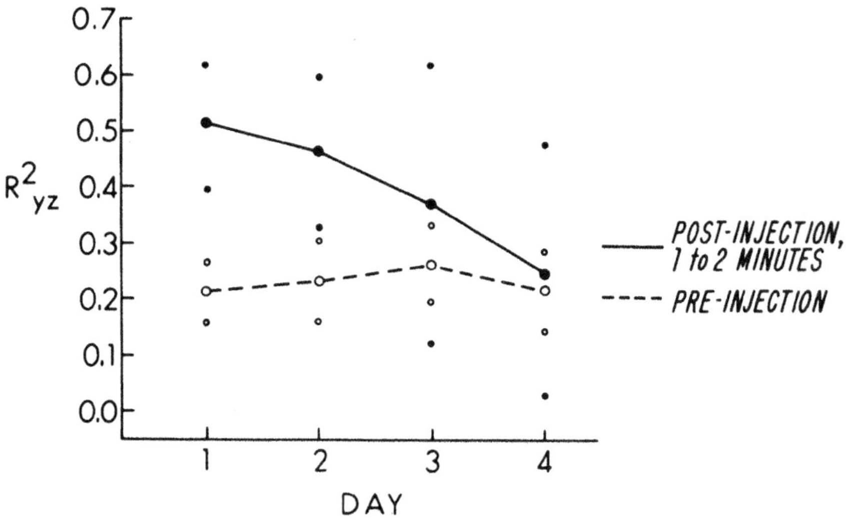

Fig. 7. Maximum squared average cross-correlation (R^2) of left amygdala (y) and left olfactory tubercle (z). Dots are standard deviation

Possible norepinephrine, dopamine, and acetylcholine effects on cocaine spindles were examined. Eight chronically-implanted cats, Group I, were pretreated with two doses of FLA-63 (40 mg/kg) i.p. 24 and 6 hr prior to cocaine, and were compared to saline-pretreated in their response to 5 mg/kg of cocaine. Two FLA-63 and two saline pretreatments were administered at weekly intervals over a 4-week period in a counterbalance order. In another study, pretreatments of apomorphine 0.2 and 0.5 mg/kg; pimozide 0.2 and 0.8 mg/kg; physostigmine 0.04 and 0.1 mg/kg; atropine 0.05 and 0.5 mg/kg; and saline were administered intravenously 10 min prior to cocaine to 8 cats in a counterbalance design. The various pretreatments were remarkably ineffective in altering the cocaine spindle response. Atropine did result in a significantly lower frequency cocaine response ($p \leq 0.01$) but without a concomitant significant increase in amplitude. A promising but nonsignificant trend was also noted in a FLA-63 pretreatment reduction of the cocaine-induced frequency. Since increased synchronization might be directly related to the early development of the seizure process, the spindle maximum squared average correlation for the various limbic nuclei were compared for cocaine plus FLA-63 versus cocaine alone. No significant differences were noted.

Development of Mesolimbic Discharges with Repeated Injections

In a continuing study on Group II, we tested the effects of various dose levels of cocaine (including the original 5 mg/kg) following a 3-month drug-free period. Of the 8 original cats, the 6 which had catheterizable veins were tested; 5 of these 6 animals demonstrated pre-drug high voltage discharges in the amygdala, accumbens, olfactory tubercle, and mesolimbic reticular formation. The remaining cat had low voltage discharges emanating from the hippocampus (probably electrode-injury-induced) during the pre-drug period of the first two sessions of the original set of experiments. In the animals tested after the 3-month drug-free period, the spikes in the pre-drug period often appeared when the animal was aroused, as when first placed in the cage. At other times the discharges would appear randomly or periodically throughout the pre-injection period. Figure 8 demonstrates the evolution of these discharges in one cat during the initial and subsequent Group II studies. Observation of the electrographic records of these cats demonstrates that the discharges often began in one amygdala or olfactory tubercle and subsequently spread over the period of repeated administration to the ipsilateral limbic nuclei and then to the mesencephalic reticular formation, and subsequently to the opposite amygdala and/or other nuclei. As the discharges organized, they then also became independently active in both amygdalae during the pre- and post-drug periods. Often during the post-cocaine period, discharges predominant in one amygdala would precede epileptic activity.

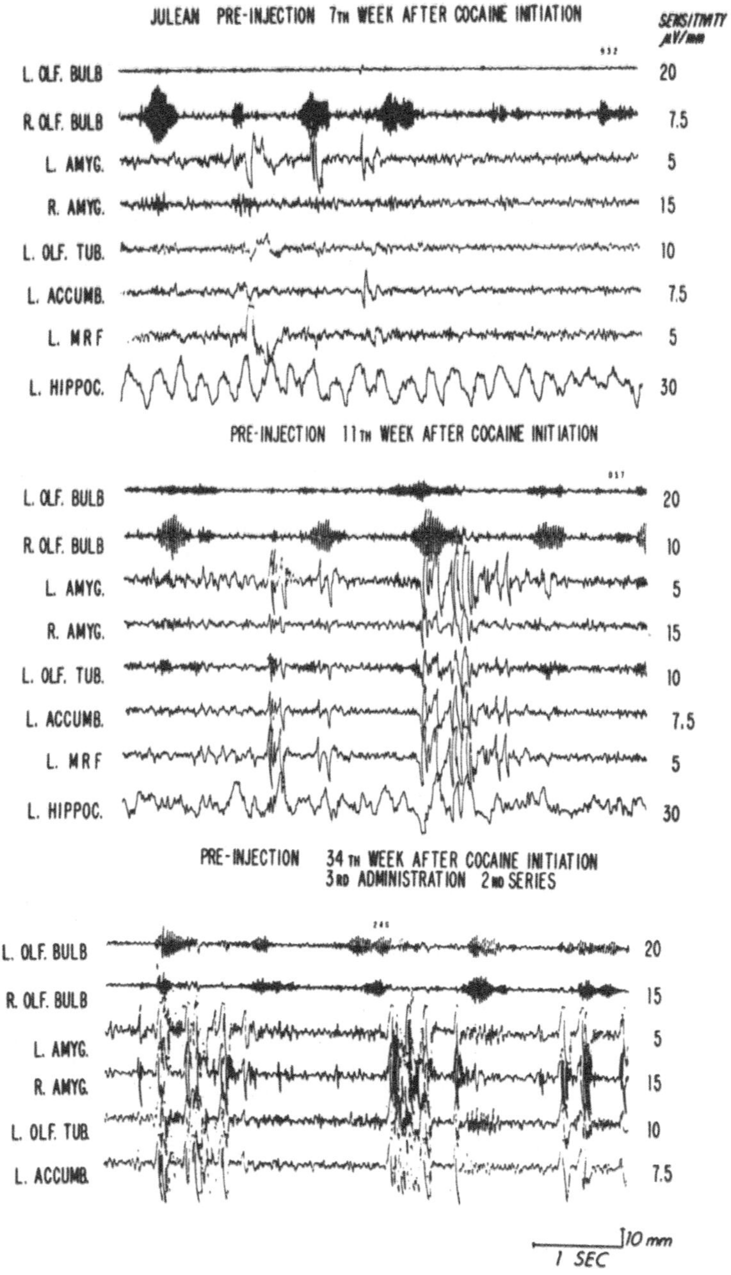

Fig. 8. Spread of pre-drug discharges over chronic intoxication period.

The organization of these discharges followed a similar spread and progression for amygdala kindled interictal discharges in the cat described by Wada and Sata (1974). Interpretation of the gradual evolution of increased discharges in the mesolimbic sites is hampered by not knowing the contribution of chronic electrode implantation to this process; this is, of course, a problem in any chronic implantation study of highly epileptogenic areas of the CNS.

DISCUSSION

In our two series of studies, it is important to separate the acute drug-induced pre-seizure effects from the more progressive chronic changes. Administered acutely, cocaine induces high-voltage, slow spindle activity in a manner almost identical to lidocaine (Ellinwood and Khoury, unpublished observations). The pre-seizure and seizure-inducing effects of the local anesthetic do not appear to have any robust relationship to norepinephrine, dopamine, or acetylcholine mechanisms. deOliveira and Bretas (1974) have demonstrated that pretreatment with 5-hydroxytryptophan lowers the cocaine CD_{50} in both cats and mice. Pretreatment with p-chlorophenylalanine increased the cocaine CD_{50}. Serotonin thus may have a role in the cocaine-induced seizure, but whether this is an effect on the pre-seizure phase or on the phase of increasing spread and synchrony leading to the convulsive end point is yet to be determined. The high doses of 5-hydroxytryptophan necessary to produce an effect indicate that the serotonin role is not a major specific or direct mechanism. In the present study, which involved acetylcholine, norepinephrine, and dopamine mechanisms, the convulsive end point was not tested; the pre-seizure events, especially as measured by the spindle parameters, did not appear to have any major relationship to these neurotransmitter mechanisms.

One of the more stable dependent measures in our studies is a derived measure of synchrony between two nuclei, the averaged cross-correlogram. Cross-correlation and derived methods are currently the best methods for analyzing the mutual functional relationship between different brain sites. Accurate information on the frequencies and phases of observed EEG activity can be obtained. The difficulty with these methods is the relatively complicated techniques (Matousek, 1973; Barlow and Freeman, 1959). In our method, we used digitized samples of spindle and pre-spindle activity identified by recognition programs. The spindle-averaged cross-correlograms are remarkably consistent and stable across days for the pre-drug period. Not only the time-shift (i.e., the ΔT for the peak nearest to the zero delay) but also the maximum cross-correlation coefficient (the value of the previously-mentioned peak) is remarkably stable for the pre-drug period.

The reduction of cross-correlation between the olfactory tubercle and the amygdala across days of cocaine administration may have a relationship to the developing epileptic discharges and polyspikes; that is, the decreased synchrony may be associated with an increase in discharges. Intravenous anesthetics have both convulsant as well as anticonvulsant properties. Lidocaine at synchronizing dose levels (2 mg/kg) abolishes the post-stimulatory epileptiform cortical afterdischarge elicited by cortical stimulation (Bernhard and Bohm, 1955). Similarly, French, Livingston, Konigsmark, and Richland (1957) noted that seizures could not be elicited electrically from even the most highly epileptogenic zones in monkeys up to 30 min after an intravenous injection of procaine or lidocaine. Local anesthetics have also been successful in reducing epileptic attacks in humans and interrupting status epilepticus (Bernhard and Bohm, 1965). We have pilot observations that small doses of cocaine also protect against subsequent injections of convulsant doses of cocaine. We are currently investigating these rather paradoxical separate actions of local anesthetics and whether limbic spindle synchrony is positively or negatively correlated with discharge activity. A finding consistent with a negative relationship is the marked cocaine-induced amygdala spikes and polyspikes at 6-9 min post-injection noted in animals with packed nares which blocked the initial spindling and hypersynchrony response.

Since systemically-administered local anesthetics, but not focal micro-injection, preferentially excite the amygdala (Tuttle and Elliott, 1969), deJong (1970) argues for a pacemaker which drives synaptic or related structures but is not easily excited itself. Our cross-correlation data demonstrate that the olfactory bulb has a leading phase relationship to the olfactory tubercle, which in turn has a phase leading to the amygdala, pre-drug as well as post-drug. As indicated above, this phase relationship is remarkably stable for a given cat across days, and although cocaine administration produces a marked increase in the cross-correlation coefficient, the lag time with respect to cross-correlogram remains quite constant. Brazier (1972) calculated the coherence between a variety of nuclei in humans and noted that there was a dominant 6 cycle/sec theta rhythm in the amygdala and septum with a consistent coherence between the two nuclei. Furthermore, the amygdala consistently led the septal waves in phase, the average displacement being a lead time of approximately 15 msec between peaks. The differences in this human study may reflect either different frequency patterns or species differences. The lower correlation--even in the pre-drug period--between the olfactory bulb and amygdala as well as olfactory tubercle in comparison to the amygdala and tubercle is surprising in view of the phase relationship as well as the abolishment of all spindle activity with obstructed nasal air flow. These effects may be interpreted that the olfactory bulb is the predominant pacing mechanism, and that local anesthetics make amygdala to olfactory tubercle more susceptible to synchronization to the olfactory bulb.

One of the most intriguing questions to be answered in the chronic stimulant model of psychosis is the nature of the CNS mechanism underlying the increasing behavioral reorganization noted in: 1) the gradual evolution of stereotypies to hyperreactive behaviors and dyskinesias in monkeys and cats (Ellinwood, 1971; Ellinwood and Kilbey, 1975); 2) the elicitation of chronic drug end-stage behaviors by inducing either stress or excitement or by low doses of amphetamine in cats subsequently made abstinent; 3) re-creation of psychotic behavior in typically abstinent human patients with only moderately high doses of amphetamine (Kramer, 1969; Bell, 1973; Ellinwood, 1973) and/or stress (Utena, 1974); 4) psychological residua in humans, e.g. delusions, stereotypies, or mannerisms that persist long after the chronic stimulant abuse has ceased; and 5) reverse tolerance to seizure threshold with chronic cocaine intoxication. The nature of these changes argues for a neuronal or receptor reorganization similar to that hypothesized in chronic schizophrenia (Fish, 1961) that persists long after the pharmacological or metabolic insult is over.

There are several possible hypotheses to account for the long-term reorganizational changes: 1) Kindling may be an explanatory mechanism for the "reverse tolerance" operating for the psychotic mechanisms in chronic amphetamine intoxication and, at least for cocaine, for the seizure threshold. The same kindling-like mechanism may have explanatory value for the lowered threshold of end-stage behaviors in cats and monkeys that are at least partially analogous to the psychotic behaviors in humans. 2) There is considerable evidence that conditioning mechanisms are operative in the reintroduction of bizarre behaviors, especially in experimental animals where these behaviors can be triggered by stimuli associated with the amphetamine injection. State-dependent mechanisms associated with arousal could certainly be operative. 3) A variety of events in the chronic pharmacological intoxication could result in a supersensitive state. These include neuronal damage, as previously noted by Escalante and Ellinwood (1970), as well as CNS damage secondary to vascular changes, as noted by Rumbaugh (1976). More specifically, there is evidence of chronic dopamine depletion, as described by Seiden, Fischman, and Schuster (1976), along with evidence by Escalante and Ellinwood (1970) that areas of greatest neuronal chromatolysis were in areas with catecholamine neurons. Such changes would more than likely result in associated receptor supersensitivity. 4) Finally, chronic dopamine depletion, as described by Seiden et al. (1976), and other possible chronic neurotransmitter changes, e.g. norepinephrine depletion with chronic stimulant intoxication, may result in altered neurotransmitter ratios within certain nuclei leading to chronic reorganization.

The kindling hypothesis is consistent with the data from our laboratory presented by Stripling (Stripling and Ellinwood, 1976) and the data presented by Post (1976). The gradual organization and spread of pre-drug or interictal epileptic discharges reported in this paper is also consistent with a kindling-like mechanism, even though the interval between drug administrations is not the optimal one for kindling. A progression of spike discharges in our chronic cocaine study similar to the development of discharges in a kindling paradigm by Wada and Sata (1974) was also noted. Wada and Sata (1974) also report that the development of the final convulsion stage was coincident with a phenomenal increase in the afterdischarge amplitude in the basal ganglia bilaterally, in the ipsilateral midbrain reticular formation, and in the contralateral amygdala.

In a study by Ellinwood, Sudilovsky, and Grabowy (1973) examining the effects of disulfiram and amphetamine-induced limbic seizures, a 10 to 20 cycle/sec afterdischarge, or--alternatively--a very high voltage 10 to 20 cycle/sec rhythm in the substantia nigra immediately preceded the stage of generalized seizure induction. This generalized seizure appeared to form as a gradual recruitment of seizure activity into or superimposed on the afterdischarges or the high voltage mesencephalic rhythms. Wada and Sata (1974) also report that, although the interictal discharges diminish after the convulsive stage, they then persist unchanged for more than 12 months following the completion of the convulsive seizure stage.

Observations in this study of persistent interictal discharge also raise the question of relatively permanent effects of chronic cocaine administration. The generalized seizures themselves may contribute to a state of supersensitivity to subsequent introduction of catecholamine-enhancing drugs. Modigh (1975) has reported that repetitive ECT sensitizes mice to the hyperactivity induced by apomorphine and clonidine. One could speculate that even the active epileptic foci without the introduction of generalized seizures cause supersensitivity to catecholamines. Thus an interaction between abnormally-electrically-active limbic nuclei and either pharmacologically-induced or arousal-induced catecholamine release is one possible explanation for some of the residual changes noted after chronic stimulant intoxication. Future studies relating the functional electrophysiological reorganization to abnormal sensitivity to neural transmitters may provide additional explanations for some of the residual changes associated with chronic stimulant intoxication.

ACKNOWLEDGMENT

This research was supported by NIDA Grant DA-00057.

REFERENCES

Appelbaum, M.I.: The MANOVA Manual: Complete Factorial Design (Research Memorandum Number 44 of the L.L. Thurstone Psychometric Laboratory). Chapel Hill, N.C.: The L.L. Thurstone Psychometric Laboratory of the University of North Carolina, 1974.

Arnold, P.S., Racine, R.J., and Wise, R.A.: Effects of atropine, reserpine, 6-hydroxydopamine, and handling on seizure development in the rat, Expl Neurol. 40, 457-470 (1973).

Balster, R.L., Kilbey, M.M., and Ellinwood, E.H.: Methamphetamine self-administration in the cat, Psychopharmacologia 46, 229-233 (1976).

Barlow, J.S. and Freeman, M.Z.: Comparison of EEG activity recorded from analogous locations on the scalp by means of autocorrelation and cross-correlation analysis, Quarterly Progress Report (M.I.T. Research Laboratory of Electronics) 54, 173-181 (1959).

Bell, D.S.: The experimental reproduction of amphetamine psychosis, Archs gen. Psychiat. 29, 35-40 (1973).

Bernhard, C.G. and Bohm, E.: The action of local anesthetics on experimental epilepsy in cats and monkeys, Br. J. Pharmacol. 10, 288-295 (1955).

Bernhard, C.G. and Bohm, E.: Local Anesthetics and Anticonvulsants: A Study on Experimental and Clinical Epilepsy. Stockholm: Almqvist and Wiksell, 1965.

Brazier, M.A.B.: Interactions of deep structures during seizures in man. In: Synchronization of EEG Activity in Epilepsia. Petsche, H. and Brazier, M.A.B., Eds., pp. 409-424. Vienna: Springer-Verlag, 1972.

Corcoran, M.E., Fibiger, H.C., McCaughran, J.A., and Wada, J.A.: Potentiation of amygdaloid kindling and metrazol-induced seizures by 6-hydroxydopamine in rats, Expl Neurol. 45, 118-133 (1974).

Eidelberg, E., Lesse, H., and Gault, F.P.: An experimental model of temporal lobe epilepsy: Studies on the convulsant properties of cocaine. In: EEG and Behavior. Gilbert, H. and Glaser, G.H., Eds., pp. 272-283. New York: Basic Books, 1963.

Eidelberg, E., Neer, H.M., and Miller, M.K.: Anticonvulsant properties of some benzodiazepine derivatives, Neurology, Minneap. 15, 223 (1965).

Ellinwood, E.H.: Effect of chronic methamphetamine intoxication in rhesus monkeys, Biol. Psychiat. 3, 25-32 (1971).

Ellinwood, E.H.: Amphetamine and stimulant drugs. In: Drug Use in America: Problem in Perspective (Second Report of the National Commission on Marihuana and Drug Abuse), pp. 140-157. Washington: U.S. Government Printing Office, 1973.

Ellinwood, E.H., Sudilovsky, A., and Grabowy, R.S.: Olfactory forebrain seizures induced by methamphetamine and disulfiram, Biol. Psychiat. 7, 89-99 (1973).

Ellinwood, E.H.: Behavioral and EEG changes in the amphetamine model of psychosis. In: Neuropsychopharmacology of Monoamines and Their Regulatory Enzymes. Usdin, E., Ed., pp. 281-297. New York: Raven Press, 1974a.

Ellinwood, E.H.: Physiological aspects of cocaine. Paper presented at NIDA conference on cocaine research, Washington, D.C., 1974b.

Ellinwood, E.H., Sudilovsky, A., and Nelson, L.: Behavior and EEG analysis of chronic amphetamine effect, Biol. Psychiat. 8, 169-176 (1974).

Ellinwood, E.H. and Kilbey, M.M.: Amphetamine stereotypy: The influence of environmental factors and prepotent behavioral patterns on its topography and development, Biol. Psychiat. 10, 3-16 (1975).

Escalante, O.D. and Ellinwood, E.H.: Central nervous system cytopathological changes in cat with chronic methedrine intoxication, Brain Res. 21, 151-155 (1970).

Fish, F.J.: A neurophysiological theory of schizophrenia, J. ment. Sci. 107, 828 (1961).

Flor-Henry, P.: Psychosis and temporal lobe epilepsy: A controlled investigation, Epilepsia 10, 363-395 (1968).

French, J.D., Livingston, R.V., Konigsmark, B., and Richland, K.J.: Experimental observations on the prevention of seizures by intravenous procaine injections, J. Neurosurgery 14, 43-54 (1957).

Goddard, G.V.: Development of epileptic seizures through brain stimulation at low intensity, Nature, Lond. 214, 1020-1021 (1967).

Grabowy, R.S. and Ellinwood, E.H.: On-line detection of EEG spindle activity, Decus Spring Symposiums, 42-45 (1971).

deJong, R.H. and Walts, L.F.: Lidocaine induced psychomotor seizures in man, Acta Anaesth. scand., Suppl. 23, 598-604 (1966).

deJong, R.H.: Local anesthetic seizures, Anesthesiology 30, 5-6 (1969).

deJong, R.H.: Physiology and Pharmacology of Local Anesthesia. Springfield, Ill.: Charles C. Thomas, 1970.

Kramer, J.C.: Introduction to amphetamine abuse, J. Psychedelic Drugs 2, 1-16 (1969).

Matousek, M.: Frequency and correlation analysis. In: Handbook of Electroencephalography and Clinical Neurophysiology. Remond, A., Ed., Vol. 5, Part A. Amsterdam: Elsevier Scientific Publishing Company, 1973.

McCall, R.B. and Appelbaum, M.I.: Bias in the analysis of repeated-measure designs: Some alternative approaches, Child Dev. 44, 401-415 (1973).

Modigh, K.: Electroconvulsant shock in post-synaptic catecholamine effects: Increased psychomotor stimulant action of apomorphine and clonidine in reserpine pretreated mice by ECT, J. Neural Transm. 36, 19-32 (1975).

deOliveira, L.F. and Bretas, A.D.: Effects of 5-hydroxytryptophan, ipromazid and p-chlorophenylalanine on lidocaine seizure threshold of mice, Eur. J. Pharmacol. 29, 5-9 (1974).

Pinel, J.P.J., Phillips, A.G., and MacNeil, B.: Blockage of highly-stable "kindled" seizures in rats by antecedent footshock, Epilepsia 14, 29-37 (1973).

Post, R.M.: Progressive changes in behavior and seizures following chronic cocaine administration: Relationship to kindling and psychosis. In: Cocaine and Other Stimulants. Ellinwood, E.H. and Kilbey, M.M., Eds. New York: Plenum Press, 1976.

Riblett, L.A. and Tuttle, W.W.: Investigation of the amygdaloid and olfactory electrographic response in the cat after toxic dosages of lidocaine, Electroenceph. clin. Neurophysiol. 38, 601-608

Rumbaugh, C.L.: Small vessel cerebral vascular changes following chronic amphetamine intoxication. In: Cocaine and Other Stimulants. Ellinwood, E.H. and Kilbey, M.M., Eds. New York: Plenum Press, 1976.

Sanders, H.D.: Procaine and pentylenetetrazol, Archs int. Pharmacodyn. Thér. 170, 115-177 (1967).

Seiden, L.S., Fischman, M.W., and Schuster, C.R.: Changes in brain catecholamines induced by long-term methamphetamine administration in rhesus monkeys. In: Cocaine and Other Stimulants. Ellinwood, E.H. and Kilbey, M.M., Eds. New York: Plenum Press, 1976.

Stripling, J.S. and Ellinwood, E.H.: Sensitization to cocaine following chronic administration in rats. In: Cocaine and Other Stimulants. Ellinwood, E.H. and Kilbey, M.M., Eds. New York: Plenum Press, 1976.

Tuttle, W.W. and Elliott, H.W.: Electrographic and behavioral study of convulsants in the cat, Anesthesiology 30, 48-64 (1969).

Utena, H.: On relapse-liability, schizophrenia, amphetamine psychosis and animal model. In: Biological Mechanisms of Schizophrenia and Schizophrenia-like Psychoses. Mitsuda, H. and Fukuda, T., Eds., p. 285. Tokyo: igaku Shoin, 1974.

Wada, J.A. and Sata, M.: Generalized convulsive seizures induced by daily electrical stimulation of the amygdala in cats: Correlative electrographic and behavioral features, Neurology, Minneap. 24, 565-574 (1974).

Wagman, I.H., deJong, R.H., and Prince, D.A.: Effect of lidocaine on central nervous system, Anesthesiology 28, 155-172 (1967).

Wagman, I.H., deJong, R.H., and Prince, D.A.: Effects of lidocaine on spontaneous cortical and subcortical electrical activity: Production of seizure discharges, Archs Neurol., Chicago 18, 277 (1968).

SENSITIZATION TO COCAINE FOLLOWING CHRONIC ADMINISTRATION IN THE RAT

Jeffrey S. Stripling and Everett H. Ellinwood, Jr.

Behavioral Neuropharmacology Section, Department of Psychiatry, Box 3838, Duke University Medical Center, Durham, North Carolina 27710

Reports of an augmented behavioral response to cocaine with repeated administration in laboratory animals have existed for some time. The earliest of these described an enhancement of both the psychomotor stimulant action (Downs and Eddy, 1932a; Tatum and Seevers, 1929) and convulsant effect (Downs and Eddy, 1932b; Tatum and Seevers, 1929) of cocaine. More recent studies have documented this sensitization with more quantitative measures, particularly with regard to the locomotor activity and stereotyped behavior associated with the psychomotor stimulant properties of cocaine (Kilbey and Ellinwood, 1976; Post, 1976; Ho, Taylor, Estevez, Englert, and McKenna, 1976). Other psychomotor stimulants, such as amphetamine, have also been shown to produce an increased response following chronic administration (Kilbey and Ellinwood, 1976; Klawans, Crossett, and Dana, 1975; Magos, 1969; Segal and Mandell, 1974). This sensitization and its underlying mechanisms are of particular interest because of their possible relationship to the gradual evolution of psychosis seen in humans during chronic use of these drugs (Ellinwood, 1967; Connell, 1958; Lewin, 1931; Ellinwood, Sudilovsky, and Nelson, 1973).

The studies reported in this paper were designed to examine the nature of the changes that occur with chronic administration of a constant dose of cocaine in the rat. More specifically they were designed to assess the behavioral changes that evolve, their persistence, and their relationship to cocaine's electrophysiological effects.

EXPERIMENT 1

The first experiment (unpublished observations) concentrated on cocaine's electrophysiological effects. Cocaine in high doses produced large-amplitude spindles (envelopes of sinusoidal activity) in the olfactory forebrain at a frequency of 20-60 Hz (Eidelberg, Lesse, and Gault, 1963; Ellinwood, Kilbey, Castellani, and Khoury, 1976; unpublished observations). The spindles can be recorded in various areas of the forebrain, including the olfactory bulb, amygdala, prepyriform cortex, olfactory tubercle, and nucleus accumbens (Ellinwood et al., 1976; Eidelberg, Neer, and Miller, 1965). This effect is quite striking, and suggests a possible explanation for the progressive sensitization to the behavioral effects of cocaine that occurs with chronic administration. This explanation is related to the kindling phenomenon first reported by Goddard and his co-workers (Goddard, 1967; Goddard, McIntyre, and Leech, 1969). Briefly, kindling consists of an enhanced behavioral and electrophysiological response to low-intensity electrical stimulation of the brain with repeated administration. If the proper parameters are used, electrical stimulation that initially elicits no obvious electrophysiological or behavioral effect can, with repetition at regular intervals, produce: a) electrical afterdischarges at the site of stimulation, b) a progressive increase in the amplitude and duration of these afterdischarges, c) a progressive augmentation of the propagation of these afterdischarges from the site of stimulation to other areas of the brain, and d) a behavioral response, which progresses from brief movements of the head or forelimbs to a full clonic convulsion. The kindling effect is most easily obtained in areas of the limbic system, with the amygdala being the most susceptible site. The pronounced electrophysiological activity produced by cocaine in this area, if repeated daily, may produce an effect similar to that of repeated electrical stimulation. Such an effect would result in an enhanced electrophysiological response to the drug. Furthermore, such a change, if it occurred, might underlie the progressive behavioral changes reported to occur with chronic cocaine.

Method

Male Sprague-Dawley rats were implanted with electrodes in the left and right amygdala. After recovery all animals were injected intraperitoneally with 40 mg/kg cocaine hydrochloride and divided into three groups balanced for their electrophysiological and behavioral response to the drug. After a two-day waiting period, the three groups, designated as SAL, 20C and 40C, received a daily intraperitoneal injection for 13 days of either saline or 20 or 40 mg/kg cocaine, respectively. On Days 1 and 13 of the chronic injection series, the behavioral and electrophysiological responses to the injection were analyzed. Ten seconds of electrical activity were recorded immediately prior to injection and once per minute for 15 minutes following injection. The behavioral response to the drug was measured at the same times.

The behavioral response was scored on a rating scale previously developed in our laboratory for assessing the response to psychomotor stimulants (Ellinwood and Balster, 1974). Using this scale, behavior was rated from 1 to 8 as follows: 1) asleep (lying down, eyes closed); 2) inactive (lying or sitting, eyes open); 3) in place activity (grooming, eating); 4) normal exploratory activity; 5) fast exploratory activity; 6) stereotyped locomotor activity, such as circling the cage perimeter; 7) fast stereotyped locomotor activity; and 8) stereotyped head movements without locomotor activity.

The electrophysiological response to cocaine was quantified by an amplitude measure, defined as the maximum peak-to-peak amplitude occurring during each ten-second period. Since the drug-induced spindles are of considerably greater amplitude than the electrical activity normally present, this measure should accurately reflect the effect of cocaine. Recordings were made with field-effect transistors mounted at the animal's head to eliminate movement-generated cable artifact which might otherwise contribute to the amplitude measure.

Following the termination of the 13-day injection series, all animals received daily a brief electrical stimulation of low intensity of the left amygdala to determine if the chronic cocaine administration had altered susceptibility to the kindling process. Stimulation was continued for each animal until that animal exhibited a fully developed behavioral convulsion in response to stimulation or until it reached the 26th day of stimulation without having developed convulsions. Each animal was then administered 40 mg/kg cocaine to determine if the response to the drug had been altered by the experimental manipulations. This administration of cocaine was designated as the Test injection.

Results

Table 1 illustrates for each group the change in the behavioral response to injection from Day 1 to Day 13 of the chronic injection series. There was a highly significant difference among the groups, indicating that the drug treatment reliably produced stereotyped behavior. In addition, there was a significant change across days, and a significant Group x Days interaction. The nature of these changes over time was pinpointed using individual comparisons. The SAL group showed a significant habituation of activity across days while the 40C group showed a significant increase in response to cocaine. The increase in the 20C group was not significant.

TABLE 1

EXPERIMENT 1. MEAN BEHAVIORAL RATING ± S.E.M. ON DAYS 1 AND 13 OF THE CHRONIC INJECTION SERIES. THE VALUES ARE POOLED ACROSS THE 15-MINUTE POST-INJECTION PERIOD FOR EACH DAY

Group	N	Day 1	Day 13
Saline	8	3.59 ± 0.10	3.32 ± 0.16
20 mg/kg cocaine	6	6.02 ± 0.17	6.44 ± 0.39
40 mg/kg cocaine	5	6.24 ± 0.30	7.15 ± 0.05

Analysis of Variance (two factors with repeated measures on one factor).

Factor	DF	F ratio	p value
Group	2/16	96.44	< 0.01
Days	1/16	5.90	< 0.05
G x D	2/16	5.56	< 0.05

Sandler's A test for matched samples: Comparisons between Day 1 and Day 13 (Runyon and Haber, 1971).

Group	DF	A	p value
Saline	7	0.27	< 0.05, two-tailed
20 mg/kg	5	0.77	--
40 mg/kg	4	0.28	< 0.05, two-tailed

The electrophysiological data for the SAL, 20C, and 40C groups on Days 1 and 13 are presented in Tables 2, 3, and 4, respectively. For the purpose of analysis the 15-minute post-injection period was divided into three 5-minute periods. The SAL group exhibited no significant change in amplitude following injection and a small but highly significant decline in amplitude from Day 1 to Day 13. There was a highly significant increase in amplitude following injection in the 40C group, reflecting the onset of cocaine-induced spindles. Furthermore, there was a highly significant increase in amplitude from Day 1 to Day 13, indicating an augmentation of the spindle response with chronic treatment.

The results in the 20C group were puzzling. There was no increase in amplitude following injection, indicating that spindles were not produced at this dose. However, in the left amygdala there was a highly significant decline in amplitude from the pre- to the post-injection periods, perhaps related to the unusually high pre-injection amplitude at this site. In addition there was a small but highly significant increase in amplitude from Day 1 to Day 13 in the right amygdala, and a similar trend in the left amygdala. Such changes, and the increase in the pre-injection amplitude of the 40C group across days, may reflect effects of chronic cocaine on intrinsic neural activity in this area of the brain in addition to its augmentation of cocaine-induced spindles (Ellinwood et al., 1976). These possibilities can be adequately evaluated only by further investigation.

The first phase of the experiment was successful in its basic goals, demonstrating an augmentation of the behavioral and electrophysiological responses to cocaine with chronic treatment. However, the next phase of the experiment did not provide an unequivocal assessment of the kindling hypothesis. A current intensity below that required to elicit electrical afterdischarges was chosen for electrical stimulation of the left amygdala with the intention of determining whether chronic cocaine administration would lower the afterdischarge threshold. Due to this unusually low current intensity, the kindling achieved was slow and unreliable, with the majority of animals in the experiment failing to reach criterion within the 26 day limit. The mean number of days to reach the kindling criterion was 23.8 for the SAL group, 18.2 for the 20C group, and 19.0 for the 40C group. This difference was not significant ($F = 2.02$, $df = 2/15$, $p > 0.10$). Nor was there any significant difference among the groups in the development of electrical afterdischarge. Thus no statement can be made on the possibility that the chronic cocaine treatment produced a neuronal reorganization similar to that caused by the kindling process. During this phase of the experiment one animal in the 40C group dislodged its electrodes, and consequently the size of this group is reduced by one on the Test injection data.

TABLE 2

EXPERIMENT 1. MEAN MAXIMUM AMPLITUDE (IN MICROVOLTS OF AMYGDALOID ELECTRICAL ACTIVITY ± S.E.M. FOR THE SALINE GROUP ON DAYS 1 AND 13 OF THE CHRONIC INJECTION SERIES. THE POST-INJECTION DATA ARE POOLED INTO THREE BLOCKS OF FIVE MINUTES EACH

	Pre-Injection	Minutes Post-Injection		
		1-5	6-10	11-15
Saline (N=8)				
L. Amygdala				
Day 1	193 ± 16	198 ± 14	197 ± 14	189 ± 12
Day 13	182 ± 15	171 ± 9	179 ± 11	176 ± 8
R. Amygdala				
Day 1	176 ± 13	168 ± 8	171 ± 8	174 ± 9
Day 13	159 ± 14	156 ± 8	152 ± 5	163 ± 5

Analysis of Variance: (two factors with repeated measures on each factor).

Factor	DF	F ratio	p value
L. Amygdala			
Minutes	3/49	0.49	-
Days	1/49	21.30	< 0.01
M x D	3/49	0.84	-
R. Amygdala			
Minutes	3/49	0.52	-
Days	1/49	7.90	< 0.01
M x D	3/49	0.12	-

TABLE 3

EXPERIMENT 1. MEAN MAXIMUM AMPLITUDE (IN MICROVOLTS) OF AMYGDALOID ELECTRICAL ACTIVITY ± S.E.M. FOR THE 20 MG/KG COCAINE GROUP ON DAYS 1 AND 13 OF THE CHRONIC INJECTION SERIES. THE POST-INJECTION DATA ARE POOLED INTO THREE BLOCKS OF FIVE MINUTES EACH

	Pre-Injection	Minutes Post-Injection		
20 mg/kg Cocaine (N=6		1-5	6-10	11-15
L. Amygdala				
Day 1	225 ± 35	177 ± 11	175 ± 6	171 ± 8
Day 13	237 ± 17	188 ± 12	195 ± 12	186 ± 11
R. Amygdala				
Day 1	162 ± 9	157 ± 9	156 ± 11	156 ± 12
Day 13	185 ± 9	177 ± 14	182 ± 18	170 ± 15

Analysis of Variance: (two factors with repeated measures on each factor).

Factor	DF	F ratio	p value
L. Amygdala			
Minutes	3/35	5.46	< 0.01
Days	1/35	1.92	-
M x D	3/35	0.03	-
R. Amygdala			
Minutes	3/35	0.52	-
Days	1/35	10.66	< 0.01
M x D	3/35	0.13	-

TABLE 4

EXPERIMENT 1. MEAN MAXIMUM AMPLITUDE (IN MICROVOLTS) OF AMYGDALOID ELECTRICAL ACTIVITY ± S.E.M. FOR THE 40 MG/KG COCAINE GROUP ON DAYS 1 AND 13 OF THE CHRONIC INJECTION SERIES. THE POST-INJECTION DATA ARE POOLED INTO THREE BLOCKS OF FIVE MINUTES EACH

	Pre-Injection	Minutes Post-Injection		
40 mg/kg Cocaine (N=5)		1-5	6-10	11-15
L. Amygdala				
Day 1	168 ± 7	170 ± 15	206 ± 24	200 ± 14
Day 13	213 ± 32	189 ± 24	287 ± 62	309 ± 49
R. Amygdala				
Day 1	168 ± 9	176 ± 17	201 ± 23	217 ± 26
Day 13	204 ± 12	194 ± 15	299 ± 39	314 ± 33

Analysis of Variance: (two factors with repeated measures on each factor).

Factor	DF	F ratio	p value
L. Amygdala			
Minutes	3/28	5.42	< 0.01
Days	1/28	14.90	< 0.01
M x D	3/28	1.43	-
R. Amygdala			
Minutes	3/28	9.49	< 0.01
Days	1/28	20.53	< 0.01
M x D	3/28	2.26	-

Table 5 shows the behavioral response to the Test injection that followed the kindling phase of the experiment. There was a significant difference among the three groups. Both cocaine-pretreated groups had a higher rating than the SAL group, but individual comparisons indicated that only the 20C group was significantly higher than the SAL group.

The electrophysiological response to the Test injection is shown in Table 6. At both electrode sites there was a highly significant increase in amplitude following injection, reflecting the onset of cocaine-induced spindles. In the right amygdala (the site not stimulated during kindling), there was no significant difference among the groups, but there was a significant Group x Minutes interaction. Inspection of the data indicates that the interaction reflects similar pre-injection levels in the three groups, but a greater response to the drug in the 40C group than in the other two. This indicates a significant persistence of the augmented electrophysiological response in the 40C group an average of 20 days beyond the termination of chronic cocaine administration. In the left amygdala (the site of electrical stimulation), there was a significant difference among the groups but no significant interaction. The 40C group again exhibited the greatest response to cocaine, but this response appears superimposed upon an elevated amplitude present during the pre-injection period, perhaps produced by the electrical stimulation. Furthermore, the other two groups show a greater drug response in the left amygdala than in the right amygdala. These differences may reflect a drug activation of abnormal activity produced by the electrical stimulation as well as the appearance of drug-induced spindles. Any such effects of the electrical stimulation on the response to cocaine would appear confined to the left amygdala, and consequently the findings in the right amygdala offer strong support for the persistence of the augmented electrophysiological response to cocaine produced by chronic administration.

EXPERIMENT 2

The objective of the second experiment (unpublished observations) was to examine in detail the changes in the psychomotor stimulant and convulsant effects of cocaine produced by chronic administration and the persistence of these changes. Part 1 was designed to determine the intensity of chronic cocaine treatment required to produce sensitization. In Part 2 an effective treatment schedule was chosen and the persistence of the sensitization was assessed at several intervals after the termination of treatment.

TABLE 5

EXPERIMENT 1. MEAN BEHAVIORAL RATING ± S.E.M. FOLLOWING THE TEST INJECTION (40 MG/KG COCAINE). THE VALUES ARE POOLED ACROSS THE 15-MINUTE POST-INJECTION PERIOD

Group	N	Rating
Saline	8	6.38 ± 0.14
20 mg/kg Cocaine	6	7.29 ± 0.28
40 mg/kg Cocaine	4	7.13 ± 0.40

Analysis of Variance

Factor	DF	F ratio	p value
Group	2/15	4.51	< 0.05

Dunnett's t: Comparison of each experimental group with the saline group (Winer, 1962).

Group	t	p value
20 mg/kg Cocaine	2.81	< 0.05, two-tailed
40 mg/kg Cocaine	2.05	--

TABLE 6

EXPERIMENT 1. MEAN MAXIMUM AMPLITUDE (IN MICROVOLTS) OF AMYGDALOID ELECTRICAL ACTIVITY ± S.E.M. FOLLOWING THE TEST INJECTION (40 MG/KG COCAINE). THE POST-INJECTION DATA ARE POOLED INTO THREE BLOCKS OF FIVE MINUTES EACH

	N	Pre-injection	Minutes Post-Injection		
			1-5	6-10	11-15
L. Amygdala					
Saline	8	189 ± 17	167 ± 12	182 ± 23	211 ± 24
20 mg/kg	6	190 ± 18	182 ± 16	211 ± 21	242 ± 24
40 mg/kg	4	248 ± 29	233 ± 16	285 ± 46	305 ± 43
R. Amygdala					
Saline	8	150 ± 10	146 ± 9	143 ± 15	165 ± 23
20 mg/kg	6	158 ± 10	153 ± 21	165 ± 17	172 ± 15
40 mg/kg	4	161 ± 9	168 ± 24	244 ± 51	236 ± 52

Analysis of Variance: (two factors with repeated measures on one factor).

Factor	DF	F ratio	p value
L. Amygdala			
Group	2/15	4.07	< 0.05
Minutes	3/45	9.04	< 0.01
G x M	6/45	0.60	-
R. Amygdala			
Group	2/15	2.31	-
Minutes	3/45	4.96	< 0.01
G x M	6/45	2.56	< 0.05

PART 1

Method

Part 1 had three stages: an initial injection series, a waiting period, and a test injection series. There were five groups of male Sprague-Dawley rats. Two of them, designated as 20C and 40C, received daily intraperitoneal injections of 20 or 40 mg/kg cocaine for 10 days. Two other groups, designated as CONV (1) and CONV (3), were given daily cocaine injections of increasing dosage. Each animal in these groups was injected until it experienced one or three convulsions, respectively. The fifth group, designated as SAL, was injected with saline; half of these animals were injected for 10 days and half were matched with animals in the CONV (1) and CONV (3) groups for number of injections. Following the initial injection series there was a waiting period of seven days, followed in turn by a test injection series. The purpose of the test injection series was to assess the sensitivity of the various groups to the convulsant effects of cocaine, which was determined by the number of injections in the series required to produce a convulsion. The seventeen-day injection series began at a dose of 45 mg/kg cocaine, which was increased in the following way: second day (50 mg/kg), third day (55 mg/kg), tenth day (60 mg/kg), fifteenth day (65 mg/kg). This schedule permitted differentiation between animals on the basis not only of the dose at which they convulsed, but also of the number of days for which the dose was administered before convulsion, intended to reflect the sensitization to cocaine with chronic treatment. On the first day of the test injection series the behavioral response to 45 mg/kg cocaine was rated for 15 minutes following injection as in Experiment 1.

Results

Table 7 shows the behavioral response to cocaine on the first day of the test injection series. There was a highly significant difference among the groups. Individual comparisons revealed that the 40C group exhibited a significantly greater effect than any of the other groups. No other comparisons were significant.

Table 8 shows the mean number of injections required to produce a convulsion during the test injection series. Four of the five groups contained an animal that did not convulse during this injection series, and to solve this problem the animal with the largest number of injections in each group was discarded for the purpose of this analysis. Because of the uneven spacing of the dose increases in the test injection series, the data were analyzed with the use of non-parametric statistics. Individual comparisons with the SAL group indicated that the 40C and CONV (1) groups

TABLE 7

EXPERIMENT 2 PART 1. MEAN BEHAVIORAL RATING ± S.E.M. FOLLOWING THE INJECTION OF 45 MG/KG COCAINE ON THE FIRST DAY OF THE TEST INJECTION SERIES. THE VALUES ARE POOLED ACROSS THE 15-MINUTE POST-INJECTION PERIOD

Group	N	Rating
SAL	10	5.93 ± 0.16
20 C	10	6.73 ± 0.13
40 C	9	7.41 ± 0.24
Conv (1)	8	6.51 ± 0.21
Conv (3)	8	6.26 ± 0.41

Analysis of Variance

Factor	DF	F ratio	p value
Group	4/40	5.92	< 0.01

Newman-Keuls: Pair-wise comparisons among groups (Winer, 1962). Only significant comparisons are shown.

Comparison	r	q	p value
40 C vs Sal	5	6.33	< 0.05
40 C vs Conv (3)	4	4.92	< 0.05
40 C vs Conv (1)	3	3.85	< 0.05
40 C vs 20 C	2	2.91	< 0.05

TABLE 8

EXPERIMENT 2 PART 1. MEAN NUMBER OF INJECTIONS ± S.E.M. REQUIRED TO PRODUCE A CONVULSION DURING THE TEST INJECTION SERIES

Group	N	Injections to Convulsion
SAL	9	7.56 ± 1.47
20 C	9	6.56 ± 1.47
40 C	8	3.75 ± 1.05
Conv (1)	7	2.71 ± 0.47
Conv (3)	7	3.86 ± 0.74

Kruskal-Wallis: Analysis of variance by ranks (Siegel, 1956).

Factor	DF	H	p value
Group	4	11.95	< 0.02

Mann-Whitney U Test: Comparison of each experimental group with the SAL group (Siegel, 1956).

Group	U	p value
20 C	33.0	--
40 C	12.5	< 0.05, two-tailed
Conv (1)	7.0	< 0.02, two-tailed
Conv (3)	12.5	< 0.10, two-tailed

convulsed significantly earlier in these test injection series than the SAL group, and the CONV (3) group approached significance. These results suggest that a lowered convulsive threshold to cocaine can be produced not only by treatment with a convulsive dose of cocaine, but also by chronic administration of a high subconvulsive dose. However, it should be noted that three animals in the 40C group had a brief convulsion during the initial injection series, and thus this was not strictly a subconvulsive treatment.

PART 2

Method

Part 2 was designed to explore in more detail the effect of chronic administration of a high subconvulsive dose of cocaine. Like Part 1, it consisted of three parts: an initial injection series, a waiting period, and a test injection series. Five groups of male Sprague-Dawley rats were used. Four of these received 40 mg/kg cocaine once per day for ten days. The fifth group (SAL) received saline. During the waiting period the four cocaine groups, designated as 40C-4, 40C-8, 40C-16, and 40C-32, were not injected for 4, 8, 16, or 32 days, respectively. The SAL group was divided into four sub-groups which were matched to the four cocaine groups for duration of the waiting period. Following the waiting period all animals began an identical test injection series, which began at 45 mg/kg cocaine and increased each day by 2.5 mg/kg. On the first day of this series the behavioral response to cocaine was rated every three minutes for the first 15 minutes post-injection, and for every 15 minutes thereafter until 120 minutes post-injection.

Results

Table 9 shows the behavioral response to cocaine on the first day of the test injection series. The data are pooled into three blocks (Minutes 3-12, 15-60, and 75-120) intended to reflect the onset of the effect, its maximum level, and its offset. Two animals were discarded from this analysis: one in the 40C-32 group that convulsed, and one in the 40C-4 group that failed to respond to the injection, receiving a mean rating over the first hour of 2.38 in comparison to 5.50 received by the next lowest animal in the experiment. There was a significant difference among the groups in each block. Individual comparisons with the SAL group indicated that all of the cocaine groups were significantly higher than the SAL group in the first block (onset), all but the 40C-8 group were significantly higher in the second block (maximal level), and none differed signicantly from the SAL group in the third block (offset). Inspection of the third block indicates that the significant overall effect

TABLE 9

EXPERIMENT 2 PART 2. MEAN BEHAVIORAL RATING ± S.E.M. FOLLOWING THE INJECTION OF 45 MG/KG COCAINE ON THE FIRST DAY OF THE TEST INJECTION SERIES. THE VALUES ARE POOLED INTO THREE BLOCKS INTENDED TO REFLECT ONSET, MAXIMAL LEVEL, AND OFFSET OF THE BEHAVIORAL EFFECT

		Rating: Minutes Post-Injection		
Group	N	3-12	15-60	75-120
SAL	16	6.16 ± 0.18	6.56 ± 0.20	5.70 ± 0.26
40 C - 4	11	7.11 ± 0.20	7.52 ± 0.14	4.98 ± 0.40
40 C - 8	12	7.17 ± 0.19	7.31 ± 0.34	5.06 ± 0.32
40 C - 16	12	7.15 ± 0.21	7.46 ± 0.20	5.88 ± 0.35
40 C - 32	11	6.91 ± 0.20	7.39 ± 0.18	6.39 ± 0.24
Analysis of Variance				
F		5.75	3.59	3.18
DF		4/57	4/57	4/57
p		< 0.01	< 0.05	< 0.05

Dunnett's t: Comparison of each experimental group with the saline group (Winer, 1962).

Group	t values		
40 C - 4	3.57 **	3.10 *	-1.67
40 C - 8	3.87 **	2.48	-1.51
40 C - 16	3.79 **	2.97 *	0.41
40 C - 32	2.81 *	2.66 *	1.58

* $p < 0.05$, two tailed
** $p < 0.01$, two-tailed

reflects a monotonic increase in the mean rating from the 40C-4 to the 40C-32 group, with the SAL group falling near the middle. The pattern of results in the first and second blocks suggest that the augmentation of the behavioral response to cocaine persists for at least 33 days after the termination of chronic administration. The pattern in the third block is puzzling, however. An explanation can be found in Table 10, which shows the behavioral response to cocaine for the SAL group broken down by subgroups. This table indicates that the SAL subgroups did not differ significantly over the first and second blocks, but did differ in the third block, and in a manner very similar to that of the four 40C groups. Thus the animals tested at the longest retention intervals exhibited the slowest offset of the drug effect, regardless of whether they were pre-treated with saline or cocaine. These changes suggest that the rate of offset is related to age or body weight rather than drug treatment. In addition, while not significant, the trends in the first and second blocks for the SAL subgroups resemble the significant effect in the third block. If there is an age-related increase in the onset and maximal level of the behavioral response, this may have contributed to the significant persistence seen at the longer delay intervals. Thus the duration of the persistence cannot be determined with certainty.

Table 11 illustrates the dose at which the animals convulsed during the test injection series. As in Part 1, a few animals failed to convulse during the series, which was terminated at 77.5 mg/kg. To solve this problem the highest score per group was discarded for this analysis. Under these conditions there is a highly significant difference among the groups (Table 11A). Individual comparisons indicate that the 40C-4, 40C-8, and 40C-32 groups convulsed at a significantly lower dose than the SAL group, while the 40C-16 group was not significantly lower. However, six animals in the various 40C groups convulsed during the initial injection series, and thus these results are not solely attributable to a subconvulsive treatment. If the animals that convulsed are discarded, there is still a significant overall difference among the groups (Table 11B). However, the probability levels of the individual comparisons are reduced, with only the 40C-8 group convulsing at a significantly lower dose than the SAL group. If one-tailed statistical tests are used, which is reasonable in view of the directional nature of the hypothesis being tested (that sensitization will occur following chronic cocaine treatment), then the 40C-4 and 40C-32 groups are again significantly more sensitive to the convulsant effect of cocaine than the SAL group.

Table 12 gives the dose at convulsion for the SAL subgroups. There is no significant difference among the subgroups, and inspection of the data reveals no age-related trend as was present in the behavioral ratings. Thus the convulsant effect of cocaine does not

TABLE 10

EXPERIMENT 2 PART 2. MEAN BEHAVIORAL RATING ± S.E.M. FOR THE SALINE SUBGROUPS FOLLOWING THE INJECTION OF 45 MG/KG COCAINE ON THE FIRST DAY OF THE TEST INJECTION SERIES. THE VALUES ARE POOLED INTO THREE BLOCKS INTENDED TO REFLECT ONSET, MAXIMAL LEVEL, AND OFFSET OF THE BEHAVIORAL EFFECT

		Rating Minutes Post-Injection		
	N	3-12	15-60	75-120
Saline Subgroups				
Sal - 4	4	5.94 ± 0.39	6.38 ± 0.38	5.44 ± 0.44
Sal - 8	4	5.88 ± 0.13	6.06 ± 0.21	4.75 ± 0.35
Sal - 16	4	6.38 ± 1.38	6.69 ± 0.47	6.00 ± 0.35
Sal - 32	4	6.44 ± 0.50	7.13 ± 0.43	6.63 ± 0.52
F		0.60	1.39	3.62
DF		3/12	3/12	3/12
p		--	--	< 0.05

TABLE 11

EXPERIMENT 2 PART 2. MEAN DOSE IN MG/KG COCAINE AT WHICH A CONVULSION OCCURRED DURING THE TEST INJECTION SERIES. A SHOWS THE RESULTS WITH ANIMALS WHICH CONVULSED DURING THE INITIAL INJECTION SERIES RETAINED IN THE ANALYSIS, AND B THE RESULTS WITH THOSE ANIMALS DISCARDED

Group	N	Dose at Convulsion	Dunnett's t	p value
A. Animals which convulsed during the initial injection series; retained.				
SAL	15	62.50 ± 1.73	x	x
40C-4	11	54.09 ± 1.44	3.37	< 0.01, two-tailed
40C-8	11	53.41 ± 1.27	3.64	< 0.01, two-tailed
40C-16	11	59.32 ± 2.31	1.28	-
40C-32	11	55.68 ± 2.16	2.73	< 0.05, two-tailed

Analysis of Variance

Factor	DF	F ratio	p value
Group	4/54	4.80	< 0.01

Group	N	Dose at Convulsion	Dunnett's t	p value
B. Animals which convulsed during the initial injection series; discarded.				
SAL	15	62.50 ± 1.73	x	x
40C-4	8	55.94 ± 1.41	2.35	< 0.10, two-tailed
40C-8	9	54.44 ± 1.30	3.00	< 0.05, two-tailed
40C-16	11	59.32 ± 2.31	1.26	-
40C-32	10	56.00 ± 2.36	2.50	< 0.10, two-tailed

Analysis of Variance

Factor	DF	F ratio	p value
Group	4/48	3.12	< 0.05

TABLE 12

EXPERIMENT 2 PART 2. MEAN DOSE IN MG/KG OF COCAINE AT WHICH A CONVULSION OCCURRED DURING THE TEST INJECTION SERIES FOR THE SALINE SUBGROUPS

Saline Subgroups	N	Dose at Convulsion
SAL-4	4	60.00 ± 3.06
SAL-8	4	65.00 ± 2.70
SAL-16	4	63.13 ± 5.72
SAL-32	4	66.25 ± 4.39

Analysis of Variance

Factor	DF	F ratio	p value
Group	3/12	0.43	-

seem to be influenced by age or body weight over the range covered by this experiment.

DISCUSSION

In the preceding experiments the repeated daily administration of cocaine produced sensitization to three of its effects in the rat: stereotyped behavior, convulsions, and hypersynchronous electrical activity in the basal forebrain. In addition, the sensitization to each of these effects persisted well beyond the termination of chronic cocaine treatment.

Stereotyped behavior was produced by both 20 and 40 mg/kg cocaine. In the present experiments only the higher dose of cocaine reliably produced sensitization to this effect with chronic treatment (Experiment 1; Experiment 2, Part 1). However, the lower dose showed a trend towards sensitization, and other experiments have demonstrated sensitization with doses in this range (Kilbey and Ellinwood, 1976; Post, 1976; Ho et al., 1976). Experiment 2, Part 2, in which behavior was rated over a longer period of time following injection, demonstrated that the sensitization is not simply a more rapid onset of the effect, but an elevation of the maximum level as well. Evidence for the persistence of the augmented response was obtained in each experiment. Based on Experiment 2, there is strong evidence that the augmentation persists for 8 to 9 days after the termination of chronic cocaine administration, and there is some evidence for persistence at intervals of 33 days or more.

According to Experiment 2, Part 1, chronic administration of 40, but not 20, mg/kg cocaine produced an augmentation of the convulsant effect of cocaine, as did convulsive doses of the drug. Experiment 2, Part 2, confirmed that 40 mg/kg could produce this effect, even if data of animals that convulsed during the initial treatment were discarded. This demonstrates clearly that the sensitization is due to cocaine itself, and not to convulsions produced by the drug. This point is important, since convulsions produced by a number of agents have been demonstrated to produce a lowered convulsive threshold (Adler, Sagel, Kitagawa, Segawa, and Maynert, 1976; Mason and Cooper, 1972; Prichard, Gallagher, and Glaser, 1969). The lowered convulsive threshold due to cocaine was shown to persist for 8 or 9 days at a minimum, with evidence for persistence at 33 days or longer.

The electrophysiological findings are of interest, since augmentation of cocaine-induced spindles has not previously been demonstrated. The spindles were produced only by the higher dose of cocaine, and their augmentation appeared to persist for 20 days or more.

The mechanism underlying these effects of chronic cocaine administration is not known. Repeated administration results in a shorter half-life of cocaine in the blood and the brain (Mulé and Misra, 1976; Ho et al., 1976). Any change in the intensity of the behavioral response to cocaine which might result from this alteration would be in the opposite direction of that observed. However, Ho et al. (1976) have reported elevated brain levels of cocaine shortly after injection following chronic treatment, suggesting that some change in the pharmacokinetics of cocaine may be involved in the augmentation of response. Angel and Roberts (1966) found that chronic pretreatment with tricyclic antidepressants resulted in higher brain levels of cocaine following injection. This is of interest since cocaine shares with the tricyclic antidepressants the effect of blocking the uptake of norepinephrine. Other possible mechanisms include conditioning effects or changes in receptor sensitivity or in the ratios of various neurotransmitters. These possibilities have been discussed in detail elsewhere (Stripling and Ellinwood, in press; Ellinwood, Stripling, and Kilbey, in press). Another hypothesis of interest is that cocaine's electrophysiological effects in the basal forebrain produce a kindling-like effect, as outlined in the beginning of this paper. The test of this hypothesis in Experiment 1 was inconclusive due to technical problems, but we are currently engaged in further tests of this possibility.

The behavioral correlates, if any, of the cocaine-induced spindles are uncertain. In these experiments the spindles do not appear to reflect the mechanism responsible for the behavioral stereotypies produced by cocaine, since in Experiment 1 both 20 and 40 mg/kg cocaine produced stereotyped behavior, while only the higher dose induced spindles. In addition, the stereotypies continued for an hour or more after injection, while the spindles lasted only about 20 minutes. Finally, local anesthetics other than cocaine that do not produce stereotyped behavior also produce a similar electrophysiological effect (Riblet and Tuttle, 1970; Wagman, de Jong, and Prince, 1976, 1968). The spindles may well be associated with the convulsant effect of cocaine, but they can occur in quite pronounced form without being accompanied by convulsions. In cats receiving chronic methamphetamine (Ellinwood and Sudilovsky, 1973; Ellinwood et al., 1973) or cocaine (Ellinwood, unpublished observations), we have noted the development of hyperreactive behavior that may be analogous to certain fearful or paranoid symptoms that can develop in humans with chronic psychomotor stimulant use (Connell, 1958; Ellinwood and Sudilovsky, 1973). Ellinwood (1974) reported that in cats treated with methamphetamine, reactive behavior was often associated with the presence of spindles in the amygdala and other areas. We are currently involved in assessing the possible relationship between quantitative measures of behavioral reactivity to sensory stimuli and the cocaine-induced spindle.

ACKNOWLEDGMENTS

This research was supported by National Institutes of Health Grants DA 00057 and MH 08394.

REFERENCES

Adler, M.W., Sagel, S., Kitagawa, S., Segawa, T., and Maynert, E.W.: The effects of repeated flurothyl-induced seizures on convulsive thresholds and brain monoamines in rats, Archs int. Pharmacodyn. Thér. 170, 12-21 (1967).

Angel, C. and Roberts, A.J.: Effect of electroshock and anti-depressant drugs on cerebrovascular permeability to cocaine in the rat, J. nerv. ment. Dis. 142, 376-380 (1966).

Connell, P.H.: Amphetamine Psychosis (Maudsley Monographs Number 5). London: Oxford University Press, 1958.

Downs, A.W. and Eddy, N.B.: The effect of repeated doses of cocaine on the dog, J. Pharmac. exp. Ther. 46, 195-198 (1932a).

Downs, A.W. and Eddy, N.B.: The effect of repeated doses of cocaine on the rat, J. Pharmac. exp. Ther. 46, 199-200 (1932b).

Eidelberg, E., Lesse, H., and Gault, F.P.: An experimental model of temporal lobe epilepsy: Studies of the convulsant properties of cocaine. In: EEG and Behavior. Glaser, G.H., Ed., pp. 272-283. New York: Basic Books, 1963.

Eidelberg, E., Neer, H.M., and Miller, M.K.: Anticonvulsant properties of some benzodiazepine derivatives, Neurology, Minneap. 15, 223-230 (1965).

Ellinwood, E.H.: Amphetamine psychosis: I. Description of the individuals and process, J. nerv. ment. Dis. 144, 273-283 (1967).

Ellinwood, E.H.: Behavioral and EEG changes in the amphetamine model of psychosis. In: Neuropsychopharmacology of Monoamines and Their Regulatory Enzymes. Usdin, E., Ed., pp. 281-297. New York: Raven Press, 1974.

Ellinwood, E.H. and Balster, R.L.: Rating the behavioral effects of amphetamine, Eur. J. Pharmacol. 28, 35-41 (1974).

Ellinwood, E.H., Kilbey, M.M., Castellani, S., and Khoury, C.: Amygdala hyperspindling and seizures induced by cocaine. In: Cocaine and Other Stimulants. Ellinwood, E.H. and Kilbey, M.M., Eds. New York: Plenum Press, 1976.

Ellinwood, E.H., Stripling, J.S., and Kilbey, M.M.: Chronic changes with amphetamine intoxication: Underlying processes. In: Neuroregulators and Hypotheses of Psychiatric Disorders. Usdin, E. and Barchas, J., Eds. London: Oxford University Press, in press.

Ellinwood, E.H. and Sudilovsky, A.: Chronic amphetamine intoxication: Behavioral model of psychosis. In: Psychopathology and Psychopharmacology. Cole, J.O., Freedman, A.M., and Friedhoff, A.J., Eds., pp. 51-70. Baltimore: Johns Hopkins University Press, 1973.

Ellinwood, E.H., Sudilovsky, A., and Nelson, L.M.: Evolving behavior in the clinical and experimental amphetamine (model) psychosis, Am. J. Psychiat. 130, 1088-1093 (1973).

Goddard, G.V.: Development of epileptic seizures through brain stimulation at low intensity, Nature 214, 1020-1021 (1967).

Goddard, G.V., McIntyre, D.C., and Leech, C.K.: A permanent change in brain function resulting from daily electrical stimulation, Exp. Neurol. 25, 295-330 (1969).

Ho, B.T., Taylor, D.L., Estevez, V.S., Englert, L.F., and McKenna, M.L.: Behavioral effects of cocaine - metabolic and neurochemical approach. In: Cocaine and Other Stimulants. Ellinwood, E.H. and Kilbey, M.M., Eds. New York: Plenum Press, 1976.

Kilbey, M.M. and Ellinwood, E.H.: Chronic administration of stimulant drugs: Response modification. In: Cocaine and Other Stimulants. Ellinwood, E.H. and Kilbey, M.M., Eds. New York: Plenum Press, 1976.

Klawans, H.L., Crossett, P., and Dana, N.: Effect of chronic amphetamine exposure on stereotyped behavior: Implications for pathogenesis of l-DOPA-induced dyskinesias, Adv. Neurol. 9, 105-112 (1975).

Lewis, L.: Phantastica. Narcotic and Stimulating Drugs. Translated by P.H.A. Wirth. New York: E.P. Dutton, 1931.

Magos, L.: Persistence of the effect of amphetamine on stereotyped activity in rats, Eur. J. Pharmacol. 6, 200-201 (1969).

Mason, C.R. and Cooper, R.M.: A permanent change in convulsive threshold in normal and brain-damaged rats with repeated small doses of pentylenetetrazol, Epilepsia 13, 663-674 (1972).

Mulé, S.J. and Misra, A.L.: Physiological disposition and biotransformation of ^{3}H-cocaine in acute and chronically-treated animals. In: Cocaine and Other Stimulants. Ellinwood, E.H. and Kilbey, M.M., Eds. New York: Plenum Press, 1976.

Post, R.M.: Progressive changes in behavior and seizures following chronic cocaine administration: Relationship to kindling and psychosis. In: Cocaine and Other Stimulants. Ellinwood, E.H. and Kilbey, M.M., Eds. New York: Plenum Press, 1976.

Prichard, J.W., Gallagher, B.B., and Glaser, G.H.: Experimental seizure-threshold testing with flurothyl, J. Pharmac. exp. Ther. 166, 170-178 (1969).

Riblet, L.A. and Tuttle, W.W.: Investigation of the amygdaloid and olfactory electrographic response in the cat after toxic dosage of lidocaine, Electroenceph. clin. Neurophysiol. 28, 601-608 (1970),

Runyon, R. and Haber, A.: Fundamentals of Behavioral Statistics. Reading, Mass.: Addison-Wesley, 1971.

Segal, D.S. and Mandell, A.J.: Long-term administration of d-amphetamine: Progressive augmentation of motor activity and stereotypy, Pharmacol. Biochem. Behav. 2, 249-255 (1974).

Siegel, S.: Nonparametric Statistics for the Behavioral Sciences. New York: McGraw-Hill, 1956.

Stripling, J.S. and Ellinwood, E.H.: Cocaine: Physiological and behavioral effects of acute and chronic administration. In: Cocaine: Chemical, Biological, Clinical, Social, and Treatment Aspects. Mulé, S, Ed. Cleveland: CRC Press, in press.

Tatum, A.L. and Seevers, M.H.: Experimental cocaine addiction, J. Pharmac. exp. Ther. 36, 401-410 (1929).

Wagman, I.H., de Jong, R.H., and Prince, D.A.: Effects of lidocaine on the central nervous system, Anesthesiology 28, 155-169 (1967).

Winer, B.J.: Statistical Principles in Experimental Design. New York: McGraw-Hill, 1962.

PROGRESSIVE CHANGES IN BEHAVIOR AND SEIZURES FOLLOWING CHRONIC COCAINE ADMINISTRATION: RELATIONSHIP TO KINDLING AND PSYCHOSIS

Robert M. Post

Section on Psychobiology, Adult Psychiatry Branch

National Institute of Mental Health, 9000 Rockville Pike

Bethesda, Maryland 20014

In this paper we will focus on the effects of repetitive cocaine administration on a variety of neurological, behavioral, and biochemical parameters. We will pay selective attention to the data suggesting that repetitive administration may be associated with increased effects on a variety of parameters, and will not review data suggesting that cocaine may produce tolerance in some systems. While we will present our findings of the effects of repetitive cocaine administration in laboratory animals, particularly the rat and rhesus monkey, they also appear relevant to the effects of stimulants in man. It has been reviewed in detail elsewhere that chronic administration of amphetamine-like stimulants may produce a paranoid psychosis difficult to distinguish from paranoid schizophrenia (Ellinwood, 1972; Connell, 1958; Snyder, 1973; Angrist, Gershon, 1970; Griffith, Cavanaugh, Held, Oates, 1970; Ånggard, Jonsson, Hogmark, Gunne, 1973). Initial or lower doses of stimulants in a variety of patient populations, on the contrary, appear to elicit predominantly affective responses in the euphoric-dysphoric spectrum (Post, Kotin, Goodwin, 1974; Post, 1975; Resnick, Schwartz, Kestenbaum, Freedman, 1975). An adequate exposition of the mechanisms involved in the transition from predominantly affective symptoms to those in the schizophreniform spectrum with chronic stimulant administration, has not been adequately given.

We began to explore the effects of chronic, repetitive, cocaine administration in animals under a variety of conditions in the hopes of more carefully dissecting the behavioral, physiological, and pharmacological mechanisms involved, both acutely and chronically.

The effects of chronic lidocaine administration on behavior and convulsions in rats will also be examined in an attempt to separate out the local anesthetic as compared to the stimulant properties of cocaine's progressive effects. Like cocaine, lidocaine produces prominent spindle--and afterdischarge activity in limbic system structures (Eidelberg, Lesse, Gault, 1963; Wagman, De Jong, Prince, 1968; Riblet, Tuttle, 1970), but is not a psychomotor stimulant (Post, Kopanda, Lee, 1975).

On the basis of studies suggesting increased sensitivity to cocaine seizures with chronic administration (Downs, Eddy, 1932; Post, Kopanda, 1975) and increased responsiveness on a variety of behavioral parameters (Post, Kopanda, Black, in press), we suggested that one potentially important mechanism by which the stimulants may produce reverse tolerance-like effects was "pharmacological kindling" (Post et al., 1975; Post, Kopanda, 1975, in press). Kindling refers to the increasing effects of repetitive electrical stimulation in a variety of subcortical structures, particularly in the limbic system, on electrical and convulsive activity (Goddard, McIntyre, Leech, 1969; Racine, 1972; Wada, Sata, 1974; Pinel, Van Oot, in press). With repetitive stimulation, progressive increases in electrical afterdischarges and seizures in subcortical sites occur; and, associated with progressive spread of this activity into other anatomical sites, the animal begins to demonstrate major motor convulsions to a stimulus which previously had no effect on electrical activity or behavior (Goddard et al., 1969; Racine, 1972; Wada, Sata, 1974; Pinel, Van Oot, in press). Repetitive cocaine and lidocaine treatments, which have similar progressive temporal effects on seizures and have prominent effects on limbic electrical activity (Eidelberg et al., 1963; Wagman et al., 1968; Riblet, Tuttle, 1970), may, in part, be kindling the limbic system. Alternate biochemical and behavioral explanations of the progressive effects of cocaine will be explored also.

METHODS

In the chronic studies reported here cocaine and lidocaine were injected at a constant mg/kg dose intraperitoneally, once daily, five times weekly except in several rhesus monkeys which received cocaine injections twice daily at approximately 9 a.m. and 4 p.m. Both monkeys and rats were weighed one to three times a week, were maintained in twelve hour light-dark cycles, and received their injections at the same time each day. Rats were housed in groups of three or four, and were removed from their home cages to a plexiglas cage mounted on top of Motron motility meters. After 20 minutes of baseline recording of horizontal and vertical activity counts, eight rats were then injected with cocaine, 10 mg/kg i.p., and studied for ninety minutes. Eight control animals were treated in an identical fashion except that they received daily injections of equal volumes of saline. In the experimental group maintained on chronic cocaine administration, two saline injections were substituted on days 25 and 29 in order to detect the possible effects of conditioning.

In a second series, rats were administered the same dose of cocaine (40-60 mg/kg i.p.) on a once daily, five times weekly basis to study the possible effects of high dose cocaine on development of seizures. A third group of 21 rats received lidocaine (60 mg/kg i.p.) on a similar basis, as described in detail elsewhere (Post et al., 1975). In addition to these animals' being closely observed for the development of seizures, a variety of objects were tested to determine lidocaine's effect on eating behavior. Pieces of straw, gauze, paper, plastic, rubber, and desiccated feces were placed in animals' cages prior to chronic lidocaine or saline administration in six control animals.

A constant dose of cocaine (10-17 mg/kg i.p.) was administered to 13 rhesus monkeys weighing 4-6 kg for periods up to six months (Post et al., in press). In a subset of seven animals, the dose of cocaine was gradually increased to that sufficient to produce seizures, and a dose just below the convulsive dose was chosen to be administered chronically. Two additional monkeys were treated with chronic saline injections for more than 3-1/2 months following identical procedures. All animals were rated on a 5-point scale for a variety of cocaine-induced excitatory and inhibitory behaviors, including stereotypic movements, hyperactivity, tremors, rapid continuous shifts of visual fields (checking behavior), degree of motor inhibition, catalepsy, staring, and apparent visual tracking consisting of slow searching, hallucinatory-like visual patterns. In addition animals were also rated for the degree of anorexia, response to threat, and dyskinesias (Post et al., in press).

In the rhesus monkeys 4 ml samples of cisternal CSF were obtained before and 10 hours after probenecid administration (100 mg/kg i.p.), during saline control drug-free intervals as well as during acute and chronic cocaine administration. CSF was analyzed for 5-hydroxyindole-acetic acid (5HIAA), homovanillic acid (HVA), and 3-methoxy-4-hydroxy-phenethylene-glycol (MHPG) by previously described methods (Post et al., in press). In collaboration with Richard Hawks, levels of cocaine in blood and CSF were measured at frequent intervals following acutely and chronically treated monkeys.

RESULTS

Cocaine-Induced Behavior in the Rat

Repetitive administration of cocaine (10 mg/kg i.p.) resulted in increasing amounts of horizontal and vertical hyperactivity and stereotypy scores. As illustrated in Table 1 for vertical activity, after the first cocaine injections, rats demonstrated moderate amounts of activity and little stereotypy; however, with repetition, the same dose of cocaine produced marked hyperactivity and marked stereotypy. With chronic cocaine administration, there was both an increase in the amount and duration of activity. On day 1 both horizontal and vertical hyperactivity returned to normal by the end of the 90 minute testing interval, while on day 20 activity was still near its peak at this time.

Conditioning phenomena as suggested by Tilson and Rech (1973) do not appear to account for the progressive increases in hyperactivity and stereotypy. Animals pretreated with repetitive cocaine

TABLE 1

INCREASING EFFECT OF REPETITIVE COCAINE INJECTIONS ON VERTICAL ACTIVITY IN THE RAT

INJECTION #	SALINE, N = 8	COCAINE (10 mg/kg), N = 8
1	17 ± 7	33 ± 15
5	8 ± 3	56 ± 12
10	20 ± 8	164 ± 20
15	42 ± 16	207 ± 22
CONTROL SALINE INJECTION (25)	60 ± 16	78 ± 10
28	50 ± 13	261 ± 30

Values = Activity counts/minutes ± SEM

Increasing effect of cocaine; significant by two-way analysis of variance for repeated measures, $p < 0.001$

Difference between control injection (#25) in chronic cocaine animals and saline controls not significant

administration received saline injections on days 25 and 29; these eight experimental animals showed hyperactivity and stereotypy levels comparable to those seen in the eight saline control animals (Table 1).

With results similar to those of Downs and Eddy (1932), a subgroup of rats treated with repetitive high dose cocaine (60 mg/kg) appeared to become increasingly susceptible to cocaine-induced convulsions and lethality. Six of eight animals eventually died in convulsions, while two animals survived for an average of 80 injections. The six rats received an average of 20 cocaine injections prior to their first seizure (20 ± 7) and an average of 21 injections before they died during a convulsion. (As noted by others [Eidelberg et al., 1963], different groups of rats, similar in strain, sex, weight, and environmental housing, show differences in convulsive threshold; and many other animals receiving lower doses of cocaine [40-50 mg] died in convulsions on the first dose.) As rats were chronically treated with high-dose cocaine, behavior changed such that they increasingly manifested repetitive sniffing and stereotypic head nodding patterns in one corner of their cage.

Effects of Repetitive Lidocaine Administration

In contrast to animals receiving cocaine, lidocaine treated rats demonstrated ataxia and sedation rather than hyperactivity and stereotypy. Following this phase animals engaged in a variety of abnormal eating patterns and eventually began to demonstrate lidocaine-induced convulsions. Figure 1, as previously reported (Post et al., 1975), illustrates that animals manifest an increasing frequency of convulsions with repetitive lidocaine administration. Animals received an average of 16 injections of lidocaine (60 mg/kg) prior to their first convulsion. The second convulsion occurred after an average of only two further lidocaine injections and subsequent convulsions occurred with increasing frequency and regularity. The duration of seizures also showed a progressive increase with chronic administration. Initially, lidocaine-induced seizures lasted for one minute or less, but increased to as long as 45 minutes in intermittent episodes with chronicity. The seizures likewise began to occur earlier after a lidocaine injection, 1-2 minutes instead of 10-15 minutes initially required.

The pattern of seizures was highly similar to that demonstrated by Goddard et al., (1969) and Wada and Sata (1974) following electrically-kindled seizures. While animals initially had seizures with rearing and falling, with chronicity they began to demonstrate an increased pattern of intermittent, clonic convulsive movements limited to the head, trunk, and forepaws while maintaining a sitting posture on their haunches.

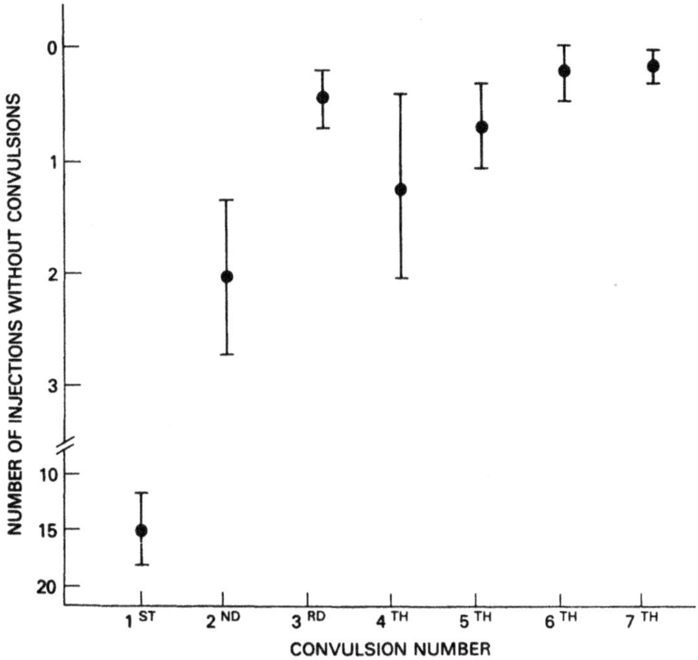

Fig. 1. Progressive increase in frequency of lidocaine convulsions in 13 rats.

Animals maintained on chronic lidocaine administration also demonstrated increasing amounts of coprophagia with chronicity (Fig. 2). This occurred after the sedative-ataxic phase or after the animals ceased convulsing. Individual animals that initially showed no coprophagic activity eventually demonstrated this behavior with increasing consistency following repetitive lidocaine administration. Experimental animals also ate more straw and gauze than saline controls.

Effects of Chronic Cocaine Administration in Rhesus Monkeys

Rhesus monkeys treated with once or twice daily intraperitoneal injections of the same dose of cocaine demonstrated increases in a variety of behaviors and neurological sequelae over a 20 week period (Post et al., in press). In eight of 13 animals prominent hyperactivity and stereotypies were observed during the first 4 to 6 weeks of cocaine administration (Fig. 3). These consisted of repetitive movements of limbs, trunk, head, and especially repetitive gnawing on

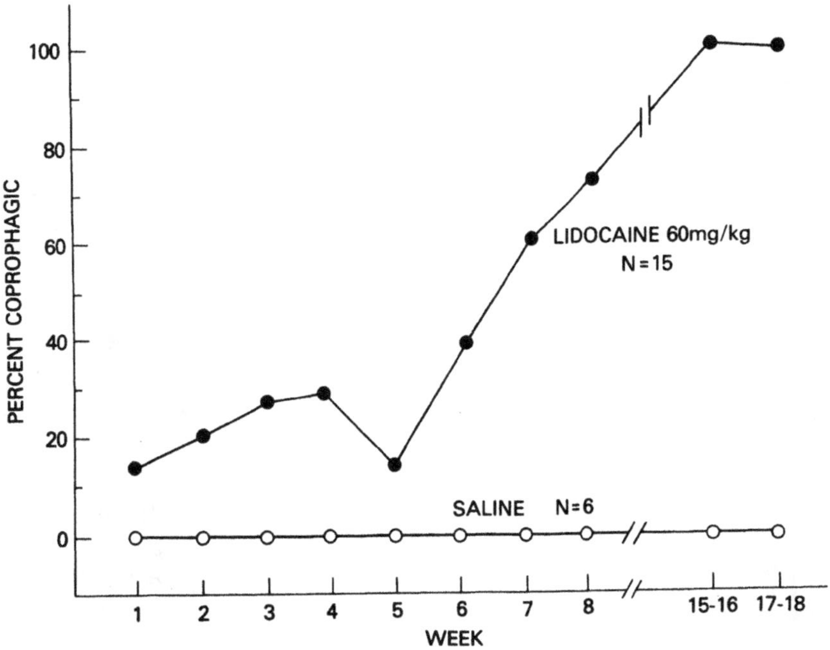

Fig. 2. Time course of lidocaine-induced coprophagia in the rat.

water bottles. As this behavior decreased during the second month of cocaine administration, prominent inhibitory behaviors emerged with increasing intensity. Monkeys remained essentially immobilized following an injection. They also became increasingly cataleptic, maintaining an abnormal posture set by the experimenters for several minutes but in some cases for periods up to one hour. Occasionally animals would maintain a posture that would involve holding a limb against gravity for prolonged periods of time. As part of this inhibitory syndrome, animals not only stared blankly at objects for prolonged periods but also engaged in visual tracking of apparently nonexistent objects about the laboratory. This appeared to be hallucinatory behavior as, in several instances, animals reached out, apparently to grab at these imaginary objects. Five monkeys did not demonstrate prominent stereotypies during the first weeks of cocaine administration and, from the onset, showed increasing severity of inhibitory behaviors.

Four of 13 animals studied developed prominent oral-buccal-lingual dyskinesias after approximately two months of chronic cocaine

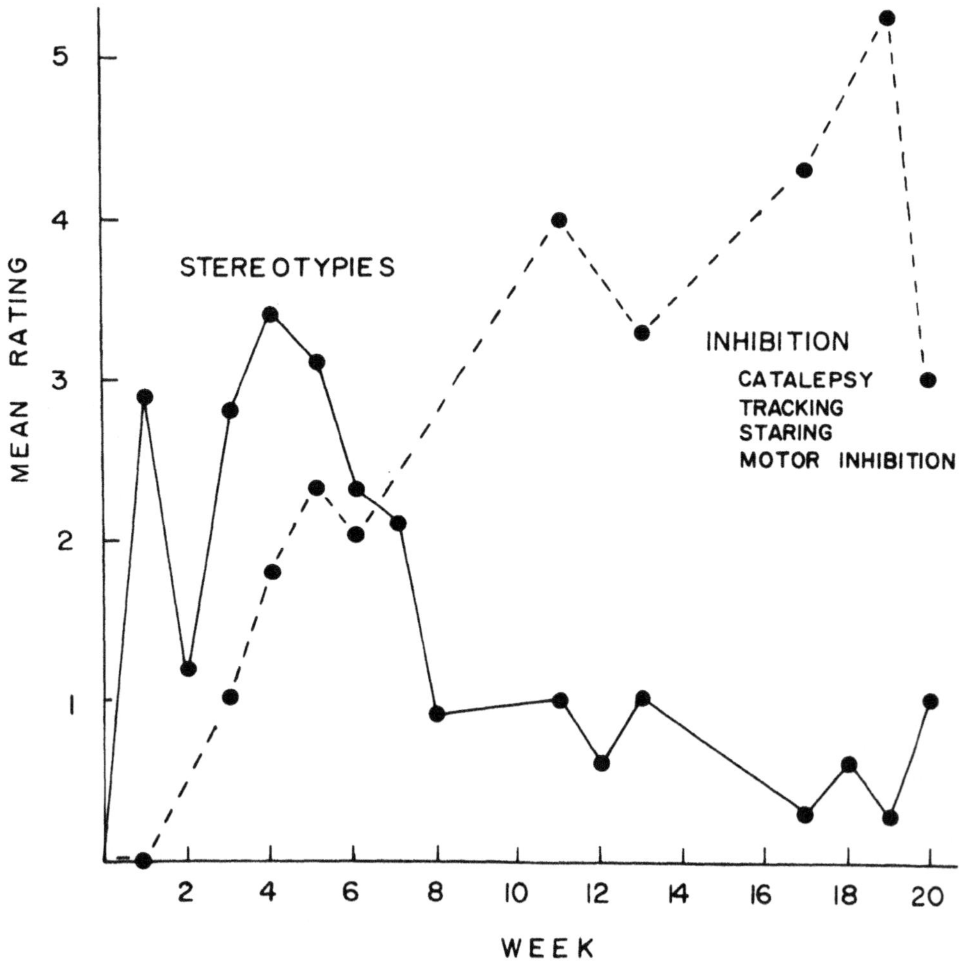

Fig. 3. Progressive development of inhibitory behavior in initially stereotypic monkeys, N = 8.

TABLE 2

COCAINE-INDUCED CHANGES IN ACID AMINE METABOLITES IN CISTERNAL CSF OF RHESUS MONKEYS

BASELINE LEVELS			
	PLACEBO (8)	ACUTE COCAINE (7)	CHRONIC COCAINE (5)
HVA	178 ± 17	289 ± 27***	265 ± 17***
5HIAA	77 ± 5	95 ± 9	79 ± 10

PROBENECID-INDUCED ACCUMULATIONS			
	PLACEBO (12)	ACUTE COCAINE (12)	CHRONIC COCAINE (9)
HVA	598 ± 50	811 ± 128*	897 ± 158*
5HIAA	184 ± 22	258 ± 24**	267 ± 37*

Data from Post et al., in press.

Values = means in mg/ml ± SEM; N in parentheses.

*p < 0.01, **p < 0.05, ***p < 0.01, paired T-test, two tailed

administration. These manifest increasing severity through the 20 weeks of study.

Figure 4 demonstrates the increasing susceptibility to cocaine-induced convulsions with chronic cocaine administration. The figure illustrates that the mean duration between convulsions decreased (ordinate) as the number of convulsions increased (abscissa). In contrast to other parameters, cocaine-induced "checking" behavior (rapid shifts in visual fields) and anorexia remained relatively stable over the course of five months. At peak cocaine effect, animals refused routine food, apples, or raisins even during chronic injections.

Baseline levels of the dopamine metabolite, HVA, increased following both acute and chronic cocaine injections (Table 2). A similar borderline statistically significant trend was observed for probenecid-induced increases in HVA, suggesting that both acute and chronic cocaine administration may be associated with increased turnover of dopamine. While accumulations of 5HIAA also increased, MHPG decreased non-significantly in five of six animals.

DISCUSSION

These data suggest that both low and high dose, repetitive cocaine administration may be associated with increasing effects on a variety of behaviors and neurological sequelae. Low doses of cocaine (10 mg/kg) in the rat are associated with progressive increases in horizontal and vertical hyperactivity and stereotypy. Higher doses appear to be associated with an increased frequency of seizures in some animals and eventually death as in the work of Downs and Eddy (1932). Repetitive administration of a given dose of cocaine to rhesus monkeys (10-17 mg/kg i.p.) is also associated with increasingly progressive effects on behavior: in this instance, the development of prominent motor inhibition, catalepsy, staring, and visual tracking behavior. After the initial weeks of cocaine administration, during which there was a non-significant trend for cocaine-induced hyperactivity and stereotypy to increase, bizarre inhibitory behaviors began to predominate. Temporally associated with the decrease in hyperactivity and stereotypy was the onset of oral-lingual-buccal dyskinesias. The monkeys also became increasingly susceptible to cocaine-induced convulsions. Thus, repetitive administration of cocaine to both rats and rhesus monkeys on a once or twice daily basis, five times a week, appears to be associated with reverse tolerance in many parameters rather than the more typically reported findings that chronic stimulant administration is associated with a development of tolerance.

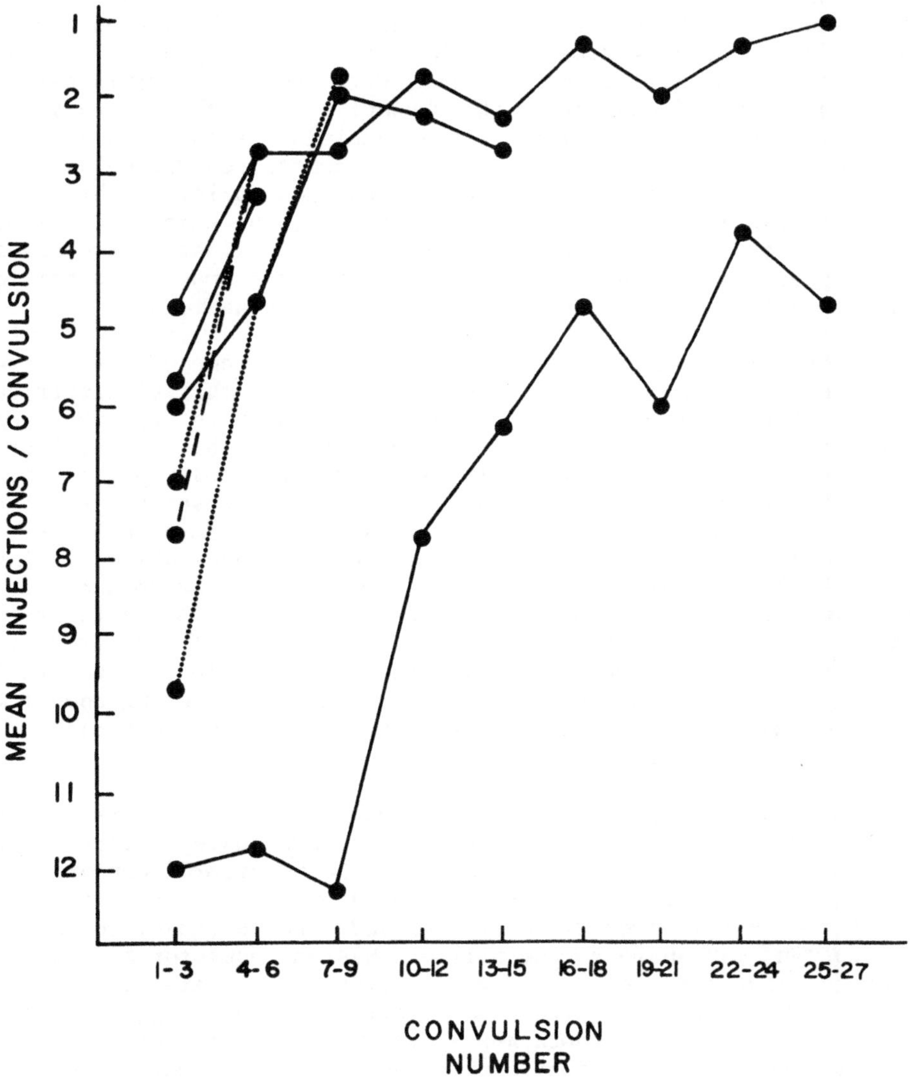

Fig. 4. Increasing susceptibility to convulsions during chronic cocaine administration in rhesus monkeys.

These data in the rat are highly similar to those reported by Klawans and Margolin (1975) and Segal and Mandell (1974) with repetitive amphetamine administration. Similarly, Ellinwood et al. (1972) and Ellinwood and Kilbey (1975) have reported the development of an amphetamine-induced syndrome with chronic, increasing doses of amphetamine very much like that observed with repetitive administration of the same dose of cocaine in the present study. These data might lead to the suggestion that repetitive administration of cocaine- or amphetamine-like stimulants in some circumstances may be associated with reverse tolerance manifestations on a variety of bizarre behaviors, dyskinesias, and seizures; however, the effects of lidocaine on abnormal eating patterns and seizures suggest that classes of compounds other than the psychomotor stimulants may be associated with progressive effects on seizures and other behaviors.

A potentially unifying mechanism to explain some of the progressive phenomena might involve a process similar to that of electrical kindling of the nervous system which could occur with repetitive drug administration (pharmacological kindling) (Post et al., 1975; Post, Kopanda, 1975). Particularly with lidocaine, not only is the time course of development of seizures similar to that observed with electrical kindling but also the quality of seizures themselves (i.e., clonic intermittent convulsions of trunk and forepaws while sitting on haunches) (Post et al., 1975). Moreover, both cocaine and lidocaine, in high doses, produce prominent alterations in limbic system spindles, afterdischarges, and seizure activity (Eidelberg et al., 1963; Wagman et al., 1968; Riblet, Tuttle, 1970). Thus, repetitive stimulant or local anesthetic administration may be acting upon limbic system mechanisms capable of reacting with increased effects to repetitive stimulation.

One might speculate that while a number of drugs and treatments are capable of progressively increasing seizure susceptibility, perhaps by some common mechanism (Table 3), the behavioral concomitants might vary according to the neuroanatomical loci and neurotransmitter systems predominantly involved. For example, cocaine and lidocaine may share a common limbic system focus for electrical discharges, but cocaine's psychomotor stimulant effects mediated by catecholamines are associated with a very different progressive behavioral syndrome than lidocaine, a drug without major effects on catecholamine systems. Thus, cocaine administration may be associated with increases in catecholamine related excitatory-stereotypic behavior as well as later development of bizarre, hallucinatory-like, and catatonic-like behavior. The non-stimulant, lidocaine, on the other hand, is associated with increases in other behaviors, such as omniphagia and coprophagia. It is noteworthy that Arieti (1974) reports that the most chronic, end-stage schizophrenic patients also engage in omniphagia and coprophagia. This behavior is also reminiscent of one component of the Kluver-Bucy (1937) syndrome produced by bilateral temporal-hippocampal lesions.

TABLE 3

SELECTIVE REVIEW OF TREATMENTS ASSOCIATED WITH PROGRESSIVE EFFECTS ON BEHAVIOR OR SEIZURES IN SOME CIRCUMSTANCES

DRUG	ANIMAL	EFFECT	
Cocaine	Rat	Hyperactivity, Stereotypy Seizures	Downs and Eddy (1932) Post and Rose, unpub. data
	Dog	Hyperthermia	Zapata-Ortiz (1944)
		Catalepsy,	Guiterrez-Noriega (1950)
		Seizures	Tatum and Seevers (1929)
	Monkey	Catalepsy, Bizarre visual behavior, Dyskinesias, Seizures	Post and Kopanda (in press)
Lidocaine	Rat	Coprophagia, Seizures	Post et al. (1975)
Amphetamine	Rat	Hyperactivity, Stereotypy,	Segal and Mandell (1974)
		Disruption of learning	Ranje and Ungerstedt (1974)
	Guinea Pig	Stereotypy, Dyskinesias	Klawans and Margolin (1975)
	Monkey	Stereotypy,	Ellinwood et al. (1972)
		Dyskinesias	Ellinwood and Kilbey (1975)
	Man	Reactivation of psychosis,	Kramer (1972)
		Increased mood effects	Griffith, personal communition (1975)
Apomorphine (following chronic amphetamine)	Rat	Stereotypy	Klawans and Margolin (1975)
Flurothyl ether	Rat Mice, Guinea Pig	Seizures	Prichard et al. (1969)
Metrazol	Rat	Seizures	Pinel and Van Oot (in press) Mason and Cooper (1972)
Carbacol (intracerebral)	Rat	Seizures	Vosu and Wise (1975)
Electroshock	Rat	Seizures	Pinel and Van Oot (in press) Modigh (1975)

TABLE 3 (continued)

DRUG	ANIMAL	EFFECT	
Audiogenic stimulation	Mice	Seizures	Leech (1971)
Intracranial electrical stimulation (kindling)	Rat Cat Monkey	Seizures	Goddard et al. (1969) Racine (1972) Wada and Sata (1974) Pinel and Van Oot (in press)

Table 3 summarizes the variety of treatments that have been associated with increasing frequency of convulsions upon repetitive application. It should be emphasized that most treatments have been given on a daily basis; intermittant rather than continuous stimulation, as in electrical kindling, may be critical to the reverse tolerance effects. The variety of stimuli administered repetitively which produce this effect suggest that the central nervous system may have a basic capability for synaptic reorganization or neuroplasticity in response to repetitive stimulation. We have suggested elsewhere (Post, Kopanda, in press) that a kindling-like mechanism might also be activated by psychological stresses and be important in the development of a variety of psychopathological behaviors in man by this process. Lesse et al. (1955) have reported the production of limbic spindle activity occurring upon recollection of stressful experience. Clearly, speculation regarding a kindling mechanism requires careful documentation, but may be heuristically valuable in conceptualizing potential mechanisms to integrate the effects of repetitive neurophysiological, biochemical, or psychological stimulation on the central nervous system.

Mechanisms other than kindling to account for the progressive effects also need to be carefully explored and in some cases ruled out. Our preliminary evidence studied in collaboration with Richard Hawks (unpublished data) suggests that alterations in the blood or CSF level of cocaine with chronic administration are not sufficient to account for the progressive effects on behavior or seizures. Cocaine levels in CSF (Fig. 5) and blood reach approximately similar peaks and have similar half-lives during both initial and chronic cocaine injections. These data are consistent with those of Nayak et al. (1976), suggesting that peak plasma or brain levels of cocaine in rats are not substantially different after one or 21 days of cocaine administration. Conditioning phenomena also do not appear to be an adequate explanation of the phenomena. When either rats or monkeys that have been chronically pretreated with cocaine are given intermittent injections of saline, the typical cocaine syndromes are either minimally manifest or nonexistent. These data are consistent with those of Segal and Mandell (1974), suggesting that, while conditioning effects may be important under some experimental paradigms (Tilson, Rech, 1973), they do not provide sufficient explanation for the progressive phenomena.

Klawans and Margolin (1975) have suggested that repetitive amphetamine administration may be associated with receptor supersensitivity since animals so pretreated are more susceptible than controls to the effects of a dopamine receptor stimulating agent such as apomorphine. Ellinwood and collaborators (Ellinwood, Escalante, 1970; Escalante, Ellinwood, 1970) have also documented neurochromatolysis with repetitive stimulant administration. Thus, receptor supersensitivity, either on an innervation or denervation basis, should be considered as a potential explanation for the progressive effects on behavior and seizures. Moreover, Roth and co-workers (1975) have recently suggested that both increases and decreases in impulse flow in dopaminergic neurons may be associated with increases in tyrosine hydroxylase activity. Such increases in presynaptic enzymes' synthetic mechanisms could potentially mediate some of the progressive effects of behavior, although the elevated HVA levels and accumulations following probenecid in our study were not significantly higher during chronic as compared to acute cocaine administration. Another potential mechanism could involve the prolonged development of the slow excitatory post-synaptic potential which has been demonstrated upon administration of dopamine (Libet, Tosaka, 1970). A variety of other biochemical mechanisms, including alterations in the balance or activation of two kinds of dopamine receptor mechanisms (Cools, Hendriks, Korten, 1975; Costall, Naylor, 1975) with chronic administration as well as alterations in the agonist-antagonist dopamine receptor conformation (Creese, Burt, Snyder, 1975) may be postulated. Recently Groves, Wilson, Young, and Rebec (1975) suggested that a positive nigra-neostriatal feedback loop and self-inhibition by dopaminergic neurons could be involved in the increasing responses to chronic amphetamine intoxication. Although the progressive increases in the variety of pharmacological effects discussed here may be mediated by several different mechanisms, it is noteworthy that many of the suggested biochemical mechanisms are not inconsistent with a kindling-like process.

Since chronic administration of the psychomotor stimulants in man is associated with a paranoid psychosis resembling paranoid schizophrenia, mechanisms potentially involved in the mediation of these progressive behavioral changes take on an added import. Exploration and elucidation of the behavioral, biochemical, and neurophysiological parameters associated with chronic cocaine administration in animals and man may yield important clues to the understanding of alterations in the reactivity and sensitivity of the central nervous system to a variety of stimuli and, ultimately, to a better understanding of the functional psychoses.

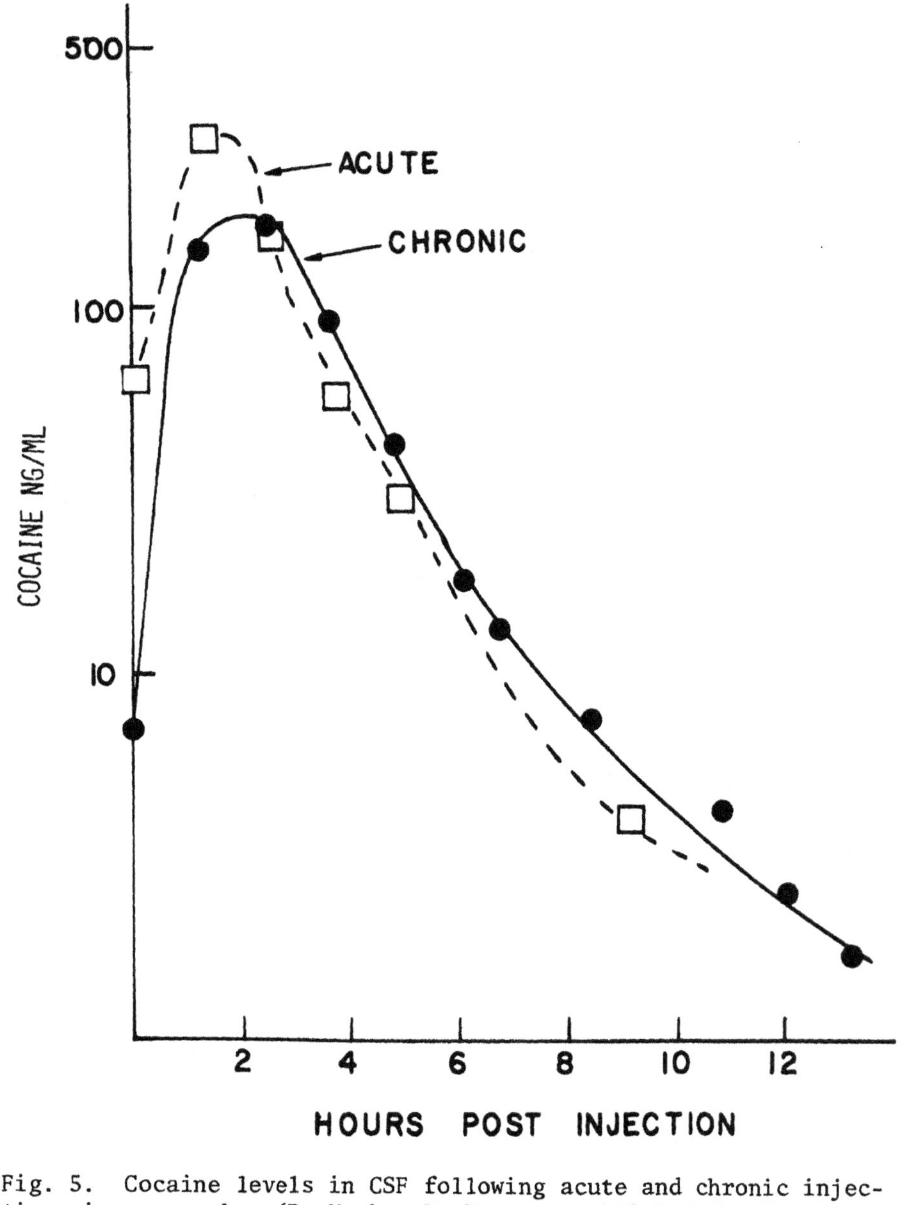

Fig. 5. Cocaine levels in CSF following acute and chronic injections in one monkey (R. Hawks, R. Post, unpublished data).

REFERENCES

Änggard, E., Jonsson, L.E., Hogmark, A.L. and Gunne, L.M.: Amphetamine metabolism in amphetamine psychosis, Clin. Pharmacol. Therap. 14, 870-880 (1973).

Angrist, B. and Gershon, S.: The phenomenology of experientially induced amphetamine psychosis: Preliminary observations, Biol. Psychiat. 2, 95-107 (1970).

Arieti, S.: Interpretation of Schizophrenia. Pp. 423-433. New York: Basic Books, 1974.

Connell, P.H.: Amphetamine Psychosis. New York: Oxford University Press, 1958.

Cools, A.R., Hendriks, G., and Korten, J.: The acetylcholine-dopamine balance in the basal ganglia of rhesus monkeys and its role in dynamic, dystonic, dyskinetic, and epileptoid motor activities, J. Neural Trans. 36, 91 (1975).

Costall, B. and Naylor, R.: Neuroleptic antagonism of dyskinetic phenomena, Eur. J. Pharmacol. 33, 301-312 (1975).

Creese, I., Burt, D.R., and Snyder, S.H.: Dopamine receptor binding: Differentiation of agonist and antagonist states with ^{3}H-dopamine and ^{3}H-Haloperidol, Life Sci. 17, 993-1002 (1975).

Downs, A.W. and Eddy, N.B.: The effect of repeated doses of cocaine on the rat, J. Pharmac. exp. Ther. 46, 199-200 (1932).

Eidelberg, E., Lesse, H., and Gault, F.P.: Experimental model of temporal lobe epilepsy: Studies of convulsant properties of cocaine. In: EEG and Behavior. Glaser, G.H., Ed., pp. 272-283. New York: Basic Books, 1963.

Ellinwood, E.H.: Amphetamine psychosis: Individuals, settings, and sequences. In: Current Concepts on Amphetamine Abuse. Ellinwood, E.H. and Cohen, S., Eds., pp. 143-157. Washington: U.S. Government Printing Office, 1972.

Ellinwood, E.H. and Escalante, O.: Chronic amphetamine effect on the olfactory forebrain, Biol. Psychiat. 2, 189-203 (1970).

Ellinwood, E.H. and Kilbey, M.M.: Amphetamine stereotypy: The influence of environmental factors and prepotent behavioral patterns on its topography and development, Biol. Psychiat. 10, 3-16 (1975).

Ellinwood, E.H., Sudilovsky, A., and Nelson, L.: Behavioral analysis of amphetamine intoxication, Biol. Psychiat. 3, 215-230 (1972).

Escalante, O.D. and Ellinwood, E.H.: CNS cytopathological changes in cats with chronic methedrine intoxication, Brain Res. 21, 151-155 (1970).

Feinberg, G. and Irwin, S.: Effects of chronic methamphetamine administration in the cat, Fed. Proc. 20, 396 (1961).

Goddard, G.V., McIntyre, D.C., and Leech, C.K.: A permanent change in brain function resulting from daily electrical stimulation, Exp. Neurol. 25, 295-330 (1969).

Griffith, J.D., Cavanaugh, J.H., Held, J., and Oates, J.A.: Experimental psychosis induced by the administration of d-amphetamine. In: Amphetamines and Related Compounds. Costa, E. and Garattini, S., Eds., pp. 897-904. New York: Raven Press, 1970.

Groves, P.M., Wilson, C.J., Young, S.T., and Rebec, G.V.: Self-inhibition of dopaminergic neurons, Science 190, 522-529 (1975).

Gutierrez-Noriega, C.: Inhibition of central nervous systems produced by chronic cocaine intoxication, Fed. Proc. 9, 280 (1950).

Klawans, H.L. and Margolin, D.I.: Amphetamine-induced dopaminergic sensitivity in guinea pigs, Arch. gen. Psychiat. 32, 725-732 (1975).

Kluver, H. and Bucy, P.C.: Psychic blindness and other symptoms following bilateral temporal lobectomy in rhesus monkeys, Am. J. Physiol. 119, 352-353 (1937).

Kramer, J.C.: Introduction to amphetamine abuse. In: Current Concepts on Amphetamine Abuse. Ellinwood, E.H. and Cohen, S., Eds., pp. 177-184. Washington: U.S. Government Printing Office, 1972.

Leech, C.K.: Sound-induced kindling resulting from daily bursts of loud noise presented to seven strains of mouse. Paper presented at Canadian Psychological Association Meeting, St. John's, Newfoundland, June 3, 1971.

Lesse, H., Heath, R.G., Mickle, W.A., Munroe, R.R., and Miller, W.H.: Rhinencephalic activity during thought, J. nerv. ment. Dis. 122, 433-440 (1955).

Libet, B. and Tosaka, T.: Dopamine as a synaptic transmitter and modulator in sympathetic ganglia: A different mode of synaptic action, Proc. natn. Acad. Sci. U.S.A. 67, 667-673 (1970).

Mason, C.R. and Cooper, R.M.: A permanent change in convulsive threshold in normal and brain damaged rats with small repeated doses of pentylenetetrazol, Epilepsia 13, 663-674 (1972).

Modigh, K.: Electroconvulsant shock and postsynaptic catecholamine effects: Increased psychomotor stimulant action of apomorphine and clonidine in reserpine pretreated mice by repeated FCS, J. Neural Trans. 36, 19-32 (1975).

Nayak, P.K., Misra, A.L., and Mulé, S.: Physiological disposition and biotransformation of (^{3}H) cocaine in acutely- and chronically-treated rats, J. Pharmac. exp. Ther. 196, 556-569 (1976).

Pinel, J.P.J. and Van Oot, P.H.: Generality of the kindling phenomenon: Some clinical implications, Can. J. Neurosci., in press.

Post, R.M.: Cocaine psychoses: A continuum model, Am. J. Psychiat. 132, 225-231 (1975).

Post, R.M. and Kopanda, R.T.: Cocaine, kindling, and reverse tolerance, Lancet i, 409-410 (1975).

Post, R.M. and Kopanda, R.T.: Cocaine, kindling, and psychosis, Am. J. Psychiat., in press.

Post, R.M., Kotin, J., and Goodwin, F.K.: The effects of cocaine on depressed patients, Am. J. Psychiat. 131, 511-517 (1974).

Post, R.M., Kopanda, R.T., and Lee, A.: Progressive development of coprophagia and seizures during chronic lidocaine administration: Relationship to kindling and psychosis, Life Sci. 17, 943-950 (1975).

Post, R.M., Kopanda, R.T., and Black, K.E.: Progressive effects of cocaine on behavior and central amine metabolism in rhesus monkeys, Biol. Psychiat., in press.

Prichard, J.W., Gallagher, B.B., and Glaser, G.H.: Experimental seizure-threshold testing with flurothyl, J. Pharmac. exp. Ther. 166, 170-178 (1969).

Racine, R.J.: Modification of seizure activity by electrical stimulation. II. Motor seizure, Electroenceph. clin. Neurophysiol. 32, 281-294 (1972).

Ranje, C. and Ungerstedt, U.: Chronic amphetamine treatment: Vast individual differences in performing a learned response, Eur. J. Pharmacol. 29, 307-311 (1974).

Resnick, R.B., Schwartz, L.K., Kestenbaum, R.S., and Freedman, A.M.: Cocaine dose-response curves in man. Paper presented at the Annual Meeting of the Society of Biological Psychiatry, New York, 1975.

Riblet, L.A. and Tuttle, W.W.: Investigation of the amygdaloid and olfactory electrographic response in the cat after toxic dosage of lidocaine, Electroenceph. clin. Neurophysiol. 28, 601-608 (1970).

Roth, P.H., Walters, J.R., Murrin, L.C., and Morgenroth, V.H.: Dopamine neurons: Role of impulse flow and presynaptic receptors in the regulation of tyrosine hydroxylase. In: Pre- and Post-Synaptic Receptors. Usdin, E., and Bunney, W.E., Eds., pp. 5-48. New York: Marcel Dekker, 1975.

Segal, D.S. and Mandell, A.J.: Long-term administration of d-amphetamine: Progressive augmentation of motor activity and stereotypy, Pharmac. Biochem. Behav. 2, 249-255 (1974).

Snyder, S.H.: Amphetamine psychosis: A "model" schizophrenia mediated by catecholamines, Am. J. Psychiat. 130, 61-67 (1973).

Tatum, A.L. and Seevers, M.H.: Experimental cocaine addiction, J. Pharmac. exp. Ther. 36, 401-410 (1929).

Tilson, H.A. and Rech, R.H.: Conditioned drug effects and absence of tolerance to d-amphetamine-induced motor activity, Pharmac. Biochem. Behav. 1, 149-153 (1973).

Vosu, H. and Wise, R.A.: Cholinergic seizure kindling in the rat: Comparison of caudate, amygdala, and hippocampal, Behav. Biol. 13, 491-495 (1975).

Wada, J.A. and Sata, M.S.: Generalized convulsive seizures induced by daily electrical stimulation of the amygdala in cats, Neurology, Minneap. 24, 565-574 (1974).

Wagman, I.H., DeJong, R.H., and Prince, D.A.: Effects of lidocaine on spontaneous cortical and subcortical electrical activity, Arch. Neurol. 18, 277-290 (1968).

Zapata-Ortiz, V.: Modificaciones psicológicas y fisiológicas producidas par la coca y la cocaína en los coqueros, Revta. Med. exp. 3, 132-161 (1944).

COCAINE: DISCUSSION ON THE ROLE OF DOPAMINE IN THE BIOCHEMICAL MECHANISM OF ACTION

Jorgen Scheel-Krüger, Claus Braestrup, Mogens Nielson,

Krystyna Golembiowska,* and Ewa Mogilnicka*

Psychopharmacological Research Laboratory, Sct. Hans

Hospital, Department E, Roskilde, Denmark

*Polish Academy of Sciences, Department of Pharmacology,

Krakow, Poland

INTRODUCTION

The central stimulant effect of cocaine is generally considered related to its potentiating effect on biogenic amines. However, the individual role and significance of the amines involved in various stimulant effects of cocaine are still a controversial topic. Cocaine is a potent inhibitor of noradrenaline uptake (Hertting, Axelrod, and Whitby, 1961; Ross and Renyi, 1967; Langer and Enero, 1974; Azzaro, Ziance, and Rutledge, 1974), dopamine uptake (Fuxe, Hamberger, and Malmfors, 1967; Ross and Renyi, 1967; Harris and Baldessarini, 1973; Heikkila, Orlansky, Mytilineou, and Cohen, 1975), and serotonin uptake (Ross and Renyi, 1969; Friedman, Gershon, and Rotrosen, 1975). High affinity uptake of tryptophan into synaptosomes is also inhibited (Knapp and Mandell, 1972). *In vivo* studies have shown that cocaine induces a short-lasting uptake inhibition into brain tissues of noradrenaline (Schanberg and Cook, 1972), dopamine (Fuxe, Hamberger, and Malmfors, 1967), and serotonin (Ross and Renyi, 1969).

Ross and Renyi (1969) considered cocaine as a more potent inhibitor of serotonin than of dopamine and noradrenaline uptake. Furthermore, cocaine inhibits uptake in dopamine and noradrenaline nerve terminals at approximately the same concentrations (Hamberger, 1967; Ross and Renyi, 1967; 1969). The effect of cocaine on brain dopamine might be responsible for the differences in several behavioral experiments between cocaine and tricyclic antidepressant drugs of the imipramine type, since the latter drugs in general are considered as appreciably less potent on the dopamine uptake mechanism than cocaine (Ross and Renyi, 1967; Hamberger, 1967).

The association of brain dopamine to some cocaine behavioral effects has previously been hypothesized in studies on motility in mice and rats (van Rossum and Hurkmans, 1964), since cocaine induces an amphetamine-like stereotyped locomotor and/or head bobbing response in the cat (Wallach and Gershon, 1972) and the dog (Willner, Samach, Angrist, Wallach, and Gershon, 1970). However, Christie and Crow (1971) found, as a difference from amphetamine, that cocaine *per se* did not induce turning in rats with a unilateral lesion of the dopamine nigro-neostriatal pathway but only following pretreatment with a monoamine oxidase inhibitor (nialamide).

Some differences between amphetamine and cocaine have also been found in the chicken (Wallach, Friedman, and Gershon, 1972; Schrold, 1972; Schrold, personal communication) in which cocaine showed several similarities to the tricyclic antidepressant drugs. Rats pretreated with cocaine show two phases of excitation following the injection of Ro 4-1284, a reserpine analogue. The first excitatory phase is a typical amphetamine-like excitation; the second phase excitation is a typical desipramine-like stimulation (Matussek and Rüther, 1965; Scheel-Krüger and Jonas, 1973). Cocaine exhibits several similarities to amphetamine in studies on self-administration (Schuster and Wilson, 1972; Pickens, Thompson, and Yokel, 1972), conditioned behavior (Goldberg, 1973; MacPhail and Seiden, 1975), and drug discriminative studies (Winter, 1975). Similarities on EEG effects also have been found (Wallach and Gershon, 1971). In humans, amphetamine can produce psychoses, often indistinguishable from certain forms of schizophrenia, especially the paranoid form (Matthysse, 1973; Randrup, Munkvad, and Scheel-Krüger, 1973; Randrup, Munkvad, Fog, and Ayhan, 1975; Snyder, 1972). Similarly, the chronic misuse of cocaine may also induce psychoses with several similarities to schizophrenia. For discussion and extensive review see Post (1975).

In the present study on cocaine we focused our experiments on some points which have not been made clear by the available literature; i.e., detailed information of cocaine on stereotyped behavior in the rat in comparison with the effect of the stimulant amphetamines; the effect of drugs affecting dopamine, noradrenaline, serotonin, and acetylcholine mechanisms on cocaine stimulation; the role of different intraneuronal catecholamine pools; and, finally, the role of catecholamine release versus re-uptake inhibition in cocaine stimulation.

METHODS

Stereotyped Behavior

Male Wistar rats weighing 200-300 g were used in all experiments in the present communication. The behavioral excitatory effect after stimulant amphetamines is, in our laboratory, considered to be stereotyped if the behavioral repertoire is strongly restricted in variation and consists of continuous repetition of one or few items of behavior. Varied normal behavior, such as eating, drinking, grooming, social behavior, etc., is absent.

The stereotyped sniffing after amphetamine or apomorphine is characteristically shown as a persistent, continuous sniffing that only covers a small area of the cage, usually of either the lower part of the wall or of the floor. During this stereotyped sniffing, the nose of the rat touches the wire nettings of the cage. Following higher doses of amphetamine/apomorphine, the concomitant appearance of continuous licking of the cage wire is seen and, following still higher doses, in addition, biting and gnawing activities are seen.

Cocaine and Stereotypy

A major conclusion of the present study is that, although the behavioral elements of amphetamine/apomorphine-induced stereotypy, sniffing, licking, and biting, can be induced by cocaine, these elements never attained the characteristically compulsive, continuous, and restrictive stereotyped performance. We, therefore, decided to use extensive descriptions of the cocaine-behavioral effects instead of attempting to use arbitrary rating scales previously used for several amphetamine analogues (Scheel-Krüger, 1971, 1972).

In studies on "stereotypy" after cocaine, the rats were kept in individual wire netting cages for at least 3 to 4 days and preferably for one week before the experiments. This adaption period was most important to facilitate the appearance of "stereotypic periods" after cocaine administration. The stereotyped behaviors after apomorphine, amphetamine, and various dopaminergic drugs have also been found to develop more strongly and more reproducibly in familiar home cages (Mogilnicka and Scheel-Krüger, unpublished data), and a similar finding has been reported by Sahakian and Robbins (1975) on amphetamine stereotypy in guinea pigs.

Biochemical Analyses

The dopamine metabolites, homovanillic acid (HVA) and 3,4-dihydroxyphenylacetic acid (DOPAC), were assayed in one half of a whole rat brain according to a gaschromatographic procedure (Andersen, Braestrup, and Randrup, 1975; Braestrup, Andersen, and Randrup, 1975) The major noradrenaline metabolites, free plus conjugated 3-methoxy-4-hydroxyphenylglycol (MOPEG) and 3,4-dihydroxyphenylglycol (DOPEG), were also estimated by gaschromatographic methods (Braestrup, 1973; Nielsen and Braestrup, personal communication). ^{3}H-noradrenaline and free plus conjugated ^{3}H-MOPEG and ^{3}H-DOPEG formed after intraventricularly injected ^{3}H-tyrosine were estimated according to Nielsen (1975; personal communication). In all our biochemical experiments, vehicle-treated control rats were analyzed in parallel to drug-treated animals, and values in the tables are expressed as the drug-treated group in per cent of the control group.

RESULTS

Cocaine-Induced Motility

The locomotor stimulant effect of cocaine in doses of 10, 25, or 35 mg/kg i.p. was surprisingly weak and unpredictable when given to the rats housed singly in their familiar cages. The effects of cocaine were mainly an alerting reaction, increased rearing, and many up and down head movements (see later description of cocaine-induced "stereotypy"). Even a sudden noise or tactile stimulation only induced an abrupt, short-lasting but rapid locomotor stimulation. However, when the rats were placed in a novel environment, a large open-field cage, or in the photocell activity cages, they showed high and intense locomotor activity.

For motility studies we then used the rats directly from the big colony cages housing about 20 to 30 rats each. The rats were placed individually in the photocell cages. A period of only 30 min was used for adaption before the cocaine injection to reduce the non-drug dependent explorative behavior. The preliminary studies showed that 10 mg/kg intraperitoneal cocaine induced only weak motility whereas 25 and 35 mg/kg i.p. cocaine induced a remarkably high and pronounced motility which we never have seen in rats housed individually in familiar home cages.

Effect of Drugs on Cocaine-Induced Motility

The following experiments indicate that the cocaine-induced (35 mg/kg i.p.) locomotor activity depends on both noradrenaline and dopamine receptor activity. The noradrenaline antagonist phenoxybenzamine (20 mg/kg i.p., 3 hr before cocaine) or the dopamine antagonist pimozide (0.30 mg/kg s.c., 3 hr before cocaine) antagonized almost completely the cocaine-induced motility (Fig. 1). Pimozide, 0.15 mg/kg, (3 hr before cocaine) induced only partial antagonism of the motility.

Pimozide, 0.30 mg/kg, antagonized in addition the cocaine-induced "stereotypy"; i.e., head movements up and down ("head bobbing") and sniffing in the air. Pimozide (0.15 mg/kg) or phenoxybenzamine did not antagonize these behavioural activities. In later experiments on stereotypy in familiar cages, we found that phenoxybenzamine increased the cocaine-induced "stereotypy" (see later results). Cocaine-induced "stereotypy" was rather resistant to pimozide antagonism since the pretreatment with pimozide (0.15 mg/kg s.c., 3 hr) did not antagonize the head bobbing/sniffing in the air of a lower dose of cocaine, 25 mg/kg i.p. (5 rats tested).

Making a comparison to *d*-amphetamine, we found that cocaine, 35 mg/kg i.p., induced stronger intensity of the motility than 2.5 mg/kg s.c. *d*-amphetamine, HCl. The pretreatment of pimozide (0.15 mg/kg s.c., 3 hr) antagonized all signs of stimulation after *d*-amphetamine (Fig. 2). Phenoxybenzamine (10 and 20 mg/kg) also antagonizes almost completely the locomotor activity induced by *d*-amphetamine in doses of 1 to 2.5 mg/kg (Rolinski and Scheel-Krüger, 1973).

An experiment with α-methyltyrosine and reserpine showed that the cocaine-induced motility, in contrast to *d*-amphetamine, is not dependent on newly synthesized catecholamines but on catecholamines stored in a reserpine-sensitive pool. Cocaine resembles, thus, in this respect, the stimulant amphetamine analogues: methylphenidate, pipradrol, amfonelic acid (NCA), and nomifensine (Scheel-Krüger, 1971; Braestrup and Scheel-Krüger, unpublished data).

Cocaine, 35 mg/kg i.p., was found remarkably resistant to antagonism by α-methyltyrosine since the pretreatment with 250 mg/kg 1 hr or 5 hr before cocaine did not produce any antagonism in the time interval 0 to 60 min after cocaine (Fig. 3). The pretreatment with α-methyltyrosine (250 mg/kg, 5 hr), which decreases brain dopamine to 25 to 35% of the controls and noradrenaline to 40 to 50% of the controls, induced only an antagonism in the time interval 60 to 75 min after 35 mg/kg cocaine (Fig. 3). However, a more extensive catecholamine depletion induced by α-methyltyrosine (2 x 250 mg/kg given 22 and 4 hr, respectively, before cocaine) or reserpine (7.5 mg/kg s.c., 18 hr before cocaine) induced a strong antagonism of the 35 mg/kg cocaine-induced motility (Fig. 4).

It was remarkable, however, that the rats, even after extensive catecholamine depletion, were able to show locomotor stimulation

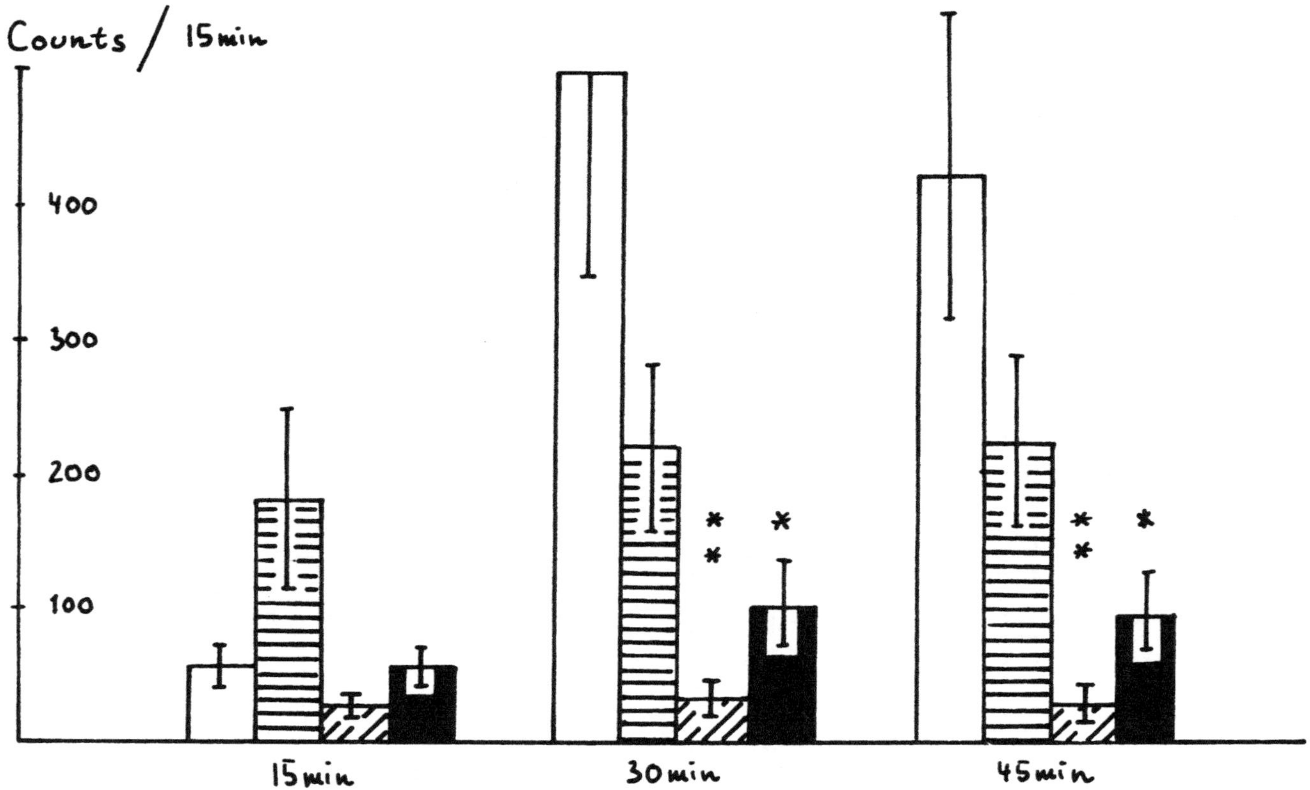

Fig. 1 The effect of pimozide and phenoxybenzamine on cocaine-induced motility. ▭ = saline; ▤ = 0.15 pimozide; ▨ = 0.3 pimozide; ■ = PBZ. The rats were pretreated with the following drugs: Pimozide 0.15 or 0.30 mg/kg s.c., 3 hr; phenoxybenzamine, 20 mg/kg i.p., 3 hr or saline 3 hr.. All rats received 35 mg/kg cocaine, HCl i.p. immediately before the photocell countings. *$p < 0.025$; **$p < 0.01$.

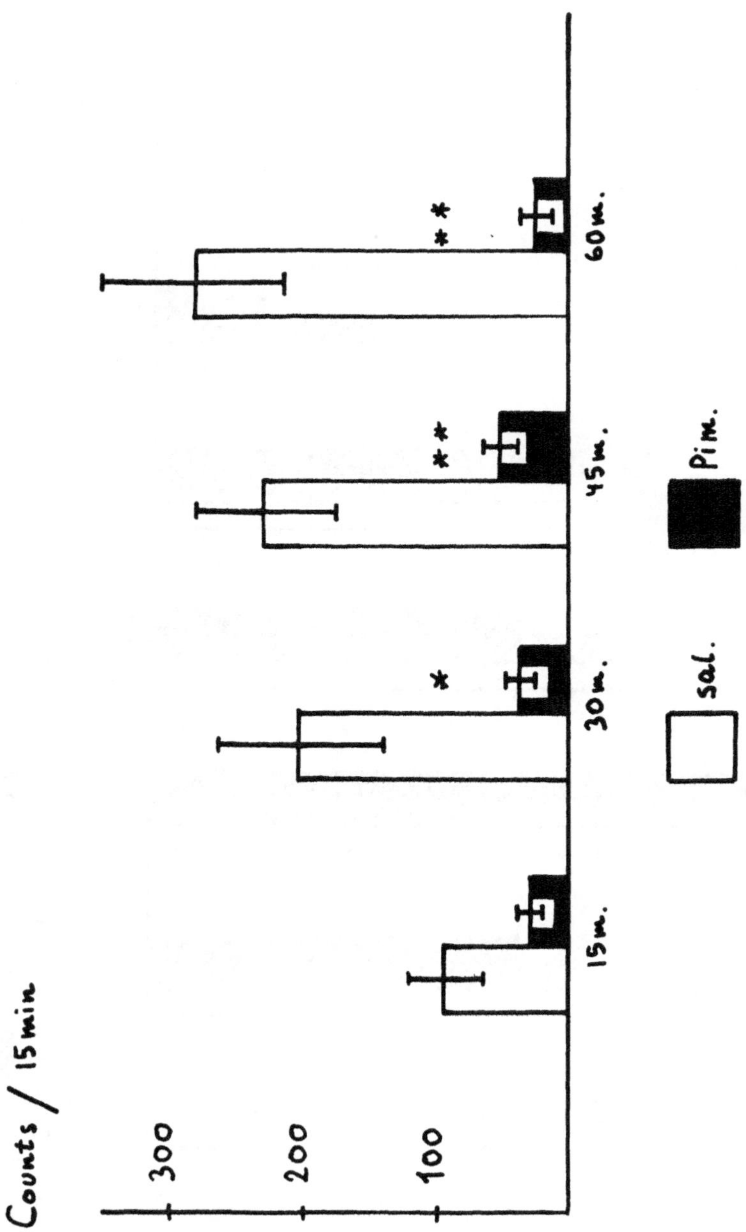

Fig. 2. The effect of pimozide on amphetamine-induced motility. Pimozide 0.15 mg/kg s.c. was injected 3 hr before 2.5 mg/kg s.c. d-amphetamine, HCl. The photocell countings were initiated immediately after the amphetamine injection. $*P < 0.05$; $**P < 0.01$.

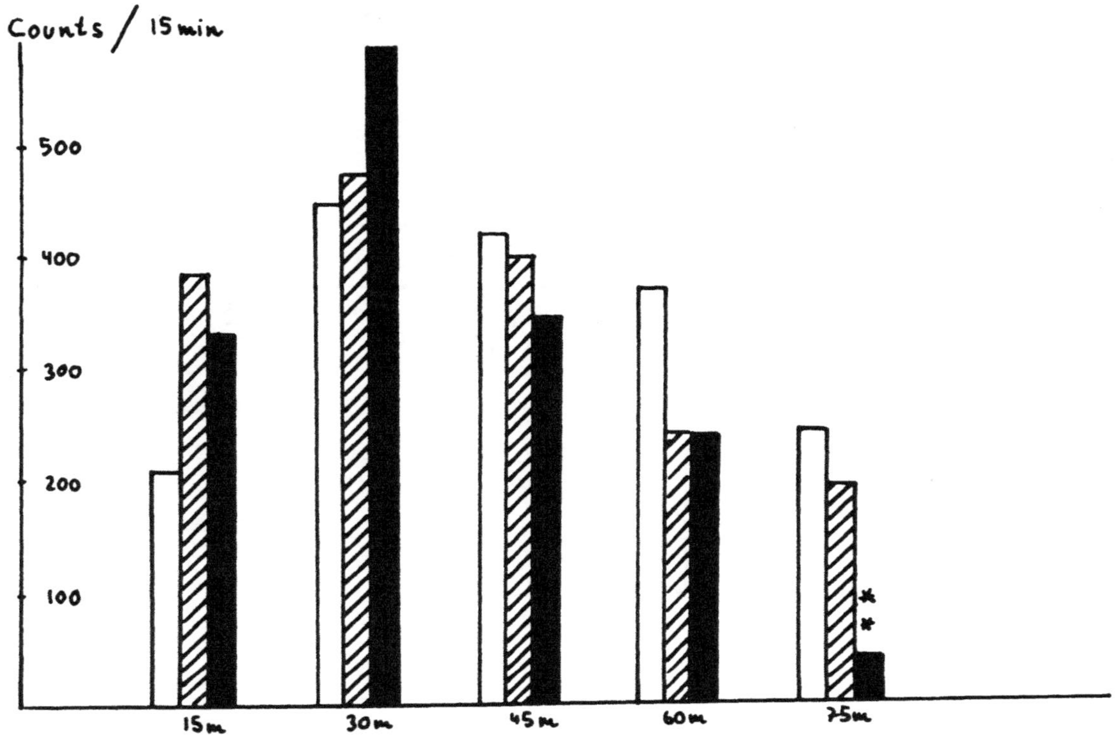

Fig. 3. The effect of α-methyltyrosine on cocaine-induced motility. α-methyltyrosine methylester (H 44/68, 250 mg/kg i.p.) was injected 1 hr or 5 hr before cocaine 35 mg/kg i.p. ** $p < 0.01$. □ = saline; ▨ = αMT, 1 hr; ■ = αMT, 5 hr.

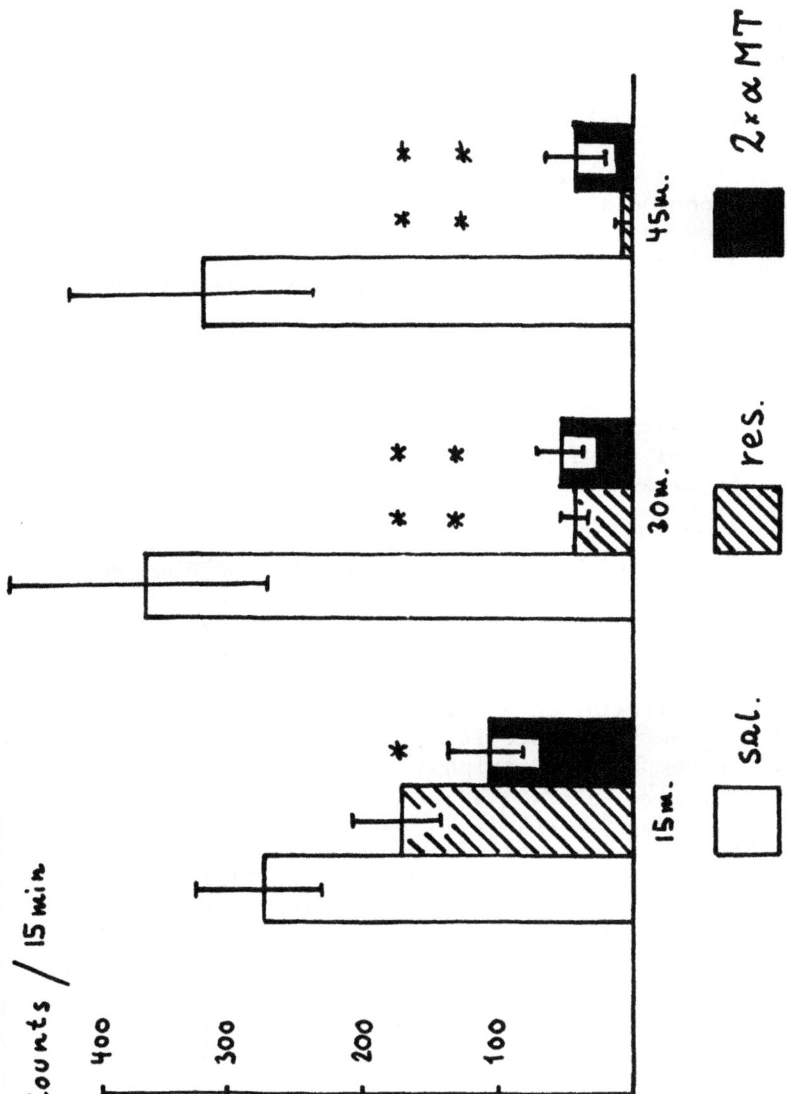

Fig. 4. The effect of extensive catecholamine depletion on cocaine-induced motility. The rats were pretreated with reserpine (7.5 mg/kg s.c., 18 hr) or α-methyltyrosine methylester (H 44/68, 2 x 250 mg/kg, 22 hr and 4 hr) or saline before the injection of 35 mg/kg cocaine, i.p. Photocell countings started immediately after the cocaine injection. $*p < 0.025$; $**p < 0.01$.

for 5 to 10 min in the first period after the injection of 35 mg/kg cocaine. We found in other experiments that the combined pretreatment with reserpine (7.5 mg/kg, 18 hr) and α-methyltyrosine (250 mg/kg, 3 hr) antagonized completely all locomotor and other stimulant effects of 35 mg/kg cocaine. These data may thus indicate that cocaine does not act directly on catecholamine receptors but depends on a critical small pool of catecholamines. Cocaine in a smaller dose, 25 mg/kg i.p., is completely antagonized by pretreatment with reserpine, 7.5 mg/kg s.c., given 3 hr or 18 hr before cocaine (5 rats on each time interval have been tested).

The pretreatment with α-methyltyrosine, given 5 hr before 25 mg/kg cocaine, produced also almost complete antagonism of cocaine-induced motility or head movements, whereas the 1 hr pretreatment with 250 mg/kg α-methyltyrosine induced no significant changes of the 25 mg/kg stimulation (5 rats tested on each time interval).

Figure 5 shows that a large depletion of brain serotonin by p-chlorophenylalanine methyl ester (Koe and Weissman, 1966) (H 69/17, 3 x 100 mg/kg) given at 24 hr intervals with the last dose 24 hr before cocaine (35 mg/kg), induced a potentiation of the cocaine-induced motility in the time interval 0 to 15 min after cocaine and nonsignificant increases in the subsequent time intervals.

Studies on Stereotyped Behavior After Various Amphetamines

In Table 1 is summarized the equivalent dose levels for stereotyped licking/biting activity which is typically produced by several amphetamine analogues and apomorphine. Dextroamphetamine sulphate induces stereotyped licking in a dose of 5 mg/kg s.c. (approximately ED_{50} for licking), whereas concomitant stereotyped biting appears at 10 mg/kg s.c. Levoamphetamine sulphate induces licking in a few rats at 30 mg/kg s.c. (2/17), whereas 50 mg/kg induces licking and/or biting in all rats tested (12/12). Apomorphine, HCl induces discontinuous licking in a few rats after 0.25 mg/kg s.c. (6/30 rats) and typical stereotyped licking after 0.50 mg/kg (32/43 rats). Typically stereotyped licking and biting are seen after 1 mg/kg s.c. apomorphine (10 rats). In general it can be stated that all the stimulant amphetamines induced continuously increased locomotor and rearing activity in the prephase to the occurrence of the typically stereotyped phase. Apomorphine induced the lowest degree of locomotor and rearing activity, which was mainly seen in the dose interval 0.25 to 0.50 mg/kg.

Cocaine and "Stereotyped" Behavior in the Rat

Cocaine induced, in comparison with the central stimulant amphetamine analogues, only a weak "stereotypic" response following

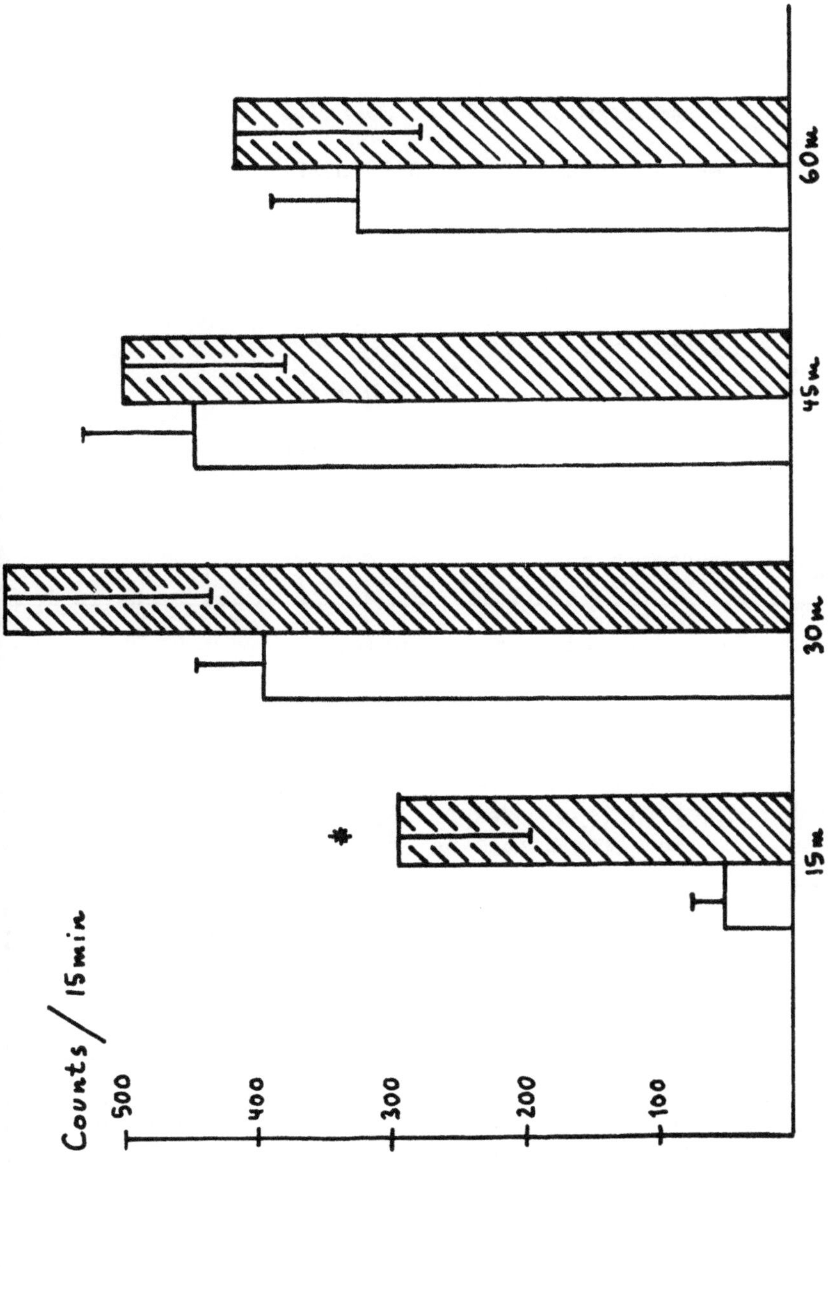

Fig. 5. The effect of serotonin depletion on cocaine-induced motility. The rats were pretreated with p-chlorophenylalanine methylester (H 69/17) 3 x 100 mg/kg i.p. given 72, 48, and 24 hr before cocaine 35 mg/kg i.p. Photocell countings started immediately after the cocaine injection. □ = saline; ▨ = PCPA. $*p < 0.05$.

TABLE 1

Equivalent Doses Of Various Stimulants For Stereotyped Licking/Biting Activity

d-amphetamine	5 to 10 mg/kg
l-amphetamine	30 to 50 mg/kg
methamphetamine	5 to 10 mg/kg
phentermine	50 mg/kg
phenmetrazine	50 mg/kg
pipradrol	50 mg/kg
methylphenidate	50 mg/kg
nomifensine	30 mg/kg
NCA, amfonelic acid	5 mg/kg
apomorphine	0.5 to 1 mg/kg

All stimulants were injected subcutaneously.

TABLE 2

The Effect of Various Doses Of Cocaine On Sniffing And Licking/Biting Activity

		Sniffing		Licking or Biting
Cocaine doses given i.p.	(n)	in the air	at wall or bottom	
10 mg/kg	(5)	0	0	0
25 mg/kg	(20)	100	0	0
35 mg/kg	(15)	100	100	0
50 mg/kg	(5)	100	80	0

The results are presented as percentage of rats showing the activity.

intraperitoneal administration (Table 2). Cocaine (10 mg/kg i.p.) induced mainly an alerting effect, much hind leg scratching, but no constant, typically stereotyped sniffing. Enhanced reactivity to auditory and tactile stimulation was observed. Cocaine (25 mg/kg i.p.) induced much up and down head movement ("head bobbing"), discontinuous sniffing (mainly in the air), and a frequent standing up and down on the hind legs; i.e., rearing activity.

The highest motility, especially rearing activity, was induced by 35 mg/kg cocaine i.p. in the rats kept singly in their familiar cages. About 45 to 60 min after the injection, these rats showed decreasing motor and rearing activities and increasing periodical amphetamine-like sniffing (almost continuous and stereotyped) towards the bottom and lower wall of the cages. No licking/biting activity was observed. Fifty mg/kg cocaine i.p. induced convulsions in 2/5 rats and apparently illness in the others. Following recovery, 20 to 30 min after the injection, the rats showed frequent side to side movements of the head and almost continuous sniffing towards the lower part of the wall. The cocaine stimulation was relatively short-lasting (30 min after a 10 mg/kg dose and about 75 min after a 35 mg/kg dose).

An additional dose of cocaine given 1 hr after the first injection induced a weak further increase in the "stereotypic" response (Table 3). However, weak and periodical licking and biting were observed about 40 min after the second dose of 35 or 50 mg/kg.

TABLE 3

The Effect of Various Doses of Cocaine on Sniffing and Licking/Biting Activity

		Sniffing		Licking or Biting
Cocaine doses given at intervals of 1 hr	(n)	in the air	at wall or bottom	
2 x 10 mg/kg	(5)	0	0	0
2 x 25 mg/kg	(12)	100	25	0
2 x 35 mg/kg	(10)	100	100	10
2 x 50 mg/kg*	(5)	80	80	20

The results are presented as percentage of rats showing the activity.
*One rat died after the second dose.

Summarizing: The "stereotypy" after cocaine is of much weaker intensity than that seen after central stimulant amphetamine analogues or apomorphine. The extreme forms of stereotypy; i.e., continuous licking and biting stereotypy, was not seen after an intraperitoneal injection of cocaine given in even toxic doses. The sniffing effect of cocaine (i.e., "the stereotypic response") after doses of 25 to 35 mg/kg i.p. is similar to that of apomorphine in the dose range of 0.10 to 0.25 mg/kg s.c. or *d*-amphetamine in doses of 1.5 to 2.5 mg/kg s.c.

Stereotyped Behavior After Subcutaneously Injected Cocaine

Cocaine induced the strongest and most characteristically stereotyped behavior after subcutaneous injection but only after extremely high doses (100 to 600 mg/kg). The subcutaneous injection of cocaine induces undoubtedly a local vasoconstrictor effect (Simon, Sultan, Chermat, and Boissier, 1972) that retards the absorption of the drug. The central stimulant effect of cocaine developed slowly. A highly characteristic, amphetamine-like stereotyped sniffing (continuous and performed at only a small constricted area of the floor or lower wall) had developed after a time lag of 3 hr. This behavior was seen in all rats after cocaine in doses of 100 (5 rats), 300 (10 rats), and 600 (10 rats) mg/kg s.c. This stereotyped sniffing lasted approximately 2 to 3 hr after 100 mg/kg s.c. but for more than 24 hr after the 600 mg/kg s.c. dose of cocaine.

The rats were observed continuously for 9 hr after the injection. Episodical and discontinuous licking occurred after a time lag of 6 to 9 hr after the injection in 3/10 rats after the 300 and 600 mg/kg doses and in a total of 6/10 rats from each group after 24 hr. Continuous licking and biting was observed in only one rat after the 600 mg/kg, but with a duration for more than 16 hr. Another rat on the 600 mg/kg dose showed a short-lasting biting 9 hr after the injection. No other rats showed biting or gnawing. The results are summarized in Table 4.

Characteristically for cocaine (and in sharp contrast to the amphetamine/apomorphine-induced stereotypy), a sudden noise or a close approach by the observer to the experimental cage almost completely abolished all sniffing or licking activities. The rats showed then either a "freezing" reaction or a pronounced, strong locomotor and jumping response. All the rats survived the 100 and 300 mg/kg doses of cocaine whereas 4/10 rats were found dead 24 hr after the 600 mg/kg dose.

TABLE 4

Cocaine-induced Licking After Subcutaneous Injection

Cocaine dose	Time after injection				
	Number of rats showing licking*				
	0-6 h	6-9 h	14 h	24 h	0-24 h (total)
100 mg/kg s.c. (5)	0/5	0/5	0/5	0/5	0/5
300 mg/kg s.c. (10)	0/10	3/10	3/10	0.10	6/10
600 mg/kg s.c. (10)**	0/10	0/10	3/10	3/10	6/10

*The licking was mainly performed discontinuously and episodically in all rats. Two rats showed a short-lasting (30 min) continuous licking after 300 mg/kg, whereas one rat showed a long-lasting (more than 16 hr) continuous licking/biting after 600 mg/kg.

**4 rats were found dead 24 hr after 600 mg/kg.

TABLE 5

The Effect Of Various Drugs On Licking/Biting Activities In Nialamide-Cocaine-Treated Rats

Further pretreatment (mg/kg)	Sniffing	Licking/biting
Saline, 25 rats	100	0
Phenoxybenzamine (20), 10 rats	70	40
Methergoline (1), 10 rats	100	30
p-Chlorophenylalanine (3 x 100), 10 rats	100	0
Scopolamine (3), 5 rats*	100	0

All rats received 100 mg/kg nialamide i.p. 1 hr before 25 mg/kg i.p. cocaine. The results are presented as percentage of rats showing the activity.

*For further details on behaviour, see text.

Effect of Various Drugs on the Cocaine-Induced "Stereotypy"

The very weak and infrequent development of licking and biting stereotypy after intraperitoneally injected cocaine was an unexpected finding. In the following experiments we tested the effects of various drugs that, according to our previous experience, have been found to increase licking/biting stereotypy after various amphetamines and apomorphine (see discussion).

The pretreatment with phenoxybenzamine (20 mg/kg i.p., 3 hr, 5 rats) or scopolamine, HCl (3 mg/kg s.c., ½ hr, 5 rats) induced no licking or biting stereotypy following the subsequent injection of cocaine (35 mg/kg i.p.). Phenoxybenzamine antagonized almost completely the cocaine-induced motility but not the "head bobbing" movements. Scopolamine alone induced the typical anticholinergic stimulation in the rats: increased motility and much rearing. The sniffing was increased but discontinuous and not stereotyped. The scopolamine pretreatment induced a strong increase in cocaine-induced motility and especially rearing activity which was performed with a very high up and down frequency. However, scopolamine did not increase the cocaine-induced "stereotypy" with respect to performance of sniffing, licking, or biting.

However, the pretreatment with the serotonin antagonist methergoline (1 mg/kg s.c. given 3 hr before cocaine, 35 mg/kg i.p.) induced episodes of licking and biting activities in 2/5 rats and increased in addition the cocaine-induced motility.

The Effect of Various Drugs on Nialamide-Cocaine-Induced "Stereotypy"

In the following experiments the rats were pretreated with the monoamine oxidase inhibitor nialamide (100 mg/kg i.p.) 1 hr before cocaine. This pretreatment was found to induce side to side movements of the head and almost continuous sniffing at the bottom and the lower part of the wall of the cages in the period 30-60 min. after 25 mg/kg cocaine. However, no licking or biting was observed in a total of 25 rats tested. Two rats placed in one cage performed the typical "bizarre social behavior" previously described by van Rossum (1970) after 1-DOPA or amphetamine. The 25 mg/kg dose of cocaine was selected for further experiments, since the 35 mg/kg cocaine dose given i.p. after nialamide was found toxic.

The results summarized in Table 5 show that antagonism of noradrenaline receptors with phenoxybenzamine or serotonin receptors with methergoline induced biting and licking activity in the nialamide-cocaine-treated rats. The pretreatment with methergoline induced in addition, mainly during the first 10 min after the cocaine injection, a clearcut increase in motility and rearing in comparison with the rats receiving nialamide-cocaine.

However, depletion of brain serotonin with p-chlorophenylalanine methylester (PCPA, 3 doses of 100 mg/kg i.p. given at intervals of 24 hr, last dose 24 hr before cocaine) did not facilitate performance of licking/biting activity following the cocaine injection. The PCPA pretreatment induced instead a remarkable increase in locomotor and rearing activities for 90 min after the cocaine injection. Constant and intense sniffing activities directed towards the upper part of the cage walls were observed.

The pretreatment with scopolamine, HCl (3 mg/kg s.c. ½ hr before cocaine) induced in these nialamide-cocaine-treated rats a strong behavioral reaction: Within 5-10 min after the cocaine (25 mg/kg/ i.p.) injection, the rats showed an intense, compulsive, forward locomotion, large, very stereotyped side to side movements of the head (head weaving), (frequently a rapid head twitch may proceed to a shake including the whole body ["wet dog shake"]); and increased squeaking, especially during handling; but no aggressiveness or social interaction appeared when placing two rats in one cage. Tremor, hind leg abduction, and frequent episodes of "piano playing" with the forelegs appeared also. However, no licking or biting activity occurred.

Biochemical Results

The effects of various doses of cocaine injected intraperitoneally on the major dopamine metabolites are summarized in Table 6.

Cocaine induced only minor effects of HVA and a small but significant increase was found 1 hr after 35 mg/kg. DOPAC was significantly decreased after 15 mg/kg, 1 hr and 35 mg/kg, ½ hr after cocaine. Benztropine (25 mg/kg), an uptake inhibitor of dopamine, induced no change in HVA but a decrease in DOPAC.

Cocaine (25 mg/kg i.p.) showed clearcut similarities to desipramine (2.5 mg/kg s.c.) on the ^{3}H-noradrenaline metabolites ^{3}H-MOPEG and ^{3}H-DOPEG formed from ^{3}H-noradrenaline after intraventricularly injected ^{3}H-tyrosine: ^{3}H-MOPEG and ^{3}H-DOPEG were significantly decreased. Amphetamine (10 mg/kg showed, in comparison, a stronger decrease in ^{3}H-DOPEG than in ^{3}H-MOPEG and, in addition, a decrease in ^{3}H-noradrenaline. The effect of cocaine on ^{3}H-noradrenaline metabolism corresponds closely to the effect that we previously have found after some tricyclic antidepressant drugs and not to the characteristic effect of various amphetamines (Nielsen, 1975; Nielsen, personal communication; Scheel-Krüger, Braestrup, and Nielsen, 1975).

The results on endogenous MOPEG and DOPEG showed that cocaine, like desipramine, did not increase MOPEG but showed a decrease in DOPEG (conjugated), the catechol-deaminated metabolite of noradrenaline (a major noradrenaline metabolite, Nielsen and Braestrup, personal communication).

TABLE 6

The Effect of Cocaine and Benztropine on the Brain Dopamine Metabolites

Drugs and doses	HVA		DOPAC	
Cocaine, 15 mg/kg i.p., 1 hr	93 ± 3.6	(4)	68 ± 1.7	(4)**
Cocaine, 25 mg/kg i.p., 1 hr	114 ± 8.8	(4)	89 ± 9.0	(4)
Cocaine, 2 x 25 mg/kg i.p. 1 and 2 hr	121 ± 14	(3)	101 ± 19	(3)
Cocaine, 35 mg/kg i.p., ½ hr	110 ± 6.6	(9)	84 ± 3.5	(9)**
Cocaine, 35 mg/kg i.p., 1 hr	122 ± 5.6	(10)**	99 ± 3.0	(10)
Benztropine, 25 mg/kg s.c., 2 hr	100 ± 5.0	(4)	78 ± 2.5	(3)

The mean values ± s.e.m. are presented as percentage of saline-treated rats.

*$p < 0.05$; **$p < 0.02$.

TABLE 7

The Effect of Cocaine, Desipramine, and Amphetamine on Brain ^{3}H-Noradrenaline Accumulation and Metabolism

Drugs and doses	(n)	^{3}H-NA	^{3}H-MOPEG	^{3}H-DOPEG	^{3}H-Tyr
		Brain levels in % of controls			
Cocaine 25 mg/kg i.p.	(6)	91 ± 4.6	82 ± 5.1*	74 ± 5.9*	111 ± 9
Desipramine 2.5 mg/kg s.c.	(5)	105 ± 6.4	72 ± 3.7*	62 ± 5.1**	110 ± 7
d-Amphetamine 10 mg/kg s.c.	(5)	58 ± 8.0	76 ± 16	43 ± 7.0*	171 ± 16*

Cocaine was injected 10 min and desipramine and *d*-amphetamine 30 min before the intraventricular injection of ^{3}H-tyrosine (50 μCi). The rats were killed 30 min after ^{3}H-tyrosine. The mean values ± s.e.m. are expressed as percentages of a corresponding number (n) of control rats receiving saline only. The absolute values (in d.p.m./total brain tissue and not corrected for recovery) in saline-treated rats are ^{3}H-NA 55749 ± 2255; ^{3}H-MOPEG (free + conjugated) 7392 ± 137; ^{3}H-DOPEG-SO_4 4095 ± 104; ^{3}H-tyrosine 4.85 ± 0.92 x 10^{6}.

The statistical analyses were performed according to Student's t-test:

*$p < 0.02$; **$p < 0.001$.

TABLE 8

The Effect Of Cocaine And Desipramine On Endogenous Brain MOPEG And DOPEG, The Major Noradrenaline Metabolites

Doses and time schedules	MOPEG (free + conjugated)	DOPEG (conjugated)
	Brain levels in % of controls	
Cocaine 25 mg/kg, 1 hr	103 ± 7.1 (4)	82.5 ± 3.7* (4)
Cocaine 35 mg/kg, 1 hr	96 ± 9.0 (3)	77.6 ± 4.5 (5)
Cocaine 2 x 25 mg/kg, 1 hr interv.	89 ± 6.3 (4)	90 ± 5.8 (4)
Desipramine 2.5 mg/kg, 2½ hr	111 ± 11.6 (4)	61 ± 2.6** (4)

Cocaine was injected i.p. and desipramine s.c. The mean values ± s.e.m. are expressed as percentages of corresponding numbers of control rats receiving saline only.

*$P < 0.025$; **$P < 0.01$.

However, following pretreatment with nialamide, cocaine showed clearcut similarities to the central stimulant amphetamines (see also Scheel-Krüger, 1971; 1972) since cocaine, 25 mg/kg, and especially 2 x 25 mg/kg, significantly increased NM (normetanephrine) and MT (3-methoxytyramine), the major noradrenaline and dopamine metabolities following inhibition of monoamine oxidase.

TABLE 9

The Effect Of Cocaine, *d*- and *l*-Amphetamine On the Accumulation Of Dopamine, Noradrenaline And Their O-Methylated Metabolites (MT And NM, Respectively)

Drugs and doses	(n)	Brain Levels In % Of Controls			
		NA	NM	DA	MT
Cocaine, 25 mg/kg	(3)	79±4.5*	133±6.6	86± 7	106±25
Cocaine, 2 x 25 mg/kg	(6)	84±2.5*	164±19**	80± 6	192±18**
l-Amphetamine 10 mg/kg	(5)	68±5.0**	310±31**	96±10	245±30**
d-Amphetamine 10 mg/kg	(5)	55±3.5**	380±61**	80± 5	415±33**

$^{*}P < 0.05$; $^{**}P < 0.01$

All rats received nialamide, 200 mg/kg s.c., 30 min before the stimulant drugs. The divided dose of cocaine 2 X 25 mg/kg was given 1 and 2 hr before the rats were decapitated. The rats were decapitated 2½ hr after nialamide. Each value in the table represents the mean ± s.e.m. expressed as a percentage of the controls.

DISCUSSION

Cocaine-induced Motility

The stimulant effects of cocaine are most interestingly contrasted to the behavioral profile of action of apomorphine in the rat: apomorphine induces only a moderate locomotor stimulant effect, especially seen after lower doses (0.10-0.50 mg/kg) and particularly in young rats (Grabowska and Michaluk, 1974; results, present study; Buus Lassen, in press) but is very potent in inducing extreme forms of stereotypy; i.e., intense, continuous licking/biting activity. Amphetamine shares behavioral effects of both drugs: a strong effect on motility in the dose range of 1-2.5 mg/kg s.c. *d*-amphetamine sulfate (in our rats) and the apomorphine-like stereotypic licking and/or biting effect after higher doses in the range of 5-10 mg/kg s.c.

On the background of the present state of knowledge these findings invite the hypothesis that cocaine might interact with mesolimbic dopaminergic structures in the brain in preference for the nigra-neostriatal dopamine structures.

A considerable body of evidence has shown that nucleus accumbens septi in the mesolimbic dopamine system seem most significantly involved in the motility induced by amphetamine or dopaminergic stimulants including apomorphine (Pijnenburg and van Rossum, 1973; Pijnenburg, Honig, and van Rossum, 1975a, b; Roberts, Zis, and Fibiger, 1975; Kelly, Seviour and Iversen, 1975).

The role of the mesolimbic dopamine system in amphetamine- (and apomorphine-) induced stereotyped licking/biting behavior is presently a more controversal topic (Costall and Naylor, 1974a, b; 1975), but several investigators consider the nigro-striatal dopamine structures as more significant for these extreme forms of stereotypy (Asher and Aghajanian, 1974; Kelly et al., 1975; Iversen, in press; Creese and Iversen, 1975; Fog, Randrup, and Pakkenberg, 1970).

A 6-OH-dopamine lesion of the nigro-striatal dopamine system changes the amphetamine-induced stereotypy (sniffing directed towards a localized area of the floor, licking, and biting) to a more cocaine-like stimulation; i.e., sniffing mainly in the air, absence of licking and biting. A lesion of nucleus accumbens septi antagonized both the cocaine or amphetamine locomotor response (Kelly et al., 1975; Iversen, in press).

The hypermotility induced by cocaine and amphetamine may be considered as an animal model providing some information on the stimulant and possibly also psychotic effects of these drugs in the human clinic. Several years ago the antagonism of amphetamine hypermotility was suggested by van Rossum (1965, 1967, 1970) as a useful animal model for the evaluation and classification of antipsychotic drugs with antidopaminergic effects.

Recently, Buus Lassen (in press) concluded in a study on the hypermotility induced by small doses of apomorphine (0.25-0.5 mg/kg) in the rat that the antagonism of apomorphine motility is a useful model for the evaluation of antipsychotic drugs (including thioridazine and clozapine) and the antagonism may be due to selective blockade of some dopamine receptors possibly localized in mesolimbic structures.

The above-mentioned points of view have been cited because, during recent years, there has been a considerable interest in potential screening tests for the evaluation of new antipsychotic drugs in addition to the most widely used test: the antagonism of amphetamine- or apomorphine-stereotyped licking and biting stereotypy (Randrup et al., 1973; Randrup et al., 1975; Matthysse, 1973).

The importance of dopaminergic mechanisms for cocaine motility has been suggested by van Rossum and Hurkmans (1964). Creese and Iversen (1975) have also shown that a 6-hydroxydopamine lesion of the dopaminergic cell bodies in substantia nigra antagonized the cocaine- (and amphetamine-) induced motility. Wilner et al. (1970) found that haloperidol, a dopamine antagonist, inhibited the cocaine- (and amphetamine-) stereotyped running and circling behavior in the dog. Studies with mice and rats have shown that the cocaine- (and amphetamine-) induced motility is antagonized by dopamine antagonists (van Rossum, 1965, 1967, 1970; Simon, Sultan, Chermat, and Boissier, 1972; Rolinski and Scheel-Krüger, 1973; result, present study).

However, the cocaine- or amphetamine-induced locomotor activity is a complex model in mechanism of action (just as extreme forms of stereotypy, see later discussion), since the motility also is inhibited by noradrenaline depletion or noradrenaline antagonists (Maj, Przegalinski and Wielosz, 1968; Rolinski and Scheel-Krüger, 1973; Galambos, Pfeifer, György, and Molnar, 1967; Pfeifer, Galambos, and György, 1966; results, present study). Furthermore, inhibitory cholinergic and serotonergic mechanisms seem also involved in the cocaine- and amphetamine-induced motility (Arnfred and Randrup, 1968; Galambos et al., 1967; Breese, Cooper, and Mueller, 1974; Scheel-Krüger, 1970; Scheel-Krüger and Hasselager, 1974; Schelkunov, 1967; Samanin and Garattini, 1975; van Rossum, 1970).

Cocaine- and Amphetamine-induced Stereotypy - the Role of Various Neurotransmitter Systems

The amphetamine- or apomorphine-induced licking and/or biting stereotypy in the rat is absolutely dependent on a dopaminergic mechanism. However, recently evidence for an inhibitory noradrenergic mechanism (Mogilnicka and Braestrup, in press; Braestrup, personal communication) influencing stereotypy has been found. The ratio between dopamine and noradrenaline receptor activity seems significant in the qualitative expression of different behavioral elements of stereotypy; i.e., in the transfer of stereotyped sniffing behavior into licking/biting activity as well as to the expression of motility. The present experiments of the influence of phenoxybenzamine on the nialamide-cocaine-induced stereotypy provide, thus, additional support for this hypothesis.

The inhibitor of serotonin synthesis, p-chlorophenylalanine (PCPA), increased the cocaine- or nialamide-cocaine-induced locomotor and rearing activities but did not, in contrast to methergoline, induce licking/biting activity. This apparently contradictory finding seems presently hard to explain. Methergoline seems to be a potent long-lasting and specific serotonin antagonist (Beretta, Ferrini, and Glasser, 1965; Ferrini and Glasser, 1965; Hawson and Whittington, 1970), but it must be emphasized that our present knowledge of central serotonin antagonists is most limited, (e.g., Haigler and Aghajanian, 1974).

In other studies we have found that methergoline but not PCPA increased the intensity of sniffing stereotypy and facilitated the occurrence of licking/biting after some amphetamine-like dopaminergic drugs (Mogilnicka and Scheel-Krüger, unpublished data) in agreement with studies by Weiner, Goetz, Westheimer, and Klawans (1973), suggesting the existence of an inhibitory serotonergic mechanism influencing the amphetamine-like licking/biting elements of stereotypy.

Unexpectedly, the anticholinergic drug scopolamine had very weak influence on the cocaine-induced "stereotypy". No typical amphetamine or apomorphine-like continuously stereotyped sniffing restricted to a small area of the bottom or the roof of the cage occurred. Neither did scopolamine induce licking/biting after cocaine. Licking/biting activities have previously been observed to increase following various amphetamines and apomorphine in combination with central anticholinergic drugs (Arnfred and Randrup, 1968; Scheel-Krüger, 1970). Scopolamine did, however, increase and facilitate a very strong standing up and down ("stereotypy"?) of very high frequency when given together with 35 mg/kg cocaine.

When scopolamine pretreatment was applied to rats receiving both cocaine and nialamide, a most remarkable stimulation was induced:

a constant, compulsive forward locomotion, and very stereotyped, large side to side movements of the head. (For details see results section). This remarkable behavioral syndrome has previously been described by others in mice or rats receiving monoamine oxidase inhibitors and tryptophan - LSD also induced this syndrome - and has also been seen in our laboratory (Scheel-Krüger, unpublished data; Corrodi, 1966; Grahame-Smith, 1971; Grahame-Smith and Green, 1974; Green and Grahame-Smith, 1974; Modigh and Svensson, 1972; Squires and Buus Lassen, 1975). This behavioral snydrome seems mainly dependent on the cooperation of brain dopamine and serotonin. Inhibitors of serotonin uptake facilitate this nialamide-tryptophan snydrome (Modigh and Svensson, 1972; Buus Lassen, Petersen, Kjellberg, and Olsson, 1975), and it seems, therefore, reasonable to assume that in the present experiments the inhibitory effect of cocaine on the reuptake of serotonin (Ross and Reny, 1969) is directly involved in addition to the catecholamine effect.

Mechanisms of Actions of Cocaine

Cocaine interaction with catecholamine pools. Amphetamine and its congeners may be classified in at least two groups according to inhibition of the behavioral stimulation by reserpine or α-methyltyrosine: the amphetamine group (consisting of *d*-amphetamine, *l*-amphetamine, methamphetamine, and phenmetrazine) is not antagonized by high doses of reserpine. The methylphenidate group (consisting of methylphenidate, pipradrol, NCA amfonelic acid, and nomifensine) is in contrast completely antagonized by high doses of reserpine (7.5 mg/kg or more), but is less sensitive to antagonism by α-methyltyrosine than the amphetamine group (Scheel-Krüger, 1971; Braestrup and Scheel-Krüger, unpublished data; van Rossum and Hurkmans, 1964). Our results clearly emphasize that cocaine corresponds in this respect to the methylphenidate group.

The dose-dependent inhibition of cocaine stimulation by reserpine has previously been shown (Kobinger, 1958; Simon et al., 1972; van Rossum, van Schoot, and Hurkmans, 1962; Wallach and Gershon (in the cat), 1972). Concerning the inhibitory effect of α-methyltyrosine on cocaine lomomotion, Simon et al. (1972) found no significant effect and Wallach and Gershcn (1972) found only weak inhibition. In our studies on motility cocaine was remarkably resistant to antagonism by α-methyltyrosine even when considered in comparison with drugs belonging to the methylphenidate group. However, antagonism was found after extensive catecholamine depletion induced by repeated doses of α-methyltyrosine or by reserpine in combination with α-methyltyrosine.

These data may indicate that cocaine does not act directly on catecholamine receptors as has been suggested by some investigators working with peripheral organs but which later studies have challenged (see Trendelenburg, Graefe, and Eckert, 1972). The early studies by van Rossum and Hurkmans (1964) in which the reserpine-induced inhibition of cocaine-induced motility was restored by *l*-DOPA also indicate that cocaine does not act directly on dopamine receptors.

Cocaine: The effects on catecholamine release and uptake mechanism. In our biochemical studies cocaine has been compared with various types of drugs; i.e., benztropine and desipramine, that inhibit the uptake of dopamine and noradrenaline, respectively (Scheel-Krüger, 1972), and *d*-amphetamine, methylphenidate, and some other amphetamines: drugs that produce release and uptake inhibition of dopamine and noradrenaline (Scheel-Krüger, 1971, 1972; Scheel-Krüger et al., 1975). According to our experimental schedule, cocaine *per se* mainly showed similarities to both benztropine and desipramine; whereas, following pretreatment with a monoamine oxidase inhibitor, nialamide, cocaine showed clearcut similarities to the amphetamines. Cocaine seems thus mainly to influence the uptake of dopamine and noradrenaline but a certain minor catecholamine releasing component seems also to be present.

Our biochemical studies on the major dopamine metabolites, HVA and DOPAC, showed that cocaine only in very high doses (2 x 25 or 35 mg/kg) induced a small increase in HVA (which effect may be indicative of dopamine release (Braestrup, personal communication), whereas DOPAC only was decreased at some doses or time schedules. Cocaine is thus biochemically different from the methylphenidate group (including pipradrol, NCA, and nomifensine) which increases HVA considerably and also DOPAC, although to a smaller extent than the HVA increase (Braestrup, personal communication). Cocaine is also different from amphetamine which increases HVA and decreases DOPAC and apomorphine which decreases both HVA and DOPAC (Braestrup, personal communication). The effect of cocaine showed a close similarity to benztropine, which decreased DOPAC but did not change the HVA level.

Concerning noradrenaline, cocaine *per se* showed a closer similarity to desipramine than to *d*-amphetamine. This conclusion was reached in our *in vivo* studies on the measurement of ^{3}H-noradrenaline and its major metabolites ^{3}H-MOPEG (total) and ^{3}H-DOPEG-SO_4 following intraventricular injection of ^{3}H-tyrosine or following the measurement of endogenous MOPEG (total) and DOPEG-SO_4 after cocaine, desipramine, and *d*-amphetamine (Tables 7,8). Amphetamine induces also, in contrast to cocaine, a strong increase in MOPEG (total) (Mogilnicka and Braestrup, in press). Some recent *in vitro* studies which in particular have focused on the relative role of release versus uptake inhibition have reached the conclusion that cocaine in noradrenaline terminals (Azzaro et al., 1974) and dopamine terminals (Heikkila et al., 1975) mainly affects the uptake mechanism but, in addition, has a weak but significant effect on catecholamine release.

The pretreatment with a monoamine oxidase inhibitor seems to facilitate the occurrence of some amphetamine-like components of cocaine: the stereotypic response is increased (see results section), and following nialamide pretreatment cocaine induces a turning in rats with a unilateral lesion of the dopamine system (Christie and Crow, 1971). In nialamide pretreated rats (Table 9) cocaine increases O-methylated dopamine and noradrenaline. This provides evidence that cocaine also induces release of dopamine and noradrenaline in addition to the well-known reuptake inhibitory properties. In this biochemical model (nialamide pretreatment), cocaine thus shows clearcut similarities to the central stimulant amphetamines (including the stimulants belonging to both the amphetamine group and the methylphenidate group) and a clearcut difference to the imipramine-like antidepressant drugs or benztropine, which have no effect on normetanephrine or 3-methoxytryamine after nialamide (Scheel-Krüger, 1971, 1972).

In summary, cocaine has been compared to the stimulant amphetamines and apomorphine in the rat. All these drugs induce stimulation, including locomotion and stereotyped behavior. These activities appear dependent on brain catecholamines and probably most significantly on dopamine. The behavioral profile of action of these drugs is, however, different: apomorphine is very potent in inducing extreme forms of stereotyped behavior including licking and biting, while cocaine is a very potent locomotor stimulant and surprisingly weak in inducing the licking/biting stereotypies. The strongest degree of locomotion or stereotypies appears at different time intervals after the injection of cocaine (and the amphetamines) and these behavioral effects may not in the present situation be considered as mutually competitive. These behavioral results of cocaine are discussed in relation to a preferential interaction with the mesolimbic contra the nigra-neostriatal dopamine systems.

The weak induction of the extremely stereotyped elements of licking/biting after cocaine may, however, be transformed into more amphetamine- or apomorphine-like effects by pharmacological manipulations; i.e., pretreatment with noradrenaline or serotonin blocking drugs, pretreatment with a monoamine oxidase inhibitor, nialamide, or, following an extremely prolongated exposure to cocaine, after a subcutaneous injection of very high doses (300-600 mg/kg s.c.). In the treatment with scopolamine-nialamide, cocaine induced the characteristic "monoamine oxidase inhibitor-tryptophan syndrome." The studies on motility and "stereotypy" showed that the cocaine stimulation depends on a reserpine sensitive pool of catecholamines, whereas cocaine is very insensitive to antagonism by α-methyltyrosine, an inhibitor of catecholamine synthesis.

The biochemical profile of cocaine was investigated on catecholamine metabolites. Cocaine exhibited a profile of action resembling both the dopamine uptake inhibitor, benztropine, and the noradrenaline uptake inhibitor, desipramine. Cocaine showed only to a minor degree similarities to amphetamine-like drugs on catecholamine metabolites. This effect of cocaine was most clearly found following pretreatment with a monoamine oxidase inhibitor, nialamide. Cocaine seems thus mainly to influence the dopamine and noradrenaline uptake mechanisms and has in addition a smaller but significant effect on the release mechanism.

ACKNOWLEDGMENTS

This investigation was supported by a NIH research grant no. DA 00023 from the National Institute on Drug Abuse, and a grant from Foundations' Fund for Research in Psychiatry.

REFERENCES

Andersen, H., Braestrup, C., and Randrup, A.: Apomorphine-induced stereotyped biting in the tortoise in relation to dopaminergic mechanisms, Brain, Behav. and Evol. 11, 365-373 (1975).

Arnfred, T. and Randrup, A.: Cholinergic mechanism in brain inhibiting amphetamine-induced stereotyped behavior, Acta Pharmac. Tox. 26, 384-394 (1968).

Asher, I.M. and Aghajanian, G.K.: 6-Hydroxydopamine lesions of olfactory tubercles and caudate nuclei: Effect on amphetamine-induced stereotyped behavior in rats, Brain Res. 82, 1-12 (1974).

Azzaro, A.J., Ziance, R.J., and Rutledge, C.O.: The importance of neuronal uptake of amines for amphetamine-induced release of ^{3}H-norepinephrine from isolated brain tissue, J. Pharm. exp. Ther. 189, 110-118 (1974).

Beretta, C., Ferrini, R., and Glässer, A.H.: 1, 6-dimethyl-8 β-carbobenzyloxy-aminomethyl-10α-ergoline, a potent and long-lasting 5-hydroxytryptamine antagonist, Nature 207, 421-422 (1965).

Breese, G.R., Cooper, B.R., and Mueller, R.A.: Evidence for involvement of 5-hydroxytryptamine in the actions of amphetamine, Br. J. Pharmacol. 52, 307-314 (1974).

Braestrup, C.: Identification of free and conjugated 3-methoxy-4-hydroxyphenylglycol (MOPEG) in rat brain by gas chromatography and mass fragmentography, Anal. Biochem. 55, 420-431 (1973).

Braestrup, C., Andersen, H., and Randrup, A.: The monoamine oxidase B inhibitor deprenyl potentiates phenylethylamine behavior in rats without inhibition of catecholamine metabolite formation, Eur. J. Pharmacol. 34, 181-187 (1975).

Buus Lassen, J., Petersen, E., Kjellberg, B., and Olsson, S.: Comparative studies of a new 5HT-uptake inhibitor and some tricyclic thymoleptics, Eur. J. Pharmacol. 32, 108-115 (1975).

Buus Lassen, J.: Inhibition and potentiation of apomorphine-induced hypermotility in rats by neuroleptics, Eur. J. Pharmac. (In press).

Christie, J.E. and Crow, T.J.: Possible role of dopamine-containing neurones in the behavioural effects of cocaine, Br. J. Pharmacol. 42, 643P-645P (1971).

Corrodi, H.: Blockade of the psychotic syndrome caused by nialamide in mice, J. Pharm. Pharmac. 18, 197-198 (1966).

Costall, B. and Naylor, R.J.: Extrapyramidal and mesolimbic involvement with the stereotypic activity of *d*- and *l*-amphetamine, Eur. J. Pharmacol. 25, 121-129 (1974a).

Costall, B. and Naylor, R.J.: Mesolimbic involvement with behavioral effects indicating antipsychotic activity, Eur. J. Pharmacol. 27, 46-58 (1974b).

Costall, B. and Naylor, R.J.: The behavioural effects of dopamine applied intracerebrally to areas of the mesolimbic system, Eur. J. Pharmacol. 32, 87-92 (1975).

Creese, I. and Iversen, S.D.: The pharmacological and anatomical substrates of the amphetamine response in the rat, Brain Res. 83, 419-436 (1975).

Ferrini, R. and Glässer, A.: Antagonism of central effects of tryptamine and 5-hydroxytryptophan by 1,6-dimethyl-8 β-carbobenzyloxyaminomethyl-10α-ergoline, Psychopharmacologia (Berl.) 8, 271-276 (1965).

Fog, R., Randrup, A., and Pakkenberg, H.: Lesions in corpus striatum and cortex of rat brains and the effects on pharmacologically induced stereotyped, aggressive and cataleptic behavior, Psychopharmacologia 18, 346-356 (1970).

Foldes, A. and Costa, E.: Relationship of brain monoamine and locomotor activity in rats, Biochem. Pharmacol. 24, 1617-1621, (1975).

Friedman, E., Gershon, S., and Rotrosen, J.: Effects of acute cocaine treatment on the turnover of 5-hydroxytryptamine in the rat brain, Br. J. Pharmacol. 54, 61-64 (1975).

Fuxe, K., Hamberger, B., and Malmfors, T.: The effect of drugs on accumulation of monoamines in tubero-infundibular dopamine neurons, Eur. J. Pharmacol. 1, 334-341 (1967).

Galambos, E., Pfeifer, A.K., György, L., and Molnár, J.: Study on the excitation induced by amphetamine, cocaine and α-methyltryptamine, Psychopharmacologia (Berl.) 11, 122-129 (1967).

Goldberg, S.R.: Comparable behavior maintained under fixed-ratio and second-order schedules of food presentation, cocaine injection or *d*-amphetamine injection in the squirrel monkey, J. Pharmacol. exp. Ther. 186, 18-30 (1973).

Grabowska, M. and Michaluk, J.: On the role of serotonin in apomorphine-induced locomotor stimulation in rats, Pharmacol. Biochem. Behav. 2, 263-266 (1974).

Grahame-Smith, D.G.: Studies *in vivo* on the relationship between brain tryptophan, brain 5-HT synthesis and hyperactivity in rats treated with a monoamine oxidase inhibitor and l-tryptophan, J. Neurochem. 18, 1053-1066 (1971).

Grahame-Smith, D.G. and Green, A.R.: The role of brain dopamine in the hyperactivity syndrome produced in rats after administration of l-tryptophan and a monoamine oxidase inhibitor, Br. J. Pharmac. Chemother. 50, 442-443 (1974).

Green, A.R. and Grahame-Smith, D.G.: The role of brain dopamine in the hyperactivity syndrome produced by increased 5-hydroxytryptamine synthesis in rats, Neuropharmacol. 13, 949-959 (1974).

Haigler, H.J. and Aghajanian, G.K.: Peripheral serotonin antagonists: Failure to antagonize serotonin in brain areas receiving a prominent serotonergic input, J. Neural Transm. 35, 257-273 (1974).

Hamberger, B.: Reserpine-resistant uptake of catecholamines in isolated tissues of the rat. A histochemical study, Acta Physiol. Scand., Suppl. 295, (1967).

Harris, J.E. and Baldessarini, R.J.: Uptake of [^{3}H]-catecholamines by homogenates of rat corpus striatum and cerebral cortex: Effects of amphetamine analogues, Neuropharmacol. 12, 669-679 (1973).

Heikkila, R.E., Orlansky, H., Mytilineou, C., and Cohen, G.: Amphetamine: Evaluation of d- and l-isomers as releasing agents and uptake inhibitors for ^{3}H-dopamine and ^{3}H-norepinephrine in slices of rat neostriatum and cerebral cortex, J. Pharm. exp. Ther. 194, 47-56 (1975).

Hertting, G., Axelrod, J., and Whitby, L.G.: Effect of drugs on the uptake and metabolism of ^{3}H-norepinephrine, J. Pharm. exp. Ther. 134, 146-153 (1961).

Iversen, S.D.: Neural substrates mediating amphetamine responses. In: Cocaine and Other Stimulants. Ellinwood, E.H. and Kilbey, M.M., Eds. New York: Plenum Press, 1976.

Kelly, P.H., Seviour, W., and Iversen, S.: Amphetamine and apomorphine responses in the rat following 6-OHDA lesions of the nucleus accumbens septi and corpus striatum, Brain Res. 94, 507-522 (1975).

Knapp, S. and Mandell, A.J.: Narcotic drugs: Effects on the serotonin biosynthetic systems of the brain, Science 177, 1209-1211 (1972).

Kobinger, W.: Differentiation between the sedative actions of 5-hydroxytryptamine and reserpine in mice by means of two stimulating substances, Acta Pharmac. Tox. 14, 138-147 (1958).

Koe, B.K. and Weissman, A.: p-Chlorophenylalanine: A specific depletor of brain serotonin, J. Pharm. exp. Ther. 154, 499-516 (1966).

Langer, S.Z. and Enero, M.A.: The potentiation of responses to adrenergic nerve stimulation in the presence of cocaine: Its relationship to the metabolic fate of released norepinephrine, J. Pharm. exp. Ther. 191, 431-443 (1974).

Macphail, R.C. and Seiden, L.S.: Time course for the effects of cocaine on fixed-ratio water-reinforced responding in rats, Psychopharmacologia (Berl.) 44, 1-4 (1975).

Maj, J., Przegaliński, E., and Wielosz, M.: Disulfiram and the drug-induced effects of motility, J. Pharm. Pharmac. 20, 247-248 (1968).

Matthysse, S.: Antipsychotic drug actions: A clue to the neuropathology of schizophrenia, Fed. Proc. 32, 200-205 (1973).

Matussek, N. and Rüther, E.: Wirkungsmechanismus der Reserpinumkehr mit Desmethylimipramin, Med. Pharmacol. Exp. 12, 217-225 (1965).

Mawson, C. and Whittington, H.: Evaluation of the peripheral and central antagonistic activities against 5-hydroxytryptamine of some new agents, Br. J. Pharmacol. 39, 223P-224P (1970).

Modigh, K. and Svensson, T.H.: On the role of central nervous system catecholamines and 5-hydroxytryptamine in the nialamide-induced behavioral syndrome, Br. J. Pharmacol. 46, 32-45 (1972).

Mogilnicka, E. and Braestrup, C.: Evidence for a noradrenergic involvement in stereotyped behavior induced by amphetamine, J. Pharm. Pharmac. (in press).

Nielsen, M.: The influence of desipramine and amitriptyline on the accumulation of ^{3}H-noradrenaline and its two major metabolities formed from ^{3}H-tyrosine in the rat brain, J. Pharm. Pharmac. 27, 207-209 (1975).

Pfeifer, A.K., Galambos, E., and György, L.: Some central nervous properties of diethyldithiocarbamate, J. Pharm. Pharmac. 18, 254 (1966).

Pickens, R., Thompson, T., and Yokel, R.A.: Characteristics of amphetamine self administration by rats. In: Current Concepts on Amphetamine Abuse. Ellinwood, E.H. and Cohen, S., Eds., pp. 43-48. Washington, D.C.: U.S. Government Printing Office, 1972.

Pijnenburg, A.J.J. and van Rossum, J.M.: Stimulation of locomotor activity following injection of dopamine into the nucleus accumbens, J. Pharm. Pharmac. 25, 1003-1005 (1973).

Pijnenburg, A.J.J., Honig, W.M.H. and van Rossum, J.M.: Inhibition of d-amphetamine-induced locomotor activity by injection of haloperidol into the nucleus accumbens of the rats, Psychopharmacologia (Berl.) 41, 87-95 (1975a).

Pijnenburg, A.J.J., Honig, W.M.H., and van Rossum, J.M.: Effects of antagonists upon locomotor stimulation induced by injection of dopamine and noradrenaline into the nucleus accumbens of nialamide-pretreated rats, Psychopharmacologia (Berl.) 41, 175-180 (1975b).

Post, R.M.: Cocaine psychoses: A continuum model, Am. J. Psychiat. 132, 225-231 (1975).

Randrup, A., Munkvad, I., and Scheel-Krüger, J.: Mechanisms by which amphetamines produce stereotypy, aggression and other behavioural effects. In: Psychopharmacology, Sexual Disorders and Drug Abuse. Ban, T., Boissier, J., Gessa, G., Heimann, H., Hollister, L., Lehmann, H., Munkvad, I., Steinberg, H., Sulser, F., Sundwall, A., and Vinar, O., Eds., pp. 659-673. Amsterdam: North-Holland Publishing Company, 1973. Prague: Avicenum Czechoslovak Medical Press, 1973.

Randrup, A., Munkvad, I., Fog, R., and Ayhan, I.H.: Catecholamines in activation, stereotypy, and level of mood. In: Catecholamines and Behavior. Friedhoff, A.J., Ed., pp. 89-107. New York: Plenum Press, 1975.

Roberts, D.C.S., Zis, A.P., and Fibiger, H.C.: Ascending catecholamine pathways and amphetamine-induced locomotor activity: Importance of dopamine and apparent non-involvement of norepinephrine, Brain Res. 93, 441-454 (1975).

Rolinski, Z. and Scheel-Krüger, J.: The effect of dopamine and noradrenaline antagonists on amphetamine induced locomotor activity in mice and rats, Acta Pharmac. Tox. 33, 385-389 (1973).

Ross, S.B. and Renyi, A.L.: Inhibition of the uptake of tritiated catecholamines by antidepressant and related agents, Eur. J. Pharmacol. 2, 181-186 (1967).

Ross, S.B. and Renyi, A.L.: Inhibition of the uptake of tritiated 5-hydroxytryptamine in brain tissue, Eur. J. Pharmacol. 7, 270-277 (1969).

Sahakian, B.J. and Robbins, T.W.: The effects of test environment and rearing condition on amphetamine-induced stereotypy in the guinea pig, Psychopharmacologia 45, 115-117 (1975).

Samanin, R. and Garattini, S.: The serotonergic system in the brain and its possible functional connections with other aminergic systems, Life Sci. 17, 1201-1210 (1975).

Schanberg, S.M. and Cook, J.D.: Effects of acute and chronic methamphetamine on brain norepinephrine metabolism. In: Current Concepts on Amphetamine Abuse. Ellinwood, E.H. and Cohen, S., Eds., pp. 87-95. Washington, D.C.: U.S. Government Printing Office, 1972.

Scheel-Krüger, J.: Central effects of anticholinergic drugs measured by the apomorphine gnawing test in mice, Acta Pharmac. Tox. 28, 1-16 (1970).

Scheel-Krüger, J.: Comparative studies of various amphetamine analogues demonstrating different interactions with the metabolism of the catecholamines in the brain, Eur. J. Pharmacol. 14, 47-59 (1971).

Scheel-Krüger, J.: Behavioural and biochemical comparison of amphetamine derivatives, cocaine, benztropine and tricyclic antidepressant drugs, Eur. J. Pharmacol. 18, 63-73 (1972).

Scheel-Krüger, J., Braestrup, C., and Nielsen, M.: Feedback regulation of brain noradrenaline synthesis and release *in vivo* after treatment with amphetamines and tricyclic antidepressant drugs. In: Chemical Tools in Catecholamine Research. Almgreen, O., Carlsson, A., and Engel, J., Eds., pp. 227-234. Amsterdam: North-Holland Publishing Company, 1975.

Scheel-Krüger, J. and Jonas, W.: Pharmacological studies on tetrabenazine-induced excited behaviour of rats pretreated with amphetamine or nialamide, Arch. int. Pharmacodyn. 206, 47-65 (1973).

Scheel-Krüger, J. and Hasselager, E.: Studies of various amphetamines, apomorphine and clonidine on body temperature and brain 5-hydroxytryptamine metabolism in rats, Psychopharmacologia (Berl.) 36, 189-202 (1974).

Schelkunov, E.L.: Integrated effect of psychotropic drugs on the balance of cholino-, adrenö-, and serotoninergic processes in the brain as a basis of their gross behavioural and therapeutic actions, Act. Nerv. Super. (Praha) 9, 207-217 (1967).

Schrold, J.: Behavioural effects of *d*-amphetamine alone and in combination with antidepressants, antihistamines or other psychotropic drugs in young chicks, Psychopharmacologia (Berl.) 23, 115-124 (1972).

Schuster, C.R. and Wilson, M.L.: The effect of various pharmacological agents on cocaine self administration by rhesus monkeys. In: Current Concepts on Amphetamine Abuse. Ellinwood, E.H. and Cohen, S., Eds., pp. 37-41. Washington, D.C.: U.S. Government Printing Office, 1972.

Simon, P., Sultan, Z., Chermat, R., and Boissier, J-R.: La cocaine, une substance amphétaminique? Un problème de psychopharmacologi experimentale, J. Pharmacol. (Paris) 3, 129-142 (1972).

Snyder, S.H.: Catecholamines in the brain as mediators of amphetamine psychosis, Arch. gen. Psychiat. 27, 169-179 (1972).

Squires, R.F. and Buus Lassen, J.: The inhibition of A and B forms of MAO in the production of a characteristic behavioural snydrome in rats after l-tryptophan loading, Psychopharmacologia (Berl.) 41, 145-151 (1975).

Trendelenburg, U., Graefe, K-H., and Eckert, E.: The prejunctional effect of cocaine on the isolated nictitating membrane of the cat, Naunyn-Schmiedeberg's Arch. Pharmacol. 275, 69-82 (1972).

van Rossum, J.M.: Different types of sympathomimetic α-receptors, J. Pharm. Pharmac. 17, 202-216 (1965).

van Rossum, J.M.: The significance of dopamine-receptor blockade for the action of neuroleptic drugs. In: Neuropsychopharmacology. Brill, H., Cole, J.O., Deniker, P., Hippius, H., and Bradley, P.B., Eds., pp. 321-329. Amsterdam: Exerpta Medica Foundation (International Congress Series No. 129), 1967.

van Rossum, J.M.: Mode of action of psychomotor stimulant drugs, Int. Rev. Neurobiology 12, 307-383 (1970).

van Rossum, J.M., van Schoot, J.B., and Hurkman, J.A.T.M.: Mechanism of action of cocaine and amphetamine in the brain, Experientia 18, 229-230 (1962).

van Rossum, J.M. and Hurkman, J.A.T.M.: Mechanism of action of psychomotor stimulant drugs, Int. J. Neuropharmacol. 3, 227-239 (1964).

Wallach, M.B., Friedman, E., and Gershon, S.: Behavioral and neurochemical effects of psychotomimetic drugs in neonate chicks, Eur. J. Pharmacol. 17, 259-269 (1972).

Wallach, M.B. and Gershon, S.: A neuropsychopharmacological comparison of *d*-amphetamine, l-DOPA and cocaine, Neuropharmacol. 10, 743-752 (1971).

Wallach, M.B. and Gershon, S.: The induction and antagonism of central nervous system stimulant-induced stereotyped behavior in the cat, Eur. J. Pharmacol. 18, 22-26 (1972).

Weiner, W.J., Goetz, C., Westheimer, R., and Klawans, H.L.: Serotonergic and antiserotonergic influences on amphetamine-induced stereotyped behavior, J. Neurol. Sci. 20, 373-379 (1973).

Willner, J.H., Samach, M., Angrist, B., Wallach, M.B., and Gershon, S.: Drug-induced stereotyped behavior and its antagonism in dogs, Commun. Behav. Biol. 5, 135-141 (1970).

Winter, J.C.: The effects of 2,5-dimethoxy-4-methylamphetamine (DOM), 2,5-dimethoxy-4-ethylamphetamine (DOET), *d*-amphetamine, and cocaine in rats trained with mescaline as a discriminative stimulus, Psychopharmacologia (Berl.) 44, 29-32 (1975).

CHRONIC ADMINISTRATION OF STIMULANT DRUGS: RESPONSE MODIFICATION

M. Marlyne Kilbey and Everett H. Ellinwood, Jr.

Behavioral Neuropharmacology Section

Department of Psychiatry, Duke University Medical Center

Durham, North Carolina 27710

Tolerance, lack of tolerance, and reverse tolerance of physiological and behavioral responses have been reported to develop with multiple administrations of stimulant drugs (Magos, 1969; Klawans, Corsett, and Dana, 1975; Kalant, Le Blanc, and Gibbins, 1971; Kosman and Unna, 1968; and Schuster, Dockens, and Woods, 1966). Stimulants that have been investigated include cocaine, amphetamine in its various isomers and analogs, and methylphenidate. Dosages have been used that produce sustained normal activity, hyperactivity, stereotyped behavior, anorexia, and hyperthermia. Changes in these measures with multiple administrations have been evaluated in man, monkey, cat, guinea pig, and mouse. As work in this area has developed, it has become increasingly apparent that a multiplicity of drug-, subject-, behavioral-, and environmental factors, as well as the interactions of these factors, must be specified if one hopes to correlate the observed changes in response to drug with changes in biological parameters in order to elucidate neurochemical mechanisms.

The studies in this area that are most relevant to the investigations reported in this paper are those that have looked at multiple administrations of d-amphetamine as a factor in amphetamine-induced-stereotyped-behavior (AISB). Stereotyped behavior refers to repetitive sniffing, biting, gnawing, circling, ritualized motor pattern, swaying of the head, rearing, or digging which may be observed after drug administration. Magos (1969) has shown that a single injection of 6 mg/kg d-amphetamine potentiates stereotyped responding when rats are retested after two- or five-week intervals.

In this experiment sniffing and two intensities of licking and gnawing were the categories used to characterize the drug-induced behavior. Animals that had previously received amphetamine showed stereotyped licking, gnawing, paw-chewing, and mock bar-biting while control Ss showed stereotyped sniffing (Magos, 1969).

Segal and Mandell (1974) use Schiørring's (1971) description of amphetamine-induced behavior which distinguishes a "prephase" of increased activity, a "stereotypy phase" characterized by an absence of locomotion, and an "after phase" of increased activity. These investigators report that 2.5 mg/kg d-amphetamine administered for 15 days reduced locomotion significantly, suggesting a concomitant increase in AISB. With doses of 5.0 and 7.5 mg/kg administered daily for 36 days, the primary result was an increase in activity in the "after phase". When Ss were retested with 1.0 to 7.5 mg/kg seven days after cessation of the original treatment, the 7.5 mg/kg group was significantly more active in the "post-stereotypy" period. Thus, the main result of chronic treatment with both low and high doses of d-amphetamine in this study was prolonged hyperactivity although there was some augmentation of stereotypy, described as the absence of activity, in the 1.0 and 2.5 mg/kg groups.

Klawans et al. (1975) report that, after treatment with seven to ten mg/kg d-amphetamine for one or five weeks, 4.0 mg/kg amphetamine, which is normally subthreshold in the guinea pig, elicited stereotyped behavior characterized as intense gnawing. These investigators report similar potentiation of responding to subthreshold doses of apomorphine (.15 to .20 mg/kg). While they reported that stereotypies had a more rapid onset after pretreatment, no statistical evaluation was given to substantiate this observation.

These studies, which indicate the development of reverse tolerance (Segal and Mandell, 1974) and response potentiation after treatment (Segal and Mandell, 1974; Magos, 1969; Klawans et al., 1975), can be contrasted with those of other investigators also using chronic administration of stereotypy-eliciting doses of amphetamine. Lewander (1971) and Lu, Ho, and McIsaac (1972) found no change in behavior, while Gunne and Lewander (1966) reported diminished behavioral responses in rats treated for six days.

Many techniques have been used to measure behavioral responses to amphetamine, including rating of sniffing, licking, and gnawing components (Fog, Randrup, and Pakkenberg, 1967); rating of the intensity of a single component (Ernest, 1969); measuring the latency of onset and/or duration of stereotypy (Lal and Sourkes, 1972); photocell crossings; rearings; and observation of stereotypy (Segal and Mandell, 1974). In previous work we have shown a significant relationship between increasing doses of d- and l-amphetamine and increasing stereotypies, using a nine point rating scale (Ellinwood and Balster, 1974). The scale recognizes four normal and five abnormal behaviors described in Table 1. Using the scale, we have investigated the effects of multiple administrations of amphetamine or cocaine on stereotyped behavior.

In work with cats we have described the ontogeny of AISB which initially is strongly influenced by environmental contingencies and the primary arousal effects of amphetamine. After repeated episodes of intoxication, more constricted stereotyped behaviors develop and even later reactive and dyskinetic behaviors are seen (Ellinwood and Sudilovsky, 1973 a,b; Ellinwood and Kilbey, 1975a). The correlation between behavioral effects of chronic amphetamine administration in several species and the development of stimulant psychoses in man (Ellinwood, 1967, 1968, 1971) has been reviewed recently (Ellinwood and Kilbey, 1975b). One difficulty in determining the biochemical and anatomical substrates of abnormal behavior in rodents in stimulant models of psychoses has been the lack of a measure sensitive to possible

Table One

Rating scale for the behavioral effects of psychomotor stimulants in rats

Score		Definition
1	Asleep	Lying down, eyes closed
2	Inactive	Lying down, eyes open
3	Inplace activities (Grooming, consummatory)	Normal grooming, chewing cage litter, eating or drinking
4	Normal, alert, active	Moving about cage, sniffing rearing
5	Hyperactive	Running movement characterized by rapid changes in position (jerky)
6	Slow patterned	Repetitive exploration of the cage at normal levels of activity
7	Fast patterned	Repetitive exploration of the cage with hyperactivity
8	Restricted	Remaining in same place in cage with fast repetitive head and/or foreleg movement (includes licking, chewing, and gnawing stereotypies)
9	Dyskinetic-reactive	Backing up, jumping, seizures, abnormally maintained postures, dyskinetic movements

NOTE: Score represents activity which predominates in 20" interval, except for 8, which is scored only when observed for entire 20" interval

transitions in stereotyped behavior occurring as a function of chronic treatment. Thus, our major purpose in these studies was to determine if shifts in stereotyped behavior are found when Ss are given multiple administrations of stimulants at doses that originally produce hyperactivity (rating of 5) or patterned stereotypies (ratings of 6 or 7). We also wanted to determine the duration of any changes produced by multiple treatments and, thus, readministered drug after a period of abstinence.

Method

Three experiments are reported that examined the effects of chronic administration of d-amphetamine or cocaine on stereotyped behavior. One experiment is reported that utilized a dopamine-beta-hydroxylase inhibitor to lower norepinephrine (NE) levels prior to administration of d-amphetamine in order to evaluate the role of NE in stereotyped behavior. The subjects were female, Sprague-Dawley rats (Zivic Miller, Pittsburgh, Penna.) weighing approximately 120-130 grams at the beginning of each experiment. The Ss were isolated in a private room and housed in plastic cages, 16 x 8 x 8 inches, with food and water ad lib. For Experiments One and Two, the light-dark cycle was controlled manually with an approximate 8-hour light phase from 8 a.m. to 5 p.m. In Experiments Three and Four, the cycle was controlled automatically with a light period from 7 a.m. to 7 p.m. Rats were weighed every two or three days throughout an experiment. Cocaine and d-amphetamine were administered as aqueous solutions in saline. Bis (4-methyl-1-homopiperazinyl-thiocarbonyl) disulfide (FLA-63) was suspended in saline with Tween-80. All injections were i.p. at a volume of 1 cc/kg. Behavior ratings were made periodically on the basis of 20 seconds observations of each S. Throughout the experimental series, ratings were made by the same observer who was not informed of the experimental treatments. In Experiments One and Two ratings were done in the morning; in Three and Four, in the afternoon.

Experiment One

Twenty rats were randomly assigned to two equal groups. Group 1 received d-amphetamine, once daily, in the a.m. at the following doses: 4.0, 4.4, 4.8, 5.3, 5.9, 6.4, 7.1, 7.8, 8.6, and 9.4 mg/kg. On the 11th day, they received 4.0 mg/kg, and behavior was rated at 5 minutes pre- and post-injection and every 5 minutes thereafter through 45 minutes post-injection and then every 30 minutes through 150 minutes post-injection. Data were analyzed using a two-way ANOVA with one repeated measure (Winer, 1962).

Results of Experiment One

This analysis showed that there were no significant differences between the groups as a function of pretreatment ($F_{1,240} = 1.5$, $p > 0.10$). Thus, in these Ss treated once a day with amphetamine at doses from 4.0 to 9.4 mg/kg, there is no evidence for tolerance or reverse tolerance in terms of mean level of stereotypy induced by 4.0 mg/kg d-amphetamine. There was a significant time effect, as expected, ($F_{12,216} = 46.7$, $p \leq 0.01$) and a significant interaction between the pretreatment and time factors ($F_{12,216} = 4.8$, $p \leq 0.01$), reflecting the earlier onset and offset of maximum AISB in the Ss that had received ten previous administrations of amphetamine.

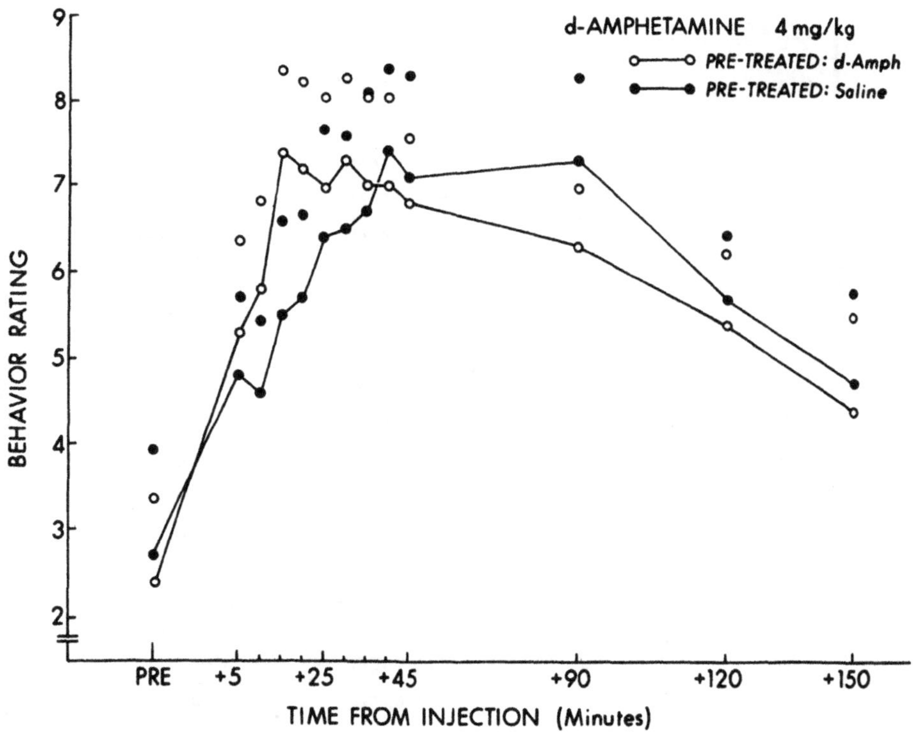

Fig. 1. Mean behavioral ratings and standard deviation on day 11.

Experiment Two

Experiment Two utilized 18 Ss randomly assigned to two groups of nine each. The experimental paradigm is presented in Table 2. Behavioral ratings were made in the morning after Administrations 1, 11, 12, and 13 at five minutes pre-injection, 5 minutes post-injection, and every 5 minutes thereafter through 45 minutes post-injection. In addition, behavior was rated at 90 minutes post-injection and at 30 minute intervals thereafter through 210 minutes post-injection.

Table Two

Administration	Group 1 d-Amphetamine	Group 2 Saline
One	7.0 mg/kg*	1 cc/kg
TWO-DAY INTERVAL - NO TREATMENT		
Two	4.0 mg/kg	1 cc/kg
Three	4.7 mg/kg	1 cc/kg
Four	4.8 mg/kg	1 cc/kg
Five	6.3 mg/kg	1 cc/kg
Six	7.0 mg/kg	1 cc/kg
TWO-DAY INTERVAL - NO TREATMENT		
Seven	7.0 mg/kg	1 cc/kg
Eight	8.0 mg/kg	1 cc/kg
Nine	9.0 mg/kg	1 cc/kg
Ten	10.0 mg/kg	1 cc/kg
Eleven	7.0 mg/kg	1 cc/kg
FOUR-DAY INTERVAL - NO TREATMENT		
Twelve	7.0 mg/kg*	d-Amphetamine 7.0 mg/kg
FOUR-DAY INTERVAL - NO TREATMENT		
Thirteen	7.0 mg/kg*	7.0 mg/kg

*Dose administered once per day (a.m.). All other days, dose administered twice per day (a.m. and p.m.).

Results of Experiment Two

Data for each group were analyzed using a two-way analysis of variance (ANOVA) with repeated measures (Winer, 1962). For Group One the behavior ratings following drug Administrations 1, 11, 12, and 13 were analyzed. These data, presented in Fig. 2, indicate a significant change in stereotyped behavior during the course of the experiment. To evaluate this further, a Dunnett's T test (Winer, 1962) was done comparing all means with the mean behavioral rating for Administration 1. This is shown in Table 3. Behavior after Administration 11 was not significantly different from that following Administration 1 which indicates that, during a period in which Ss received increasing doses of d-amphetamine twice daily, neither tolerance nor reverse tolerance developed ($p > 0.05$) for the maximum level of stereotypy induced by 7 mg/kg, d-amphetamine. However, after four days' abstinence from drug, Ss were

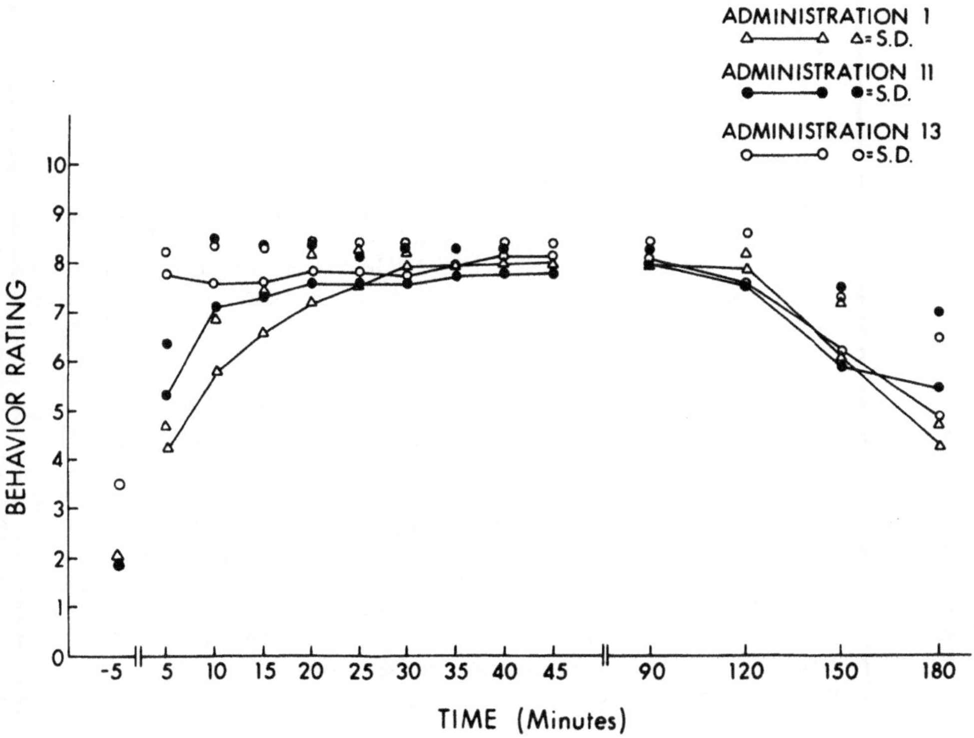

Fig. 2. Mean behavioral ratings and standard deviation for Group 1 following Administrations 1, 11, and 13.

Table Three

Outcomes of ANOVA and Comparisons of Successive Test Days: Behavioral Ratings for Nine Rats Tested with d-Amphetamine (7.0 mg/kg i.p.)

Factor	F Ratio	p Value
Test Day	$F_{3,495} = 14.89$	$p \leq 0.01$
Time	$F_{13,495} = 144.40$	$p \leq 0.01$
Test Day by Time	$F_{39,495} = 3.36$	$p \leq 0.01$
Comparison	**Dunnett's T**	**p Value**
Test on Day 1 vs Day 11	1.7	$p > 0.05$
Test on Day 1 vs Day 12	3.4	$p \leq 0.01$
Test on Day 1 vs Day 13	6.4	$p \leq 0.01$

retested with the same dose and potentiation of stereotypy was observed ($p \leq 0.01$) which was still present when Ss were again tested after an additional four days of abstinence ($p \leq 0.01$). The data for Treatment 13 (i.e., the 10th day after original treatment had stopped) are shown in Fig. 2. As Treatment 12 data (i.e., the 5th day after original treatment stopped) are very similar, they are not presented graphically.

Analysis of the behavior ratings for Group Two after Administrations 1 (saline), 11, 12, and 13 (amphetamine) also reached significance ($p \leq 0.01$), reflecting the increase in stereotyped behavior with d-amphetamine administration. This is shown in Fig. 3. The Tukey A test (Winer, 1962) demonstrated no significant differences among the mean levels of stereotyped behavior for the three amphetamine test days. A decrease in the latency of onset of stereotyped behavior is apparent between Treatment 11 and Treatment 13 and is reflected in the significant interaction of day and time factors ($p \leq 0.01$). Thus, as in Experiment One, the groups manifested a faster onset of stereotypy with repeated drug administrations even though, for Group Two, this amounts to only three injections, each separated by four days.

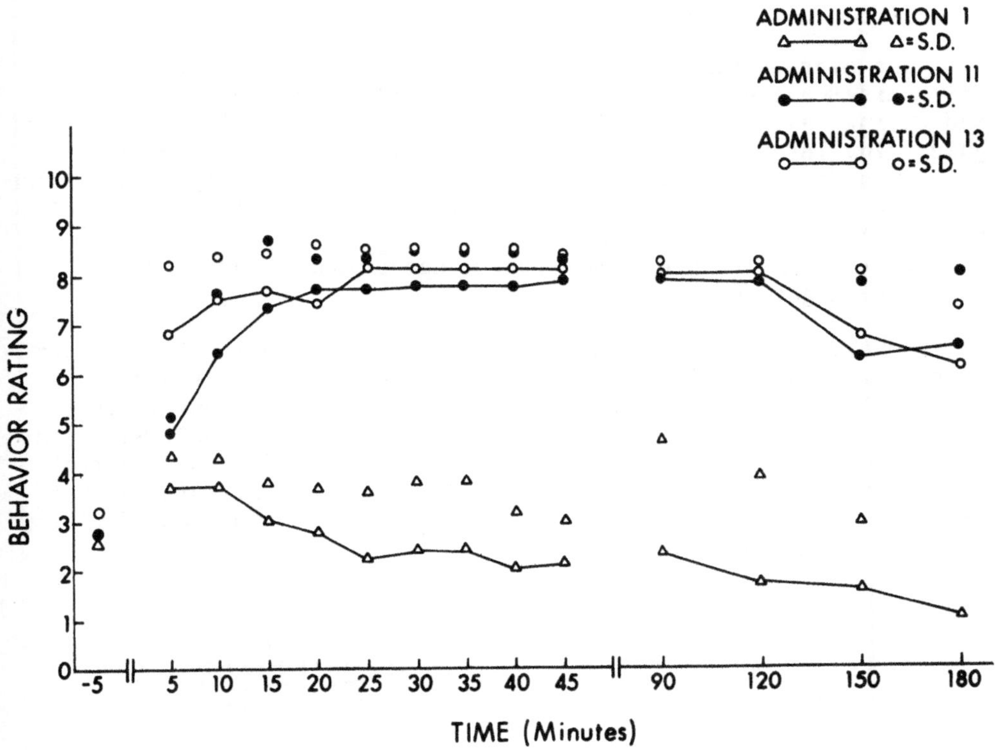

Fig. 3. Mean behavioral ratings and standard deviation for Group 2 following Administrations 1, 11, and 13.

Experiment Three

Experiment Three was designed to determine the effect of chronic administration of cocaine on cocaine-induced stereotyped behavior (CISB). Thirty rats were divided randomly into two groups. Group One received daily injections of 15 mg/kg cocaine: and Group Two, 40 mg/kg for 14 days. Behavioral ratings were made on Day 1 (Test 1), Day 4 (Test 2), Day 8 (Test 3), and Day 13 (Test 4) during daily treatment. Following cessation of daily administrations, cocaine was readministered on post-treatment Days 5, 12, 19, 26, and 54 (Tests 5, 6, 7, 8, and 9); and behavior was rated. All drug administrations were done mid-day.

Results of Experiment Three

The average daily weight gain for the two groups during the daily treatment period was not significantly different ($p > 0.05$), indicating that cocaine did not have a dose-related effect on weight gain. The intensity of stereotyped behavior induced by 40 mg/kg cocaine i.p. upon initial administration was significantly greater than that induced by 15 mg/kg ($F_{1,23} = 18.4$, $p \leq 0.01$). The dose level by time factor was significant also ($F_{18,414} = 3.6$, $p \leq 0.01$), showing that the stereotyped behavior had a longer duration in Ss given the higher dose.

Behavioral ratings were analyzed for each dose level as a function of four successive tests in which each test point represented the total stereotypy score for two test days at each post-injection time. A two-way ANOVA for repeated measures (Winer, 1962) was used and the mean behavioral ratings are shown in Fig. 4. As data from Tests 7 and 8 were very similar to Tests 5 and 6, they are not presented graphically. The results of statistical evaluation of these data are shown in Table 4.

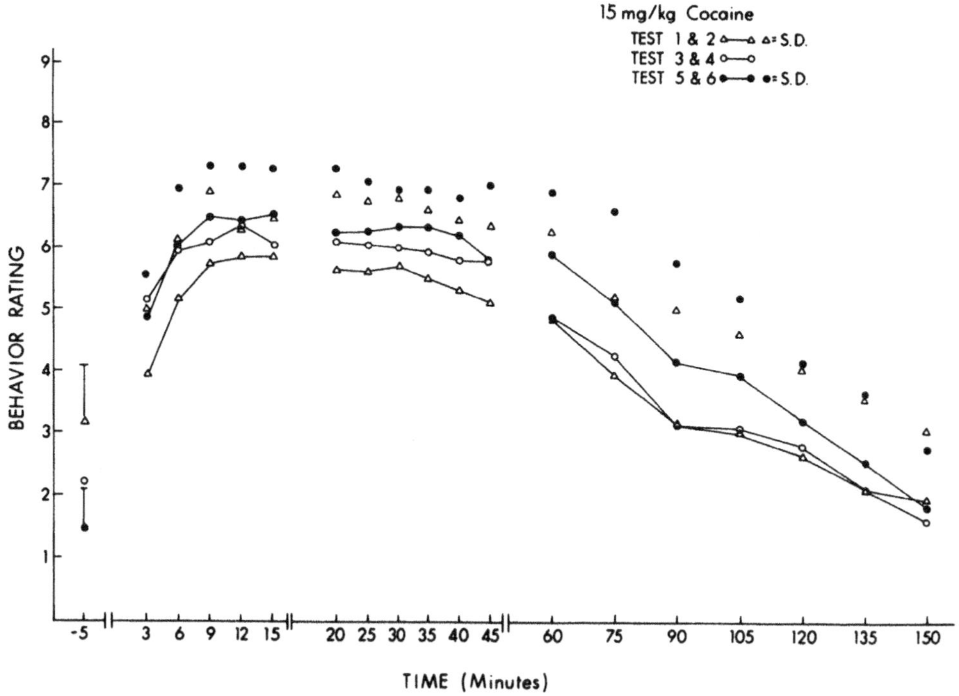

Fig. 4. Mean behavioral ratings and standard deviation for the 15 mg/kg group for Tests 1 through 6.

Table Four

Outcome of ANOVA and Comparisons of Successive Test Days: Behavioral Ratings for Rats Treated with Cocaine (15 mg/kg: 14 Ss)

Factor	F Ratio	p Value
Test	$F_{3,975} = 43.87$	$p \leq 0.01$
Time	$F_{18,975} = 231.40$	$p \leq 0.01$
Test x Time	$F_{54,975} = 1.36$	$p \leq 0.05$
Comparison	**Dunnett's T**	**p Value**
Tests 1 & 2 vs Tests 3 & 4	4.9	$p \leq 0.01$
Tests 1 & 2 vs Tests 5 & 6	9.4	$p \leq 0.01$
Tests 1 & 2 vs Tests 7 & 8	10.0	$p \leq 0.01$

Tests 1, 2, 3, 4 were done during 14-day drug administration period. Tests 5, 6, 7, 8 were done at 5, 12, 19, and 26 days post treatment.

Data for Group One (15 mg/kg) show that potentiation for stereotyped behavior was seen during the course of daily treatment. The combined data for Tests One and Two, however, represent a drop in the average behavioral rating on the second test. The behavioral ratings rose during the second week (Tests 3 and 4), indicating greater stereotypy and the combined data reached significance in the individual comparison test (Table 4). Response potentiation is significant, also, when cocaine is re-administered after daily treatment ceases. This effect is similar to that seen in Experiment Two with d-amphetamine. This is illustrated by data from Test Nine, completed at 54 days post-treatment. These data continue to reflect significant response potentiation in comparison with the initial test, illustrated in Fig. 5.

The data for Group Two (40 mg/kg) (Fig. 6) and statistical evaluation (Table 5) indicate potentiation of the maximum response during and after treatment. The data from Tests 7 and 8 are not presented graphically as they are very similar to those for Tests 5 and 6. Likewise, the statistical outcome from Test 9, which indicated significantly potentiated response in comparison with

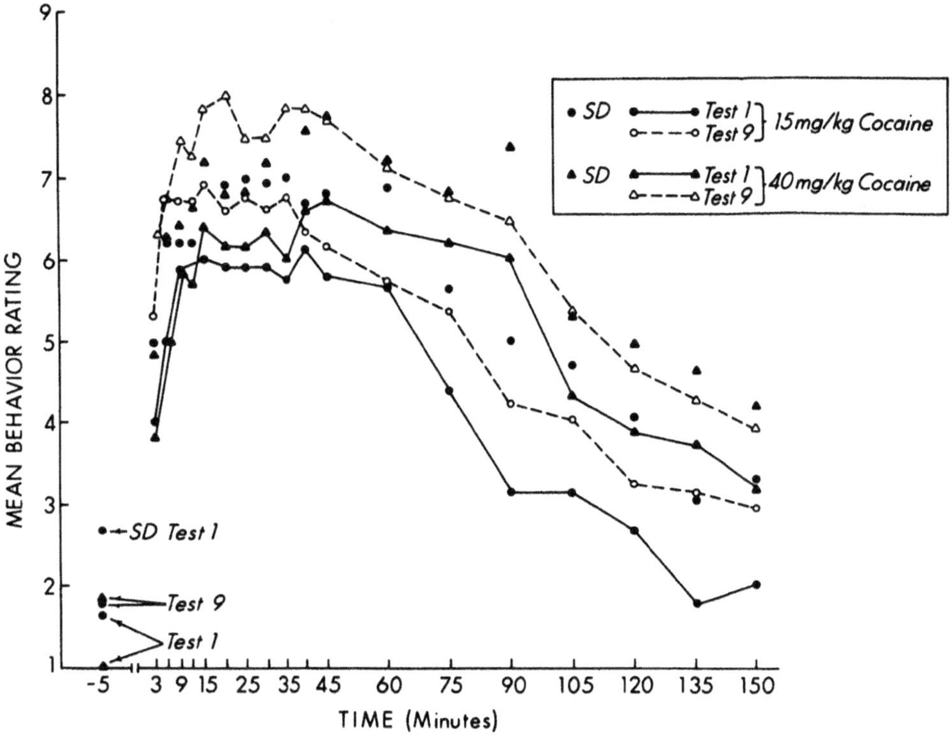

Fig. 5. Mean and standard deviation of behavior ratings following initial administration of cocaine at two dose levels and 54 days following cessation of 14 daily administrations.

Day One, is not included in Table 5, but is illustrated in Fig. 5. The significantly more rapid onset of stereotyped behavior at both cocaine dose levels is similar to that seen with d-amphetamine, while the steady augmentation of maximum response has been seen during treatment with cocaine only. Response augmentation, however, followed re-administration of both stimulants.

Experiments One, Two, and Three have shown that, as a result of initial injections of d-amphetamine or cocaine, subsequent injection leads to more rapid onset of stereotyped behaviors. In Experiments Two and Three, stimulant treatment was associated with potentiation of the level of stereotyped response when drugs were readministered periodically for periods of up to 54 days. In Experiment 3, potentiation of the mean response level was seen during daily treatment with cocaine.

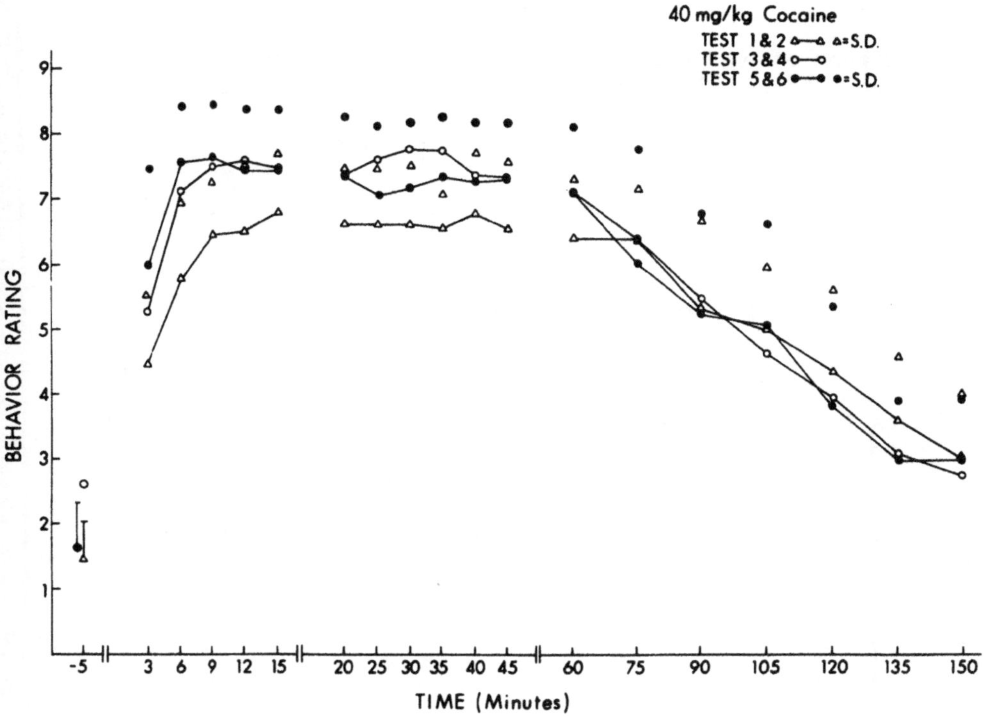

Fig. 6. Mean behavioral ratings and standard deviation for the 40 mg/kg cocaine group for Test 1 through 6.

Experiment Four

In an attempt to determine if NE mechanisms may contribute to the onset of stereotyped behavior, we tested the effects of FLA-63, a dopamine-beta-hydroxylase inhibitor, on this response. We reasoned that, if NE mechanisms contributed to the expression of AISB, reducing the synthesis of NE and lowering the amount available for release by amphetamine might delay the onset and/or decrease the level of AISB. On the other hand, if NE had an inhibitory effect on AISB, then one might expect to see a more rapid onset and/or higher level of AISB. Some support for the latter came from the finding of increased AISB in rats pretreated with disulfiram (Ellinwood and Kilbey, 1975b) or with reserpine and FLA-63 (Corrodi, Fuxe, Ljungdahl, and Ogren, 1970). Attributing these effects to NE mechanisms must be done cautiously, however, as in our study the response potentiation could have reflected disulfiram's action on dopamine mechanisms (Goldstein and Nakajima, 1967) while, in the Corrodi et al. study, behavior was recorded in a semi-quantitative manner and was not subjected to statistical analysis.

Table Five

Outcome of ANOVA and Comparisons of Successive Test Days: Behavioral Ratings for Rats Treated with Cocaine (40 mg/kg: 11 Ss)

Factor	F Ratio	p Value
Test	$F_{3,750} = 29.71$	$p \leq 0.01$
Time	$F_{18,750} = 203.78$	$p \leq 0.01$
Test x Time	$F_{54,750} = 1.77$	$p \leq 0.01$
Comparison	**Dunnett's T**	**p Value**
Tests 1 & 2 vs Tests 3 & 4	6.8	$p \leq 0.01$
Tests 1 & 2 vs Tests 5 & 6	6.0	$p \leq 0.01$
Tests 1 & 2 vs Tests 7 & 8	9.0	$p \leq 0.01$

Tests 1, 2, 3, 4 were done during 14-day drug administration period.
Tests 5, 6, 7, 8 were done at 5, 12, 19, and 26 days post treatment.

The Ss were 18 rats randomly divided into three groups of six assigned to one of three dose levels of FLA-63: 0, 10, or 25 mg/kg. Two hours after FLA-63 treatment, one of three levels of d-amphetamine (0, 3, or 12 mg/kg) was administered to each S in counterbalanced order. Dose levels of FLA-63 were chosen on the basis of work that has shown that 25 mg/kg of FLA-63 reduces NE in the rat brain to approximately 1/4th normal (Corrodi et al., 1970). Tests were given one week apart. Behavioral ratings were made periodically from 20 minutes pre-injection through 270 minutes post-injection.

Results of Experiment Four

As we were interested in the effect of FLA-63 on the early components of the amphetamine response, the behavioral ratings for each amphetamine group over the first 30 minutes were analyzed using an ANOVA for a 2-way design with one repeated measure. Administration of a NE synthesis inhibitor delayed the onset of behavioral stereotypies in the 12 mg/kg d-amphetamine group ($p \leq 0.01$) for both 10 and 25 mg/kg FLA-63 groups. However, FLA-63 had no effect on the behavioral changes associated with 3 mg/kg d-amphetamine ($p > 0.10$). Thus, while the data suggest that the more rapid onset of stereotypies we have observed may reflect more release of newly synthesized NE after chronic treatment, the failure to demonstrate a dose-response function demands that these data be considered as suggestive, only.

DISCUSSION

The major findings of these studies are that multiple injections of d-amphetamine and cocaine are associated with a more rapid onset of stereotyped behavior during drug treatment as well as when the drug is re-administered after periodic abstinence of up to 54 days. Likewise, administration of cocaine results in a potentiation of the maximum CISB during daily treatment as well as when cocaine is re-administered periodically throughout a 54 day post-drug period. In addition, re-administration of d-amphetamine after a drug-free interval results in potentiation of the maximum stereotyped response. A preliminary study suggests that a mechanism underlying the development of more rapid onset of AISB may be dependent on the release of newly synthesized NE by amphetamine as administration of FLA-63, a beta hydroxylase inhibitor, retards the onset of AISB after administration of 12 mg/kg d-amphetamine.

These experiments have implications for several current behavioral neuropharmacological problems. One concern in our laboratory has been the development of a measure of chronic drug effects in rats which reflects the range of behavioral changes similar to that we have observed in cats administered amphetamine chronically. We have quantified these effects in the cat using the behavioral rating inventory for drug-generated effects (BRIDGE) scale (Sudilovsky, Ellinwood, Dorsey, and Nelson, 1975).

In developing a scale for measuring these effects in rats, Ellinwood and Balster (1975) showed a positive dose relationship for d- and l-amphetamine reflected in increasing stereotypies and an inhibitory dose response effect for pimozide. The present studies have shown clearly that this scale is sensitive to changes in the onset of AISB and CISB that were found to occur with multiple administration of the drugs. Thus, using this scale, we have been able to replicate Klawan's observation (1975) of decreased latency in onset of stereotyped responses in guinea pigs following pretreatment with amphetamine. We have quantified the change, and shown that it endures, in the case of cocaine, for over seven weeks following cessation of daily treatment. Furthermore, we have quantified the potentiation of the maximal AISB or CISB. Previous investigators have shown changes during or following chronic amphetamine treatment that represent (1) a lowering of the threshold amount of amphetamine or apomorphine to induce stereotyped behavior

(Klawans et al., 1975); (2) an increase in amphetamine-induced activity, or, at higher doses, an increase in the post-stereotyped phase hyperactivity; or (3) an increase in stereotype measured by the absence of locomotor activity (Segal and Mandell, 1974; Segal, 1975). Similar shifts in response towards greater amphetamine-induced hyperactivity have been shown following cessation of pretreatment with α-methyl-para-tyrosine (Beuthin, Miya, Blake, and Bosquet, 1972; Dominic and Moore, 1969; Geyer and Segal, 1973) and have been attributed to supersensitivity of post synaptic receptors following extended periods during which catecholamine synthesis was suppressed. However, it has been difficult to assess contributions of various catecholamine mechanisms to these behaviors because of the question of whether or not behaviors described as normal activity, hyperactivity, slow and fast patterned stereotypies, and reactive and dyskinetic behaviors are related in any specific manner.

Showing that chronic social isolation potentiates amphetamine-induced stereotypy, but not hyperactivity, other investigators (Sahakian, Robbins, Morgan, and Iversen, 1975) have argued that different mechanisms underlie hyperactivity and stereotypy. The present studies, which show a shift from hyperactivity to slow patterned stereotypy (15 mg/kg cocaine group); from slow to fast patterned stereotypy (40 mg/kg cocaine group); and from fast patterned stereotypy to restricted stereotypy (d-amphetamine group), argue that these behaviors, even if they represent a variety of mechanisms, form a continuum as they are observed sequentially with chronic administration although category 9 (i.e., dyskinetic-reactive behavior) on our scale requires further validation. Thus, from a pragmatic viewpoint, these studies have further established a scale sensitive to a range of behaviors associated with chronic stimulant use. The scale should be appropriate for investigation of aminergic and anatomical contributions to these behaviors and thus contribute to our understanding of amphetamine-induced psychoses in man.

In terms of elucidating a mechanism or mechanisms active during the ontogeny of stimulant-induced behavior, the data of these studies are more difficult to interpret. It is generally accepted that amphetamine has two major actions: (1) release of NE and dopamine (DA) and (2) inhibition of re-uptake of these catecholamines (Iversen and Iversen, 1975). Brain levels of amphetamine reach their peak at 30 min post-injection after acute administration of doses from 0.25 to 8.0 mg/kg (Maickel, Cox, Miller, Segal, and Russell, 1969): a time course which coincides with the onset of maximum stereotyped behavior in our animals after initial administration of amphetamine. After acute cocaine administration, stereotypy reached a maximum level at 15 minutes and, after chronic administration, this peak was seen at 6 to 9 minutes. These data correlate very well with Ho's (1976) finding that, after acute treatment, unchanged cocaine in brain has a half-life of 13 minutes which is reduced to 8.5 minutes after repeated administrations.

Experiment Four suggests that release of newly synthesized NE may contribute to the initial onset of AISB as treatment with FLA-63 retarded the onset in Ss given 12 mg/kg d-amphetamine and suggest that NE may be released more rapidly after multiple administrations. Further investigation of this point is required, however, as we failed to show a dose-related effect. Also, it is now apparent that the use of an experimental design in which various levels of an agonist or antagonist plus the stimulant are repeatedly administered to a subject is not appropriate to evaluate the effects of these agents on AISB or CISB, as the behaviors change significantly as a function of as few as three administrations of stimulants (Experiment 2) separated by four days as well as during daily administration (Experiment 3). In addition, a single dose of amphetamine has been reported to potentiate responsiveness two and five weeks following treatment (Magos, 1969).

Segal (1975) has shown that striatal DA biosynthesis is depressed for 12 hours following 5.0 mg/kg amphetamine. He suggests that amphetamine will produce a potentiated response when readministered during a period of compensatorily elevated DA biosynthesis. As Seiden, Fischman, and Schuster (1976) have shown, long-term depletions of caudate DA and midbrain and frontal cortex NE follow chronic methamphetamine administration; similar depletions may underlie our observations.

The data we report--(1) a decrease in latency of AISB and CISB during and post-treatment, (2) a potentiation of maximum CISB during treatment, and (3) a potentiation of maximum AISB and CISB post-treatment--may reflect alterations in drug metabolism with chronic treatment, changes in levels of striatal DA, and altered striatal DA biosynthesis, and/or presynaptic and postsynaptic supersensitivity mechanisms.

ACKNOWLEDGMENTS

The authors wish to thank Nancy Wagoner, who rated the behavior of the animals in these studies.

This research was supported by NIDA Grants DA-00386 and DA-00057.

REFERENCES

Beuthin, F.C., Miya, R.S., Blake, D.E., and Bosquet, W.F.: Enhanced sensitivity to noradrenergic agonists and tolerance development to α-methyl-tyrosine in the rat, J. Pharmac. exp. Ther. 181, 446-456 (1972).

Corrodi, H., Fuxe, K., Ljungdahl, A., and Ogren, S-O.: Studies on the action of some psychoactive drugs on central noradrenaline neurones after inhibition of dopamine-β-hydroxylase, Brain Res. 24, 451-470 (1970).

Dominic, J.A. and Moore, K.E.: Supersensitivity to the central stimulant actions of adrenergic drugs following discontinuation of a chronic diet of methyltyrosine, Psychopharmacologia 15, 96-101 (1969).

Ellinwood, E.H.: Amphetamine psychosis: I. Description of the individuals and process, J. nerv. ment. Dis. 144, 273-283 (1967).

Ellinwood, E.H.: Amphetamine psychosis: II. Theoretical implications, J. Neuropsychiat. 4, 45-54 (1968).

Ellinwood, E.H.: Effect of chronic methamphetamine intoxication in rhesus monkeys, Biol. Psychiat. 3, 25-32 (1971).

Ellinwood, E.H. and Balster, R.L.: Rating the behavioral effects of amphetamines, Eur. J. Pharmacol. 28, 35-41 (1974).

Ellinwood, E.H. and Kilbey, M.M.: Amphetamine stereotypy: The influence of environmental factors and prepotent behavioral patterns on its topography and development, Biol. Psychiat. 10, 3-16 (1975a).

Ellinwood, E.H. and Kilbey, M.M.: Species differences in response to amphetamine. In: Psychopharmacogenetics. Eleftheriou, B.L., Ed., pp. 323-375. New York: Plenum Press, 1975b.

Ellinwood, E.H. and Sudilovsky, A.: Chronic amphetamine intoxication: Behavioral model of psychoses. In: Psychopathology and Psychopharmacology. Cole, J.O., Freedman, A.M., and Friedhoff, A.J., Eds., pp. 51-70. Baltimore: Johns Hopkins University Press, 1973a.

Ellinwood, E.H. and Sudilovsky, A.: The relationship of the amphetamine model psychosis to schizophrenia. In: Psychopharmacology, Sexual Disorders and Drug Abuse. Ban, T.A., Boissier, J.R., Gessa, G.J., Heimann, H., Hollister, L., Lehmann, H.E., Munkvad, I., Steinberg, H., Sulser, F., Sundwall, A., and Vinar, O., Eds., pp. 189-203. Amsterdam and London: North-Holland Publishing Company; Prague: Avicenum, Czechoslovak Medical Press, 1973b.

Ernest, A.M.: The role of biogenic amines in the extrapyramidal system, Acta physiol. pharmac. néerl. 15, 141-154 (1969).

Fog, R.A., Randrup, A., and Pakkenberg, H.: Aminergic mechanisms in corpus striatum and amphetamine-induced stereotyped behavior, Psychopharmacologia 11, 179-183 (1967).

Geyer, M.A. and Segal, D.S.: Differential effects of reserpine and alpha-methyl-p-tyrosine on norepinephrine and dopamine induced behavioral activity, Psychopharmacologia 29, 131-140 (1973).

Goldstein, M. and Nakajima, K.: The effect of disulfiram on catecholamine levels in the brain, J. Pharmac. exp. Ther. 157, 96-102 (1967).

Gunne, L.M. and Lewander, T.: Brain catecholamines during chronic amphetamine intoxication, Res. Publs Ass. Res. nerv. ment. Dis. 46, 106-116 (1966).

Ho, B.: Behavioral effects of cocaine: Metabolic and neurochemical approach. In: Cocaine and Other Stimulants. Ellinwood, E.H. and Kilbey, M.M., Eds. New York: Plenum Press, 1976.

Iversen, S.D. and Iversen, L.L.: Behavioral Pharmacology. New York: Oxford University Press, 1975.

Kalant, H., Le Blanc, A.E., and Gibbins, R.J.: Tolerance to, and dependence on, some non-opiate psychotropic drugs, Pharmac. Rev. 23, 135-191 (1971).

Klawans, H.L., Corsett, P., and Dana, N.: Effect of chronic amphetamine exposure on stereotyped behavior: Implications for pathogenesis of l-dopa-induced dyskinesias, Adv. Neurol. 9, 105-112 (1975).

Kosman, M.E. and Unna, K.R.: Effects of chronic administration of the amphetamines and other stimulants on behavior, Clin. Pharmacol. Therap. 9, 240-254 (1968).

Lal, S. and Sourkes, T.I.: Potentiation and inhibition of the amphetamine stereotypy in rats by neuroleptics and other agents, Archs int. Pharmacodyn. Thér. 199, 289-301 (1972).

Lewander, T.: Urinary excretion and tissue levels of catecholamines during chronic amphetamine intoxication, Psychopharmacologia 13, 394-407 (1968).

Lu, T.C., Ho, B.T., and McIssac, W.M.: Effects of repeated administration of DL-amphetamine and methamphetamine on tolerance to hyperactivity, Experientia 28, 1461 (1972).

Magos, L.: Persistence of the effect of amphetamine on stereotyped activity in rats, Eur. J. Pharmacol. 6, 200-201 (1969).

Maickel, R.P., Cox, R.H., Miller, F.P., Segal, D.S., and Russell, R.W.: Correlation of brain levels of drugs with behavioral effects, J. Pharmac. exp. Ther. 165, 216-224 (1969).

Sahakian, B.J., Robbins, T.W., Morgan, M.J., and Iversen, S.D.: The effects of psychomotor stimulants on stereotypy and locomotor activity in socially-deprived and control rats, Brain Res. 84, 195-205 (1975).

Schiørring, E.: Amphetamine induced selective stimulation of certain behaviour items with concurrent inhibition of others in an openfield test with rats, Behaviour 39, 1-17 (1971).

Schuster, C.R., Dockens, W.S., and Woods, J.H.: Behavioral variables affecting the development of amphetamine tolerance, Psychopharmacologia 9, 170-182 (1966).

Segal, D.S.: Behavioral and neurochemical correlates of repeated d-amphetamine administration. In: Neurobiological Mechanisms of Adaptation and Behavior. Mandell, A.J., Ed., pp. 247-262. New York: Raven Press, 1975.

Seiden, L.S., Fischman, M.W., and Schuster, C.R.: Changes in brain catecholamine induced by long-term methamphetamine administration in rhesus monkeys. In: Cocaine and Other Stimulants. Ellinwood, E.H. and Kilbey, M.M., Eds. New York: Plenum Press, 1976.

Sudilovsky, A., Ellinwood, E.H., Dorsey, F., and Nelson, L.: Evaluation of the Duke University Behavioral Rating Inventory for Drug Generated Effects (BRIDGE). In: Prediction in Psychopharmacology: Preclinical and Clinical Correlations. Sudilovsky, A., Gershon, S., and Beer, B., Eds., pp. 189-212. New York: Raven Press, 1975.

Winer, B.J.: Statistical Principles in Experimental Design. New York: McGraw-Hill, 1962.

DIFFERENTIAL EFFECTS OF SEROTONIN DEPLETION ON AMPHETAMINE-INDUCED LOCOMOTION AND STEREOTYPY

David S. Segal

University of California, San Diego

La Jolla, California 92093

INTRODUCTION

We have previously demonstrated that long-term administration of d-amphetamine in rats results in a progressive augmentation of stereotypy and/or locomotion, depending upon dose. Similar behavioral changes have been observed with repeated injection of l-amphetamine and methylphenidate (Segal, unpublished data). Since amphetamine has been shown to exert effects on both catecholaminergic and serotonergic systems in the brain, it is conceivable that alterations in one or more of these neurochemical systems are responsible for the chronic amphetamine-induced behavioral augmentation. In fact, some evidence indicates that brain serotonin (5-HT) may be implicated since its depletion by either parachlorophenylalanine (PCPA) (Swonger and Rech, 1972; Mabry and Campbell, 1973; Breese, Cooper, and Mueller, 1974; Neuberg and Thut, 1974) or raphe lesion (Neill, Grant, and Grossman, 1972; Costall and Naylor, 1974; Jacobs, Wise, and Taylor, 1975; Geyer, Puerto, Menkes, Segal, and Mandell, 1976a) has been reported to enhance amphetamine-induced locomotion. Although the effects of 5-HT depletion on stereotypy are somewhat more equivocal (Rotrosen, Angrist, Wallach, and Gershon, 1972; Swonger and Rech, 1972; Weiner, Goetz, Westheimer, and Klawans, 1973; Breese et al., 1974; Costall and Naylor, 1974; Baldessarini, Amatruda, Griffin, and Gerson, 1975; Weiner, Goetz, and Klawans, 1975), it is possible that the behavioral augmentation observed with repeated administration of amphetamine is due, at least in part, to a progressive decrease in the functional activity of brain 5-HT systems.

However, it is difficult to compare the alterations in the

response reported by others to result from 5-HT depletion with those we observe after chronic amphetamine administration. One reason for this is that in most previous studies locomotion and stereotypy have been assessed separately. However, if these behaviors are subserved by the action of amphetamine on different neurochemical systems, the particular behavior expressed during any interval of time might reflect the net effect of a competitive interaction between the mechanisms underlying the two behaviors. That is, facilitation of one behavior could result from its specific activation and/or from suppression of competing responses. Therefore, it is essential that both components of the amphetamine response be evaluated concurrently.

Furthermore, it has been shown that moderate to high doses of amphetamine produce a multiphasic behavioral sequence, consisting of an initial period of hyperactivity, a stereotypy phase during which both rearing and locomotion are absent, and a post-stereotypy phase of enhanced motor activity after which locomotion may be suppressed for an extended period of time, depending upon dose (Segal and Mandell, 1974; Segal, 1975a). Our previous investigations have indicated that relatively complete temporal characterization of the behavioral sequence is necessary for accurate interpretation of the effects of pretreatment procedures. Therefore, to characterize the effects of 5-HT depletion, we monitored amphetamine-induced locomotion and stereotypy continuously for at least 8 hours following injection in different groups of rats pretreated with 5-HT depleting agents (parachlorphenylalanine or parachloramphetamine) or after raphe lesion.

MATERIALS AND METHODS

Adult male Wistar rats (300-325 g) that were obtained from Hilltop Labs (Pittsburgh, PA) were used in all the experiments. After one week of housing under standard laboratory conditions, the rats were placed individually into sound-attenuated chambers (12x12x15"). Food and water were available *ad libitum* and a 12-hour bright light (6 am to 6 pm)/12-hour dim light cycle was maintained. The animals lived in the experimental chambers for at least 24 hours prior to and for the duration of experimentation. Movement from one quadrant to another (crossovers) was automatically measured through contacts in the floors of the chambers. Rearings were measured by touchplates set 5" above the floor. Both measures of locomotion were continuously monitored by a Nova 1200 computer. Viewing lenses located in each experimental chamber and a closed circuit videotape system allowed for regular observation without disturbing the animals.

Our previous observations of the animals during the various

phases of the amphetamine response indicated that the intensity of stereotypy, in the form of continuous sniffing, licking, gnawing, and repetitive movement of the head and forelimbs, is inversely related to the frequency of rearings and crossovers. Furthermore, preliminary studies showed that the qualitative features of the repetitive behaviors displayed during the stereotypy phase do not appear to be significantly altered by the pretreatment procedures employed. Therefore, in the present studies the transient decrement in locomotion and rearing typically present in the pattern of behavior elicited by moderate to high doses of amphetamine was used as an index of the onset and duration of the stereotypy phase.

RESULTS

Parachlorophenylalanine: After at least 24 hours of habituation to the experimental chambers, the rats were injected with either PCPA (300 mg/kg) or vehicle (peanut oil), followed 48 hours later with various doses of d-amphetamine (0.5, 2.5, or 4.0 mg/kg). Preliminary studies indicated that PCPA effects on the amphetamine response were minimal during the first 24 hours after injection. Because of the carryover effects previously demonstrated to occur with amphetamine (Segal and Mandell, 1974; Segal, 1975a), each animal received only one injection of amphetamine. The rats were disturbed for only 2-3 minutes each day (about 10 am) during which time they were injected and their chambers serviced.

Figure 1 illustrates the effect of PCPA pretreatment on spontaneous and low-dose amphetamine-induced motor activity. As previously described, PCPA produced a significant elevation in spontaneous activity, although the pattern of activity closely parallels that of control animals. After the initial peak increase in crossovers (49 ± 7 and 19 ± 4, respectively; $P<0.01$) which followed saline injection, crossovers in both groups declined markedly. However, the activity levels for the PCPA group remained comparatively elevated throughout the light phase (12 ± 2 and 3 ± 1 per hour, respectively; $P<0.01$). Rearings during the first hour and the remainder of the light phase were similarly affected after PCPA administration (20 ± 4 and 5 ± 2, P 0.01; and 3 ± 0.5 and 0.5 ± 0.3 per hour, respectively; $P<0.01$). These differences in activity were not simply initiated by disturbance of the animals: PCPA pretreated rats exhibited significantly greater activity than controls even when left undisturbed.

Pretreatment with PCPA also potentiated the response to the 0.5 mg/kg dose of d-amphetamine (Fig. 1). The enhanced locomotion during the 4 hours following amphetamine injection is apparent for both crossovers (509 ± 104 and 277 ± 55, $P<0.22$) and rearings (136 ± 26 and 34 ± 10, $P<0.01$). These results reveal a synergistic

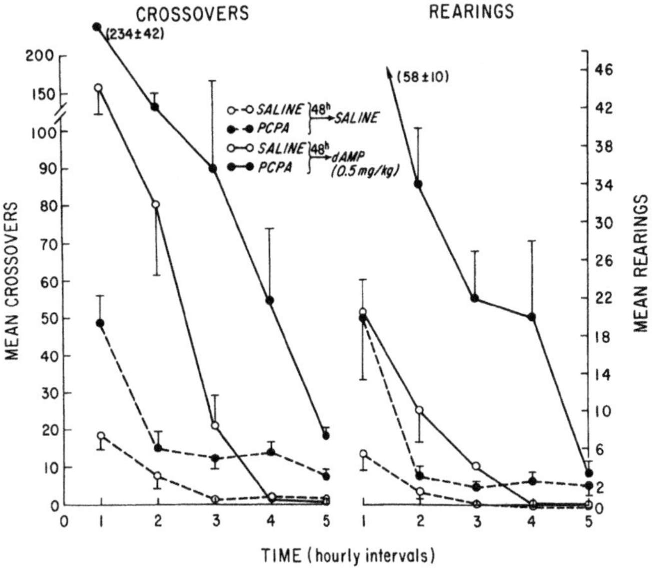

Fig. 1. Mean crossovers ± S.E.M. (left panel) and rearings ± S.E.M. (right panel) during successive hourly intervals following s.c. injection of either 0.5 mg/kg d-amphetamine or isotonic saline. Rats were previously injected (48 hours) with either PCPA (300 mg/kg, s.c.) or vehicle; N = at least 10 animals in each group. Parachlorophenylalanine pretreatment significantly increased spontaneous activity (saline group) and potentiated the locomotion evoked by 0.5 mg/kg d-amphetamine. The synergistic effects of PCPA and amphetamine are especially apparent during the fourth hour after injection. (From Segal, unpublished data)

action of the two drugs which is especially apparent during the fourth hour after injection when the behavior of non-pretreated amphetamine animals has declined to saline control levels. If the effects of the two drugs were simply additive, the activity of the PCPA-pretreated animals that received amphetamine would be expected to decline to PCPA control levels during the fourth hour. Instead, the PCPA-amphetamine group exhibited significantly greater activity than did the PCPA-saline group (crossovers: 54 ± 20 and 13 ± 3, $P<0.02$; rearings: 20 ± 8 and 3 ± 1, $P<0.05$).

The effects of PCPA pretreatment on behavior elicited by higher doses of amphetamine, i.e., 2.5 and 4.0 mg/kg, are illustrated in Figs. 2 and 3, respectively. Instead of the prolonged interval of stereotypy typically produced by a dose of 2.5 mg/kg, after PCPA pretreatment crossovers and rearings emerge as the predominant behaviors during this period (12-minute intervals 4-10, crossovers: 215 ± 36 and 12 ± 4, $p<0.01$; rearings: 68 ± 31 and 3 ± 1, $P<0.01$). Locomotor activity exhibited during the stereotypy phase is similar in appearance to that displayed by control rats during the pre- and post-stereotypy intervals. As previously described (Segal, 1975b), the locomotion is perseverative; that is, the rats tend to follow fixed patterns of movement. Parachlorophenylalanine pretreatment also elevated motor activity during the post-stereotypy intervals (hours 3-7, crossovers: 542 ± 105 and 257 ± 19, $P<0.02$; rearings: 168 ± 49 and 52 ± 6, $P<0.05$).

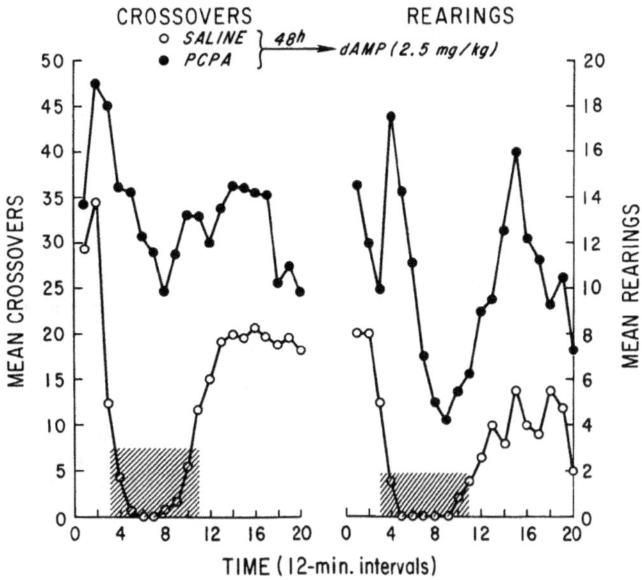

Fig. 2. Locomotor activity during successive 12-minute intervals for the first 4 hours after saline or 2.5 mg/kg d-amphetamine administration in rats injected 48 hours earlier with either PCPA (300 mg/kg) or vehicle; N = at least 10 rats/group. In controls amphetamine produces a multiphasic pattern of behavioral change (the shaded area indicates the presence of focused stereotypy during which most of the rats do not display crossovers or rearings). Locomotion emerges as the prominent behavior during the stereotypy interval when PCPA is administered 48 hours prior to amphetamine. (From Segal, unpublished data.)

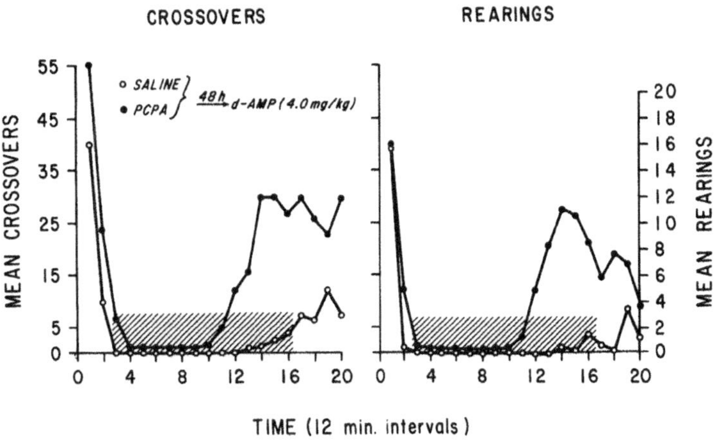

Fig. 3. Forty-eight hours after PCPA (300 mg/kg), 4.0 mg/kg d-amphetamine produces focused stereotypy (shaded area) with significantly shorter duration than for the control group; N = 8 animals/group. (From Segal, unpublished data)

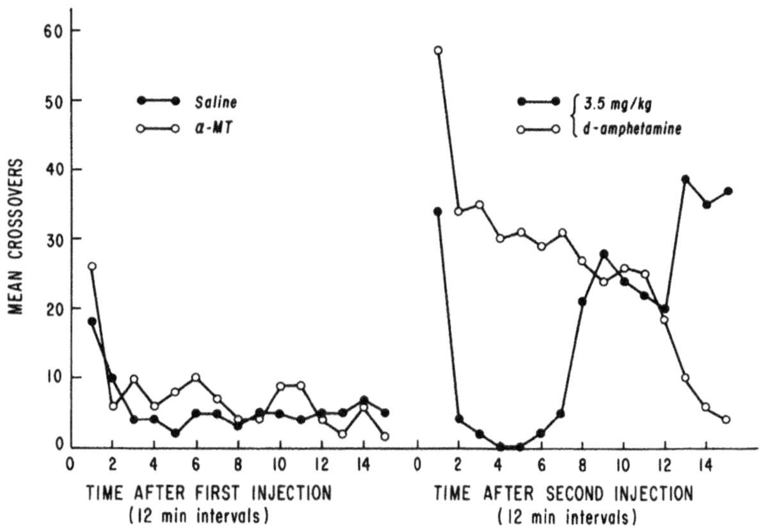

Fig. 4. Mean crossovers during successive 12-minute intervals following injection of either 100 mg/kg αMT or saline (left panel). Three hours later both groups (N = 8 animals/group) were injected i.p. with 3.5 mg/kg d-amphetamine and their behavioral activity was monitored for an additional three hours (right panel). Reprinted from Pharmac. Biochem. Behav. 2:249-255, 1974, by permission of ANKHO International Inc., C 1974.

With the higher dose of amphetamine (4.0 mg/kg) PCPA pretreatment did not completely abolish focused stereotypy (Fig. 3). The PCPA group showed a latency to onset of stereotypy which was only slightly longer than for corresponding controls; however, the duration was markedly increased (12-minute intervals 3-16, crossovers: 130 ± 23 and 10 ± 4, P<0.01; rearings: 40 ± 6 and 3 ± 2, P<0.01). In addition, as with the lower doses of amphetamine, PCPA pretreatment significantly elevated the locomotor activity during the post-stereotypy phase (hours 4-7, crossovers: 272 ± 106 and 74 ± 13, P<0.05; rearings: 69 ± 16 and 17 ± 3, P<0.01).

We have previously demonstrated that alpha-methyl-p-tyrosine (αMT) can also produce a displacement of stereotypy by locomotion (Fig. 4). However, although the stereotypy produced by 3.5 mg/kg d-amphetamine is abolished following αMT pretreatment, the duration of the amphetamine effect is also substantially diminished. Therefore, αMT appears to decrease the effective dose of amphetamine. In contrast, with both the 2.5 and 4.0 mg/kg doses of d-amphetamine, PCPA pretreatment resulted in significantly enhanced locomotion during the post-stereotypy interval. Thus, unlike those of αMT, the effects of PCPA cannot be interpreted as resulting in a shift to an effectively lower dose of amphetamine which elicits relatively less stereotypy.

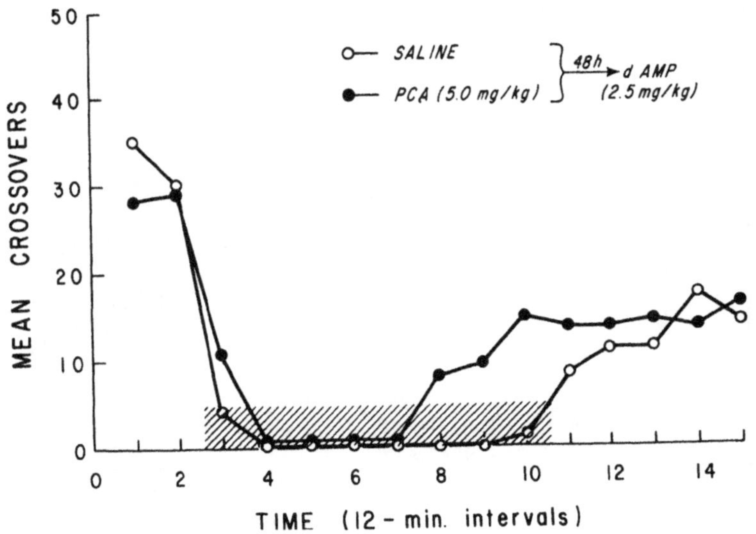

Fig. 5. Mean crossovers during the 3-hour interval following administration of d-amphetamine (2.5 mg/kg) in rats injected 48 hours previously with either saline or 5.0 mg/kg parachloramphetamine; N = 5 animals/group. Parachloramphetamine pretreatment reduced the duration of the stereotypy phase. (From Segal and Geyer, unpublished data.)

Parachloramphetamine. In order to determine whether the effects of PCPA on the various components of the amphetamine response are due to a depletion of brain 5-HT levels rather than to some idiosyncratic interaction between PCPA and amphetamine, we also examined the effects of other manipulations that have been shown to reduce brain 5-HT levels (Fig. 5). In preliminary studies (Segal and Geyer, unpublished data), we have found that 5-0 mg/kg of parachloramphetamine (PCA), which produces a long-lasting, relatively specific reduction in brain 5-HT levels (Vorhees, Schafer, and Barrett, 1975), significantly increased spontaneous activity during both the light and dark cycles. Furthermore, 48 hours after injection of PCA, when 5-HT levels are reported to be reduced by 70% (Vorhees et al., 1975), a dose of 2.5 mg/kg of d-amphetamine produces significantly less stereotypy and correspondingly more locomotion than observed in non-pretreated animals.

Raphe lesion. Further evidence that the effects of PCPA are due to its depletion of 5-HT stems from the results we have obtained

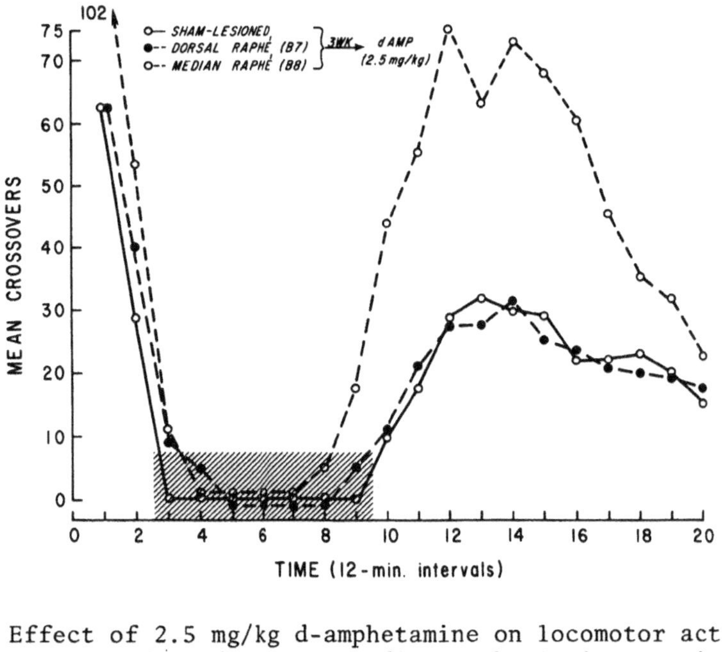

Fig. 6. Effect of 2.5 mg/kg d-amphetamine on locomotor activity in rats three weeks after dorsal or median raphe lesions or in sham controls; N = at least 10 animals/group. The duration of stereotypy (shaded area) was reduced and the post-stereotypy hyperactivity was enhanced only after lesion of the median raphe. (From Segal and Geyer, unpublished data)

following specific raphe lesions (Segal and Geyer, unpublished data). Three weeks following the lesion of median, but not dorsal, raphe, the stereotypy phase produced by a 2.5 mg/kg of d-amphetamine is shortened and the post-stereotypy hyperactivity phase is markedly enhanced (Fig. 6). However, although histofluorescence and biochemical measures (see Geyer, Puerto, Dawsey, et al., 1976b, for details of procedures) indicated that the median raphe lesions resulted in a substantial destruction of 5-HT fibers, especially in the hippocampus, the lesion-induced displacement of stereotypy by locomotor activity is not as pronounced as that observed following PCPA pretreatment. This may be due to a partial recovery of function during the three-week interval between lesion and amphetamine testing. In fact, there are some reports that behavioral effects produced by raphe lesions diminish with time after lesion (Costall and Naylor, 1974; Jacobs, Wise, and Taylor, 1974). We are currently testing this possibility by examining the behavioral response to amphetamine at shorter intervals following raphe lesion.

DISCUSSION

The results that we have obtained with both drugs and median raphe lesions indicate that progressive depletion of 5-HT cannot completely account for the pattern of behavioral change obtained with long-term amphetamine administration. However, these results do suggest that 5-HT pathways, perhaps those projecting to the hippocampus, may play a significant role in modulating the behavioral response to amphetamine.

There are several possible explanations for the apparently opposite effects of 5-HT depletion on the various behavioral components of the amphetamine response. For one, amphetamine-induced locomotion and stereotypy may be mediated by the activation of different neurochemical systems competing for behavioral expression. For example, some evidence indicates that the mesolimbic and nigrostriatal dopaminergic pathways may subserve locomotion and stereotypy, respectively (Kelly, Seviour, and Iversen, 1975). The effect of PCPA on the behavioral response to amphetamine could result from an activation of the mechanisms subserving locomotion and/or suppression of those underlying stereotypy.

It is also conceivable that enhanced locomotion and stereotypy may result from the action exerted by amphetamine on the same neurochemical systems, with other factors unrelated to the primary effect of amphetamine determining the specific behaviors expressed during any interval of time. In fact, a behaviorally nonspecific activating effect of amphetamine is consistent with the observation that a broad spectrum of behaviors can be facilitated by amphetamine administration (Teitelbaum and Derks, 1958; Hearst and Whalen, 1963;

Chance and Silverman, 1964; Clark and Steele, 1966; Rech, 1966; Randrup and Munkvad, 1970; Heise and Boff, 1971; Carey, Goodall, and Procopio, 1974; German and Bowden, 1974). Furthermore, amphetamine appears to affect locomotion and more focused behaviors, such as sniffing, biting, and licking, in a similar fashion. Amphetamine-induced locomotor patterns are markedly different from the exploratory activity typically displayed by animals placed in a novel environment. That is, the basic feature of stereotypy, continuous repetition of behavior, is apparent with doses of d-amphetamine as low as 0.5 mg/kg in the form of marked perseveration in the pattern of locomotion (Chance and Silverman, 1964; Lat, 1965; Randrup and Munkvad, 1970; Segal, 1975b).

Within the context of a general activating effect, the specific behaviors elicited by amphetamine might depend upon their relative position in a hierarchy of competing response tendencies. Under the experimental conditions employed in the present studies, locomotor activity appears to represent a dominant response in such a hierarchy. Thus, with increases in amphetamine-induced behavioral activation correspondingly greater rates of locomotion would be manifested until a limit in locomotion output capacity is reached. If the response output capacity (or "response strength ceiling," according to Storms and Broen, 1969) for locomotion is less than that for the more focused stereotyped behaviors, then with increasing doses of amphetamine the more focused forms of stereotyped behavior would become gradually more dominant. The effect of reducing activity in certain serotonergic systems might then be to elevate the ceiling that limits response output capacity. Thus, in 5-HT-depleted animals, enhanced locomotion would remain the predominant response over a higher range of amphetamine-induced activation.

ACKNOWLEDGMENT

This research is supported by USPHS Grant No. DA-00046-5 and NIMH Research Scientist Award No. MH-70183-03 to D.S.S.

REFERENCES

Baldessarini, R.J., Amatruda, T.T., III, Griffin, F.F., and Gerson, S.: Differential effects of serotonin on turning and stereotypy induced by apomorphine. Brain Res. 93, 158-163 (1975).

Breese, G.R., Cooper, B.R., and Mueller, R.A.: Evidence for involvement of 5-hydroxytryptamine in the actions of amphetamine. Br. J. Pharmac. 52, 307-314 (1974).

Carey, R.J., Goodall, E.B., and Procopio, G.F.: Differential effects of d-amphetamine on fixed ratio 30 performance maintained by food versus brain stimulation reinforcement. Pharmacol. Biochem. Behav. 2, 193-198 (1974).

Chance, M. and Silverman, A.: The structure of social behavior and drug action. In: Animal Behaviour and Drug Action. Steinberg, H., Reuck, A., and Knight, J., Eds., pp. 65-82. London: Churchill, 1964.

Clark, F.C. and Steele, B.J.: Effects of d-amphetamine on performance under a multiple schedule in the rat. Psychopharmacologia (Berl.) 9, 157-169 (1966).

Costall, B. and Naylor, R.J.: Stereotyped and circling behaviour induced by dopaminergic agonists after lesions of the midbrain raphe nuclei. Eur. J. Pharmacol. 29, 206-222 (1974).

German, D.S. and Bowden, D.M.: Catecholamine systems as the neural substrate for intracranial self-stimulation: A hypothesis. Brain Res. 73, 381-419 (1974).

Geyer, M.A., Puerto, A., Menkes, D.B., Segal, D.S., and Mandell, A. J.: Behavioral studies following lesions of the mesolimbic and mesostriatal serotonergic pathways. Brain Res., in press.

Geyer, M.A., Puerto, A., Dawsey, W.J., Knapp, S., Bullard, W.P., and Mandell, A.J.: Histologic and enzymatic studies of the mesolimbic and mesostriatal serotonergic pathways. Brain Res., in press.

Hearst, E. and Whalen, R.E.: Facilitating effects of d-amphetamine on discriminated-avoidance performance. J. comp. physiol. Psychol. 56, 124-128 (1963).

Heise, G.A. and Boff, E.: Stimulant action of d-amphetamine in relation to test compartment dimensions and behavioral measure. Neuropharmacology 10, 259-266 (1971).

Jacobs, B.L., Wise, W.D., and Taylor, K.M.: Differential behavioral and neurochemical effects following lesions of the dorsal or median raphe nuclei in rats. Brain Res. 79, 353-361 (1974).

Jacobs, B.L., Wise, W.D., and Taylor, K.M.: Is there a catecholamine-serotonin interaction in the control of locomotor activity? Neuropharmacology 14, 501-506 (1975).

Kelly, P.H., Seviour, P.W., and Iversen, S.D.: Amphetamine and apomorphine responses in the rat following 6-hydroxydopamine lesions of the nucleus accumbens septi and corpus striatum. Brain Res. 94, 507-522 (1975).

Lat, J.: The spontaneous exploratory reactions as a tool for psychopharmacological studies. In: Proceedings of the Second International Pharmacological Meeting. Mikhelson, M. and Longo, V., Eds., Vol. 1, pp. 47-66. London: Pergamon, 1965.

Mabry, P.D. and Campbell, B.A.: Serotonergic inhibition of catecholamine-induced behavioral arousal. Brain Res. 49, 381-391 (1973).

Meill, D.B., Grant, L.D., and Grossman, S.P.: Selective potentiation of locomotor effects of amphetamine by midbrain raphe lesions. Physiol. Behav. 9, 655-657 (1972).

Neuberg, J. and Thut, P.D.: Comparison of the locomotor stimulant mechanisms of action of d-amphetamine and d-amphetamine plus l-dopa: Possible involvement of serotonin. Biol. Psychiat. 8, 139-150 (1974).

Randrup, A. and Mankvad, I.: Biochemical, anatomical and psychological investigations of stereotyped behavior induced by amphetamines. In: Amphetamines and Related Compounds. Costa, E. and Garattini, S., Eds., pp. 695-713. New York: Raven Press, 1970.

Rech, R.H.: Amphetamine effects on poor performance of rats in a shuttle-box. Psychopharmacologia (Berl.) 9, 110-117 (1966).

Rotrosen, J., Angrist, B.M., Wallach, M.B., and Gershon, S.: Absence of serotonergic influence on apomorphine-induced stereotypy. Eur. J. Pharmacol. 20, 133-135 (1972).

Segal, D.S.: Behavioral and neurochemical correlates of repeated d-amphetamine administration. In: Neurobiological Mechanisms of Adaptation and Behavior, Advances in Biochemical Psycho-Pharmacology. Mandell, A.J., Ed., Vol 13 pp. 247-262. New York: Raven Press, 1975a.

Segal, D.S.: Behavioral characterization of d and l-amphetamine: Neurochemical implications. Science 190, 475-477 (1975b).

Segal, D.S. and Mandell, A.J.: Long-term administration of amphetamine: Progressive augmentation of motor activity and stereotypy. Pharmac. Biochem. Behav. 2, 249-255 (1974).

Storms, L.H. and Broen, W.E.: A theory of schizophrenic behavioral disorganization. Arch. gen. Psychiat. 20, 129-144 (1969).

Swonger, A.K. and Rech, R.H.: Serotonergic and cholinergic involvement in habituation of activity and spontaneous alterations of rats in a Y maze. J. comp. physiol. Psychol. 81, 509-522 (1972).

Teitelbaum, P. and Derks, P.: The effect of amphetamine on forced drinking in the rat. J. comp. physiol. Psychol. 51, 801-810 (1958).

Vorhees, C.V., Schaefer, G.J., and Barrett, R.J.: p-Chloramphetamine: Behavioral effects of reduced cerebral serotonin in rats. Pharmac. Biochem. Behav. 3, 279-284 (1975).

Weiner, W.J., Goetz, C., and Klawans, H.L.: Serotonergic and antiserotonergic influences on apomorphine-induced stereotyped behaviour. Acta Pharmacol. Toxicol. 36, 155-160 (1975).

Weiner, W.J., Goetz, C., Westheimer, R., and Klawans, H.L.: Serotonergic and antiserotonergic influences on amphetamine-induced stereotyped behavior. J. Neurol. Sci. 20, 373-379 (1973).

ROLE OF MONOAMINE NEURAL PATHWAYS IN d-AMPHETAMINE- AND METHYLPHENIDATE-INDUCED LOCOMOTOR ACTIVITY

George R. Breese, Alan S. Hollister, Barrett R. Cooper

Departments of Psychiatry and Pharmacology, Biological Sciences Research Center of the Child Development Institute, University of North Carolina, School of Medicine, Chapel Hill, North Carolina 27514

INTRODUCTION

Extensive efforts have been made during the past few years to correlate the pharmacological actions of d-amphetamine and other centrally-acting stimulants with neurochemical changes in brain. Initial work was directed toward the role of brain catecholamine systems in the complex actions of such centrally-acting stimulants. Studies showing that tyrosine hydroxylase inhibitors antagonized the behavioral actions of d-amphetamine led to the proposal that d-amphetamine is an indirectly acting amine and that an uninterrupted synthesis of catecholamines is required for its central actions (Weissman, Koe, and Tenen, 1966; Hanson, 1967). From experiments that utilized a dopamine-β-hydroxylase inhibitor, Randrup and Scheel-Krüger (1966) suggested that noradrenergic fibers were responsible for amphetamine-induced locomotor activity and that dopaminergic pathways were necessary for the stereotypies that occur after amphetamine administration. However, even though subsequent studies supported the view that dopamine was involved in the stereotypic behavior induced by d-amphetamine (Simpson and Iversen, 1971; Fibiger, Fibiger, and Zis, 1973), several investigators provided evidence that dopamine rather than norepinephrine release was essential for amphetamine-induced locomotor activity (Costa, Groppetti, and Naimzada, 1972; Carlsson, 1970; Breese, Cooper, and Smith, 1973; Hollister, Breese, and Cooper, 1974).

Failure of d-amphetamine to deplete brain serotonin generally discouraged speculation that serotonergic neurons were involved in its actions (Paasonen and Vogt, 1956). Nevertheless, Reid (1970) reported that d-amphetamine increased serotonin turnover and Fuxe and Ungerstedt (1970) suggested that d-amphetamine released serotonin. In spite of this work, few studies indicated a role for serotonin in the behavioral actions of d-amphetamine.

In the present manuscript, data will be presented consistent with the view that brain dopamine is important for d-amphetamine- and methylphenidate-induced locomotor activity (Breese, Cooper, and Hollister, 1974; Hollister et al., 1974; Breese, Cooper, and Hollister, 1975). Additional experiments which suggest that brain serotonin may have an inhibitory role in the modulation of the stimulant actions of these drugs also will be presented (Breese, Cooper, and Hollister, 1974a; Breese, Cooper, and Mueller, 1974b; Hollister, Breese, Kuhn, Cooper, and Schanberg, in press).

Role of Catecholamine Systems in the Locomotor Activity Induced by Central Stimulants

Effect of α-methyltyrosine and U-14,624 on d-amphetamine- and methylphenidate-induced locomotor activity. In accord with previous reports (Weissman, Koe, and Tenen, 1966; Hanson, 1967), α-methyltyrosine was found to reduce the locomotor activity produced by d-amphetamine and methylphenidate in reserpinized rats (Fig. 1). If the antagonism of these stimulants by α-methyltyrosine were related to an inhibition of norepinephrine synthesis, it was reasoned that inhibition of dopamine-β-hydroxylase to decrease norepinephrine synthesis would produce a similar effect. However, under these experimental conditions, the motor stimulation induced by both d-amphetamine and methylphenidate was not antagonized (Fig. 1; Hollister et al., 1974; Breese et al., 1975).

Effect of various 6-hydroxydopamine treatments on d-amphetamine-induced locomotor activity. The discovery that 6-hydroxydopamine could be used to reduce dopamine or norepinephrine preferentially provided an additional means to assess the role of these amines in the action of d-amphetamine (Breese and Traylor, 1970, 1971). As shown in Fig. 2, depletion of dopamine caused a drastic reduction of d-amphetamine-induced locomotor activity whereas preferential depletion of norepinephrine with 6-hydroxydopamine did not. Results qualitatively similar to these were also found to occur at 1 and 3 mg/kg of d-amphetamine (Hollister et al., 1974).

Thus, results obtained after inhibition of catecholamine synthesis or after treatment with 6-hydroxydopamine provided convincing evidence that dopaminergic systems in brain were responsible for the locomotor stimulation observed after administration of d-amphetamine or methylphenidate.

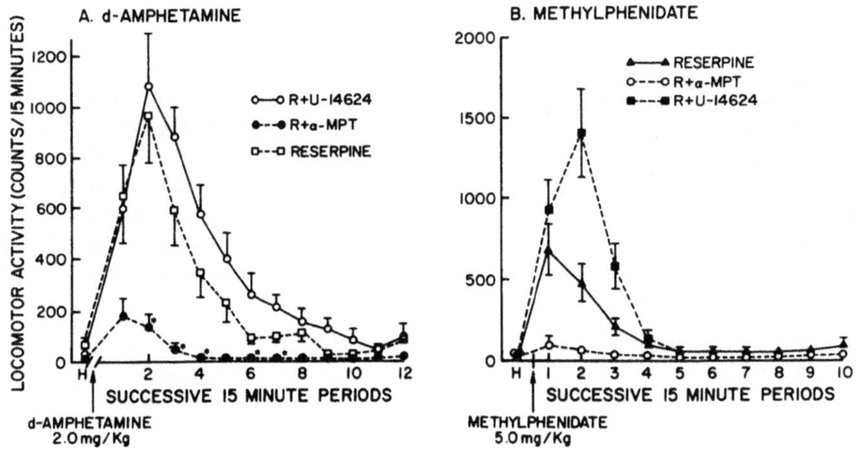

Fig. 1. Effect of α-methyltyrosine (α-MPT) and U-14,624 on (A) d-amphetamine- and (B) methylphenidate-induced motor activity in reserpinized rats. All animals received 2.5mg/kg of reserpine 24h before receiving d-amphetamine sulfate (2mg/kg) or methylphenidate HCl (5mg/kg). α-MPT (25mg/kg) or U-14,624 (75mg/kg) was administered at the beginning of the habituation (H) period, 1 h before the stimulant drugs.

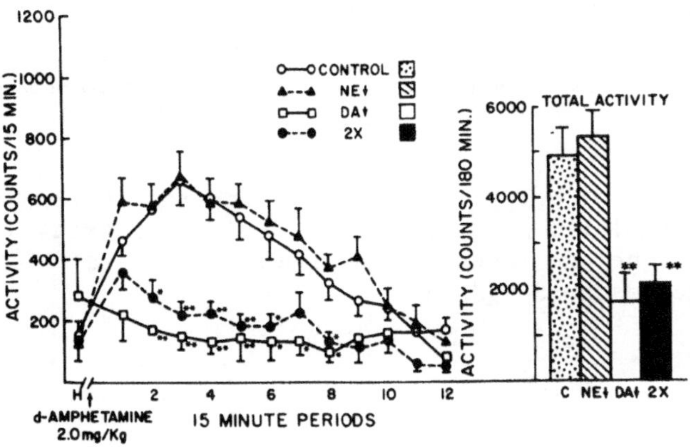

Fig. 2. Effect of various 6-hydroxydopamine treatments on d-amphetamine-induced motor activity. Treatments are those described by Hollister et al. (1974). $*p < 0.01$; $**p < 0.001$ when compared with control.

Evidence Implicating Serotonergic Pathways in the Actions of Central Stimulants

Effect of pargyline on d-amphetamine- and methylphenidate-induced locomotor activity. Administration of pargyline (50 mg/kg) 1 hour before the injection of d-amphetamine or methylphenidate was found to reduce the locomotor response to these stimulants (Fig. 3). Since the pargyline antagonism of the locomotor response to d-amphetamine and methylphenidate was found to be reversed by p-chlorophenylalanine (PCPA), it appeared that serotonergic fibers were exerting an inhibitor influence on the locomotor stimulation induced by these drugs.

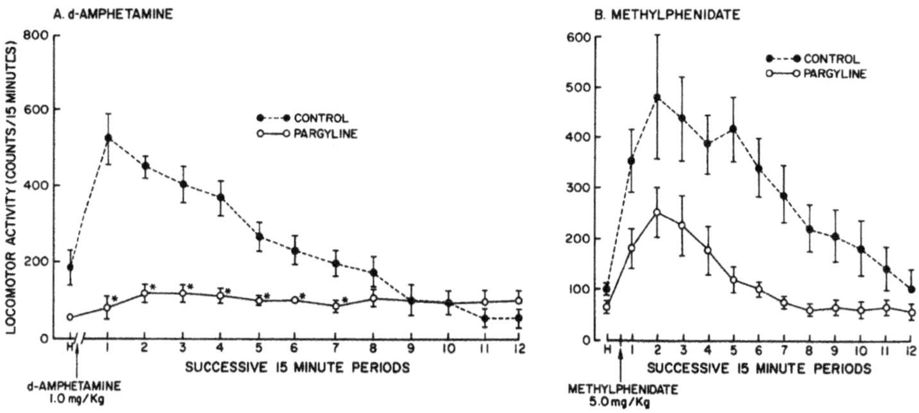

Fig. 3. Effect of pargyline on (A) d-amphetamine- and (B) methylphenidate-stimulated motor activity. Rats were treated with pargyline 1 h before receiving d-amphetamine sulfate (1 mg/kg) or methylphenidate (5 mg/kg).

Effect of PCPA on the locomotor activity induced by d-amphetamine or methylphenidate. If serotonergic neurons mediated an inhibitory action of centrally-active stimulants, it was reasoned that reduction of serotonin in brain should enhance the locomotor activity stimulated by d-amphetamine and methylphenidate. As shown in Table 1, reduction of serotonin with PCPA produced a marked potentiation of locomotor activity by these stimulants. In an additional group of experiments, PCPA-treated animals were given 5-hydroxytryptophan (75 mg/kg) 1 hour before d-amphetamine or methylphenidate to replete serotonin content. This latter treatment eliminated the potentiation of the enhanced locomotor activity observed after PCPA treatment (Breese et al., 1974b, 1975; Hollister et al., in press).

Table 1

Effect of Parachlorophenylalanine (PCPA) on d-Amphetamine- and Methylphenidate-Induced Locomotor Activity

Treatment	Locomotor Activity (cts/180 min)
d-Amphetamine	5670 ± 371
Methylphenidate	3660 ± 550
PCPA + Amphetamine	10,006 ± 1070*
PCPA + Methylphenidate	8440 ± 650*

Animals were treated with PCPA (150 mg/kg, orally) on 2 successive days before receiving d-amphetamine SO_4 (3 mg/kg) or methylphenidate (10 mg/kg). The stimulants were administered 24 h after the last dose of PCPA.

*$P < 0.01$ when compared with control.

Effect of a tryptophan-free diet on d-amphetamine-stimulated motor activity. Previous work has provided convincing data that food deprivation increases the locomotor response to d-amphetamine (Campbell and Fibiger, 1971; Simpson, 1974). Because food deprivation alters dietary tryptophan which in turn can affect serotonin synthesis in brain (Fernstrom and Wurtman, 1971), it was felt that removal of tryptophan from the diet might potentiate d-amphetamine-induced locomotor activity. In accord with this logic, rats maintained on a tryptophan-free diet exhibited an enhanced locomotor response to d-amphetamine (Fig. 4). Furthermore, administration of L-tryptophan abolished the enhanced locomotor effect of d-amphetamine in rats fed the tryptophan-free diet (Fig. 5).

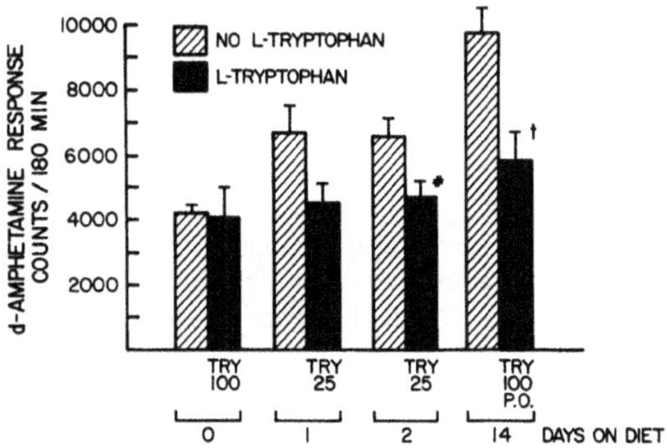

Fig. 4. Effect of tryptophan-free diet on d-amphetamine-induced motor activity. Dose of d-amphetamine sulfate was 2 mg/kg. Zero days of treatment represents the response to d-amphetamine in pair-fed controls. Solid portion of bars represents the activity accumulated for 3 h after injection of saline. *p < 0.05; **p < 0.01 when compared with control response to d-amphetamine.

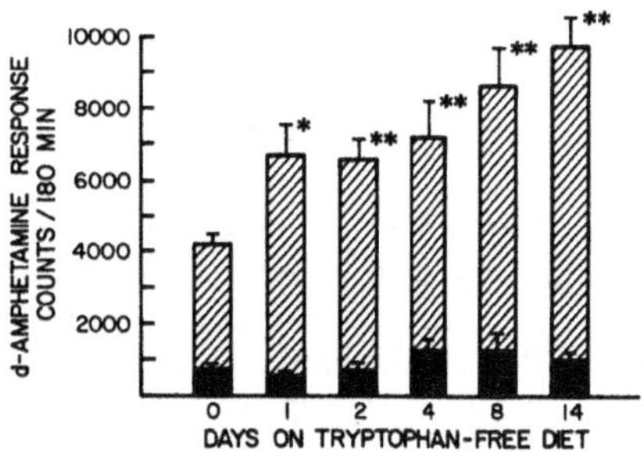

Fig. 5. Reversal of the tryptophan-free diet potentiation of d-amphetamine by L-tryptophan administration. Animals fed the tryptophan-free diet for 0, 1, 2, or 14 days received 100, 25, 25, and 100 mg/kg of L-tryptophan (TRY), respectively, 1 h before the administration of d-amphetamine sulfate (2 mg/kg). *p < 0.05; +p < 0.01 when compared with no tryptophan treatment.

DISCUSSION

The present work provides additional support for the view that intact catecholamine fibers are necessary for the locomotor stimulant actions of d-amphetamine and methylphenidate. However, in contrast to earlier assumptions (Randrup and Scheel-Krüger, 1966), the present data provides evidence that dopaminergic systems are important for the locomotor stimulant properties of these compounds. This conclusion is based upon the reduction of locomotor activity of d-amphetamine after 6-hydroxydopamine and the blockade of d-amphetamine and methylphenidate-induced activity by α-methyltyrosine but not by a dopamine-β-hydroxylase inhibitor. Thus, for the present, a role for noradrenergic fibers in the actions of d-amphetamine and methylphenidate cannot be defined. Considerable biochemical evidence is available that d-amphetamine affects noradrenergic fibers in brain (McClean and McCartney, 1961; Moore and Lariviere, 1963; Glowinski and Axelrod, 1965). Since pretreatment of reserpinized rats with U-14,624 was found to cause a significant potentiation of methylphenidate-stimulated motor activity, a possibility exists that under proper conditions noradrenergic fibers can display inhibitory actions.

In addition to data provided in this manuscript, other investigators have reported data supporting the view that dopaminergic systems are important for the stimulant properties of d-amphetamine. For example, bilateral injection of 6-hydroxydopamine into the nigro-striatal pathway or electrolytic lesions in the substantia nigra (Simpson and Iversen, 1971) have been shown to antagonize the locomotor actions of d-amphetamine (Ungerstedt, 1974; Fibiger et al., 1973). These studies, however, did not eliminate a role for noradrenergic fibers in the actions of d-amphetamine, because these procedures reduced both norepinephrine and dopamine in the forebrain (Oltmans and Harvey, 1972; Breese, 1975; Breese, Smith, Cooper, Hollister, Kraemer, and McKinney, in press). Nevertheless, lesions of the dorsal and ventral norepinephrine pathways do not alter d-amphetamine-induced locomotor activity (unpublished data), supporting the view that dopaminergic fibers play an essential role in this action of d-amphetamine. The possibility that mesolimbic rather than striatal dopaminergic neurons may mediate the locomotor activity induced by amphetamine recently gained support from the observation that bilateral administration of 6-hydroxydopamine into the nucleus accumbens septi blocked the characteristic amphetamine locomotor response (Kelly, Seviour, and Iversen, 1975). Furthermore, Kelly et al. (1975) have demonstrated that destruction of dopaminergic fibers in this area with intracerebral injection of 6-hydroxydopamine in the presence of desipramine to protect noradrenergic fibers also reduce the actions of d-amphetamine. Such findings seem consistent with the findings of Pijnenburg and van Rossum (1973) that bilateral injection of dopamine directly into the nucleus accumbens produced an enhancement of locomotor activity.

In addition to the investigations underlying the importance of dopamine systens in the actions of d-amphetamine and methylphenidate, the present work also provides convincing evidence that serotonergic pathways play a role in their actions. Confirming earlier reports (Neill, Grant, and Grossman, 1972; Mabry and Campbell, 1973; Breese et al., 1974a), d-amphetamine hyperactivity was found to be potentiated following the reduction of brain serotonin with PCPA. Hollister et al. (in press) have also found that agents that block serotonin receptors will enhance d-amphetamine-induced motor activity and, as indicated in the present work, a dietary deficiency of tryptophan will increase the locomotor response to d-amphetamine. Additional evidence for the involvement of serotonergic fibers in the actions of stimulant compounds was obtained when the inhibition of d-amphetamine- and methylphenidate-stimulated motor activity by pargyline was found to involve brain serotonin (Breese et al., 1974b). More recent evidence implicating serotonergic fibers in the actions of d-amphetamine was the demonstration that the potentiation of d-amphetamine-stimulated motor activity induced by starvation could be reversed by pretreating animals with L-tryptophan (Hollister et al., in press). Whether the inhibitory action displayed by these compounds is the consequence of a direct effect of the central stimulants on serotonergic fibers or a reflex action related to their effects on dopaminergic fibers has yet to be determined. This latter possibility as well as the potential interactions of other types of neural pathways such as cholinergic (Fibiger, Lytle, and Campbell, 1970; Thornburg and Moore, 1973) or γ-aminobutyric acid (McGeer et al. 1974) systems in the actions of central stimulants will await future research efforts.

ACKNOWLEDGMENTS

This work was supported by USPHS grants MH-16522 and HD-03110. G.R.B. is a USPHS Career Development Awardee (MH-00013). A.S.H. is a predoctoral fellow in the Neurobiology Program (MH-11107 and Sloan Foundation).

REFERENCES

Breese, G.R.: Chemical and immunochemical lesions by specific neurotoxic substances and antisera. In: Handbook of Psychopharmacology. Iversen, L.L., Iversen, S.D., and Snyder, S.H., Eds., Vol. 1, pp. 137-189. New York: Plenum Press, 1975.

Breese, G.R. and Cooper, B.R.: Behavioral and biochemical interactions of 5,7-DHT with various drugs when administered intracisternally to adult and developing rats, Brain Res. 98, 517-527 (1975).

Breese, G.R., Cooper, B.R., and Hollister, A.S.: Involvement of brain monoamines in the stimulant and paradoxical inhibitory effects of methylphenidate, Psychopharmacologia 44, 5-10 (1975).

Breese, G.R., Cooper, B.R., and Hollister, A.S.: Relationship of biogenic amines to behavior, J. Psychiat. Res. 11, 125-134 (1974a).

Breese, G.R., Cooper, B.R., and Mueller, R.A.: Evidence for involvement of 5-hydroxytryptamine in the actions of amphetamine, Br. J. Pharmac. 52, 307-314 (1974b).

Breese, G.R., Cooper, B.R., and Smith, R.D.: Biochemical and behavioral alterations following 6-hydroxydopamine administration into brain. In: Frontiers in Catecholamine Research. Usdin, E. and Snyder, S., Eds., pp. 701-706. New York: Pergamon Press, 1973.

Breese, G.R., Smith, R.D., Cooper, B.R., Hollister, A.S., Kraemer, G., and McKinney, W.T.: Use of neurocytotoxic agents in neuropsychopharmacology. In: Chemical Tools in Catecholamine Research. Malmfors, T., Jonsson, G., and Sachs, C., Eds. Amsterdam: North-Holland Publishing Co., in press.

Breese, G.R. and Traylor, T.D.: Depletion of brain noradrenaline and dopamine by 6-hydroxydopamine, Br. J. Pharmac. 42, 88-89 (1971).

Breese, G.R. and Traylor, T.D.: Effect of 6-hydroxydopamine on brain norepinephrine and dopamine: Evidence for selective degeneration of catecholamine neurons, J. Pharmac. exp. Ther. 174, 413-420 (1970).

Campbell, B.A. and Fibiger, H.C.: Potentiation of amphetamine-induced arousal by starvation, Nature 233, 424-425 (1971).

Carlsson, A.: Amphetamine and brain catecholamines. In: Amphetamines and Related Compounds. Costa, E. and Garattini, S., Eds., pp. 289-300. New York: Raven Press, 1970.

Costa, E., Gropetti, A., and Naimzada, M.: Effects of amphetamine on the turnover rate of brain catecholamines and motor activity, Br. J. Pharmac. 44, 742-751 (1972).

Fernstrom, J.D. and Wurtman, R.J.: Brain serotonin content: Physiological dependence on plasma tryptophan levels, Science 173, 149-152 (1971).

Fibiger, H.C., Fibiger, H.P., and Zis, A.P.: Attenuation of amphetamine induced motor stimulation and stereotypy by 6-hydroxydopamine in the rat, Br. J. Pharmac. 47, 683-692 (1973).

Fibiger, H.C., Lytle, L.D., and Campbell, B.A.: Cholinergic modulation of adrenergic arousal in the developing rat, J. comp. physiol. Psychol. 72, 384-389 (1970).

Fuxe, K. and Ungerstedt, U.: Histochemical, biochemical and functional studies on central monoamine neurons after acute and chronic amphetamine administration. In: Amphetamines and Related Compounds. Costa, E. and Garattini, S., Eds., pp. 257-288. New York: Raven Press, 1970.

Glowinski, J. and Axelrod, J.: Effects of drugs on the uptake, release, and metabolism of H^3-norepinephrine in the rat brain, J. Pharmac. exp. Ther. 149, 43-49 (1965).

Hanson, L.: Evidence that the central action of (+)-amphetamine is mediated via catecholamines, Psychopharmacologia 10, 289-297 (1967).

Hollister, A.S., Breese, G.R., and Cooper, B.R.: Comparison of tyrosine hydroxylase and dopamine-β-hydroxylase inhibition with the effects of various 6-hydroxydopamine treatments on amphetamine-induced motor activity, Psychopharmacologia 36, 1-16 (1974).

Hollister, A.S., Breese, G.R., Kuhn, C.M., Cooper, B.R., and Schanberg, S.M.: An inhibitory role for brain serotonin-containing systems in the locomotor effects of d-amphetamine, J. Pharmac. exp. Ther. (in press).

Kelly, P.H., Seviour, P.W., and Iversen, S.D.: Amphetamine and apomorphine responses in the rat following 6-OHDA lesions of the nucleus accumbens septi and corpus striatum, Brain Res. 94, 507-522 (1975).

Mabry, P.D. and Campbell, B.A.: Serotonergic inhibition of catecholamine induced behavioral arousal, Brain Res. 49, 381-391 (1972).

McGeer, P.H., Fibiger, H.C., Hattori, T., and McGeer, E.G.: Evidence for descending pallido-nigral GABA-containing neurons, Adv. Neurol. 5, 153-160 (1974).

McLean, J.R. and McCartney, M.: Effect of d-amphetamine on rat brain noradrenaline and serotonin, Proc. Soc. exp. Biol. Med. 107, 77-79 (1961).

Moore, K.E. and Lariviere, E.W.: Effects of d-amphetamine and restraint on the content of norepinephrine and dopamine in the rat brain, Biochem. Pharmac. 12, 1283-1288 (1963).

Neill, D.B., Grant, L.D., and Grossman, S.P.: Selective potentiation of locomotor effects of amphetamine by midbrain raphe lesions, Physiol. Behav. 9, 655-657 (1972).

Oltmans, G.A. and Harvey, J.D.: LH syndrome and brain catecholamine levels after lesions of nigrostriatal bundle, Physiol. Behav. 8, 69-78 (1972).

Paasonen, M.K. and Vogt, M.: The effect of drugs on the amounts of substance P and 5-hydroxytryptamine in mammalian brain, J. Physiol. 131, 617-626 (1956).

Pijnenburg, A.J.J. and van Rossum, J.M.: Stimulation of locomotor activity following injection of dopamine into the nucleus accumbens, J. Pharm. Pharmac. 25, 1003-1005 (1973).

Randrup, A. and Scheel-Krüger, J.: Diethyldithiocarbamate and amphetamine stereotype behavior, J. Pharm. Pharmac. 18, 752 (1966).

Reid, W.D.: Turnover rate of brain 5-hydroxytryptamine increased by d-amphetamine, Br. J. Pharmac. 40, 483-491 (1970).

Simpson, B.A. and Iversen, S.D.: Effects of substantia nigra lesions on the locomotor and stereotypic responses to amphetamine, Nature new Biol. 230, 30-32 (1971).

Simpson, L.L.: A study of the interaction between amphetamine and food deprivation, Psychopharmacologia 38, 279-286 (1974).

Thornburg, J.E. and Moore, K.E.: Inhibition of anticholinergic drug induced locomotor stimulation in mice by α-methyltyrosine, Neuropharmacology 12, 1179-1185 (1973).

Ungerstedt, U.: Brain dopamine neurons and behavior. In: The Neurosciences. Schmitt, F.O. and Worden, F.G., Eds., pp. 695-703. Cambridge, Mass.: MIT Press, 1974.

Weissman, A., Koe, B.K., and Tenen, S.S.: Antiamphetamine effects following inhibition of tyrosine hydroxylase, J. Pharmac. exp. Ther. 151, 339-352 (1966).

THE EFFECTS OF COCAINE ON THE AGGRESSIVE BEHAVIOR OF MICE, PIGEONS AND SQUIRREL MONKEYS

Ronald R. Hutchinson, Grace S. Emley, and Norman A. Krasnegor*

Foundation for Behavioral Research, Augusta, MI 49012

*National Institute on Drug Abuse, Rockville, MD 20852

Historically cocaine, a central nervous stimulant, has been associated with subjective effects of euphoria, elevation of mood, indifference to pain, and increased vigor and muscular strength (Jaffe, 1965; Byck, 1974; Maurer and Vogel, 1967). Chronic use and high doses have been associated with irritability, anxiety, paranoid delusions and violence (Maurer and Vogel, 1967; Byck, 1974). Because cocaine shares many properties with the amphetamines and several studies have shown that amphetamine can potentiate aggression, there is supposition that cocaine may influence aggressive behavior but there is limited data on cocaine and violence to support this conclusively. Most information on the effects of cocaine on human behavior are anecdotal or clinical observations of addicts (Post, Kotin, and Goodwin, 1974). The experimental literature on the effects of cocaine is also sparse. Smith (1964) administered cocaine to pigeons on a fixed interval-fixed ratio (FI-FR) schedule for food. Responding on the FI schedule was increased at the higher doses of cocaine but FR rates were depressed. Hill, Bell and Wikler (1967) report no effect of cocaine administration (10 mg/kg s.c.) to rats on lever pressing for food on a conditioned suppression procedure. Kosman and Unna (1968) report increased endurance to swimming in dogs given cocaine and Simon, Sultan, Chermat and Boissier (1972) report hyperactivity and increased explorations in rats and mice at 2-4 mg/kg with stereotyped behavior occurring at 8 mg/kg. Kosman and Unna (1968) have reported that rats working on a water-reinforced task exhibited no tolerance to chronic administration of cocaine and performance returned to control levels upon withdrawal of the drug. Chronic administration of cocaine in humans does not produce physiological addiction (Jaffe, 1965; Post et al., 1974).

The clinical and experimental literature on the effects of cocaine leaves many questions unanswered, and of particular interest to us was the more complete explanation of whether cocaine possessed unique and specific mood altering qualities. The experiments reported here were designed to study the effect of acute and chronic cocaine administration on aggression in squirrel monkeys, pigeons and mice. The experimental tests necessarily involved a sequence of independent tests of drug influence, as several major causes of aggression exist.

Research has identified a set of fundamental variables generally responsible for the production of aggressive behavior in a large variety of species including man (Hutchinson, 1973). These studies have shown that aggression is affected both by several forms of stimulation which precede, and certain types of stimulation which may follow, such behavior. The two major classes of variables are thus antecedent stimuli and consequent stimuli (Hutchinson, 1973). Each of these types of stimulation can be divided into two major subcategories. One form of antecedent stimulation which--by its introduction--causes attack, is painful, noxious, aversive, unpleasant, or negative-reinforcement-type stimulation. The other antecedent stimulus subclass producing attack includes offset or withdrawal of pleasant, beneficial, or positive-reinforcement-type events.

The subcategories of consequent or post-aggression-stimulation, which can influence the future display of aggression, include the operational reciprocals of the two forms of stimulation capable of triggering aggression when presented prior to any behavioral episodes. Thus noxious stimulation can trigger aggression directly when presented antecedently and yet also increase further occurrences of aggression when such stimulation is decreased subsequent to attack instances. In similar fashion, positive-reinforcing-type stimuli which, by their antecedent decrease, produce aggression, can produce future episodes of attack if such stimuli increase increase subsequent to attack behavior. Thus the two classes of antecedent stimulation which produce aggression directly can, by their opposite and consequent actions, function in a contingent relation to also influence attack display.

The general logic for the present experiments was to assess the effect of both acute and chronic cocaine administration upon the aggression attack sequences generated by each of the two subclasses of each of the two major types of causes of aggressive behavior. Cocaine was acutely and chronically administered to subjects attacking because of the antecedent administration of noxious stimulation and in other experiments where attack was caused by the antecedent termination of positive-reinforcement-type stimulation. Further, cocaine was acutely and chronically administered to subjects engaged in aggression attack sequences caused by attack-produced reduction of shock delivery, and in other experiments to subjects attacking because of attack-produced increases in positive reinforcement.

An important feature of the present experiments was their capacity to assess the differential influence of cocaine upon attack compared to influence upon several other behaviors generated by the same environmental conditions.

EXPERIMENT 1: EFFECTS OF ACUTE AND CHRONIC COCAINE ADMINISTRATION UPON SHOCK-PRODUCED ATTACK BY SQUIRREL MONKEYS

Subjects

The subjects were six adult male squirrel monkeys weighing 700-900 grams. The subjects were housed in individual cages in a large colony room, had free access to fluids, and were fed fruit and Wayne monkey diet.

Apparatus

A primate restraint chair (Plas Labs, Lansing, Michigan) equipped with tail electrodes and response sensors consisting of a response lever and a latex rubber bite hose mounted on the front panel was used (Fig. 1). The bite hose was connected to an Air Wave switch (Tapeswitch Corp., Farmingdale, New York) which was calibrated to record only bite attacks. The restraint chair was enclosed in a sound-attenuated, ventilated outer chamber. White noise was present in the chamber to mask extraneous noise.

Procedure

Experimental sessions of sixty-four minutes were conducted five days a week. During each session, 15 electric tail shocks (200 ms, 400 v.ac) were delivered on a four-minute, fixed-period, response-independent schedule. The shocks were delivered through brass tail electrodes resting on the distal portion of the tail, which had been shaved and prepared with electrode paste. Hose bites and lever responses were recorded on cumulative recorders and counters.

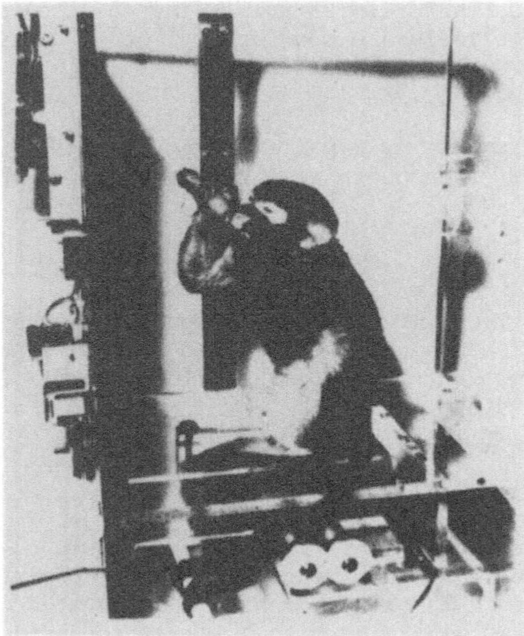

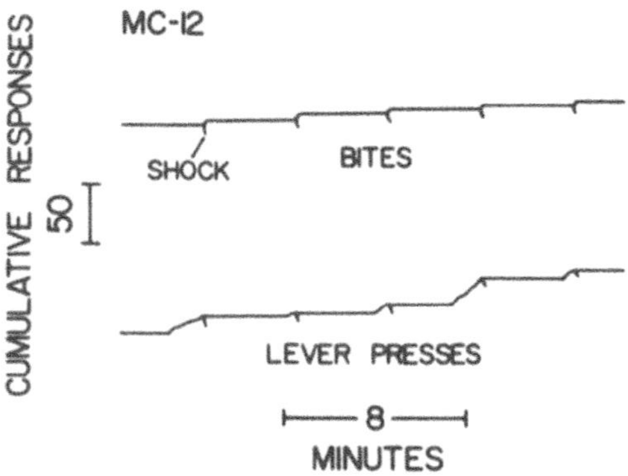

Fig. 1. A squirrel monkey subject seated in the restraint chair equipped with tail electrodes and bite hose. A portion of a cumulative record of bite and lever press responses produced by response-independent fixed-time tail shock to the squirrel monkey.

Acute Drug Administration

All injections were given subcutaneously 30 minutes prior to the experimental session. Saline control injections were given in a constant volume on four days of the week. Cocaine hydrochloride was administered in a mixed order of dosages on Wednesday of the experimental week. All drug doses below 1.25 mg/kg were given in a mixed order. The doses above 1.25 mg/kg were given in an ascending order until the highest dose was determined. Cocaine was administered acutely in the establishment of a dose-response function. Subjects were returned to control conditions prior to instatement of the chronic drug regimen.

Chronic Drug Administration

Cocaine hydrochloride was administered in the drinking water of the subjects. A graduated water bottle was mounted on the home cage for the recording of daily fluid intake. Distilled water was the control fluid for the determination of daily fluid intake for each subject. When fluid intake stabilized, drug was added to the water. The drug was added to the drinking water starting at a concentration of 0.007 mg/100 cc and increasing in a doubling function. Drug dosage was changed when behavioral responding was stable. Intake was recorded daily at 11 a.m. and fresh solutions supplied. Dosage of drug administered was based on body weight and fluid intake such that mg/kg/subject would be approximately the same. For each subject fluid intake and body weight remained consistent across the chronic regimen.

Results

The procedure of presentation of fixed-periodic, response-independent tail shock produced a temporal and topographic pattern of responding such that bites on the rubber hose occurred after the shock and responses on the lever occurred prior to the shock. The performance is illustrated in the bottom portion of Fig. 1.

The results of this experiment demonstrate the differential effect of the acute administration of cocaine (Fig. 2) on anticipatory and aggressive responses produced by response-independent, fixed-time schedule of shock presentation in the squirrel monkey. Across a range of dosages, there was a differential increase in non-attack responses. These data differ from other drug results on this paradigm (Hutchinson and Emley, 1972; Emley and Hutchinson, 1971, 1972) which are presented in summary form in Fig. 2. Figure 3 shows the effect of increasing doses of acute and chronic cocaine administration on the bite attack and lever press responses for

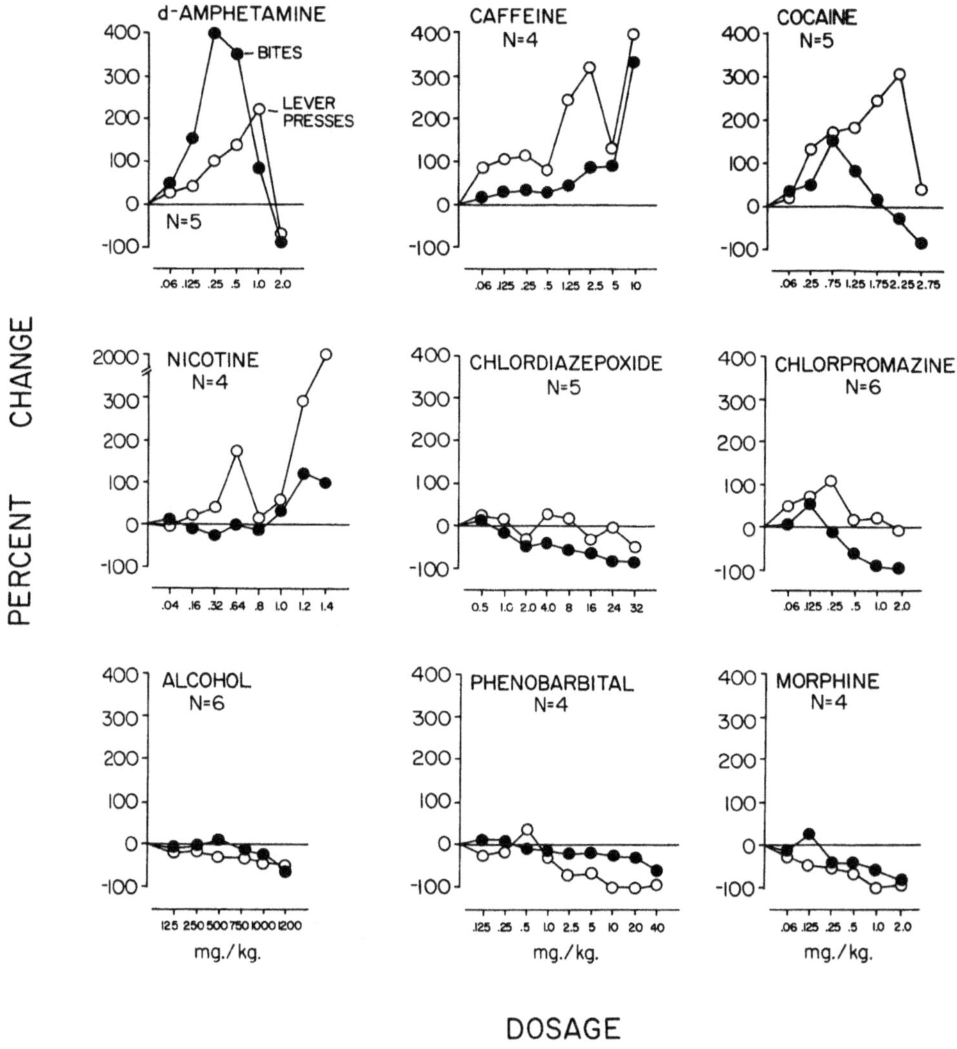

Fig. 2. Changes in lever press and bite responses produced by several drugs when administered to the squirrel monkey on the response-independent shock procedure.

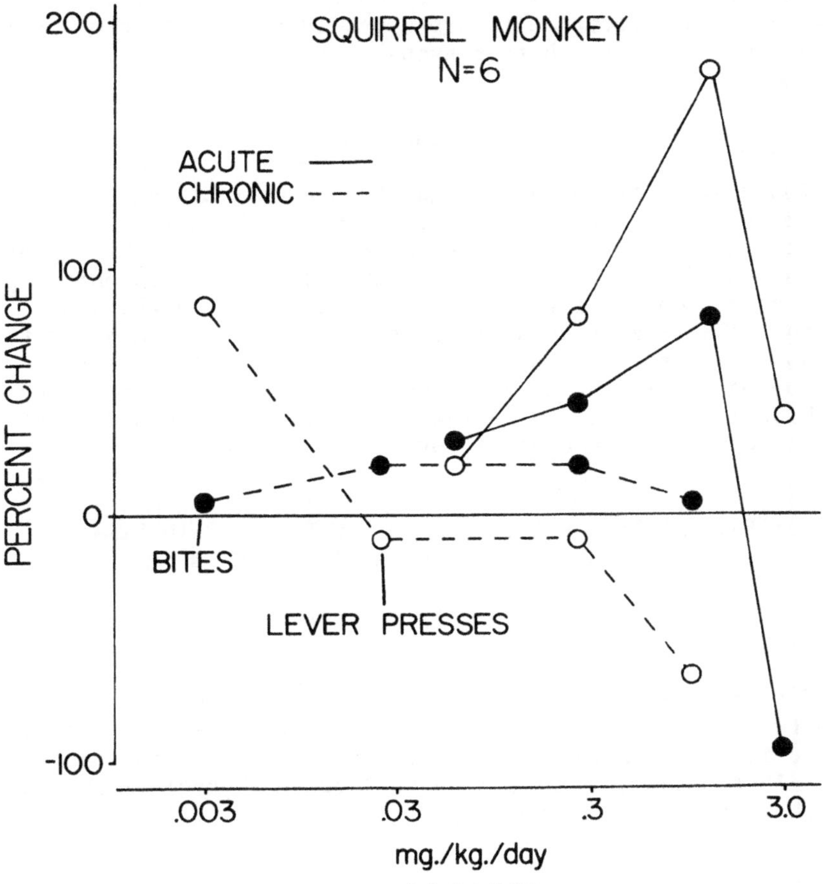

Fig. 3. Effects of acute and chronic cocaine administration on bite and lever press responses in the squirrel monkey on a response-independent shock schedule.

the six subjects. The solid line at zero indicates non-drug baseline responding and all drug points are indicated as percent change from saline control for the four days preceding the dose on the acute regimen and for the distilled water baseline on the chronic regimen. All doses are expressed as mg/kg/day. The results of the acute regimen illustrate a differential elevation of pre-shock lever press responses while the chronic regimen results illustrate a dose-dependent decrease in pre-shock lever presses and a slight increase in post-shock bite responses.

Discussion

The results of the acute and chronic cocaine regimens are consistent in that at the low dosages of the drug there is a differential increase in pre-shock behaviors and at the higher doses of the drug both behaviors decrease. On the chronic regimen the effective doses of the drug were lower than on the acute regimen. The relatively small effect of chronic cocaine on these responses may have been a result of the dosage range tested. For each subject fluid intake and body weight were consistent across the chronic regimen and withdrawal of the drug resulted in a gradual return toward control levels of responding.

EXPERIMENT 2: EFFECTS OF ACUTE COCAINE ADMINISTRATION UPON SHOCK-PRODUCED ATTACK BY MICE

Subjects

Subjects were five male mice of the Balbc/Tex strain, weighing between 35 and 55 grams. Subjects were housed individually and had free access to food (Wayne Lab Blox) and water in the home cage. In the colony room a reverse light-dark cycle was maintained such that light was on from 7 p.m. to 7 a.m.

Apparatus

The apparatus is illustrated in Fig. 4. Subjects were placed within a small plexiglas tube which was affixed in a larger test apparatus. The apparatus was equipped with tail shock electrodes and a response sensor which protruded into the plexiglas tube in front of the subject. The target was a nylon strip which was connected to a telegraph key calibrated to record biting or tugging responses by the subject. The apparatus was enclosed in a sound-attenuated, ventilated outer chamber. White noise was used to mask extraneous noise.

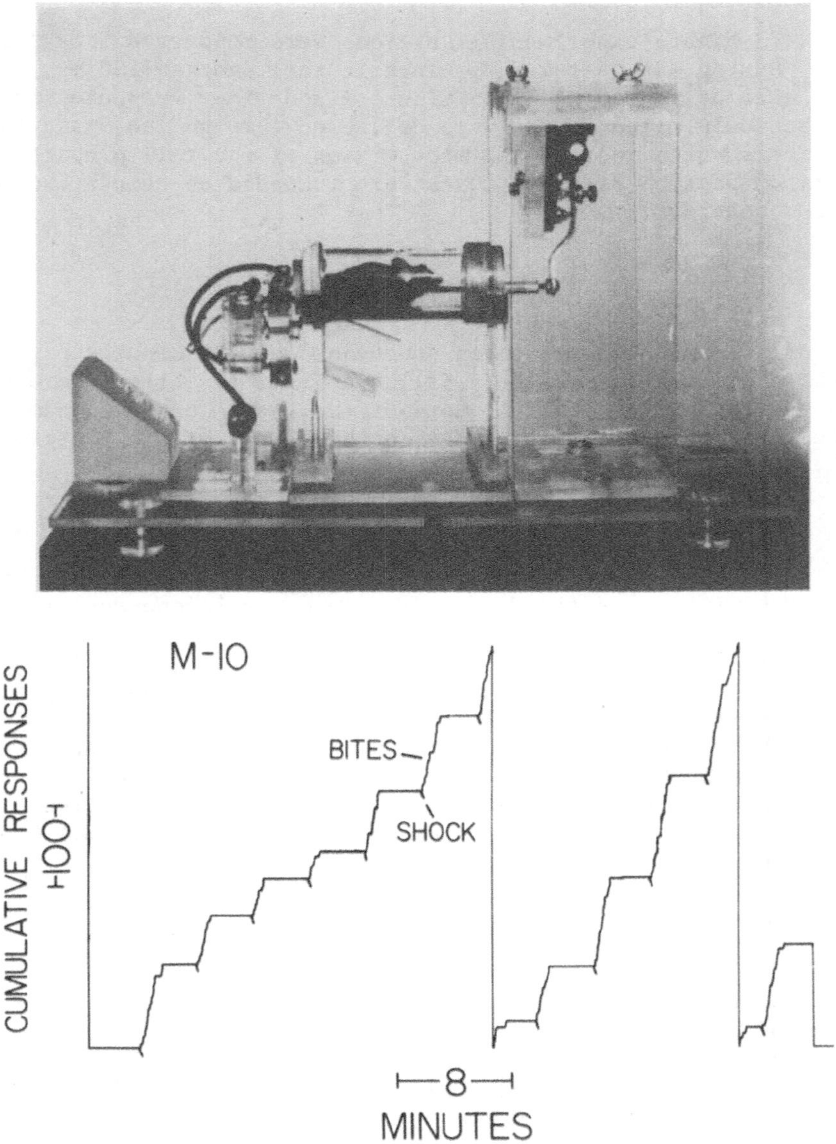

Fig. 4. (Top) Apparatus for tail shock-elicited attack in the mouse subject. (Bottom) Sample cumulative record of bite attacks in the mouse subject.

Procedure

41.5-Minute experimental sessions were conducted 5 days a week. During each session, 7 electric tail shocks (200 ms, 750 v.ac) were delivered on a 5.5-minute fixed-time, response-independent schedule. The shocks were delivered through the brass tail electrodes which rest on the mid portion of the tail prepared with electrode paste. Bite responses were recorded on cumulative recorders and counters.

Drug Administration

All injections were given subcutaneously 30 minutes prior to the experimental session. Saline control injections were given in a constant volume on four days of the week. Drug was administered in a mixed order of dosages on Wednesday of the experimental week.

Results

Presentation of fixed-periodic, response-independent tail shocks produced biting on the nylon strip after shock. This response pattern is illustrated in the lower section of Fig. 4. The effect of increasing dosages of cocaine hydrochloride on this responding is illustrated in Fig. 5. The line at zero indicates the saline control baseline and all drug points are indicated by percent change from saline control for the four days preceding that dosage. Across the dosages tested there was generally a decrease in biting. In the case of all subjects there was no topographic or temporal disruption of the behavior.

Discussion

The results of this experiment demonstrate the depressant effect of cocaine on the shock-produced attack behavior in mice. These data are similar to the results of Experiment 1, in which cocaine had a relative depressant effect on shock-produced attack behavior in the squirrel monkey.

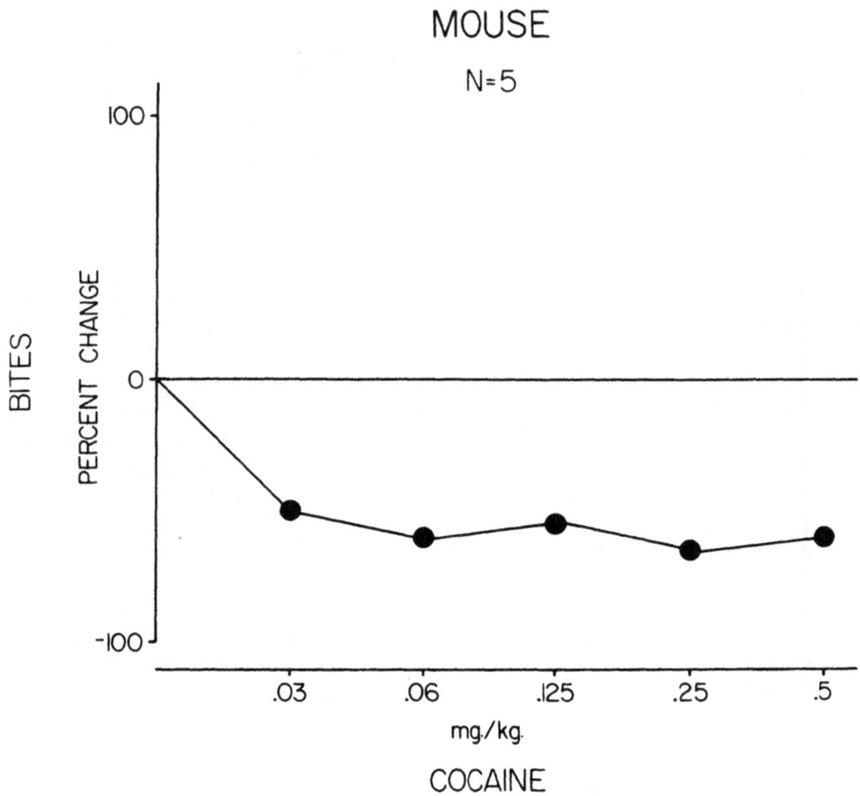

Fig. 5. Effect of acute cocaine administration on shock-elicited attack in the mouse.

EXPERIMENT 3: EFFECTS OF ACUTE AND CHRONIC COCAINE ADMINISTRATION UPON FOOD REMOVAL-PRODUCED ATTACK BY PIGEONS

Subjects

Subjects were five adult, male, naive, White Carneaux pigeons weighing 350-500 grams. Subjects were housed in individual cages and had free access to water and grit in the home cage. Subjects were fed (Purina Pigeon Chow Checkers) immediately after the experimental session to maintain 85% of free feeding weight.

Apparatus

A modified operant conditioning pigeon chamber divided into two sections by a plexiglas divider (as illustrated in Fig. 6) was used in this experiment. In one section (left side of illustration) was a taxidermically stuffed White Carneaux pigeon mounted via a pressure spring recording sensing rod suitable for the monitoring of pecking and wing beats by the subject. This target bird protruded into the other half of the chamber by approximately 2 inches. The subject bird was placed in the half of the chamber (right side of illustration) which contained a transilluminated plexiglas key mounted on the wall opposite the target bird and a feeder hopper mounted below and to the right of the response key. The entire chamber was illuminated by house lights and contained a true stimulus generator (sonoalert) in the top of the chamber. The entire chamber was enclosed in a larger, sound-attenuated, ventilated outer chamber. White noise was used to mask extraneous noise.

Procedure

Experimental sessions were conducted five days a week. The procedure was a multiple continuous reinforcement extinction program. Sessions started with a five minute extinction period and were followed by a reinforcement period of 10 food deliveries for key pecks. A tone signaled the onset of reinforcement and during this period each key peck activated the food hopper. At the completion of 10 hopper deliveries the extinction period was in effect for 5 minutes. These segments were alternated in the session until 5 extinction periods occurred. All responses on the key and the target bird during CRF and extinction were recorded on counters and cumulative recorders.

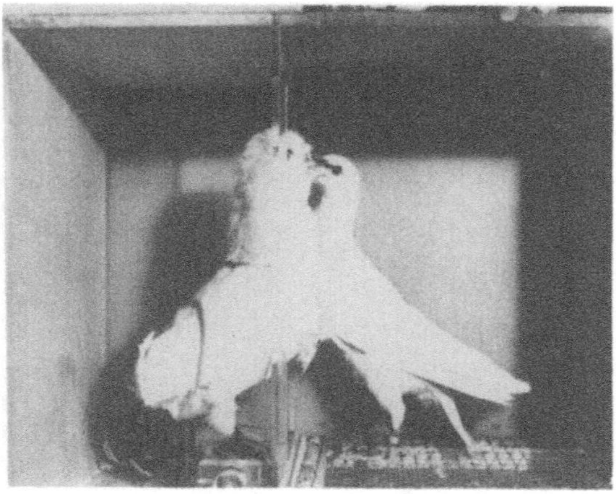

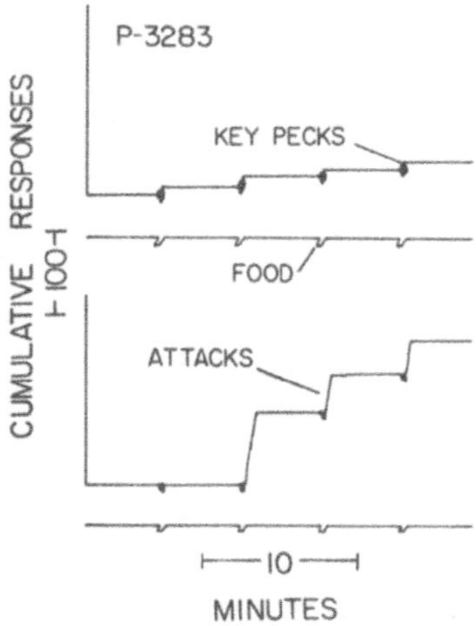

Fig. 6. (Left) Apparatus for reinforcement-extinction attack procedure with the pigeon. (Right) Sample cumulative record for key peck and attack responses in the pigeon.

Acute Drug Administration

All injections of cocaine hydrochloride were given into the pectoral muscle 30 minutes prior to the experimental session. Saline control injections were given in a constant volume on four days of the week. Drug was administered in a mixed order of dosages on Wednesday of the experimental week. All drug dosages above 1.0 mg/kg were given in an ascending order of dosages until the maximal dose was reached.

Chronic Drug Administration

Cocaine hydrochloride was administered daily in the pectoral muscle in a constant volume. On weekdays the drug was administered 30 minutes prior to the experimental session and on weekends the drug was administered at a constant time within one hour of the experimental session time. The drug dosage for the chronic regimen was chosen by taking the dosage which produced approximately a 50% decrease in responding on the acute regimen. This dose was administered for several days and then withdrawn. The next dose chosen was that dose which produced a 75% decrease in responding on the acute regimen.

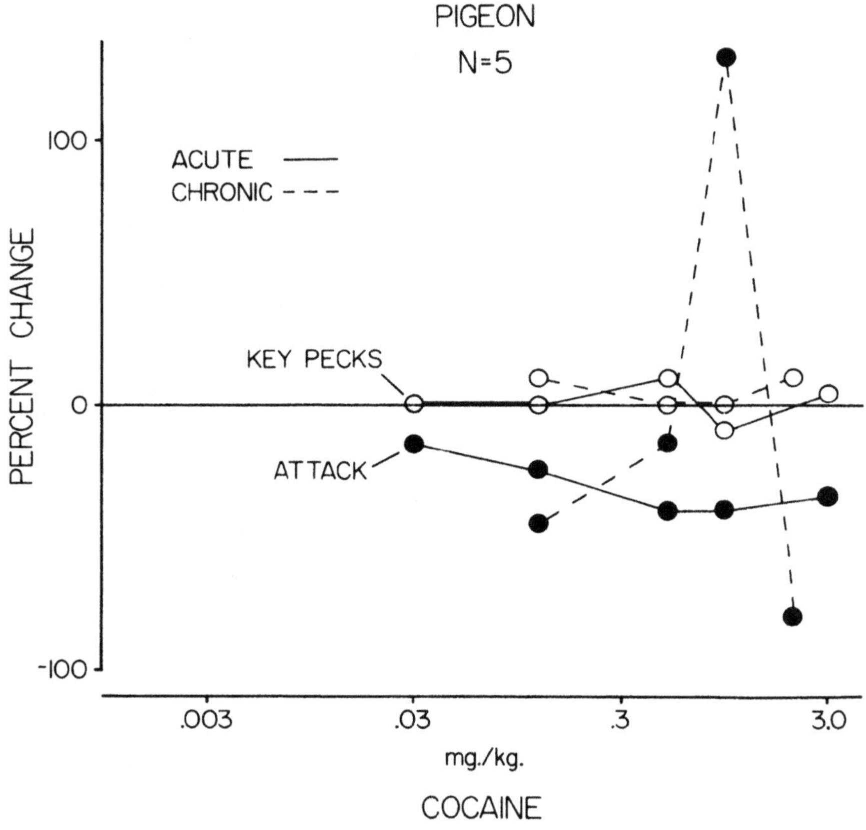

Fig. 7. Effects of acute and chronic cocaine on the key peck and attack responses of the pigeon on a multiple reinforcement-extinction schedule.

Results

The multiple reinforcement-extinction procedure of this experiment generated responding as illustrated in the right hand section of Fig. 6. The top record is of cumulative key pecks. The downward deflection of the pen indicates feeder presentations. Reinforcement periods are indicated by the deflection of the baseline pen. The bottom record shows cumulative attack responses. It can be noted that transition to periods of extinction produced attack responses on the stuffed target pigeon in the chamber. Figure 7 illustrates the effect of increasing dosages of acute and chronic cocaine on attack and food acquisition responses. The open circles represent extinction-attack responses. The line at zero represents saline control preceding that dosage.

The results of this experiment demonstrate the differential effect of cocaine on food acquisition and attack responses produced by a multiple reinforcement-extinction procedure in the pigeon. Across the range of dosages tested there was a dose dependent decrease in extinction attack responses and little or no effect on CRF key peck responses. These results are consistent across the acute and chronic drug regimens. The attack increase noted at one dosage on the chronic regimen was the result of an extreme effect for one subject.

Discussion

The results of this experiment demonstrate that the effect of cocaine on attack responses produced by food removal is the same whether the drug is given on an acute or chronic regimen. It is interesting to note that there was no withdrawal effect of the drug in that responding returned immediately to saline control baseline levels upon withdrawal of the chronic cocaine at all doses tested. The decrease in attack responses is consistent with similar effects of cocaine on aggressive responses in Experiments 1 and 2.

EXPERIMENT 4: EFFECTS OF ACUTE AND CHRONIC COCAINE ADMINISTRATION UPON SHOCK AVOIDANCE-PRODUCED ATTACK BY SQUIRREL MONKEYS

Subjects

Subjects were three adult male squirrel monkeys weighing between 700 and 900 grams. The subjects were housed in individual cages in a large colony room, had free access to fluids, and were fed fruit and Wayne monkey diet.

Apparatus

A primate restraint chair as described in Experiment 1 and illustrated in Fig. 1 was used. The front panel was modified in such a way that there was no lever.

Procedure

60-Minute experimental sessions were conducted five days a week. During each session an avoidance procedure in which tail shocks would occur every 20 seconds unless a bite response occurred was in effect. A bite postponed the shock delivery for 60 seconds. Shocks (400 v.ac, 200 ms) were delivered through the brass tail electrodes which rested on the distal portion of the tail, which had been shaved and prepared with electrode paste. Hose bites and shock deliveries were recorded on cumulative recorders and counters.

Acute Drug Administration

All injections of cocaine hydrochloride were given subcutaneously 30 minutes prior to the experimental session. Saline control injections were given in a constant volume on four days of the week. Cocaine was administered in a mixed order of dosages on Wednesday of the experimental week. All drug dosages below 1.5 mg/kg were given in a mixed order. The doses above 1.5 mg/kg were given in an ascending order. The doses above 1.5 mg/kg were given in an ascending order until the highest dose was determined.

Chronic Drug Administration

Cocaine hydrochloride was administered in the drinking water of the subjects. A graduated water bottle was mounted on the home cage for the recording of daily fluid intake. Distilled water was the control fluid for the determination of daily fluid intake for each subject. When fluid intake stabilized, drug was added to the water. The drug was added to the drinking water starting at 0.007 mg/100cc and increasing in a doubling function. Drug dosage was changed when behavioral responding was stable. Intake was recorded daily at 11 a.m. and fresh solutions supplied. Dosages of cocaine administered were based on body weight and fluid intake such that mg/kg/subject would be approximately the same.

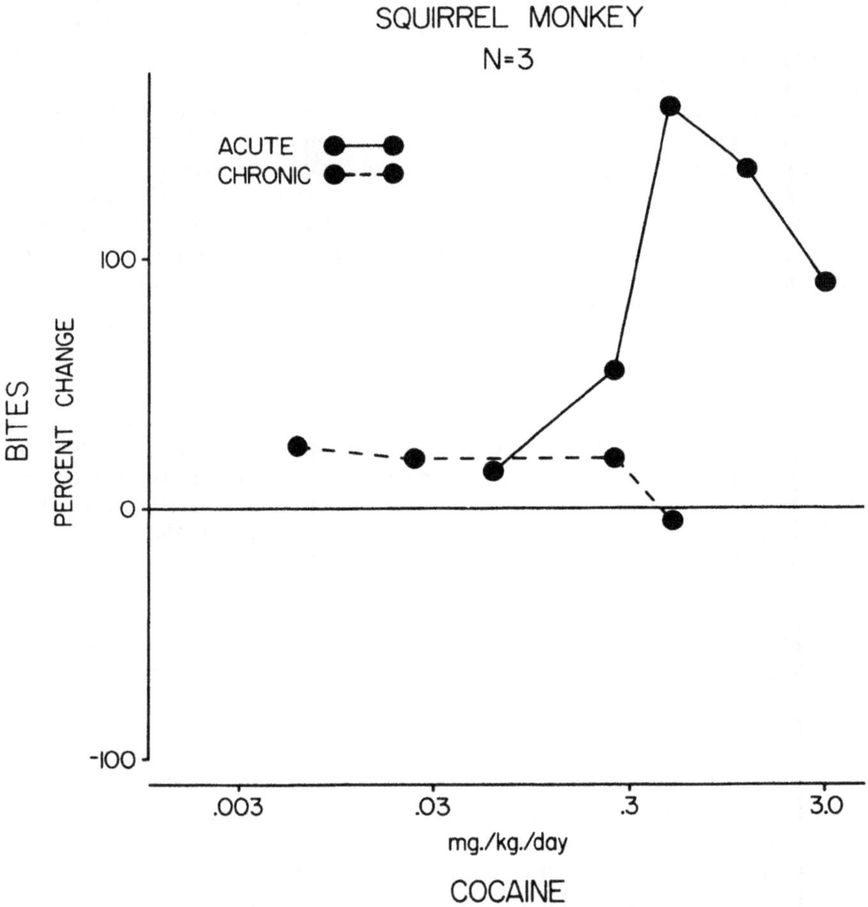

Fig. 8. Effects of acute and chronic cocaine on the bite-avoidance response in the squirrel monkey.

Results

Figure 8 illustrates the effect of increasing dosages of acute and chronic cocaine hydrochloride on the bite responses of the three subjects in this experiment. The line at zero indicates the saline control or distilled water baseline and the drug points are indicated by percent change from the saline control baseline immediately preceding the dose on the acute regimen or the distilled water control on the chronic regimen. The results show that bite responses were elevated over control at each dosage of the drug. At the highest doses on the acute regimen, two of the three subjects took several shocks and showed some disruption of performance. On the chronic regimen, subject fluid intake and body weight were consistent across the range of dosages tested, and withdrawal of the drug resulted in a gradual return toward control levels of responding.

Discussion

The data from this experiment show that the cocaine-produced effects on the bite-shock avoidance response are similar to the effect of cocaine upon the lever press pre-shock responding in Experiment 1. In these experiments, chronic and acute cocaine administration elevates pre-shock responding on both the shock-elicited biting paradigm and the bite avoidance paradigm.

EXPERIMENT 5: EFFECTS OF ACUTE AND CHRONIC COCAINE ADMINISTRATION ON FOOD ACQUISITION-PRODUCED ATTACK BY SQUIRREL MONKEYS

Subjects

Subjects were three adult male squirrel monkeys weighing between 600 and 800 grams. The subjects were housed in individual cages in a large colony room. The subjects had free access to fluids and were fed Wayne monkey diet and fruit to maintain 90% of free feeding weight.

Apparatus

A primate restraint chair (as illustrated in Fig. 1) was used. The restraint chair was equipped with a bite hose and a food cup mounted on the front panel. The feeder (Davis Model TD 109 A) mounted on the back of the front panel was adjusted to deliver 45 mg banana pellets (P.J. Noyes) into the food cup on the front of the panel. The restraint chair was enclosed in a sound-attenuated, ventilated outer chamber. White noise was present in the chamber to mask extraneous noise.

Procedure

45-Minute experimental sessions were conducted five days a week. During each session a variable-interval 90" reinforcement schedule was in effect in which the first bite response following satisfaction of the variable interval caused the feeder to deliver a 45 mg pellet into the food cup. Hose bites and pellet deliveries were recorded on cumulative recorders and counters.

Acute Drug Administration

All injections of cocaine hydrochloride were given subcutaneously 30 minutes prior to the experimental session. Saline control injections were given in a constant volume on four days of the week. Drug was administered in a mixed order of dosages on Wednesday of the experimental week.

Chronic Drug Administration

Cocaine hydrochloride was administered in the drinking water of the subject. A graduated water bottle was mounted on the home cage for the recording of daily fluid intake. Distilled water was the control fluid for the determination of daily fluid intake for each subject. When fluid intake stabilized, drug was added to the water. The drug was added to the drinking water starting at 0.007 mg/100 cc and increasing in a doubling function. Drug dosage was changed when behavioral responding was stable. Intake was recorded daily at 11 a.m. and fresh solutions supplied.

Results

Figure 9 illustrates the effect of increasing dosages of acute and chronic cocaine hydrochloride on bite responses for food pellets for three squirrel monkeys. The line at zero indicates the saline control baseline for the acute regimen and the distilled water baseline for the chronic regimen. The results for the acute regimen of cocaine administration illustrate a slight increase in responding at the low dosages with a decrease at the high dose. The decrease in responding at the high dose is characterized by a period of no responding at the beginning of the session followed by a gradual increase in responding toward the end of the session. On the chronic regimen, also, there was a slight increase in responding at the low dosages and a slight decrease at the higher doses.

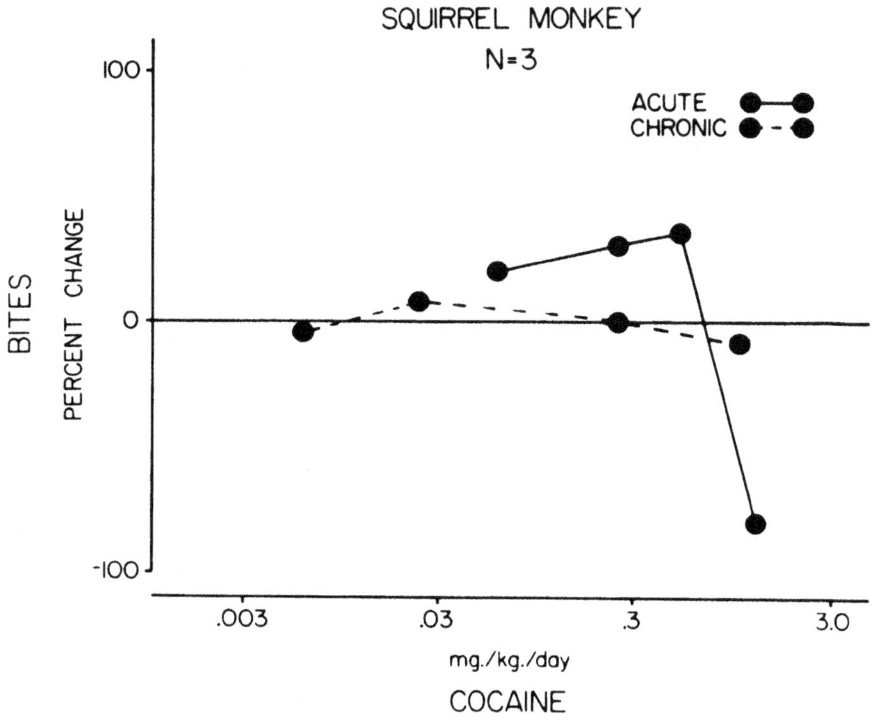

Fig. 9. Effects of acute and chronic cocaine on the bite response for food reinforcement in the squirrel monkey.

Discussion

The slight increases at low doses and decreases at higher doses of cocaine on the food acquisition-produced attack paradigm agree with drug results on other paradigms tested.

DISCUSSION

The results of the present experiments demonstrate that cocaine has neither a fundamental nor consistent potentiating effect on aggressive behavior. Experiments 1, 2 and 3 were designed to test the effect of cocaine upon the two types of antecedent stimulus-produced aggression. The results of these experiments collectively demonstrate that, in fact, the primary effect of cocaine administration is either to increase several classes of reactions and actually increase, differentially, non-aggressive responses relative to attack reactions or to differentially decrease attack behaviors while leaving non-attack performances relatively unchanged.

Experiment 1 studied the effects both of acute and chronic cocaine administration on the dual baseline of post-shock biting and pre-shock lever pressing. The acute administration of cocaine in early portions of the drug dose range tested resulted in an increase in both responses, but differential increases in pre-shock lever pressing. At higher doses biting was actually decreased almost to zero while lever pressing still continued at above control levels. Chronic oral administration of cocaine at lowest doses also caused an increase in pre-shock lever pressing while leaving biting unaffected. Little influence of the drug was seen at higher doses until at the highest dose tested; though biting was unaffected, lever pressing was actually decreased to below control levels. In retrospect, it appears that extended testing of chronic cocaine at daily dosages below the 0.003 mg/kg/day level would be warranted. Earlier work of this laboratory (Hutchinson and Emley, 1973) has demonstrated that the chronic oral administration of drug to squirrel monkeys often produces effects equivalent to 1/100 of the acute subcutaneous dose of the same compound when expressed on a mg/kg/day basis.

Experiment 2 was designed to replicate in a second species the effects of acute cocaine administration on a shock-produced biting baseline. The results of this experiment demonstrated that, throughout the range of doses tested, cocaine produced a decrease in biting attack by mice.

Experiment 3 tested in the pigeon the influence of both acute and chronic administration of cocaine on the dual baseline of key pecks for food and post-food extinction attacks against a stuffed target pigeon. With only one exception, this experiment demonstrates for both acute and chronic cocaine administration that pecking attacks are differentially reduced relative to key pecking for food throughout the range of doses tested. The single exception to this general finding for both routes of administration involves the marked increase in pecking attack relative to key pecking for food at the 1.0 mg/kg dose during chronic testing. Again it should be pointed out that this increase was the anomalous result contributed by a single subject. Each of the other subjects demonstrated the general differential decrease in pecking attack relative to key pecking for food.

In the three experiments designed to assess the effect of acute and chronic cocaine administration upon attack performances generated by antecedent stimulation, cocaine generally resulted in actual decreases in aggression or relatively greater increases in non-aggressive behavior.

Further experiments were designed to measure the effects of acute and chronic cocaine administration on attack behavior maintained by its consequences. Experiment 4 tested drug influence upon biting attack performances by squirrel monkeys which were maintained by shock avoidance, while Experiment 5 tested the effects of cocaine upon a baseline of biting attack reinforced by the presentation of food on a variable interval schedule. In Experiment 4, the acute administration of cocaine produced increases in attack behavior. Drug effects were progressively higher at higher dosages until the maximum was reached at 0.5 mg/kg. At still higher doses, though attack was increased, the increases were less than were seen at 0.5 mg/kg. In this same paradigm, the chronic oral administration of cocaine produced smaller increases in attack behavior and, at the highest dosage, did not change attack behavior. The dose-response function obtained for the acute administration of cocaine in the bite-shock avoidance paradigm of Experiment 4 is highly similar to the dose-response function obtained for similar quantities of the drug upon anticipatory pre-shock lever pressing in Experiment 1. In each experiment, identical drug administration procedures at essentially equivalent dosage levels produced comparable changes in two different topographic behaviors. A common feature, however, of these two performances is that they are maintained by temporal and related stimuli associated with the imminent delivery of shock. In Experiment 5, the effect of acute and chronic cocaine administration was tested for influence upon a baseline of biting attack maintained by the intermittent food reinforcement. Acute cocaine administration produced, at lower doses, a modest increase in food-reinforced biting attack. At the highest dosage, this performance was reduced considerably below control values. Chronic cocaine administration produced little or no change in performance in this paradigm. The minimal drug effects on performance maintained by food reinforcement observed in this experiment are similar to the observations of Experiment 3, where key pecking for food by pigeons was only slightly affected by cocaine.

Thus the results of Experiments 4 and 5 support the view that aggressive behavior may be increased by cocaine administration insofar as aggressive performances possess certain features in common with other performances. More specifically, it was shown that when aggressive sequences occur in an environment where temporal and related stimuli associated with the imminent delivery of shock are present, such aggression can be increased or decreased just as non-aggressive performances are influenced.

In conclusion, it seems apparent that cocaine does not show unique influences upon aggressive behavior as compared with several other drugs, and--further--does not selectively increase aggression relative to non-aggressive behavioral sequences. Alternatively, cocaine does, in some environmental contexts, produce relative decreases in aggressive behavior.

ACKNOWLEDGMENTS

The work upon which this publication is based was performed pursuant to Contract No. ADM-45-74-163 with the National Institute on Drug Abuse. Our thanks to E.R. Hallin, N.J. Murray, S.H. Crawford, D. Mann, I. Wing, J. Bushong, D. Santek, K. Dinzik, R. Sewell, and T. Proni for their assistance.

REFERENCES

Byck, R.: Cocaine Papers: Sigmund Freud. New York: Stonehill Publishing Co., 1974.

Emley, G.S. and Hutchinson, R.R.: Similar and selective actions of chlorpromazine, chlordiazepoxide, and nicotine on shock-produced aggressive and anticipatory responses in the squirrel monkey. In: Proceedings of the 79th Annual Convention. American Psychological Association, pp. 759-760. Washington, D.C.: American Psychological Association, 1971.

Emley, G.S. and Hutchinson, R.R.: Basis of behavioral influence of chlorpromazine, Life Sci. 11, 43-47 (1972).

Hill, H.E., Bell, E.C., and Wikler, A.: Reduction of conditioned suppression: Actions of morphine compared with those of amphetamine, pentobarbital, nalorphine, cocaine, LSD-25 and chlorpromazine, Archs int. Pharmacodyn. Thér. 165, 212-226 (1967).

Hutchinson, R.R. and Emley, G.S.: Schedule-independent factors contributing to schedule-induced phenomena. In: Schedule Effects: Drugs, Drinking and Aggression. Gilbert, R.M. and Keehn, J.D., Eds., pp. 174-202. Toronto: University of Toronto Press, 1972.

Hutchinson, R.R.: The environmental causes of aggression. In: Nebraska Symposium on Motivation. Cole, J.K. and Jensen, D.D., Eds., pp. 155-181. Lincoln, Neb.: University of Nebraska Press, 1973.

Hutchinson, R.R. and Emley, G.S.: Effects of nicotine on avoidance, conditioned suppression and aggression response measures in animals and man. In: Smoking Behavior: Motives and Incentives. Dunn, W.L., Ed., pp. 171-196. Washington, D.C.: V.H. Winston, 1973.

Jaffe, J.H.: Drug addiction and drug abuse. In: The Pharmacological Basis of Therapeutics. Goodman, L.S. and Gilman, A., Eds., 3rd edition, pp. 285-311. Toronto: Macmillan, 1965.

Kosman, M.E. and Unna, K.R.: Effects of chronic administration of the amphetamines and other stimulants on behavior, Clin. Pharmacol. Therap. 9, 240-254 (1968).

Maurer, D.W. and Vogel, V.H.: Narcotics and Narcotic Addiction. Springfield, Ill.: C.C. Thomas, 1967.

Post, R.M., Kotin, J., and Goodwin, F.: The effects of cocaine on depressed patients, Am. J. Psychiat. 131, 511-517 (1974).

Simon, P., Sultan, Z., Chermat, R., and Boissier, J.: La cocaine, une substance amphetaminique? Un probleme de psychopharmacologic experimentale, J. Pharmacol. 3, 129-142 (1972).

Smith, C.B.: Effects of d-amphetamine upon operant behavior of pigeons: Enhancement by reserpine, J. Pharmac. exp. Ther. 146, 167-174 (1964).

CHANGES IN INDIVIDUAL AND SOCIAL BEHAVIOR INDUCED BY AMPHETAMINE AND RELATED COMPOUNDS IN MONKEYS AND MAN

Erik Schiørring

Psychopharmacological Research Laboratory

Sct. Hans Hospital, Dept. E, DK-4000 Roskilde, Denmark

INTRODUCTION

Ever since Edeleano (1887) made the first synthesis of phenyl-substituted aliphatic amines, this type of compound has been an object of research. Stern (1889) initially showed that beta-tetrahydronaphtylamine caused a motoric unrest in rabbits, and Airila (1913) supported this finding in the same species with ephedrine, which later was used to treat narcolepsy by Janota (1931). Alles (1933) demonstrated that beta-phenylisopropylamine sulphate is antagonistic to hypnotics. The introduction of Benzedrine in therapy (Prinzmetal and Bloomberg, 1935) made this group of amines the object of a closer study in humans because of its peculiar effects on the central nervous system. The psychiatric literature of 1936 and 1937 contained several articles on the use of Benzedrine, both in psychotic and non-psychotic persons (Donley, 1937).

A few years after the clinical use of amphetamine had been initiated, the first cases of paranoid psychosis with a schizophreniform clinical picture were reported (Young and Scoville, 1938). At this time the first controlled, double-blind studies with low doses of amphetamine in non-psychotic volunteers were made (Bahnsen, Jacobsen, and Thesleff, 1938; Wollstein, 1938; Jacobsen, 1939; Jacobsen and Wollstein, 1939; Wollstein, 1939).

During the following decades, especially in the last twenty years, both experimental and clinical research have increased. In various animal species it has been found consistently that all mammalian species respond to the administration of amphetamine and related compounds with marked changes in the individual and social behaviors (various stereotypies and social withdrawal).

Experimental work and clinical observations have made comparative analyses possible. From such studies it is evident that the response of man to CNS-stimulants is parallel to that of other mammalian species.

Important issues in the field of amphetamine research are found in books by the following authors: Bonhoff and Lewrenz, 1954; Connell, 1958; Kalant, 1966; Efron, Holmstedt, and Kline, 1967; Romano, 1967; Wilson, 1968; Cerletti and Bové, 1969; Sjöqvist and Tottie, 1969; Costa and Garattini, 1970; Ellinwood and Cohen, 1972; Cole, Freedman, and Friedhoff, 1973; Ban, Boissier, Gessa, Heimann, Hollister, Lehmann, Munkvad, Steinberg, Sulser, Sundwall, and Vinar, 1973; Snyder, 1974; Mitsuda and Fakuda, 1975; Grinspoon and Hedblom, 1975; Eleftheriou, 1975. On cocaine, Maier (1926) is still the classical, clinical reference.

In the present paper, some of the essential data from our animal and human studies are presented. Further details will be published elsewhere (Schiørring and Hecht, unpublished observations; Schiørring, unpublished observations; Schiørring, Rylander, and Holmberg, unpublished observations). Our interest is the biological and psychological significance of any item and pattern of behavior, especially the social interaction with other individuals and the function that these behavior elements serve for the organism. Thus we systematically record, quantify, qualify, and analyze the behavioral phenomena. Our approach is ethological. This method has proved valid in relation to both animal and human research (Tinbergen, 1963; Blurton-Jones, 1967; Esser, 1968; Esser and Paluck, 1968; Hutt and Hutt, 1970). Especially, we focus on the changes in naturally occurring patterns of behavior induced by amphetamine and related compounds.

It is our opinion (based on the results presented in this paper and the scientific literature cited) that CNS-stimulants (including cocaine) produce profound psychopathological conditions. The changes in behavior induced by these agents make it relevant to retain the amphetamine-psychosis as a suitable "model-psychosis," especially in connection with those clinically well-known aberrations that we call the schizophrenias. We also find that the results are important for the considerations on addiction to these drugs and for the basic understanding of social interaction.

The possible biochemical mechanisms underlying the behavioral aberrations following the use and abuse of the amphetamines are not discussed in this paper. Theories in the biochemical field have been concerned about neurotransmitters, such as dopamine, noradrenaline, serotonin and cholinergic systems (Randrup and Munkvad, 1970; Scheel-Krüger, 1971 and this meeting; Costa and Groppetti, 1972; Duarte-Escalante and Ellinwood, 1972; Fog, 1972; Mandell and Knapp, 1972; Randrup and Munkvad, 1972; Snyder, Taylor, Coyle, and Meyerhoff, 1972; Spooner and Flaming, 1972; Welch and Welch, 1972; Randrup and Munkvad, 1974; Cools, 1975, 1976). At present it seems most probable that the theories that include a dynamic interaction between the different transmitter-systems are the most realistic.

METHODS

Experimental Data

The "OPEN-FIELD" technique was used in both the triadic and dyadic groups of green vervet monkeys (Cercopithecus aethiops). The animals were allowed to move freely in the cage with water ad libitum on a stable daily feeding-routine at 9 a.m. No conditioning of the behavior was deliberately induced by the experimenter. All experimental sessions started at 10 a.m. and lasted for exactly one hour. d-Amphetamine in doses from 0.1 mg to 0.7 mg/kg body-weight was administered non-chronically, s.c. at intervals of 7 to 10 days. Control sessions (s.c. administration of corresponding volumes of isotonic NaCl-solution [placebo])came between the amphetamine sessions.

The observations of the behavior were made either by the author plus one specially trained technician or by two such technicians. The recordings were made by semi-automatic equipment consisting of event-markers, stopwatches, and videotape and by manual notation.

Three independent experiments were made with the monkey-triad (Groups I, II, and III):

I:	16	placebo and	16	amphetamine	sessions
II:	21	" "	17	"	"
III:	15	" "	10	"	"

Two independent experiments were made with the mother/infant-dyad (Group I and II):

I:	15	placebo and	16	amphetamine	sessions
II:	48	" "	10	"	"

The groups were used as their own controls.

The adult monkeys (about 5-8 years old) were imported from Ethiopia (East Africa) via the State Serum Institute of Copenhagen, where they were examined for various tropical diseases before delivery to our laboratory.

Triadic social behavior (adult monkeys)

The experimental group-cage was constructed in a way which made it possible to separate the monkeys into three individual cages for injections and during the night. The dimension of the cage was 6 m^2 for Group I and Group II. For Group III it was enlarged to 12 m^2. The following behavior elements were recorded:

a) all social grooming combinations, b) approach/avoidance movements, c) hierarchical balance (rank order) between the male and the two females, d) sexual activity, e) location and locomotion in the experimental cage, f) aggression, g) self-grooming, h) total isolation, i) "staring" (with head and eye movements).

In all experiments, a period of three months was taken to establish a stable social pattern of interaction. The experimental sessions started after these three-month periods and lasted for approximately six months.

After 11-12 months the base line placebo behavior began to change and thus the experiments were terminated. It has been difficult to analyze whether the change in base-line behavior was caused by the non-chronic, but repeated, amphetamine injections, or was due to the restricted laboratory environmental conditions--or a combination of the two factors.

Dyadic social behavior (mother/infant)

The infants were born in our laboratory. The mother and infant were housed in a special, two-room cage (3 x 1.5 x 1 m). Except for certain experimental sessions (Table 1, Group I), mother and infant were allowed to stay together day and night. Amphetamine was administered to the mother in the main experiments, but preliminary experiments were made to observe the effect of amphetamine on the infant's behavior. The following behavior elements were recorded:

a) ventral-ventral contact (Picture 1), b) mother grooming infant, c) other physical contacts (arms, legs, body), d) approach/avoidance movements, e) eye-contact, f) mother, self-grooming.

Definition of "close-sitting": This pattern was recorded, when the animals were sitting together without grooming, if the physical distance between them was less than the length of their arms: a distance that made it possible to start mutual grooming without moving the whole body.

The experiments were made while the infant was between one month and six months old. In this period the infant was closely connected to and deeply dependent on the mother's parental care. In order to measure the strength of the binding between mother and infant a test of social cohesion was made. The infant was separated from the mother by a clear fiberglass wall. Thus the animals could see and hear each other, but could not establish physical contact (Group I, Table I). The reactions of the infant to the amphetamine-induced changes in the mother were recorded.

METHODS

Clinical data

Forty Swedish and ten Danish abusers of CNS-stimulants, who were drug-free and without abstinence symptoms, were interviewed in face-to-face dialogues. The Swedish abusers were patients at the Clinic of Forensic Psychiatry in Stockholm. The Danish abusers were clients in a group therapeutic treatment program with the author as therapist. An additional six abusers were observed during a "run" (about half an hour post injection of i.v. administration of 200-350 mg phenmetrazine of d-amphetamine). The observations were made at a police station in Stockholm and in the drug milieu in Copenhagen.

A questionnaire (see below) was developed from many preliminary discussions with CNS-stimulant abusers, and some of the questions were based on animal data made in our laboratory (referred to by Rylander, 1971, 1972). Tape recordings were also used.

Introduction to the English/American version of the questionnaire:

A great number of linguistic problems occur when drug-world lingo is translated. The questionnaire, therefore, should be corrected in accordance with the language used within the American "speed-scene" (drug culture).

In the original Swedish version the questions have a formulation that is easily understood by the abuser. In the present translation (below) the Swedish slang-word "PUNDING" is retained because Rylander (1971, 1972) introduced this term in the scientific literature in 1967.

Linguistically, the word PUND-HUVUD (huvud = head) is synonymous with BLOCK-HEAD in English. Thus PUNDING means to behave stupidly, foolishly, etc. When used by the amphetamine-abusers, PUNDING has a more specific meaning, namely, the characteristically aimless, stereotyped, repetitive behaviors that are present during the "run" and sometimes during the abstinence phase.

It seems probable that the American term KNICK-KNACKING covers the content of PUNDING (Ellinwood, 1972; Kramer, 1972; Smith, 1972). The term TO BE HUNG UP (Scher, 1966) could also be synonymous with PUNDING, but might further cover another Swedish slang-word: to INSNÖA (insnoea) = to be "SNOWED UP." To INSNÖA is used synonymously with PUNDING and to describe the peculiarly social withdrawal often experienced by the abusers.

QUESTIONNAIRE

What does "punding" mean?

Do you use other words?

Have you been punding? How often and how much?

What do you usually do when you're punding?

Is any sort of punding typical for you - something special for you? What's that?

Do you often do any sort of cleaning? Make drawings? Dismantle radios, or something similar?

If you do any of these things when you're turned on, do you do them when you're not turned on, too?

Do you think everybody is punding in their own special way - I mean that one person is always dismantling radios, others are always drawing, and others are always putting on make-up? Do boys and girls act differently?

Is it possible to pund in different ways, too, or is the special way of punding always used?

Do you have the impression that people are punding with things they usually take an interest in?

Do boys and girls stay turned on in the same way, or is it different for the two sexes?

Is it true that somebody who is turned on starts punding, if one begins?

Does it happen that one starts punding in the same way as somebody else in the group? Has it happened to you? Have you seen others to whom it has happened?

Can punding become fashionable?

Is it possible to pund together with somebody else in some sort of group-punding, for instance, dismantle the same radio-set?

Does it happen that you start punding in quite a new way after some time is spent punding in the usual way?

If you are disturbed while punding, do you then carry on in the same way afterwards - or do you start another way of punding?

Have you seen what happens to others if they're disturbed?

Are you punding in the same way when you're on high doses as when you're on low doses?

Does the punding start at once after you're turned on, or does it take some time?

Are you punding during "the downer" (here used = "coming down")? If yes, what do you then do? What do the others do?

How do you experience the punding? Nice? Not nice? Anxiety-producing or not? Unpleasant? Pleasant? Pressed? Free?

Is it possible to break the punding? By needing to go to the bathroom? By thirst? By hunger? By sexual stimulation? When offered a fix from somebody? Threat from outside? By demand for help from a friend?

How do you feel if somebody tries to break off your punding? Do you become angry? Alarmed? Is it all the same?

How do others react if their punding is broken off? Anger? Carelessness?

For how long a time does the punding usually continue for you? For others?

Is it usual or unusual that a boy and a girl "fix" each other?

Is sex-activity usual between a girl and a boy while they're turned on?

Do you become more inventive - I mean, do ways of sex-activity other than the usual ones come out?

Do you have the feeling that the sex-activity can turn into some sort of punding - something that goes on and on without orgasms?

Do you talk a lot, or are you mostly silent when you're turned on?

What about the talking when you're punding?

Do you have the feeling that the one you're talking with is listening while he or she is turned on? If yes, is he (she) punding then?

Do the others talk a lot when they're turned on, for instance, in the group?

Do you listen to the others when you're turned on?

Do you listen while you're punding?

Is it true that people are talking without listening to each other while they're turned on, for instance, in the group, just to have a good time; or is it not so? Is it so while they're punding?

Is it of any interest what the others do while one is turned on, or does it not matter at all?

What about the interest in the others' activity while you're punding?

If one is turned on, is it of any interest to come to know new people who are in the same group, for instance, or is it not so?

What about the contact with new people while one is punding, then?

Why is punding often happening in the group?

Do you always pund together with the others, or do you sometimes pund when you're on your own?

Have you observed repeated body-movements or grimaces when people are turned on? Show it, please. Have you done such movements?

Do people have their own special movements or do most of them move in the same way while they're turned on?

Do you have special movements when you're turned on?

Are girls' movements different from boys'?

Does it happen that one imitates others' movements?

Have you been imitating others' movements? Have you seen others do so?

Do these movements occur in a certain order, so that some movements start early during "the run" and other movements follow?

Have you observed people who are turned on twitching their mouth upwards or sidewards? Seen people rolling their eyes? Heard some making sniffing sounds? Licking themselves around the mouth? Walking around in circles? Twitching the arms? Staring at the fingers? Picking their hands? Heard people say the same things time and again? Seen anybody standing completely still in a corner, with the face turned against the wall?

Do you have the possibility to talk about your special interests to those who use "speed"?

RESULTS

Animal data

Some of the essential data are presented in Figs. 1 to 4 and Table 1. A more detailed analysis of the data will be published elsewhere.

Figure 1 (Group I), Fig. 2 (Group II), and Fig. 3 (Group III) show the grooming relations between three adult vervet monkeys (Cercopithecus aethiops) from three different experimental groups (each consisting of one male and two females). Table 1 (Group I) and Fig. 4 (Group II) contain some of the essential results from the mother/infant dyadic interaction. It is a fundamental feature that the parental care behavior is deeply disturbed even if small, s.c., non-chronic amphetamine doses are administered to the mother.

From the figures and the table it is seen that the groups are responding differently to the administration of amphetamine, but that the results support each other. Both in the triadic and the dyadic groups amphetamine disrupts the pattern of social interaction, even to the extreme of total social isolation (social withdrawal). When isolated by amphetamine, the animals can be preoccupied with stereotyped self-grooming or can be immobile, while "staring" into space. Also, stereotyped mutual grooming occurs (Fig. 2, Group III). In this case, the grooming is unvaried and goes on continuously for 68% of the total observation time (1 hour sessions). In placebo animals the grooming is interrupted by other activities in a varied pattern, and the mutual grooming pattern is characterized by the shifting between at least 12 different parts of the body. The amphetaminized animals show a mutual grooming pattern that is quite different. Besides the continuous appearance, the grooming is restricted to only two parts of the body: the proximal and distal locations of the back.

The triad (three adult vervet monkeys):

Changes in the rank order of the females (sexual behavior):

During the first three months without drug, a stable sexual pattern was established between the male and the two females. Usually one of the females was preferred via initial power-fights, but the male always mounted both females. Amphetamine changed this pattern. The lower ranking female could become the preferred, or the male switched his sexual interest to only one of the females. Masturbation: The male was observed masturbating, and thus he did not mount either of the females. Masturbation was never observed in our placebo experiments.

The changes induced by amphetamine are extremely important, since sex activity has proved to be essential for the establishing of a stable social interaction. In fact, our experiments have shown that, if the male cannot mount the females in an appropriate way, or if the females have not reached the age of sexual maturity, a stable social pattern will never develop.

Antagonism of well-known neuroleptics to the action of amphetamines (preliminary experiments):

Several neuroleptics in various doses were administered to the amphetaminized monkeys. None of these drugs (chlorpromazine, perphenazine, pimozide, clozapin) proved to be effective in reducing the degree of social withdrawal. These drugs antagonized only the amphetamine-induced stereotypies. Only one category of compounds antagonized the amphetamine action on social behavior: an anti-serotonin compound (MCE-methergoline Sostanza 355-255). This compound, however, did not normalize the behavior of the animals, but it broke the social withdrawal. This drug changed the social behavior in the direction of stereotyped mutual grooming (also reported with amphetamine alone, Fig. 2, Group II).

The dyad (mother/infant relation of vervet monkeys):

Eye contact (gaze-aversion):

The qualitative and quantitative measures of eye contact in monkeys are, of course, extremely difficult, but we found that a specific gaze from the mother to the infant (or vice versa) was an important cue for contact. This eye-contact was lacking when the mother was influenced by amphetamine.

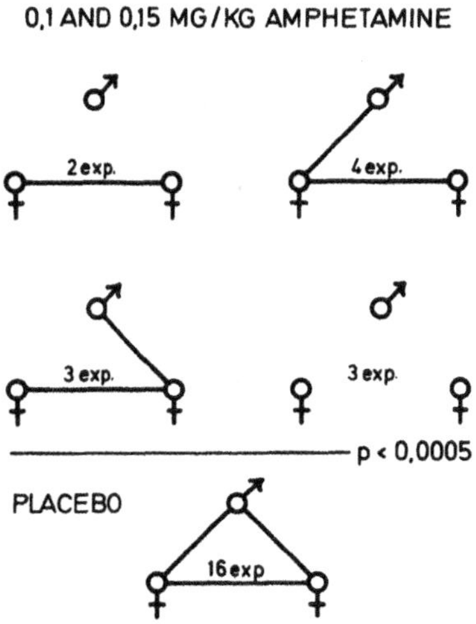

Fig. 1 (Group I): Mutual grooming. A heavy line drawn between two symbols designates that grooming occurred between the two monkeys corresponding to the two symbols connected by the line. In 16 placebo one-hour sessions all the possible mutual grooming combinations occurred and formed a stable pattern of social interaction. Of 16 amphetamine one-hour sessions, none was identical with the placebo sessions. In 4 sessions with amphetamine the grooming relations occurred, but the frequency was significantly different from placebo. In the other 12 amphetamine sessions, the social grooming was incomplete, disrupted, or abolished. The mutual grooming was replaced by stereotyped self-grooming or staring into space. Level of significance: $p < 0.0005$.

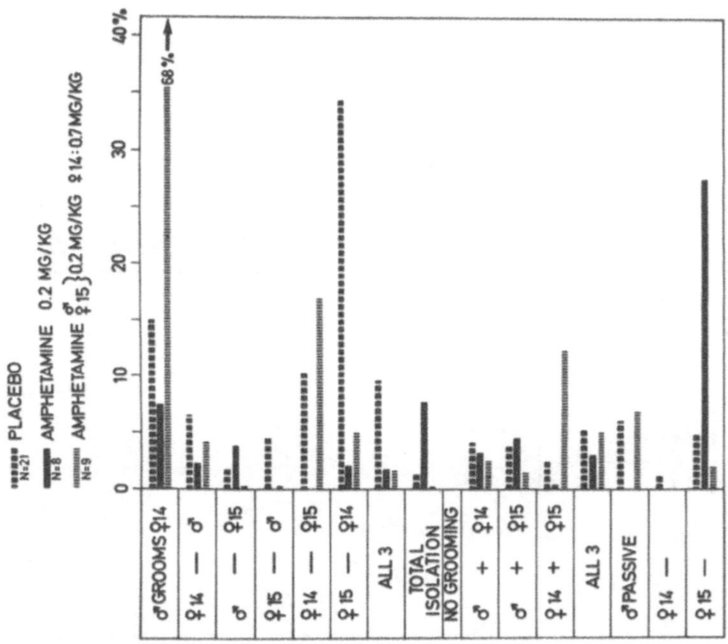

Fig. 2 (Group II): Social interaction of three vervet monkeys. Twenty-one one-hour placebo sessions and 17 one-hour amphetamine sessions were recorded. The figure shows the percent time spent in mutual grooming, total isolation, close-sitting (without grooming - see methods), and the group-interaction, where all 3 are sitting close together and the two of them are grooming while one is passive (staring or stereotyped self-grooming). The figure demonstrates the amphetamine-induced change in the social pattern of behavior. The average percentage of total observation time is indicated by the length of the columns. The recording "male grooms female No. 14" is of special interest, since this grooming pattern was present continuously in 68.5% of the total observation period. It is an example of stereotyped social behavior (see results). Also the recording "female No. 15 passive" is interesting. There is a significant increase in this social situation compared to the placebo sessions. It is an additional example of the peculiar effects of amphetamine on social behavior, which is often changed into bizarre, inappropriate patterns in which staring and stereotyped behaviors are commonly involved.

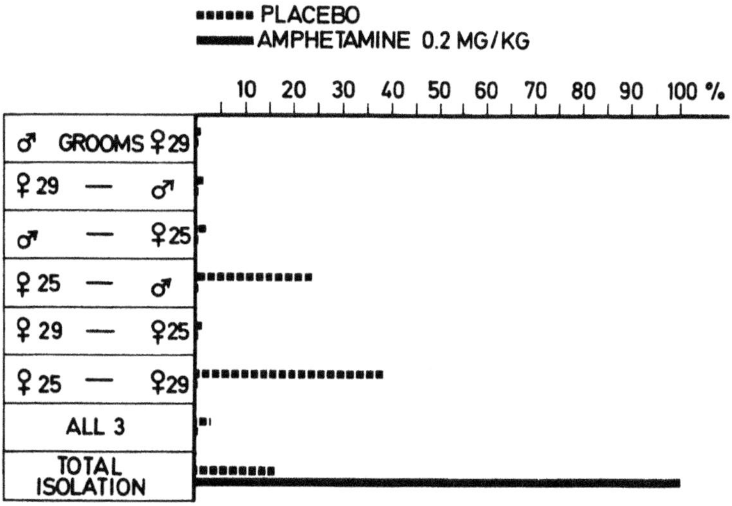

Fig. 3 (Group III): Social interaction of three vervet monkeys. In this group the total isolation induced by 0.2 mg/kg amphetamine is predominant. This experiment was made in a larger environmental setting (see methods). The difference between this environment and the environment used in Groups I and II, however, is not the explanation of the marked increase in total isolation. All three monkeys given amphetamine were sitting, immobile, on a location in the cage - which was characteristic for them - staring continuously at the one-way screen. For shorter periods they would perform stereotyped self-grooming, but the main feature of behavior was the "staring" into space. On the other hand, it might be important to investigate further the importance of spatial variables and the reaction to drugs.

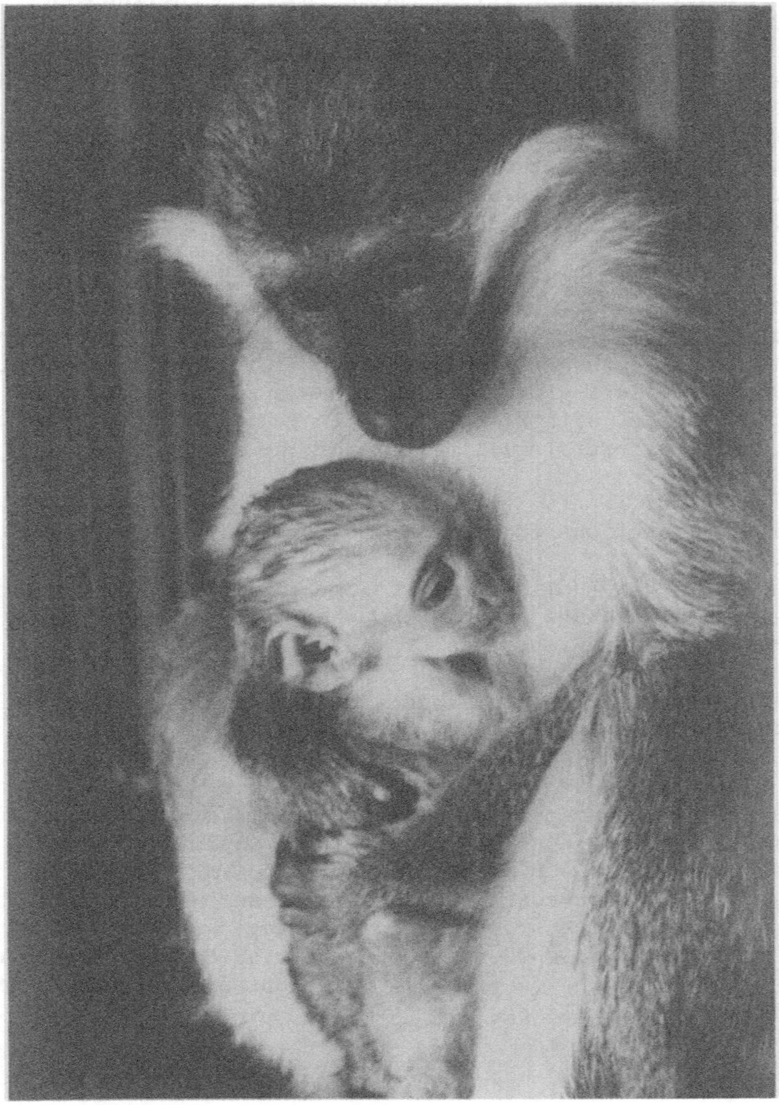

Picture 1. Characteristic parental care posture in monkeys: the ventral-ventral contact. The mother shows a specific grasping of the infant with both arms and both hands. Age of infant: two weeks. Amphetamine disrupts this fundamental element of behavior. 0.1, 0.15, and 0.2 mg/kg d-amphetamine administered s.c. non-chronically to the mother induces a social withdrawal. The mother is sitting passively "staring" into space or performing stereotyped self-grooming. In Group I (Table 1) the stereotyped self-grooming was dominating. In Group II (Fig. 4) the staring was dominating. The infant's reactions to the social withdrawal of the mother were marked (see results).

The reactions of the infant on the amphetamine-induced behavior of the mother were different in the two studies (Groups I and II). In Group I the infant increased its movements (approach-avoidance) to the mother, who reacted by active rejection. In Group II the infant sat very close to and quietly in front of the mother (a demonstrative ventral-ventral contact posture). The mother did not react to this contact-behavior. The infant thus decreased the amount of approach-avoidance movements to zero. The mother was immobile, staring into space.

In both experiments the parental care behavior pattern was disturbed. The mother lost her interest in the infant. She did not react to the calling signals of the infant, spent most of the time away from the infant (Table 1, Group I), and was preoccupied with stereotyped self-grooming. Or she was sitting, immobile, staring into space, without the specific ventral-ventral contact grasping (Fig. 4, Picture 1) in spite of the close presence of the infant.

Infants' reactions to amphetamine (preliminary experiments):

Amphetamine was administered to the infants of the two experimental groups at the age of 8 months when the main experiments were terminated. The reactions of the infants were individually different. The infant of Group I reacted to 0.2 mg/kg d-amphetamine. The calling signals were abolished and the motoric behavior was peculiarly "smooth" and lacking normal variation. Behind the clear fiberglass wall, it walked around continuously, without stopping.

The infant of Group II did not react with overt behavioral changes to the lowest dose of amphetamine. A clear-cut reaction was, however, seen to 2.0 mg/kg d-amphetamine (= 10 times the dose of infant I). On this dose it became quiet and was sitting, immobile, clinging to the front wall of the cage - "staring." No mother contact was present. When the observer entered the room, it reacted by screaming (anxiety signal), but did not run to the mother as in normal sessions.

TABLE 1
15 placebo and 15 0.2 mg/kg amphetamine one-hour sessions

GROUP I

MOTHER / INFANT
SOCIAL INTERACTION VERVET MONKEYS

% OF TOTAL SESSION TIME (1HR)

	MOTHER AWAY FROM SCREEN	MOTHER CLOSE TO SCREEN	INFANT CLOSE TO SCREEN
PLACEBO N=15	8.3	91.7	78.7
0.2 MG/ KG AMPHETAMINE TO MOTHER N=15	91.4	8.6	75.0

$P < 0.0005$

STEREOTYPES : LOOKING AT HANDS
PICKING ON LEFT HAND
BITING NAILS

SOCIAL WITHDRAWAL : NO RESPONSE TO INFANTS
CALLING-SIGNALS

This table demonstrates the response from the mother to the infant sessions in a certain experimental situation. The mother was separated from the infant by a fiberglass screen. They could easily see each other. In the placebo sessions the mother reacted adequately to the calling signals of the infant and spent 91.7% of the total observation time close (less than 10 cm) to the separating screen. After the non-chronic administration of d-amphetamine, the mother spent 91.4% of the total observation time away (more than 2 m) from the screen, preoccupied with stereotyped self-grooming, looking at her hands, picking on the left hand, and biting nails. The significance of her social withdrawal was that she stopped reacting to the infant's calling signals.

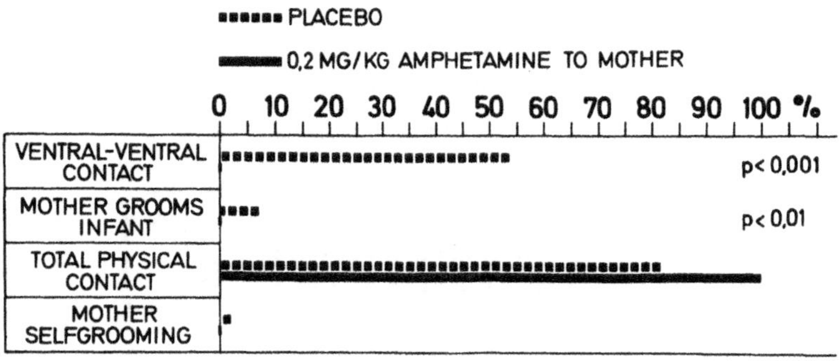

APPROACH / AVOIDANCE MOVEMENTS (AVERAGE FIGURES)

	M.appr. INF.	M.av. INF.	INF.appr. M.	INF.av.M.	SIGNIF.
N=48 PLACEBO	0,16	4,29	25,89	21,82	p<0,01
N=10 0,2 MG/KG AMPH.	0	0	0	0	

Fig. 4 (Group II): Mother/infant social interaction in vervet monkeys. In this figure it is important to notice that the ventral-ventral contact is reduced from 54.5% to zero by amphetamine and simultaneously the recording of physical contact is "increased." This feature should be understood in the following way. The two parts of the figure must be read together. From the lower part it is seen that it is the infant that defines the approach-avoidance movements between the mother and the infant. In the placebo experiments the average number of approaches is 25.89 (per hour) and the avoidance movements are 21.82 (per hour). In the amphetamine experiments the approach-avoidance movements are ZERO ($p < 0.01$). This is to be interpreted in line with what is expressed in Picture 1: the female under the influence of amphetamine shows social withdrawal with no active interest in the infant. The infant, on the other hand, tries to get into contact with the "autistic" mother by sitting close to her without the normal play pattern and the approach-avoidance movements. In Group I, (Table 1) the reactions from the infant to the "autism" of the mother were different. It induced an increased approach-avoidance frequency. Notice these two types of responses from the mother: (Group I) active rejection of the infant and no response to its calling signals; (Group II) passive staring, no reactions to the presence of the infant.

RESULTS

Human data

The results are presented in Tables 2 to 11 and in the literal examples from the interviews. Further details will be published separately.

The following amphetamine-induced changes in behavior were found:

1) Motoric, stereotyped, bizarre, choreiform movements. Repetitive, aimless activities. "Pottering," "Knick-knacking," "Punding" with various objects, including own body. Repetition of single words or phrases. Stereotyped writing, or drawing.

2) Social stereotypies: prolonged sexual intercourse without ejaculation. Collective monologues (talking without listening).

3) Social withdrawal ("autism," social isolation).

4) Paranoia.

5) Hallucinations (and illusions): auditive, visual, and tactile.

6) Micro-hallucinations (worms, insects, etc. coming out of the skin).

Both the stereotyped, overt behavior and the phenomenological reports given by the respondents point in the direction of psychotic phenomena, especially the schizophreniform and paranoid psychosis. Often the amphetamine abusers were recognized in the streets because of their odd behavior: aimless, fixed walking-patterns (in circles, up and down the same part of the street, etc.), aimless driving, continuous searching in attics or abandoned houses, repetition of certain words or phrases. In one case a motorcycle gang was stopped by the police because they had been driving 200 times around the same block of houses. Several (including the leader) were high on phenmetrazine. They could not explain why they drove in that peculiar way.

Six addicts were observed by the author during acute intoxication: four Swedish addicts at a police station in Stockholm and two Danish addicts in their drug milieu. All six addicts behaved clinically psychotically, with delusions, hallucinations (visual), paranoia, searching the room for imaginary objects. Their eye-contact (or lack of contact) was "psychotic." Two of the persons in this acute phase talked about worms coming out of their hands and body that had to be picked out of the skin. One had several scars from this kind of picking, which repeatedly started when he had taken phenmetrazine.

TABLE 2, A AND B
COMMON THEMES IN QUESTIONNAIRE RESPONSES AND PERCENT OF RESPONDENTS REPRESENTED

Table 2 a
What is "punding?"

"Punding" is a sort of behavior one gets stuck into, an activity one repeats continuously	45 %
"Punding" is an aimless activity	17.5 %
"Punding" is a kind of activity that does not have any final point, in spite of the intensive work on it	15 %
"Pottering" or "to fiddle with" is the same as "punding"	15 %

n = 50

Table 2 b
Types of "punding"

Manipulating with car engines or other technical equipment such as radio sets, various kinds of mantling and especially dismantling	44 %
Tidying up or washing of dishes	24 %
Artistic work	24 %
Collecting things in attics or abandoned houses	8 %
Walking around, aimless (up and down the street, in circles). Sometimes with the legs high, stamping	8 %
Searching for imaginary things	12 %
Odd telephone calls	5 %
Repetitious acts concerning the body (filing nails, washing hands, taking baths, putting on make-up)	12 %

All activities mentioned are performed in an unvaried, repetitive, aimless way - often continuously for hours, days, or around the clock.

n = 40

TABLE 3
IS THE TYPE OF "PUNDING" CHARACTERISTIC FOR THE INDIVIDUAL

Yes	33 %
No	27 %
In some cases	30 %
Don't know	10 %

n = 30

TABLE 4
SEX DIFFERENCES IN THE TYPE OF "PUNDING"

Sex difference pronounced	50 %
Sex difference not pronounced	47 %
Don't know	3 %

n = 30

TABLE 5
SOCIAL INTERACTION DURING "PUNDING"

	Yes	No	Don't know
a. Talkativeness during "punding"	0	97	3 %
b. Susceptibility to verbal communication during "punding"	0	94	6 %
c. Interest in other people during "punding"	0	97	3 %
d. Need of contact with other people during "punding"	7	90	3 %

n = 40

It is important to notice that during "punding" there exists a pronounced social withdrawal. When high, without "punding", this phenomenon is less pronounced, though the talkativeness seen by lower doses to some extent is characterized by lack of listening (parallel monologues).

TABLE 6
SUBJECTIVE EXPERIENCE OF "PUNDING"

	Yes	No	Sometimes	Don't know
Pleasure	76	4	18	2 %
Anxiety	6	72	22	0 %
Compulsion	57	23	20	0 %

n = 50

TABLE 7
FACTORS WHICH CAN INTERRUPT THE "PUNDING"

	Yes	No	Don't know
Sexual invitation	40	50	10 %
Demand for help from a friend	42	56	2 %
Invitation to a shot of amphetamine	72	22	6 %
Menace from the surroundings (police)	70	22	8 %

46 % postpone going to the toilet when "punding"
38 % postpone drinking during "punding"

n = 50

TABLE 8
REACTIONS TO FORCED INTERRUPTION OF THE "PUNDING"

	Yes	No	Sometimes	Don't know
Anger or irritation	60	26	6	8 %
Anxiety	50	43	0	7 %

Only few percent reports about anxiety as a direct reaction on the drug-effect. Table 8 gives, however, the impression that anxiety is easily aroused.

n = 50

TABLE 9
CHOREIFORM MOVEMENTS

Symptoms	
Chewing	17.5 %
Making faces	10 %
Setting one's teeth	7.5 %
Gnashing one's teeth	5 %
Twisting one's body	12.5 %
Twisting one's arms	10 %
Gesticulating	2.5 %
Moving one's fingers	2.5 %
Other types of jerking syndrome	12 %
No symptom	20.5 %

n = 40

TABLE 10
SEXUAL STIMULATION

Effect	
Strong	85 %
Weak	0 %
None	7 %
Different at different times	4 %

n = 40

Some abusers indicate that they have experienced impotency in relation to the effects of CNS-stimulants (about 15 %). Not all that feel a strong sex-stimulation use intercourse as a mode of reducing their sexual excitation. Many read pornographic journals while masturbating.

TABLE 11
AGE OF PERSONS AT TIME OF INTERVIEW

Number of persons	Age	
4	19	8 %
16	20-24	32 %
16	25-29	32 %
5	30-34	10 %
8	35-39	16 %
1	46	2 %

40 Swedish addicts (4 females + 36 males) plus
10 Danish addicts in the age range of 19-24 (6 males + 4 females)

All Danish addicts were connected to the rather specific youth drug-culture, while a major part of the Swedish addicts belonged to the more "classical" group of addicts. The behavioral reactions to the amphetamines, however, were identical.

About 30% of the interviewed persons claimed that one can recognize a "speed-freak" for a long time (years) after termination of the speed use. It was difficult for the respondents to explain clearly what traits in the behavior could be the cues for this. But usually they mentioned something like: "it is their way of thinking"; "it is the way they talk"; "it is something with their social contact, their suspiciousness."

In four cases (two females and two males), grimacing or certain motoric movements persisted more than one year after only two experiments with amphetamine (each time 30 mg p.o.). One twisted her foot in a special manner, another began to "clear his throat" three times before speaking.

No specific differences in the behavioral response to the CNS-stimulants (phenmetrazine and d-amphetamine) were found between the Swedish and Danish abusers. The difference in age is shown in Table 11. Furthermore, the Danish abusers never developed a speed-drug language concerning the various behavioral phenomena ("punding," "insnoea," "flumma"). Also, amphetamine use has had a different profile in Denmark. In Denmark this type of drug use was concentrated in a shorter period (1968-70), while Sweden has had a serious problem with these speed-drugs since 1966. The i.v. administration has been used more widely in Sweden, where a common daily dose among addicts has been between 400 and 1000 mg per day i.v. Danish abusers mainly have administered the drug p.p.; but, as stated above, the behavioral content of the amphetamine cycle has essentially been the same.

Psychopathology of the addicts prior to their addiction to the CNS-stimulants:

It is difficult to assess the structure of personality of these clients since they usually have lived very isolated lives in a drug sub-culture before their first admission to a hospital, prison, or other kind of institutionalized treatment program or punishment. Their emotional lives before their drug-career have been poor and many of them have abused multiple drugs. Nevertheless, 55% of the interviewed persons were classed (anamnetic record) as falling within two main categories of mental pathology: psychopaths (various character deviations) and schizoid personalities. Statistically, this 55% did not show a pattern among the reported amphetamine-induced behavioral phenomena described above. It is evident from our findings that humans without any (measurable) disposition for psychopathology will respond to amphetamines along the same lines as those with a psychopathological predisposition. On the other hand, it has been our experience that the amphetamines and the disposition in direction of a schizoid personality may act synergistically and probably prolong the recovery after cessation of the drug.

Unambiguous examples of schizophrenic thought disorder were not found in the present clinical material, but the questionnaire did not focus on this specific point. Some relatives of addicts, however, said that it was very difficult to follow the associations of the amphetamine addict. Whether such difficulties in communication were caused by thought disorder in the ordinary psychiatric and psychological sense is unknown. Associations are "speeded up" by amphetamines, and we found some traits of "concrete thinking." It is also a common phenomenon, close relatives say, that they cannot get into deeper emotional contact with the person under the influence of even small doses of amphetamine.

In one case we found that the interaction of the whole family was changed because of amphetamine abuse in one member. The father developed a paranoid psychosis. For a long time the family accepted his ideas of reference and persecution. He ordered his oldest son to march three times around the house, in order, as he said: "to prevent the invisible army with their obscure intentions" from spoiling the family. As he increased the amphetamine dose, his behavior became more and more bizarre. One night he was discovered standing in the street having a heated discussion with his car! His wife stated later (anamnetic record) that initially she was fond of his increasing talkativeness and sexual interest, but that, at the same time, she had had a feeling as if there were a glass wall between them.

EXAMPLES

Literal examples from the interviews concerning stereotypies (both individual and social), social withdrawal, and paranoia.

"I was sitting for many hours staring at the train departures - I never caught my train and missed an important date with a girl-friend."

"I am 'hung up' (insnoea) in locked postures."

"I often sit in a corner, fixed in the same position."

"I have been standing immobile for 48 hours, only moving to get another shot of the drug."

"I have been sitting for many hours staring at the same spot."

"I have been standing dead calm in front of the window - staring."

"When 'punding' you are not interested in anything else."

"When you are hung up (insnoea), you are not in contact with anybody."

"'Punding' is an autistic state."

"You are in a special world - a world of your own."

"You do not listen to anybody, when 'punding'."

"Some are 'punding' in the way that they are staring at others. They are not interested in the others, only a constant gazing."

"A heavily 'punding' human is 'insnoead' (hung up) ('snowed up'). Does not answer, when talked to. Totally autistic."

"Maybe somebody has a problem which he wants to tell about, but nobody is listening, and he doesn't feel it."

"Sometimes they answer - but not . . . the question."

"They are sitting like insane people, talking with themselves."

"I am called 'punding Benny,' because I am 'punding' so much."

"There can be ten different topics discussed at the same time - nobody is listening."

"I was playing my guitar for 3 days. My fingers were bleeding."

"I walked around in attics or abandoned houses for 2 days - searching for my identity."

"I have so many ideas myself when high, I find it difficult to follow the world of ideas of others."

"Everybody is talking for himself, without listening."

"I talk with myself - it is as if I can hear my own voice, even when I'm not speaking."

"When 'punding' they are absent-minded."

"'Punding' is an autistic phenomenon, a pure private matter."

"The higher doses you take, the more intense the 'punding' will be."

"A girl I know can tidy up her handbag in a mechanical way for many hours (even a whole day). She takes the things out and puts them back. She has done this for 6-7 years by now."

"The higher the dose, the more isolated I feel."

"One guy I know always worked with (fiddled with) cars when high. Once I saw him lying under the car at 7 p.m. A lot of engine parts were spread on the ground around him. The next morning he was still there, without having fixed the car yet."

"Once I worked as a truck-driver in the harbor, loading ships. I got the sack because I drove aimlessly around with the same goods for 4 hours."

"At the final examination I was really high on Preludin. I wrote my name a hundred times on the paper, and thought that I had solved the problem."

"I fought - even with the worms that crawled on my body."

" - those damned 'noias' I had in an unreal world - and in Paradise."

"It is almost impossible for me to get contact, and if I get it - I withdraw."

"The boyfriend is like a rabbit." (sexually)

"My first shot of phenmetrazine was a fuck pump."

" - the biggest problem was my feeling of lack of identity."

"I want to get away from that damned lack of contact."

"I had difficulties in getting into contact with other people."

"I got paranoid ideas."

"I did very well, but loneliness came, even when I was amongst other people."

"Some sort of inward anxiety forced me to try something new, all the time."

"I try to escape from everything."

"People started to speak in such a strange way and to look upon me as if they 'knew something.' The radio started to send strange programmes and the newspapers wrote subtle articles - all about me. The shadows became odd and bushes and trees changed shape . . . ."

"Later I got stuck in certain rituals. I even told myself they were meaningful."

"He's snowed up (hung up) - give up talking to him."

"Suddenly he can hear somebody call from a long distance. He answers and gets an answer back. Who is it? Where is he? Under the bed? No! In the wardrobe? No! Outside the door? No! He gets aggressive. He blows the girl up. 'You have noia,' she says, 'here is nobody else than you and me.' 'Noia, damned bullshit, I did hear him, I never get noia.'"

"Often he must throw 'the bag' away, when he feels the police are behind him."

"Why do the cops call me a pig?" - "Why do they never come in?" - "Why do they tap the line?" - "Who the hell am I?"

"He often has 'noias' - all guys look like cops, they want him because he's selling amph. They'll have to take me dead, he thinks, and starts to wear a knife."

"Couldn't even recognize my mother."

"I thought every second woman was a social worker, who wanted to get hold on me."

"One is living like in an airspace."

"There were no other feelings than sex. It was just emptiness."

" - it was just rough fucking, a complete desexualized process, could go on for hours - but it was false feelings. Chemical love."

"At last I got a better kick from the drug, by eating a good lunch, than from fucking."

"Everybody has a damned, cold, rough or tough attitude. The sexual activity is only a 'process of desexualizing.' One gets stuck into - fixed. One MUST fuck after a shot. It's a damned, cold world."

"Several people can be 'punding' in the same room, without any contact with each other."

"Lacking sense of time."

"I became rigid and egoistic, but at the same time I allowed others to trample upon me."

"I became a sort of sexmachine."

"I was tidying up a flat for 6 hours, until I was exhausted. The flat had not come to order despite all the energy I had used on it."

"I've been waiting for somebody for three days and nights."

"Hypersexual - but it was just routine."

"I just become paranoid when I shoot - completely schizophrenic."

"I felt like a rotting corpse, the sense of sickness even went to the fingertips."

"I know people who have been standing behind a curtain for many days just to write down auto-numbers."

"They could sit night after night, just listening to the sound from the cars in the area around."

DISCUSSION

The emotional and cognitive capacities of man are different from those of animals. Humans are in certain aspects more flexible, for instance, in relation to the development of social behavior, which is governed much more in humans by learning than in even the highest animal species. According to this the term "instinctive" is regarded by most human psychologists as being obsolete, while it is still relevant in animal psychology. Nevertheless, studies of the laws of animal behavior can make important contributions to the understanding of ourselves if we realize the obvious biases: the anthropomorphic interpretations of animal behavior and the zoomorphic accounts of man. Furthermore, the descriptive language can cause confusion instead of understanding if the words, terms, etc. are used incautiously.

Sometimes, however, new usages of terms can help us in the urgent task of making scientific writings more readable. Thus Abercrombie (1957) and Abercrombie, Heaysman, and Karthauser (1957) have written about the "social behavior" of cells in tissue culture, and have also used the terminology of taxes and kineses in descriptions of the orientations of cultured fibroblasts. However, these authors did not regard the social behavior or orientation of whole animals as providing proofs of propositions about the movements of cells. Also, we may refer to certain movements of a fish or a bee as "dancing" or to the signals of mating pairs as "courtship" quite harmlessly because ethologists using such descriptions, of course, do not expect to be able to regulate the "dances" of sticklebacks or bees by exposing them to foxtrots or tangos (Barnett, 1972).

Analogies can suggest testable hypotheses, but the predictive value of such hypotheses is crucial. One kind of childhood experience has in the last decade received intense experimental interest: the absence of normal mothering (Meyer, 1965; Harlow and Harlow, 1965; Jensen, Bobbit, and Gordon, 1968; Barnett and Burn, 1967; Bowlby, 1969; Ambrose, 1970; Barnett, 1972). The importance of parental care or mothering has been the direct reason for choosing the mother/infant relationship in our studies.

In this paper we have used the terms "stereotypy," "social withdrawal," "social isolation," and "autism" in the descriptions of the behavioral features observed in monkeys and man. Stereotypy is used widely in psychiatry, psychology, and pharmacology and, therefore, this term might cause some confusion. In animal psychology "stereotypy" is used in relation to normal patterns of behavior. The sequence leading to copulation in pigeons and the nest-building in birds is highly stereotyped (Fabricius and Jansson, 1963). In human (social) psychology, "stereotypy" is used about a rigid attitude directed toward other humans. In the present connection, "stereotypy" is used in relation to a pathological behavior; either produced by psychoactive drugs (especially the amphetamines) or found in naturally occurring mental diseases, such as the schizophrenias. Experimentally, Hauschild (1939) was the first to use the term "stereotyped" about the behavior of amphetaminized rats. Clinically, the term was used much earlier by Falret in 1864 in his description of schizophrenic behavior (Guiraud, 1936).

In our connection stereotypy is defined as an unvaried, selective, repetitive, fixed, aimless, restricted, often ritualized behavior (see results, literal examples of "punding"). As such, the stereotypies, found in man after administration of amphetamines, resemble the fixed patterns of behavior seen in psychiatric conditions (mania, obsessive-compulsive neurosis, the schizophrenias, and oligophrenia). The clinical pictures of the amphetamine-psychoses show psychotic symptoms displaying similarities to the schizophrenias (including social withdrawal) and not many behavioral traits that could be related to the other conditions mentioned. Initially, however, the amphetamine induced elevation of mood might have some similarities with mania.

Social isolation, social withdrawal, and autism are behavioral states that are also found in both animals and man. In the present studies such conditions are defined as a marked decrease or abolishment in the responding to relevant social stimuli. Concurrently, we often find preoccupation with stereotypies or immobile "staring" into space. This social isolation is regarded as being parallel to that of "autism." Our results from the animal experiments confirm the findings of other investigators (Kjellberg and Randrup, 1972a, 1972b, 1973; Machiyama, Utena, and Kikuchi, 1970; Crowley, Stynes, Hydinger, and Kaufman, 1974). "The behavior was bizarre, . . . repetitively, and often not in relation to current social stimuli . . . . While ethanol increased social interaction, methamphetamine produced social isolation" (Crowley et al., 1974, pp. 832, 835). Behaviors occurring frequently and apparently not in response to ambient social stimuli were called "autistic" by Bleuler (1961). And Kanner (1944) regarded two clinical features to be of particular pathognomic significance in relation to infantile autism: 1) extreme self-isolation and 2) obsessive insistence on the perseveration of sameness-criteria which are also accepted in the important behavioral studies of Hutt and Hutt (1970).

Psychopharmacologically induced stereotypies and social isolation have been reported by many investigators in both animals and humans (Angrist and Gershon, 1970, 1972; Connell, 1958; Cole et al., 1973; Ellinwood, 1971; Ellinwood and Cohen, 1972; Ellinwood, Sudilovsky, and Nelson, 1973; Ellinwood and Kilbey, 1975; Fitz-Gerald, 1967; Machiyama et al., 1970; Garver, Schlemmer, and Maas, 1973; Griffith, Cavanaugh, Held, and Oates, 1972; Redmond, Maas, and Kline, 1971; Randrup and Munkvad, 1970, 1971, 1972, 1974, 1975; Rylander, 1966, 1969, 1971; Schiørring, 1969, 1971; Schiørring and Randrup, 1971; Schiørring, 1972; Smith, 1972; Snyder, 1973).

Extreme self-isolation (autism) is of great importance because it must be regarded as a primary symptom of severe psychosis. Furthermore, it has proved to be the most difficult behavioral phenomenon to antagonize psychologically and pharmacologically. Changes in environmental variables (especially ward atmosphere) had mainly an effect on paranoid symptoms and not at all on withdrawal symptoms (Kellam, Goldberg, Schooler, Berman, and Schmelzer, 1965). And the classical deficit in simple reaction time in schizophrenics was consistently correlated with withdrawal symptoms and not with paranoid symptoms (Goldberg, Schooler, and Mattson, 1968; Goldberg, 1973). In the classification of neuroleptics, Bobon, Pinchard,

Collard, and Bobon (1972) found that "autism" was the most difficult symptom to antagonize. In our preliminary experiments with several well-known neuroleptics we found antagonism in relation to the stereotypies, while the social isolation persisted. Only one anti-serotonergic compound (see results) broke the social isolation, but in the direction of stereotyped mutual grooming. On the other hand Kjellberg and Randrup (1971) found partial antagonism with Pimozide in pairs of vervet monkeys. And clinically Angrist, Lee, and Gershon (1974) demonstrated a clear anti-psychotic effect of haloperidol in amphetamine psychosis. Thus the results are at present conflicting, but a full normalization of the social aberrations induced by amphetamines is not yet possible.

An important part of the social signalling system is the expression of emotions and other interrelations by postures and facial expressions (Darwin, 1972). Field studies of various species of primates show variation in the social behavior of the different species (DeVore, 1965; Mason, 1965 Schrier, Harlow, and Stollnitz, 1965). However, the biological processes require certain general patterns of social behavior (reproduction, parental care, play, defense). Under laboratory conditions many functions are displayed in ways that differ from displays in the natural settings. This could be the origin of severe biases. Therefore, it is of importance to estimate the resistance of the species used. In this respect the Cercopithecus monkeys, and especially C. aethiops, have a wide tolerance to impoverishment of the environment and show a great adaptiveness to different kinds of environmental conditions (Gartlan and Brain, 1968).

The amphetamine induced abolishment of reactions from the mother to the calling signals of the infant is critical. Lancaster (1971) mentions this social mechanism as a very important bond between mother and infant. Also, the social relations communicated via eye-contact are extremely important. In our experiments with the mother/infant dyad, we recorded qualitatively a lack in eye-contact. We found that a specific gaze from the mother to the infant (and vice versa) was important in relation to the maintenance of normal social interaction (parental care in particular). Under amphetamine the mother was "staring" into space and/or preoccupied with stereotyped self-grooming. The infant's reaction to this "autistic" state was anxiety expressed either by increased approach-movements or by constant "sitting-close" in ventral-ventral posture, lacking the specific grasping from the mother (Picture 1).

In humans eye-contact, besides its direct importance, also seems to be a necessary precursor to smiling (Fraiberg and Freedman, 1964). Smiling is classifiable as one social releaser which acts on the mother to bring her in the mood to stay with the child (Ambrose, 1970). The physical distance between two individuals and the frequency and duration with which they look at each other are important parameters of their social interaction (Chance, 1967; Exline, 1964; Argyle and Dean, 1965; Cranach, Frenz, and Frey, 1968). Wolff and Chess (1964), Hutt and Ounsted (1966), and Hutt and Hutt (1970) reported that autistic children avoid visual contact with other persons. A fixed stare from another person is reported to make schizophrenics panic (McLean, 1963). So, gaze-aversion - as we have observed both in the monkeys and in the clinical examples of human response to the amphetamines - seems to be of specific importance.

Normal social contacts are frequently replaced by peculiar interrelations by amphetamine. The sexual stimulation often reported (Rylander, 1972) was commonly expressed either by masturbation while reading pornographic literature or by having sexual intercourse for extended periods without ejaculation (supporting the findings reported by Scher, 1966). The verbal communication is also affected by the amphetamines, frequently in the direction of "collective monologues" (increased talking without listening). Spensley (1972) described an example of "folié a deux" in a couple where only one partner used methylphenidate; we found another case of this type. Such behaviors might be characterized as mutual or social stereotypies.

The literal examples from our interviews are parallel to those cited by other investigators. Thus Cuskey, Klein, and Krasner (1972) wrote: "Gus stared fixedly at the sidewalk and announced that he saw pearls, many and many of them, of all sizes and qualities, in the cracks in the pavement, and that he had to pick them up. He crouched down and began to scratch vigorously in the cracks, gouging out the dirt and exclaiming over the pearls. Klein began to wonder if this would continue the rest of the night" (p.10).

Some authors find that the clinical picture of amphetamine psychosis most often is of a paranoid nature (Hampton, 1961); others make classifications of the mental disorders associated with the use of central stimulants. Symptoms such as abulia, shallowness of feelings, a lonely life-style, incoherence of thoughts, audition of thoughts, delusions, hallucinations, telepathy, passivity phenomena, and catatonic states are described by Tatetsu (1972). In the discussion about the similarities of amphetamine psychosis and schizophrenias there have been rather few reports on genuine formal thought disorder. But Angrist and Gershon (1972) found examples of illogical and mutually contradictory ideas, disruption of syntax, and presence of some autistic qualities in the speech. One example showing disruption of formal elements is mentioned: a patient, who used to say that he was "feeling better 'by the power of God and Orsis,'" wrote a message on the wall: "'ATTENTION! Shape up, G.I. time. That's <u>an order</u>...Your "Spaced" Commander'" (p.200).

Fifty-five percent of the addicts in our study can be classified as psychopaths or schizophrenic personalities. This is in accordance with Ellinwood and Cohen (1972). It is, however, important that all the respondents had experienced stereotypies and various changes in social interaction. Pre-disposition of schizophrenia and the choice of amphetamines form an interesting "drug/person" affiliation (or affinity) hypothesis. Some borderline psychotics will prefer morphine because of its stimulating and anxiety-reducing properties (Schiørring and Hecht, 1974 and unpublished observations).

Most of the addicts had used i.v. doses of 400-1200 mg phenmetrazine per day. Tolerance did not develop in relation to stereotypies and changes in social behavior. Connell (1958) found that the lowest single dose that had provoked psychosis was 50 mg amphetamine. Kramer (1972) states that paranoid psychosis can develop either by a large single dose or by chronic, moderate or large doses. Griffith, Fann, and Oates (1972) find that the state following chronic abuse resembles that of paranoid schizophrenia.

In general it is interesting that the amphetamine-type of drug will often be characterized in the initial phase as the "luck-drug" and will later produce the most severe, pathological disturbances in motoric, intellectual, emotional, and social behaviors. Quite often the amphetamine addict is recognized in the streets because of his odd behavior. Other kinds of intoxication can, of course, also be striking, but it is important that the amphetamine-high has a clear consciousness and that the behavior appears more bizarre than behavior induced by most other drugs. Even the pro-drug culture itself has tried to warn against use of "speed." A statement made by Allen Ginsberg to an underground newspaper sounds: "Let's issue a general declaration to all the underground community contra speedamos ex cathedra. Speed is anti-social, paranoid making, it's a drag, bad for your body, bad for your mind, generally speaking, in the long run uncreative and it's a plague in the whole dope industry. All the nice gentle dope fiends are getting screwed up by the real horror monster Frankenstein speed-freaks who are going around stealing and bad-mouthing everybody" (cited in Pittel and Hofer, 1972, p.169).

The peculiar effects of the amphetamines and related compounds are important cues also in the considerations about the possible psychological and sociological mechanisms behind an increase in abuse of these drugs (Schiørring, 1973). There is a close connection between drug of choice, life-style, structure of personality, and the individual or group image; the drug is believed to enhance this connection. Thus, when cocaine suddenly becomes fashionable, it is not just coincidence: socio-cultural factors should also be taken into account.

Finally, one more clinical implication of our data should be mentioned. According to Cole (1972), 23.3 million prescriptions of amphetamines were made in the U.S.A. in 1967. Eighty percent of the patients receiving amphetamines for medical conditions were females. Besides the interesting considerations about sex-role-norms and efficiency-norms in the society as a probable background for this kind of use, it would be extremely important to know what effects this particular amphetamine use has had on the emotional and social relationship between the women and their children.

ACKNOWLEDGMENTS

This investigation was supported by NIH research grant no. DA 00023 from National Institute on Drug Abuse (NIDA), U.S.A.; Scottish Rite Schizophrenia Research Program, Lexington, Mass., U.S.A.; Købmand i Odense Johann og Hanne Weimann f. Seedorffs Legat, Copenhagen, Denmark; P. Carl Petersens Fond, Copenhagen, Denmark; Femte Maj Fonden, Goteborg, Sweden; Statens Laegevidenskabelige Forskningsråd, Copenhagen, Denmark.

The author also wishes to thank the members of the technical staff, who have contributed to this work with their patience and professional skill. Lene Rostén Hanse, Ulla Sørensen and Grethe Jensen made most of the observations of the monkeys; Connie Olsen took the picture of the monkeys; Annelise Stenberg Knudsen corrected and typed the manuscript and Marianne Albeck translated the questionnaire and the literal examples from Swedish.

REFERENCES

Abercrombie, M.: The directed movements of fibroblasts: A discussion, Proc. zool. Soc., Calcutta, Mookerjee Mem., 129-140 (1957).

Abercrombie, M., Heaysman, J.E.M., and Karthauser, H.M.: Social behaviour of cells in tissue culture: Mutual influence of sarcoma cells and fibroblasts, Expl Cell Res. 13, 276-291 (1957).

Airila, Y.: Über die Einwirkung verschiedener Erregungsmittel der Grosshirnrinde auf den Chloralhydratschlaf, Archs int. Pharmacodyn. Thér. 23, 453-459 (1913).

Alles, G.A.: Comparative psychological action of dl-β-phenylisopropylamines, J. Pharmac. exp. Ther. 47, 339-354 (1933).

Ambrose, J.A.: Theory and evidence on the significance of very early experiences. Cited in: Behaviour Studies in Psychiatry. Hutt, S.I. and Hutt, C., Eds., p. 116. Oxford: Pergamon Press, 1970.

Angrist, B.M. and Gershon, S.: The phenomenology of experimentally induced amphetamine psychosis: Preliminary observations, Biol. Psychiat. 2, 95-107 (1970).

Angrist, B.M. and Gershon, S.: Some recent studies on amphetamine psychosis--Unresolved issues. In: Current Concepts on Amphetamine Abuse. Ellinwood, E.H. and Cohen, S., Eds., pp. 193-204. Washington: U.S. Government Printing Office, 1972.

Angrist, B.M., Lee, H.K., and Gershon, S.: The antagonism of amphetamine-induced symptomatology by a neuroleptic, Am. J. Psychiat. 131, 817-819 (1974).

Argyle, M. and Dean, J.: Eye-contact, distance and affiliation, Sociometry 28, 289-304 (1965).

Bahnsen, P., Jacobsen, E., and Thesleff, H.: The subjective effect of beta-phenylisopropylaminesulphate on normal adults, Acta med. scand. 107, 89-131 (1938).

Ban, T., Boissier, J., Gessa, G., Heimann, H., Hollister, L., Lehmann, H., Munkvad, I., Steinberg, H., Sulser, F., Sundwall, A., and Vinar, O., (Eds.): Psychopharmacology, Sexual Disorders and Drug Abuse. Amsterdam-London: North-Holland Publishing Company; Prague: Avicenum, Czechoslovak Medical Press, 1973.

Barnett, S.A.: The ontogeny of behavior and the concept of instinct. In: Brain and Human Behavior. Karczmar, A.G. and Eccles, J.C., Eds., pp. 377-392. New York: Springer-Verlag, 1972.

Barnett, S.A. and Burn, J.: Early stimulation and maternal behaviour, Nature, Lond. 213, 150-152 (1967).

Bleuler, E.: Dementia Praecox, or, The Group of Schizophrenias. Translated by Zinkin, J. New York: International Universities Press, 1950.

Blurton-Jones, N.G.: An ethological study of some aspects of social behaviour of children in nursery school. In: Primate Ethology. Morris, D., Ed., pp. 347-368. London: Weidenfeld and Nicolson, 1967.

Bobon, J., Pinchard, A., Collard, J., and Bobon, D.P.: Clinical classification of neuroleptics, with special reference to their antimanic, antiautistic and ataraxic properties, Compr. Psychiat. 13, 123-131 (1972).

Bonhoff, G. and Lewrenz, H.: Über Weckamine. Berlin: Springer-Verlag, 1954.

Bowlby, J.: Attachment and Loss. Vol. I. London: Hogarth Press, 1969.

Cerletti, A. and Bové, F.J., (Eds.): Psychotropic Drugs. International Congress Series No. 180. Amsterdam: Excerpta Medica, 1969.

Chance, M.R.A.: Attention structure as the basis of primate rank orders, Man 2, 503-518 (1967).

Cole, J.O.: Clinical uses of the amphetamines. In: Current Concepts on Amphetamine Abuse. Ellinwood, E.H. and Cohen, S., Eds., pp. 163-168. Washington: U.S. Government Printing Office, 1972.

Cole, J.O., Freedman, A.M., and Friedhoff, A.J., (Eds.): Psychopathology and Psychopharmacology. Baltimore: The Johns Hopkins University Press, 1973.

Connell, P.: Amphetamine Psychosis. Maudsley Monographs No. 5. London: Oxford University Press, 1958.

Cools, A.R.: An integrated theory of the aetiology of schizophrenia: Impairment of the balance between certain, in series, connected dopaminergic, serotonergic and noradrenergic pathways within the brain. In: On the Origin of Schizophrenic Psychoses. van Praag, H.M., Ed., pp. 53-80. Amsterdam: De Erven Bohn, 1975.

Cools, A.R.: Basic considerations on the role of concertedly working dopaminergic, GABA-ergic, cholinergic and serotonergic mechanisms within the neo-striatum and nucleus accumbens in locomotor activity, stereotyped gnawing, turning and dyskinetic activities. In: Cocaine and Other Stimulants. Ellinwood, E.H. and Kilbey, M.M., Eds. New York: Plenum Press, 1976.

Costa, E. and Garattini, S., (Eds.): Amphetamines and Related Compounds. Amsterdam: Raven Press, 1970.

Costa, E. and Groppetti, A.: Relationships between biochemical and pharmacological responses elicited by dextro-amphetamine. In: Current Concepts on Amphetamine Abuse. Ellinwood, E.H. and Cohen, S., Eds., pp. 117-124. Washington: U.S. Government Printing Office, 1972.

Cranach, M.v., Frenz, H.G., and Frey, S.: Die "angenehmste Entfernung" zur Betrachtung soziale Objekte, Psychol. Forsch. 32, 89-103 (1968).

Crowley, T.J., Stynes, A.J., Hydinger, M., and Kaufman, I.C.: Ethanol, methamphetamine, pentobarbital, morphine, and monkey social behavior, Archs gen. Psychiat. 31, 829-838 (1974).

Cuskey, W., Klein, A.W., and Krasner, W.: Drug-Trip Abroad: American Drug-Refugees in Amsterdam and London. Philadelphia: University of Pennsylvania Press, 1972.

Darwin, C.R.: The Expression of the Emotions in Man and Animals. London: Murray, 1872.

DeVore, I.: Primate Behaviour. New York: Holt, Rinehart and Winston, 1965.

Donley, D.E.: Observations on the use of benzedrine in the psychoses, Ohio St. med. J. 33, 1229-1232 (1937).

Duarte-Escalante, O. and Ellinwood, E.H.: Effects of chronic amphetamine intoxication on adrenergic and cholinergic structures in the central nervous system: Histochemical observations in cats and monkeys. In: Current Concepts on Amphetamine Abuse. Ellinwood, E.H. and Cohen, S., Eds., pp. 97-106. Washington: U.S. Government Printing Office, 1972.

Edeleano, L.: Über einige Derivate der Phenylmetacrylsäure und der Phenylisobuttersäure, Ber. dt. chem. Ges. 20, 616a (1887).

Efron, D.H., Holmstedt, B., and Kline, N.S., (Eds.): Ethnopharmacological Search for Psychoactive Drugs (Workshop Series of Pharmacology, Psychopharmacology Research Branch, N.I.M.H., Publication 1645). Washington: U.S. Government Printing Office, 1967.

Eleftheriou, B.E., (Ed.): Psychopharmacogenetics. New York: Plenum Press, 1975.

Ellinwood, E.H.: Comparative methamphetamine intoxication in experimental animals, Pharmakopsychiatr. Neuro-Psychopharmakol. 4, 351-361 (1971).

Ellinwood, E.H.: Amphetamine psychosis: Individuals settings and sequences. In: Current Concepts on Amphetamine Abuse. Ellinwood, E.H. and Cohen, S., Eds., pp. 143-158. Washington: U.S. Government Printing Office, 1972.

Ellinwood, E.H. and Duarte-Escalante, O.: Chronic methamphetamine intoxication in three species of experimental animals. In: Current Concepts on Amphetamine Abuse. Ellinwood, E.H. and Cohen, S., Eds., pp. 59-68. Washington: U.S. Government Printing Office, 1972.

Ellinwood, E.H., Sudilovsky, A., and Nelson, L.M.: Evolving behavior in the clinical and experimental amphetamine (model) psychosis, Am. J. Psychiat. 130, 1088-1093 (1973).

Ellinwood, E.H. and Kilbey, M.M.: Species differences in response to amphetamine. In: Psychopharmacogenetics. Eleftheriou, B.E., Ed., pp. 323-375. New York: Plenum Press, 1975.

Esser, A.H.: Dominance hierarchy and clinical course of psychiatrically hospitalized boys, Child Dev. 39, 147-157 (1968).

Esser, A.H. and Paluck, R.J.: Comparable data on psychiatric patients, captive gorillas and free-ranging gibbons. Paper presented at the 23rd Annual Meeting of the Society of Biological Psychiatry, Washington, June, 1968.

Exline, R.V.: Affective phenomena and the mutual glance: Effects of evaluative feedback and social reinforcement upon visual interaction with an interviewer, Technical Report No. 11, Office of Naval Research, Group Psychology Branch (1964).

Fabricius, E. and Jansson, A.M.: Laboratory observations on the reproductive behaviour of the pigeon (Columba livia) during the preincubation phase of the breeding cycle, Anim. Behav. 11, 534-547 (1963).

Fitz-Gerald, F.: Effects of d-amphetamine upon behaviour of young chimpanzees reared under different conditions. In: Neuro-Psycho-pharmacology. Brill, H., Cole, J.O., Deinker, P., Hippius, H., and Bradley, P.B., Eds., Vol. 5, International Congress Series No. 129, pp. 1226-1227. Amsterdam: Excerpta Medica, 1967.

Fog, R.: On stereotypy and catalepsy: Studies on the effect of amphetamines and neuroleptics in rats, Acta Neurol. scand. 48, Suppl. 50 (1972).

Fraiberg, S. and Freedman, D.A.: Studies in the ego development of the congenitally blind child, Psychoanal. Study Child 19, 113-169 (1964).

Gartlan, J.S. and Brain, C.K.: Ecology and social variability in Cercopithecus aethiops and C. mitis. In: Studies in Adaptation and Variability. Jay, F., Ed., pp. 253-292. New York: Holt, Rinehart and Winston, 1968.

Garver, D.L., Schlemmer, R.F., and Maas, J.W.: A primate behavioural psychosis: A model for studying neurotransmitters and neuroleptics (abstract). Program and Abstracts, p. 346, of the Society for Neuroscience, Bethesda, Md., 1973.

Garver, D.L., Schlemmer, R.F., Maas, J.W., and Davis, J.M.: A schizophreniform behavioural psychosis mediated by dopamine, Am. J. Psychiat. 132, 33-38 (1975).

Goldberg, S.C.: Drugs and schizophrenic behaviour. In: Psychopathology and Psychopharmacology. Cole, J.O., Freedman, A.M., and Friedhoff, A.J., Eds., pp. 161-176. Baltimore: The Johns Hopkins University Press, 1973.

Goldberg, S.C., Schooler, N.R., and Mattson, N.B.: Paranoid and withdrawal symptoms in schizophrenia: Relationship to reaction time, Br. J. Psychiat. 114, 1161-1163 (1968).

Griffith, J.D., Cavanaugh, J., Held, J., and Oates, J.A.: Dextroamphetamine, Archs gen. Psychiat. 26, 97-100 (1972).

Griffith, J.D., Fann, W.E., and Oates, J.A.: The amphetamine psychosis: Experimental manifestations. In: Current Concepts on Amphetamine Abuse. Ellinwood, E.H. and Cohen, S., Eds., pp. 177-184. Washington: U.S. Government Printing Office, 1972.

Grinspoon, L. and Hedblom, P., (Eds.): The Speed Culture: Amphetamine Use and Abuse in America. Cambridge: Harvard University Press, 1975.

Guiraud, P.: Analyse de symptôme stéréotypie, Encéphale 31, 16 (1936).

Hampton, W.H.: Observed psychiatric reactions following use of amphetamine and amphetamine-like substances, Bull. N.Y. Acad. Med. II, 37(3), 167-175 (1961).

Harlow, H.F. and Harlow, M.K.: The affectional systems. In: Behavior of Nonhuman Primates. Schrier, A.M., Harlow, H.R., and Stollnitz, F., Eds., Vol. 2, pp. 287-334. London: Academic Press, 1965.

Hauschild, F.: Zur Pharmakologie des 1-phenyl-2-methylaminopropans (pervitin), Naunyn-Schmiedebergs Arch. exp. Path. Pharmak. 2, 254 (1939).

Hutt, S.J. and Hutt, C., (Eds.): Behaviour Studies in Psychiatry. Oxford: Pergamon Press, 1970.

Hutt, C. and Ounsted, C.: The biological significance of gaze aversion with particular reference to the syndrome of infantile autism, Behav. Sci. 2, 346-356 (1966).

Jacobsen, E.: Studies on the subjective effects of the cephalotropic amines in man: A comparison between β-phenylisopropylamine-sulphate and a series of other amine salts, Acta med. scand. 100, 188-202 (1939).

Jacobsen, E. and Wollstein, A.: Studies on the subjective effects of the cephalotropic amines in man: Beta-phenylisopropyl-aminesulphate, Acta med. scand. 100, 159-187 (1939).

Janota, O.: Symptomatische Behandlung der pathologischen Schlafsucht besonders der Narkolepsie, Medsche Klin. 27, 278-281 (1931).

Jensen, G.C., Bobbit, R.A., and Gordon, B.N.: Effects of environments on the relationship between mother and infant pigtailed monkeys (Macaca nemestrina), J. comp. physiol. Psychol. 66, 259-263 (1968).

Kalant, O.J.: The Amphetamines: Toxicity and Addiction. Brookside Monographs No. 5. Toronto: University of Toronto Press, 1966.

Kanner, L.: Early infantile autism, J. Pediat. 25, 211-217 (1944).

Kellam, S.G., Goldberg, S.C., Schooler, N.R., Berman, A., and Schmelzer, J.L.: Ward atmosphere and outcome of treatment of acute schizophrenia, J. psychiat. Res. 5, 145-163 (1965).

Kjellberg, B. and Randrup, A.: The effect of amphetamine and pimozide, a neuroleptic, on the social behaviour of vervet monkeys (Cercopithecus spp.). In: Proceedings of the Seventh C.I.N.P. Congress, Prague, 1970. Vinar, O., Votava, Z., and Bradley, P.B., Eds., pp. 305-310. Amsterdam: North-Holland Publishing Company, 1971.

Kjellberg, B. and Randrup, A.: Stereotypy with selective stimulation of certain items of behaviour observed in amphetamine-treated monkeys (Cercopithecus), Pharmakopsychiatr. Neuro-Psychopharmakol. 5, 1 (1972a).

Kjellberg, B. and Randrup, A.: Changes in social behaviour in pairs of vervet monkeys (Cercopithecus) produced by single, low doses of amphetamine, Psychopharmacologia, suppl. 26, 117 (1972b).

Kjellberg, B. and Randrup, A.: Disruption of social behaviour of vervet monkeys (Cercopithecus) by low doses of amphetamines, Pharmakopsychiatr. Neuro-Psychopharmakol. 6, 287-293 (1973).

Kramer, J.C.: Introduction to amphetamine abuse. In: Current Concepts on Amphetamine Abuse. Ellinwood, E.H. and Cohen, S., Eds., pp. 177-184. Washington: U.S. Government Printing Office, 1972.

Lancaster, J.B.: Play-mothering: The relations between juvenile females and young infants among free-ranging vervet monkeys (Cercopithecus aethiops), Folia primatol. 15, 161-182 (1971).

Machiyama, Y., Utena, M., and Kikuchi, M.: Behavioural disorders in Japanese monkeys produced by the long-term administration of methamphetamine, Proc. Japan Acad. 46, 738 (1970).

Maclean, P.D.: Phylogenesis. In: Expressions of the Emotions in Man. Knapp, P.H., Ed., pp. 16-35. New York: International Universities Press, 1963.

Maier, H.W.: Der Kokainismus. Leipzig: Georg Thieme Verlag, 1926.

Mandell, A.J. and Knapp, S.: Cholinergic adaptation in the brain to chronic administration of amphetamine. In: Current Concepts on Amphetamine Abuse. Ellinwood, E.H. and Cohen, S., Eds., pp. 77-86. Washington: U.S. Government Printing Office, 1972.

Mason, W.A.: Sociability and social organization in monkeys and apes, Adv. exp. soc. Psychol. 1, 278-303 (1965).

Meyer, G.W.: Other data on the effects of social isolation during rearing upon adult reproductive behaviour in the rhesus monkey (Macaca mulatta), Anim. Behav. 13, 228-231 (1965).

Mitsuda, H. and Fukada, T., (Eds.): Schizophrenia and Schizophrenia-Like Psychoses. Stuttgart: Georg Thieme Publishers, 1975.

Pittel, S.M. and Hofer, R.: The transition to amphetamine abuse. In: Current Concepts on Amphetamine Abuse. Ellinwood, E.H. and Cohen, S., Eds., pp. 169-176. Washington: U.S. Government Printing Office, 1972.

Prinzmetal, M. and Bloomberg, W.: The use of benzedrine for the treatment of narcolepsy, J. Am. med. Ass. 105, 2051 (1935).

Randrup, A. and Munkvad, I.: Biochemical, anatomical and psychological investigations of stereotyped behaviour induced by amphetamines. In: Amphetamines and Related Compounds. Costa, E. and Garattini, S., Eds., pp. 695-713. New York: Raven Press, 1970.

Randrup, A. and Munkvad, I.: Behavioural toxicity of amphetamines studied in animal experiments. In: The Correlation of Adverse Effects in Man with Observations in Animals. De C. Baker, S.B., Ed., Vol. 12, International Congress Series No. 220, pp. 6-17. Amsterdam. Excerpta Medica, 1971.

Randrup, A. and Munkvad, I.: Correlation between specific effects of amphetamines on the brain and on behaviour. In: Current Concepts on Amphetamine Abuse. Ellinwood, E.H. and Cohen, S., Eds., pp. 17-26. Washington: U.S. Government Printing Office, 1972.

Randrup, A. and Munkvad, I.: Influence of amphetamines on animal behaviour: Stereotypy, functional impairment and possible animal-human correlations, Psychiat. Neurol. Neurchir. 75, 193-202 (1972).

Randrup, A. and Munkvad, I.: Pharmacology and physiology of stereotyped behavior, J. psychiat. Res. 11, 1-10 (1974).

Randrup, A. and Munkvad, I.: Stereotyped behavior, Pharmac. Therap. 1(4), 757-768 (1975).

Redmond, D.E., Maas, J.W., and Kling, A.: Changes in primate social behaviour after treatment with alpha-methyl-para-tyrosine, Psychosom. Med. 33, 97-113 (1971).

Romano, J., (Ed.): The Origins of Schizophrenia. International Congress Series No. 151. Amsterdam: Excerpta Medica, 1967.

Rylander, G.: Addiction to preludin intravenously injected. In: Proceedings, Fourth World Congress of Psychiatry, Madrid. Lopez-Ibor, J.J., Ed., International Congress Series No. 150(3), pp. 1363-1365. Amsterdam: Excerpta Medica, 1966.

Rylander, G.: Clinical and medico-criminological aspects of addiction to central stimulating drugs. In: Abuse of Central Stimulants. Sjöqvist, F. and Tottie, M., Eds., pp. 251-273. Stockholm: Almqvist and Wiksell, 1969.

Rylander, G.: Stereotype behaviour in man following amphetamine abuse. In: The Correlation of Adverse Effects in Man with Observations in Animals. De C. Baker, S.B., Ed., Vol. 12, International Congress Series No. 220, pp. 28-31. Amsterdam: Excerpta Medica, 1971.

Rylander, G.: Psychoses and the punding and choreiform syndromes in addiction to central stimulant drugs, Folia psychiat. neurol. neurochir. neerl. 75, 203-212 (1972).

Scher, J.: Patterns and profiles of addiction and drug abuse, Archs gen. Psychiat. 15, 539-551 (1966).

Scheel-Krüger, J.: Comparative studies of various amphetamine analogues demonstrating different interactions with the metabolism of the catecholamines in the brain, Eur. J. Pharmacol. 14, 47-59 (1971).

Scheel-Krüger, J., Braestrup, C., Nielsen, M., Golembiowska, K., and Mogilnicka, E.: Cocaine: Discussion on the role of dopamine in the biochemical mechanism of action. In: Cocaine and Other Stimulants. Ellinwood, E.H. and Kilbey, M.M., Eds. New York: Plenum Press, 1976.

Schiørring, E.: Amfetamin - i focus for forskning og misbrug (Amphetamine - in focus of research and abuse), Mentalhygiejne 22, 13-20 (1969).

Schiørring, E.: Amphetamine-induced selective stimulation of certain behaviour items with concurrent inhibition of others in an open-field test with rats, Behaviour 39, 1-17 (1971).

Schiørring, E.: Social isolation and behavioural changes in a group of three vervet monkeys (Cercopithecus) produced by single, low doses of amphetamine, Psychopharmacologia, suppl. 26, 117 (1972).

Schiørring, E. and Hecht, A.: Behavioural effects of morphine in acute doses in rats and mice, J. Pharmacol. 6, suppl. 2, 90 (1974).

Schiørring, E. and Randrup, A.: Social isolation and changes in the formation of groups induced by amphetamine in an open-field test with rats, Pharmakopsychiatr. Neuro-Psychopharmakol. 4, 1-11 (1971).

Schrier, A.M., Harlow, H.F., and Stollnitz, F.: Behaviour of Nonhuman Primates. London: Academic Press, 1965.

Sjöqvist, F. and Tottie, M., (Eds.): Abuse of Central Stimulants. Stockholm: Almqvist and Wiksell, 1969.

Smith, R.C.: Compulsive methamphetamine abuse and violence in the Haight-Ashbury District. In: Current Concepts on Amphetamine Abuse. Ellinwood, E.H. and Cohen, S., Eds., pp. 205-216. Washington: U.S. Government Printing Office, 1972.

Snyder, S.H.: Amphetamine psychosis: A "model" schizophrenia mediated by catecholamines, Am. J. Psychiat. 130, 61-67 (1973).

Snyder, S.H., (Ed.): Madness and the Brain. New York: McGraw-Hill Company, 1974.

Snyder, S.H., Taylor, K.M., Coyle, J.T., and Meyerhoff, J.L.: The role of brain dopamine in behavioural regulation and the actions of psychotropic drugs. In: Current Concepts on Amphetamine Abuse. Ellinwood, E.H. and Cohen, S., Eds., pp. 3-16. Washington: U.S. Government Printing Office, 1972.

Spensley, J.: "Folié a deux" with methylphenidate psychosis, J. nerv. ment. Dis. 155, 288-290 (1972).

Spooner, C.E. and Flaming, D.: Monoamines, multiple units and various amphetamine actions. In: Current Concepts on Amphetamine Abuse. Ellinwood, E.H. and Cohen, S., Eds., pp. 27-36. Washington: U.S. Government Printing Office, 1972.

Stern, R.: Über die Wirkung der Hydronaphtylamine auf den Tierischen Organismus, Virchows Arch. path. Anat. Physiol. 115, 14-46 (1889).

Tatetsu, S.: Methamphetamine psychosis. In: Current Concepts on Amphetamine Abuse. Ellinwood, E.H. and Cohen, S., Eds., pp. 159-161. Washington: U.S. Government Printing Office, 1972.

Tinbergen, N.: On aims and methods of ethology, Z. Tierpsychol. 20, 410-433 (1963).

Welch, B.L. and Welch, A.M.: Chronic social stimulation and tolerance to amphetamine: Interaction effects of amphetamine and natural nervous stimulation upon brain amines and behavior. In: Current Concepts on Amphetamine Abuse. Ellinwood, E.H. and Cohen, S., Eds., pp. 107-116. Washington: U.S. Government Printing Office, 1972.

Wilson, C.W.M.: Adolescent Drug Dependence. New York: Pergamon Press, 1968.

Wolff, S. and Chess, W.: A behavioural study of schizophrenic children, Acta Psychiat. Scand. 40, 438-466 (1964).

Wollstein, A.: Studies on the subjective effects of the cephalotropic amines in man: The action of the cephalotropic amines on intelligence scores, Acta med. scand. 100, 203-207 (1939).

Young, D. and Scoville, W.B.: Paranoid psychosis in narcolepsy and the possible dangers of benzedrine treatment, Med. Clins N. Am. 22, 638-642 (1938).

REINFORCEMENT OF BEHAVIOR BY COCAINE INJECTIONS

S.R. Goldberg and R.T. Kelleher

Laboratory of Psychobiology, Department of Psychiatry,

Harvard Medical School, Boston, Massachusetts 02115 and

New England Regional Primate Research Center

Southborough, Massachusetts 01772

The intravenous injection of certain drugs, such as psychomotor stimulants, can function as a reinforcer to engender and maintain behavior in rats and monkeys. Such behavior has served as a laboratory counterpart to human drug-seeking and drug-taking behavior. However, the levels of behavior maintained by drug injections in experimental animals are usually lower than would be expected from observations of the extended sequences of behavior involved in the procurement, preparation, and administration of a drug by humans. The low levels of behavior may arise from the common practice of studying experimental animals under conditions in which every response or every few responses results in a drug injection during long experimental sessions lasting 3 to 24 hours. Under these conditions, mean response rates have been less than 0.1 response per second; and response rates decrease further as the dose per injection is increased above some level (e.g., Pickens and Thompson, 1968; Goldberg, Hoffmeister, Schlichting and Wuttke, 1971; Wilson, Hitomi and Schuster, 1971).

When the schedules relating behavior and consequent injection of drug permit the experimental subject to produce frequent injections within an experimental session, the reinforcing effects of a drug may be modified by its other pharmacological effects. For example, pretreatment with cocaine enhances and then at higher doses, suppresses rates of responding maintained by presentation of food or electric shock (Smith, 1964; Gonzalez and Goldberg, 1974; Woods and Tessel, 1974; Barrett, in press). Maintenance of behavior by cocaine, especially at higher doses, may be masked by such general rate-modifying properties. This paper reviews experiments on the reinforcing effects of cocaine with scheduling techniques that limited the frequency of cocaine injection in each experimental session.

PROCEDURE

Squirrel monkeys and rhesus monkeys with permanent venous catheters were studied under various schedules of cocaine injection. Short experimental sessions, lasting 60 to 100 min, were conducted once a day. During the sessions, the monkeys were seated in restraint chairs and placed in isolation chambers. Each chair was provided with a response key and different colored bulbs which, when illuminated, served as visual stimuli. The venous catheter was connected by Teflon tubing to a motor-driven syringe outside the chamber. The motor-driven syringe was controlled by automatic programming equipment. Injection duration was 200 msec; the volume of each injection was 0.18ml. Further details of catheterization techniques and apparatus have been reported previously (Herd, Morse, Kelleher, Jones, 1969; Goldberg, 1973a; Goldberg and Kelleher, 1976).

Fixed-Ratio Schedules

Under fixed-ratio schedules, drug injection follows the occurrence of a constant number of responses. As this constant number of responses may be made quickly at low response requirements, successive doses of drug can follow one another in rapid succession. The cumulative effects of successive injections can be limited by interposing timeout periods between successive injections, during which responses have no programmed consequences, or by reducing the total number of injections in each session. Responding of squirrel and rhesus monkeys was maintained in the presence of a green light under 10-response, 30-response, or 50-response fixed-ratio schedules of cocaine injection. In the squirrel monkeys, the green light went off at the completion of each ratio and an intravenous injection occurred at the onset of a 2-sec amber light; in the rhesus monkeys, the green light went off at the completion of each ratio and a white light was presented for 2 sec before, and remained on during, the intravenous injection. A 60-sec timeout period, during which the chamber was dark, followed presentation of the white or amber light. Each session ended after the 50th timeout period (rhesus monkeys) or after 100 min (squirrel monkeys).

Fixed-Interval Schedules

Under fixed-interval schedules of drug injection, the first response occurring after a fixed minimum interval of time has elapsed produces an injection. Fixed-interval schedules are particularly useful in assessing the effectiveness of drugs in maintaining behavior because the maximal frequency of drug injection is limited by the schedule parameter and is independent of the rate of responding. Squirrel and rhesus monkeys responded under a 5-min fixed-interval schedule of cocaine injection in the presence of a red (squirrel monkeys) or green (rhesus monkeys) light. In the squirrel monkeys, the red light went off at the completion of each interval and a cocaine injection occurred with the onset of a 2-sec amber light; in the rhesus monkey, the green light went off at the completion of each interval and a white light was presented for 2-sec before, and remained on during, the injection of cocaine. A 100-sec or 60-sec timeout period followed presentation of the white or amber light. Each session ended after the 10th or 15th timeout period.

Multiple Fixed-Ratio Fixed-Interval Schedules

A squirrel monkey was studied under a multiple schedule comprising a 30-response fixed-ratio component in the presence of a green light and a 5-min fixed-interval component in the presence of a red light. Each component ended with an injection of cocaine at the onset of a 2-sec amber light, which was followed by a 60-sec timeout period. Each session began with a fixed-interval component, and fixed-interval and fixed-ratio components alternated throughout the session. The session ended after the 30th timeout period.

Rhesus monkeys were studied under a multiple schedule comprising a 10-response fixed-ratio component in the presence of a green light and a 5-min fixed-interval component in the presence of an amber light. Each component ended with a white light presented for 2 sec before, and remaining on during, an injection of cocaine. A 100-sec timeout period followed presentation of the white light. Each session began with a fixed-ratio component, and fixed-ratio and fixed-interval components alternated throughout the session. The session ended after the 15th timeout period.

Second-Order Schedules

Simple fixed-ratio and fixed-interval schedules can be used as components of more complex second-order schedules. Under second-order schedules, a pattern of responding resulting from the operation of one schedule is treated as a unitary response that is itself reinforced according to a second schedule. Under one type of schedule, studied in both squirrel and rhesus monkeys, every fixed-ratio component completed during a fixed minimum interval of time produced a 2-sec light; the first fixed-ratio component completed after the time interval had elapsed produced both the light and intravenous injection of cocaine. The time interval was varied. In one experiment the interval was increased to 60 min and each daily session consisted of only one 60-min interval; consequently, cocaine was injected only at the end of the session. This schedule is a fixed-ratio schedule of stimulus presentation which is itself maintained under a fixed-interval schedule of cocaine injection. Under a second type of schedule, studied only in squirrel monkeys, responding under a 5-min fixed-interval schedule resulted in 2-sec presentations of a light; after 10 fixed intervals were completed, the light was accompanied by cocaine injection and followed by a 100-sec timeout period. Each session ended after the first or the third timeout period. The second-order schedules of cocaine injection, in which cocaine is injected only at the end of each session, allow a complete separation of cocaine's reinforcing effects from its other effects on behavior.

Drugs

Cocaine hydrochloride was dissolved in saline (0.9% NaCl). All doses are expressed as the salt.

RESULTS AND DISCUSSIONS

The schedule of reinforcement is the prime determinant of the relation between the rate and pattern of responding and the event that is consequent on responding. Comparable schedule-controlled patterns of responding can be maintained under diverse conditions and in different species by a variety of consequent events, including presentation of food, water, or electric shock (e.g., Kelleher and Morse, 1964, 1968; McKearney, 1968, 1969). Under fixed-ratio schedules, at fixed ratio parameter values of less than 60, performance is generally characterized by a brief pause before the initial response in each ratio, followed by a sustained high rate of responding until the ratio is completed. Under fixed-interval schedules, over a wide range of fixed-interval parameter values, performance is generally characterized by an initial period of no responding, followed by acceleration of responding to a final rate that is maintained until the end of the interval. Usually, only one-quarter of the total responses in each interval have been emitted when 50% or more of the time in the interval has elapsed (quarter life) (Herrnstein and Morse, 1957; Gollub, 1964). In the present experiments, these characteristic performances were maintained by intravenous injections of cocaine under various schedules. These experiments have been previously described in greater detail by Goldberg (1973a, b), Goldberg and Kelleher (1976), and Goldberg, Kelleher and Morse (1975).

Fixed-Ratio Schedules

Characteristic fixed-ratio patterns of responding were maintained by cocaine injections in both rhesus and squirrel monkeys.

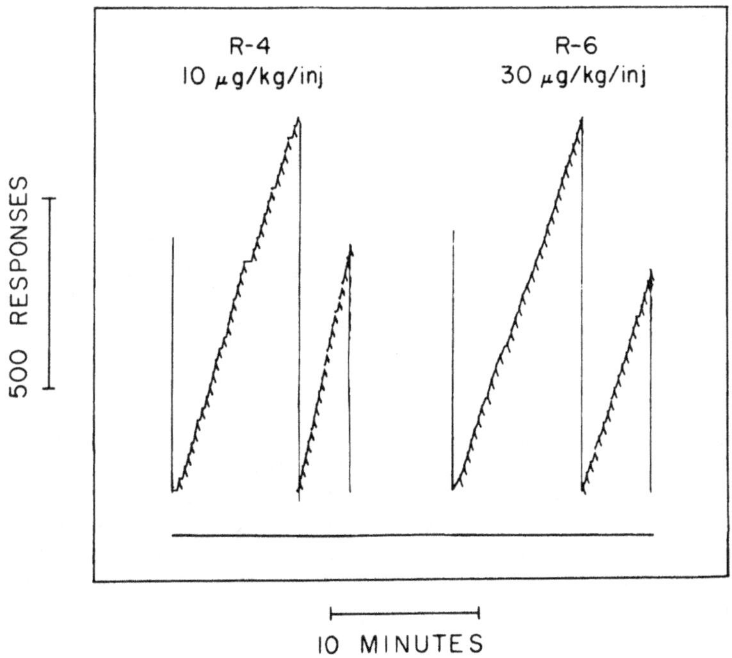

Fig. 1. Representative performances of rhesus monkeys (R-4 and R-6) under a 30-response fixed-ratio schedule of intravenous cocaine injection with 60 sec timeout periods following each injection. Ordinate: cumulative responses. Abscissa: time. The recording pen reset to the baseline whenever 1100 responses had accumulated and at the end of each experimental session. Short diagonal strokes on the records indicate cocaine hydrochloride injections; the recorder stopped during the 60-sec timeout period after each injection. (From Goldberg and Kelleher {1976} with permission. Copyright 1976 by the Society for the Experimental Analysis of Behavior, Inc.)

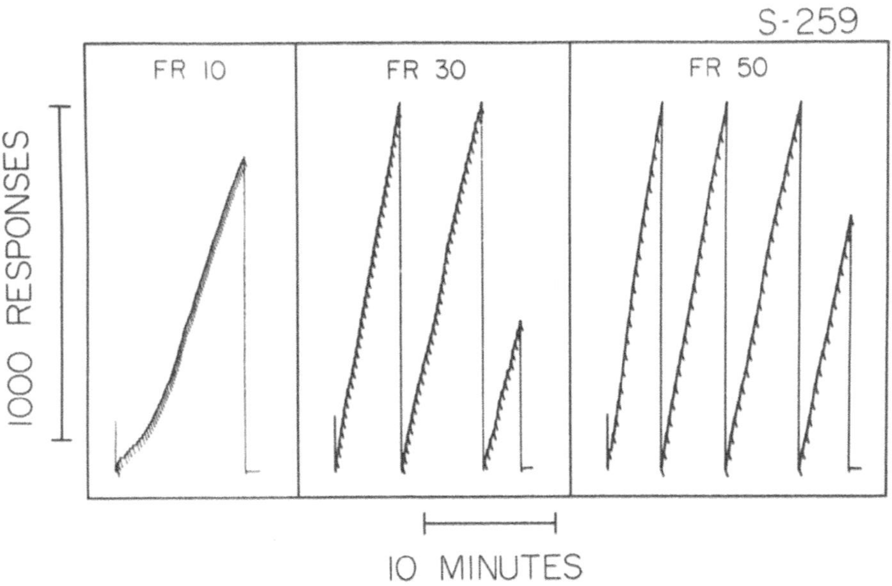

Fig. 2. Representative performances of a squirrel monkey (S-259) maintained by 12 μg/kg injections of cocaine hydrochloride under three different fixed-ratio (FR) response requirements. Recordings are as in Fig. 1. (From Goldberg {1973a} with permission.)

In the rhesus monkeys, high mean rates of responding (1.2 and 1.3 responses per sec) were maintained throughout each daily session at doses of 10 or 30 μg/kg/injection (Fig. 1). An initial brief pause was followed by an abrupt change to a high rate of responding in each fixed-ratio component. In the squirrel monkeys, high response rates and characteristic patterns of fixed-ratio responding were maintained at three fixed-ratio parameters (Fig. 2). At response requirements of 30 or 50, rates of responding exceeding two per sec were maintained by 12 μg/kg injections of cocaine. In both rhesus monkeys and squirrel monkeys, characteristic fixed-ratio patterns and rates of responding were maintained in the presence of the green light, but responding seldom occurred during timeout periods, indicating stimulus control of behavior.

In squirrel monkeys, the dose of cocaine was varied systematically under 10-response and 30-response fixed-ratio schedules (Goldberg, 1973a; Goldberg and Kelleher, 1976). As the dose of cocaine was increased, mean rates of responding increased and then decreased, with maximal rates of responding usually maintained at 25 μg/kg/injection (Fig. 3). The decreases in responding at

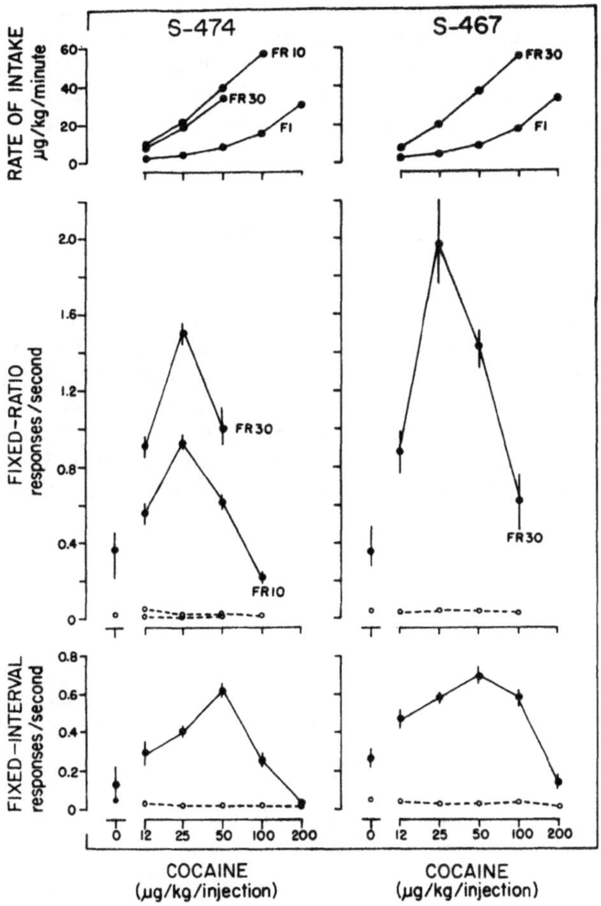

Fig. 3. Effects of dose of cocaine on rate of cocaine intake and rate of responding of squirrel monkeys (S-474 and S-467) under fixed-ratio (FR) or fixed-interval (FI) schedules of intravenous cocaine injection. Abscissa: dose of cocaine hydrochloride per injection, log scale. Ordinate of upper panel: rate of cocaine intake. Ordinate of middle and lower panels: rate of responding. Each point is the mean of three observations; vertical lines indicate range of observations. Solid-circles: rates of responding when schedule was in effect; open circles: rates of responding during timeout periods. Note that the rate of cocaine intake was directly related to dose under both schedules, that the maximal rates of responding under fixed-ratio schedules were greater than and to the left of those under fixed-interval schedules, and that responding was near zero during timeout periods. (From Goldberg and Kelleher {1976} with permission. Copyright 1976 by the Society for the Experimental Analysis of Behavior, Inc.)

higher doses usually resulted from periods of no responding which became longer as each session progressed. Since rate of cocaine intake was directly related to dose over the range of doses studied, decreases in response rates at higher doses may result from direct rate-decreasing effects of cumulated doses of cocaine within the session.

Fixed-Interval Schedules

Characteristic fixed-interval patterns of responding were maintained by cocaine injections in both rhesus and squirrel monkeys. In the rhesus monkey, an initial pause was followed by increasing responding in each interval, at a dose of 30 μg/kg/injection (Fig. 4). The mean quarter-life value was more than 60%. In squirrel monkeys, similar fixed-interval patterns of responding were maintained and mean quarter-life values ranged from 56% to 65% (Fig. 5). Again, in both rhesus and squirrel monkeys, characteristic

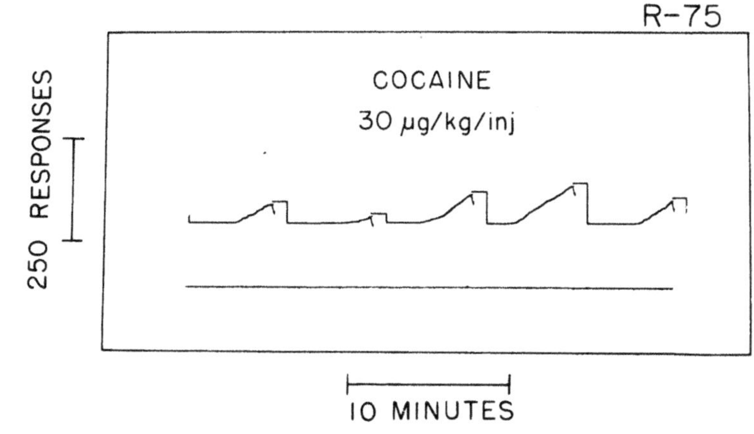

Fig. 4. Representative performance of rhesus monkey R-75 under a 5-min fixed-interval schedule of cocaine injection. Ordinate: cumulative responses. Abscissa: time. Short diagonal strokes on the record indicate cocaine hydrochloride injections (30 μg/kg). The recording pen reset to the baseline at the end of the 60-sec timeout period after each injection. (From Goldberg and Kelleher {1976} with permission. Copyright 1976 by the Society for the Experimental Analysis of Behavior, Inc.)

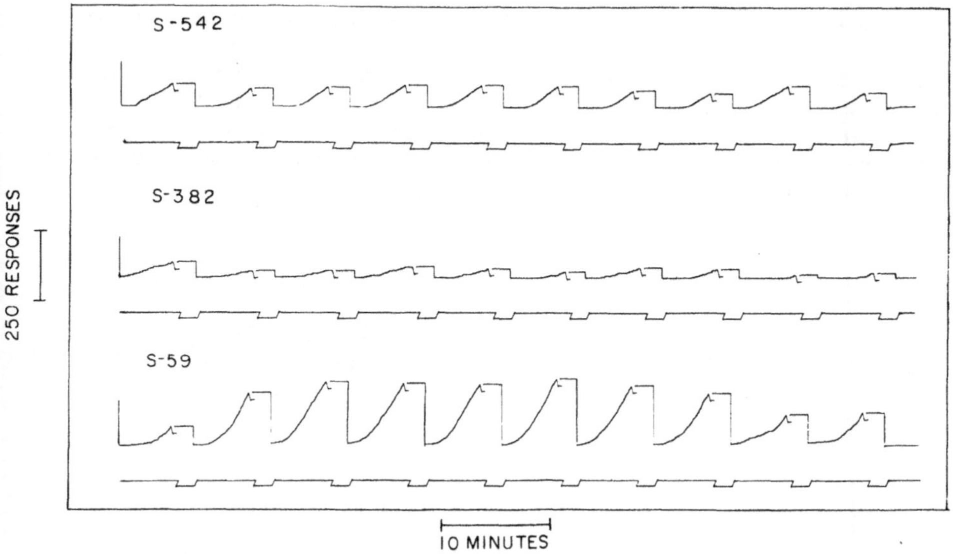

Fig. 5. Representative performances of squirrel monkeys (S-542, S-382, and S-59) under a 5-min fixed-interval schedule of cocaine injection. Ordinate: cumulative responses. Abscissa: time. The recording pen was offset during the injection of 100 μg/kg (S-542) or 30 μg/kg (S-382 and 2-59) of cocaine hydrochloride, and it reset to the baseline at the end of the timeout period which followed injection of cocaine. The event pen was offset during each 100-sec timeout period. (From Goldberg and Kelleher {1976} with permission. Copyright 1976 by the Society for the Experimental Analysis of Behavior, Inc.)

fixed-interval patterns of responding were maintained in the presence of the red or green lights; but responding seldom occurred during timeout periods, indicating that behavior was under stimulus control.

The dose of cocaine has been varied systematically under the 5-min fixed-interval schedule in two squirrel monkeys (Goldberg and Kelleher, 1976). As dose was increased, mean rates of responding increased and then decreased, with maximal rates of 0.6 to 0.7 responses per sec at 50 μg/kg/injection (Fig. 3). However, fixed-interval responding appeared less sensitive to changes in cocaine dose than fixed-ratio responding, and characteristic fixed-interval performance was maintained over a wider range of doses than characteristic fixed-ratio responding. Under the fixed-interval schedules, frequency of injection was relatively independent of response rate and could reach a maximum of only one injection per six min, whereas, under the fixed-ratio schedule, frequency of injection was directly related to rate of responding up to a maximum of almost one injection per min. The greater sensitivity of fixed-ratio responding to changes in the dose of cocaine at these parameter values probably depends in part on the greater dependence of rate of cocaine intake on rate of responding.

Multiple Fixed-Ratio Fixed-Interval Schedules

Under the multiple schedule of cocaine injection, the different performances characteristic of each component schedule alternated

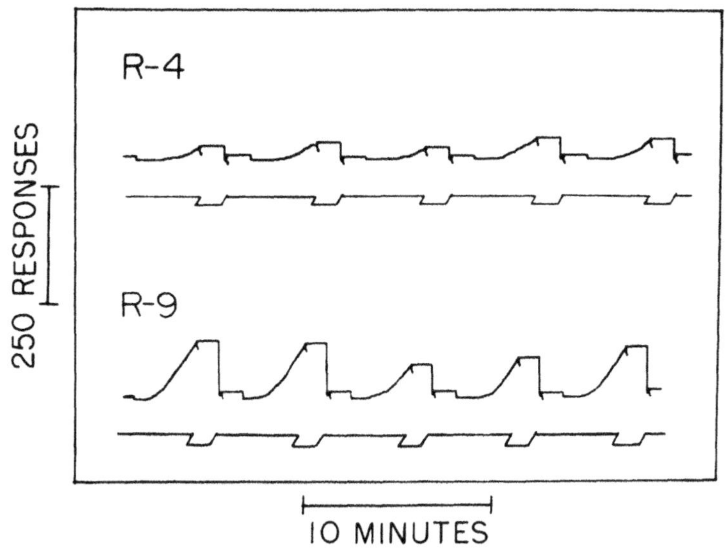

Fig. 6. Representative performances of rhesus monkeys (R-4 and R-9) under a multiple 10-response fixed-ratio 5-min fixed-interval schedule of cocaine injection. Ordinate: cumulative responses. Abscissa: time. Short diagonal strokes on the cumulative record indicate injections of cocaine hydrochloride (30 μg/kg). Each injection was followed by a 100-sec timeout period. The recording pen reset to the baseline at the end of the timeout period. The event pen remained offset during the timeout period after each fixed-interval component and during the next fixed-ratio component.

repeatedly within each session, indicating both stimulus control and schedule control of responding (Fig. 6). When the discriminative stimuli associated with the fixed-ratio schedule were present, high steady rates of responding were maintained; when the discriminative stimuli associated with the fixed-interval schedule were present, moderate rates of responding were maintained, and performance was characterized by an initial pause followed by acceleration of responding to a final rate that was maintained until the end of the interval. As the dose of cocaine was varied, characteristic performances were maintained under the multiple schedule at 30 or 100 μg/kg/injection with monkey R-4 and at 30 to 300 μg/kg/injection with monkey R-6. At higher doses rates of responding decreased, with fixed-ratio performance being more markedly disrupted than fixed-interval performance (Goldberg and Kelleher, 1976).

Similar performances were maintained under a multiple schedule of cocaine injection in squirrel monkey S-467. As the dose of cocaine was increased, mean rates of responding increased and then decreased, with maximal response rates maintained under both schedule components at 50 μg/kg/injection (Fig. 7). Although the alteration of fixed-interval and fixed-ratio components under the multiple schedule ensures the same average rate of cocaine intake under each schedule component, fixed-ratio rates of responding were again more markedly affected than fixed-interval rates of responding by changes in the dose of cocaine. This suggests that schedule factors other than rate of cocaine intake may be important in determining the dose-response functions.

Second-Order Schedules

Responding of squirrel monkeys was developed and maintained under the simple fixed-ratio schedule described earlier. Subsequently, the schedule was changed to a second-order schedule in which every 20- or 30-response fixed-ratio component completed during a 5-min fixed interval produced only a brief 2-sec light; the first fixed-ratio component completed after the 5-min interval elapsed produced both the brief light and an intravenous injection of cocaine. As in the previously described fixed-interval experiments, each injection was followed by a 60-sec timeout period and each session ended after the 15th timeout period. Under these conditions, high rates of responding were maintained throughout each daily session at a cocaine dose of 100 μg/kg/injection (Fig. 8). From 400 to 1000 responses preceded each injection of cocaine and mean rates of responding exceeded one per sec. When the dose of cocaine was varied, maximal response rates were maintained at doses of 100 to 200 μg/kg/injection (Fig. 9).

Although injection frequency was virtually identical in the

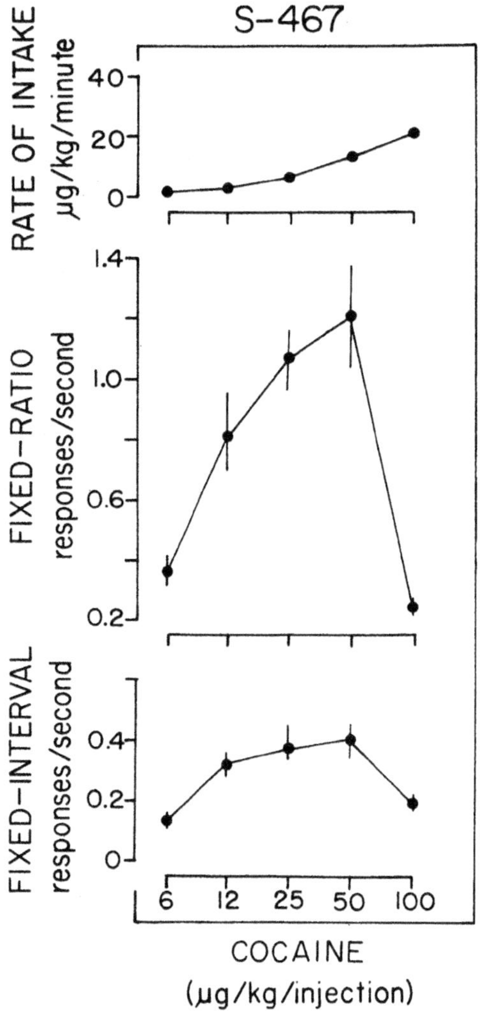

Fig. 7. Effects of cocaine dose on rates of cocaine intake and rates of responding under fixed-ratio and fixed-interval components of a multiple schedule of cocaine injection (squirrel monkey S-467). Abscissa: dose of cocaine hydrochloride per injection, log scale. Ordinate of upper panel: rate of cocaine intake. Ordinate of middle and lower panels: rate of responding. Each point is the mean of three observations; vertical lines indicate range of observations. Note that the dose-response curve is flatter for fixed-interval than for fixed-ratio responding. (From Goldberg and Kelleher {1976} with permission. Copyright 1976 by the Society for the Experimental Analysis of Behavior, Inc.)

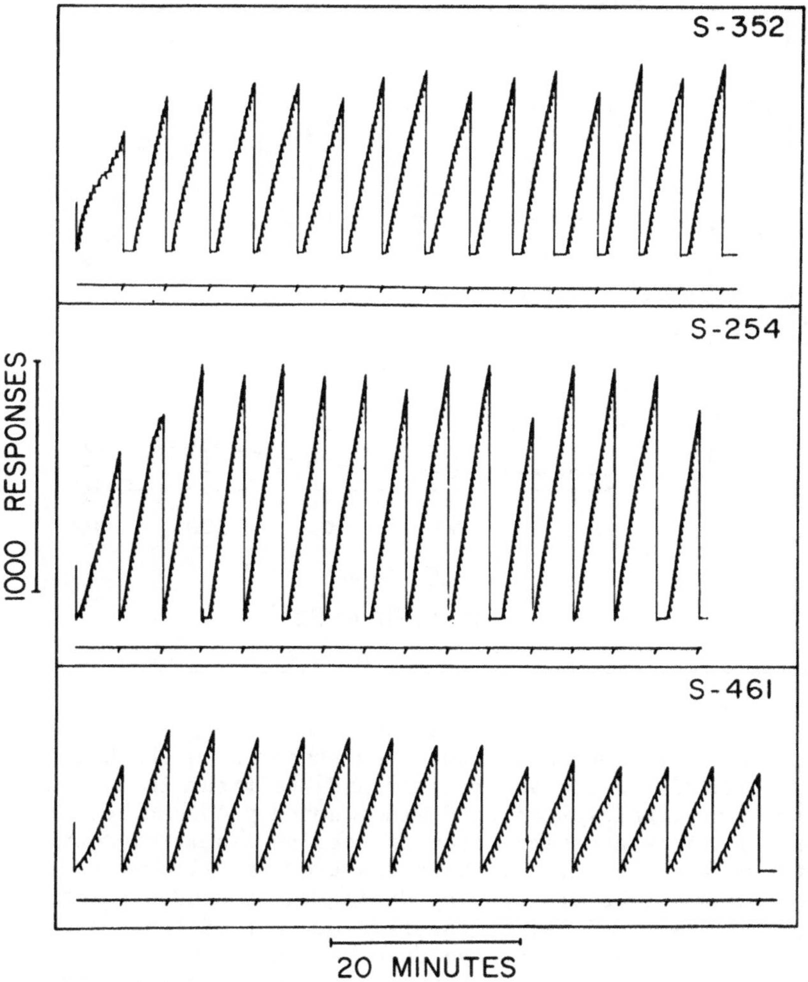

Fig. 8. High rates of responding maintained in three squirrel monkeys (S-352, S-254, and S-461) under a second-order schedule in which the first 30-response fixed-ratio component completed after 5 min produced an intravenous injection of cocaine. Ordinate: cumulative responses. Abscissa: time. Short diagonal strokes on the cumulative records indicate 2-sec presentations of an amber light at the completion of each fixed-ratio component. Diagonal strokes on the event record and the resetting of the recording pen indicate intravenous injections of 100 μg/kg of cocaine hydrochloride. After each injection there was a 60-sec timeout period. The recorder was stopped during presentations of the amber light and during timeout periods. (From Goldberg {1937b} with permission.)

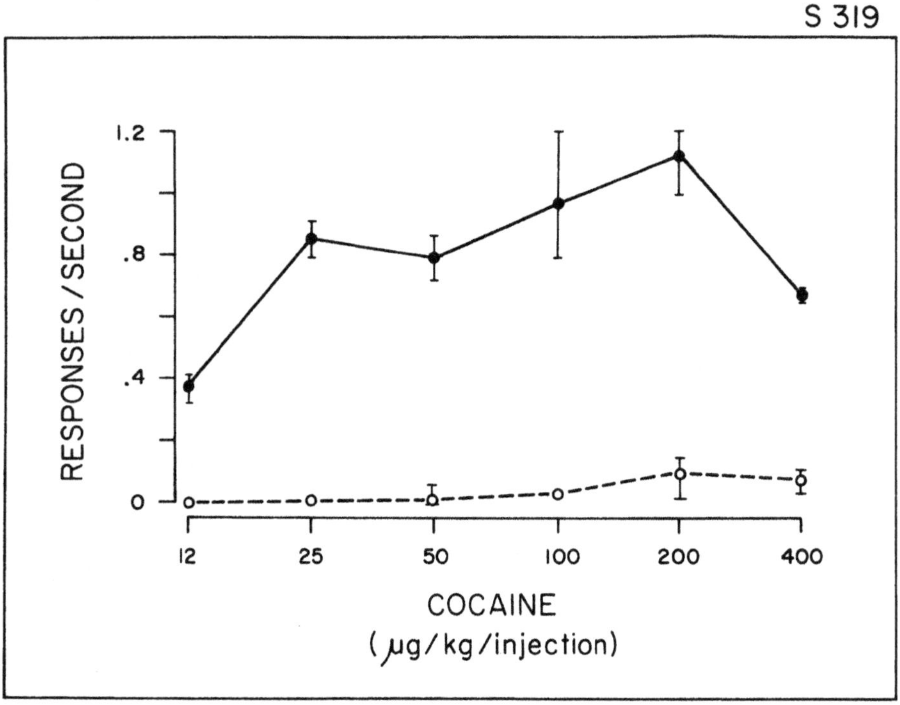

Fig. 9. Effects of dose of cocaine hydrochloride per injection on rate of responding under a second-order schedule in which every 20th response produced a 2-sec amber light and the first 20-response fixed-ratio component completed after 5 min elapsed produced both the light and an intravenous injection of cocaine (squirrel monkey S-319). After each cocaine injection, there was a 60-sec timeout period. Ordinate: mean rate of responding during the second-order schedule (filled points, solid line) or the time-out period (open points, dashed line). Abscissa: cocaine dose per injection. Each session ended after the 15th timeout period. Each point is the mean of results from the last three of four sessions at each dose; brackets indicate the range. (Modified from Goldberg {1973a} with permission.)

squirrel monkeys under the 5-min fixed-interval schedule described earlier and the present second-order schedule, the doses of cocaine that maintained optimal performance were larger and the rates of responding were much higher under the second-order schedule. The briefly presented stimuli appeared to be very important in maintaining the behavior since they controlled characteristic patterns of fixed-ratio responding and rates of responding markedly decreased when the stimuli were not presented (Goldberg, 1971, 1973b).

Another illustration of the effectiveness of second-order schedules with brief stimulus presentations in enhancing the control of behavior by cocaine injections was provided in an experiment with a rhesus monkey (Fig. 10). Responding of monkey R-259 under a 10-min fixed-interval schedule was maintained at only low rates by intravenous injections of 30 μg/kg of cocaine although responding was well maintained by this dose of cocaine in a different monkey under a 5-min fixed-interval schedule (see Fig. 4). An amber stimulus light was presented for 2 sec before and remained on during each injection. The schedule then was changed to a second-order schedule in which every 10-response or 3-response fixed-ratio component completed during the 10-min interval produced the 2-sec amber light; the first fixed-ratio component completed after the 10-min interval elapsed produced both the brief light and an injection of 30 μg/kg of cocaine. Response rates increased slightly when the fixed-ratio requirement was ten responses and then more markedly when the requirement was reduced to three responses (second panel, Fig. 10). Subsequently, high rates of responding (more than one response per sec) were maintained under the second-order schedule with either 3-response or 10-response fixed-ratio components (third and fourth panels, Fig. 10). This schedule modification did not alter the maximum frequency of cocaine injection, but it markedly altered responding within a short period of time. High rates of responding and characteristic fixed-ratio patterns of responding were maintained throughout each 10-min interval.

Second-order schedules of cocaine injection with fixed-interval components have also been studied. Responding of squirrel monkeys was developed and maintained under the 5-min fixed-interval schedule described earlier. Subsequently, the schedule of intravenous cocaine injection was changed to a second-order schedule in which completion of each 5-min fixed-interval component produced only a 2-sec amber light; the completion of every 10th fixed-interval component produced both the light and an intravenous injection of 100 μg/kg cocaine. Each cocaine injection was followed by a 100-sec timeout period and each session ended after the third timeout period. Although the maximum frequency of cocaine injection was less than one per 50 min under this schedule, repeated sequences of characteristic fixed-interval responding were maintained throughout each daily session (Fig. 11). The rates and patterns of responding controlled by the brief stimuli under this second-order schedule were almost identical to those controlled by cocaine injections under the simple fixed-interval schedules (see Fig. 5). Clearly, stimuli associated with cocaine injection can powerfully modulate the control of drug-maintained behavior.

Second-order schedules with fixed-ratio or fixed-interval components extend the range of conditions and the parameters under which

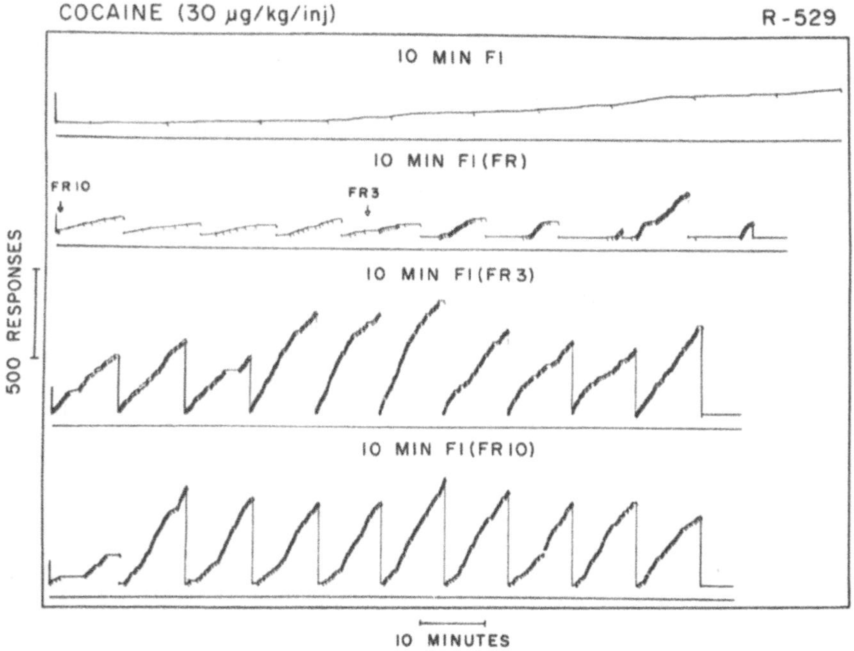

Fig. 10. Increases in responding after the transition from a 10-minute fixed-interval schedule of cocaine injection to a second-order schedule of cocaine injection with fixed-ratio components (rhesus monkey R-529). Ordinate: cumulative responses. Abscissa: time. First panel: performance under a 10-min fixed-interval schedule of cocaine injection. Each short diagonal stroke on the record indicates 2-sec presentation of an amber light accompanied by an injection of cocaine hydrochloride. Second panel: first session under second-order schedule. Each short diagonal stroke indicates a 2-sec presentation of the amber light alone under a 10-response (FR 10) or a 3-response (FR 3) fixed-ratio schedule. The presentation of the amber light accompanied by an injection of cocaine is indicated by the resetting of the pen to the baseline. Third panel: second session under second-order schedule with FR 3 components; recording as in second panel. Fourth panel: subsequent performance under second-order schedule with FR 10 components; recording as in second panel. A 100-sec timeout period followed each injection and the recorder stopped during timeout periods. (From Kelleher, in press, with permission).

drug-maintained behavior can be maintained. These schedules limit the frequency of drug injection since injection occurs only after

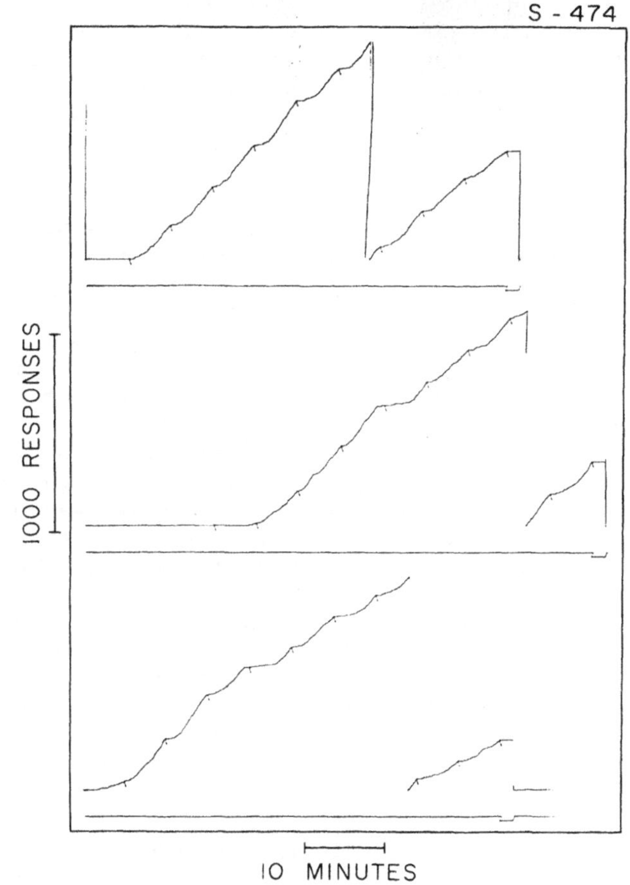

Fig. 11. Representative performances of a squirrel monkey (S-474) under a second-order schedule in which every 10th completion of a 5-min fixed-interval produced an intravenous cocaine injection. The completion of each fixed-interval produced a 2-sec amber light. Short diagonal strokes on the cumulative record indicate presentations of the light. The downstrokes on the event record indicate intravenous injections of 100 μg/kg of cocaine hydrochloride and the beginning of a 100-sec timeout period during which the event pen remained down. This figure shows a complete experimental session comprising three sequences (from top to bottom), each terminating in a cocaine injection and a timeout period. The recording pen reset to the bottom of the record whenever 1100 responses had cumulated and at the end of each sequence. Note the characteristic fixed-interval pattern of responding in most components. (From Goldberg, Kelleher and Morse {1975} with permission.)

the subject has completed a sequence of fixed-ratio or fixed-interval components. Thus, long and orderly sequences of behavior can be maintained and moment to moment control can be exerted over rates and patterns of responding at times when the direct effects of the drug are minimal or absent. In recent experiments, for example, the parameter values of both types of second-order schedules have been arranged so that cocaine injection occurred only at the end of an experimental session.

Representative performances of squirrel monkeys under second-order schedules in which cocaine was injected only at the end of each daily session are shown in Fig. 12. Under one type of schedule (upper record of Fig. 12), every 10-response fixed-ratio component completed during a 60-min interval of time produced only a 2-sec light; the first fixed-ratio component completed after the 60-min interval ended produced 15 consecutive presentations of the light, each accompanied by an injection of 100 μg/kg of cocaine. These presentations were spaced 10 sec apart so that the monkey received a total of 1.5 mg/kg of cocaine over 140 sec. Although cocaine was injected only at the end of the session, responding was maintained at high rates for most of the 60-min interval. Characteristic fixed-ratio patterns of responding were controlled by brief presentations of the light; there was a pause in responding after each light presentation, followed by an abrupt change to a high rate of responding until the light was produced again. Similar high rates and fixed-ratio patterns of responding have been maintained in both squirrel and rhesus monkeys under comparable second-order schedules in which large intravenous doses of morphine (1.5 to 5.0 mg/kg) were injected at the end of each daily session (Goldberg, in press): so, these effects are not limited to cocaine.

Under a second-type of schedule (lower record of Fig. 12), the completion of each 5-min fixed-interval component produced only a 2-sec light; at the completion of the 10th fixed-interval component, a 4-sec presentation of the light was accompanied by 10 rapidly pulsed injections of 60 μg/kg cocaine (a total of 0.6 mg/kg of cocaine). Characteristic patterns of fixed-interval responding were maintained throughout most of the 60-min interval. There was a pause in responding after each light presentation, followed by an acceleration of responding to a final rate that was maintained until the light was produced again.

These results demonstrate that long sequences of behavior comprising successive patterns of either fixed-ratio or fixed-interval responding can be maintained by intravenous injections of cocaine even when cocaine is injected only at the end of the session. Second-order schedules of cocaine injection in which drug is injected only at the end of each experimental session: (1) provide a complete separation of the reinforcing effects of cocaine from its other

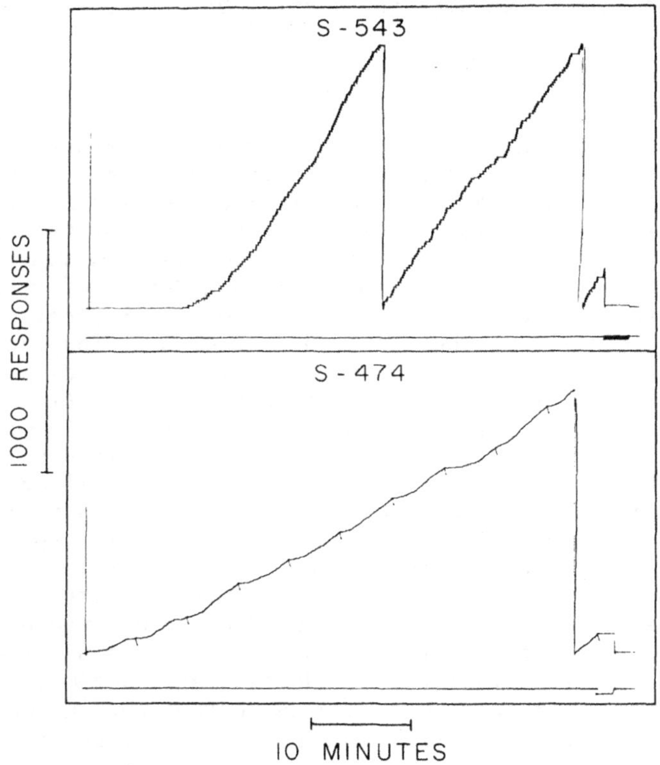

Fig. 12. Representative performances under second-order schedules comprising fixed-ratio components (upper frame) or fixed-interval components (lower frame) under conditions in which cocaine is injected only at the end of each daily session (squirrel monkeys S-543 and S-474). Ordinate: cumulative responses. Abscissa: time. Short diagonal strokes on the cumulative records indicate 2-sec presentations of an amber light at the completion of each component schedule. Upper panel: the first completion of a 10-response fixed-ratio schedule after 60 min produced 15 consecutive intravenous injections of 100 μg/kg of cocaine hydrochloride over 140 sec (total dose 1.5 mg/kg). Each diagonal stroke on the event record indicates a cocaine injection. Lower panel: the tenth completion of a 5-min fixed-interval schedule produced 10 consecutive injections of 60 μg/kg of cocaine hydrochloride (total dose 0.6 mg/kg). The downstroke of the event pen indicates the start of the period of cocaine injection. The recording pen reset to the bottom of the record whenever 1100 responses had cumulated and at the end of the session.

pharmacological effects, and (2) illustrate the role of both cocaine injections and environmental stimuli associated with cocaine injections in the maintenance of drug-seeking behavior.

SUMMARY

In the present experiments, the reinforcing effects of cocaine were separated from its other rate-modifying effects on behavior by using scheduling techniques that limited the maximal possible frequency of cocaine injection within each experimental session. Under appropriate conditions, rates and patterns of responding maintained in squirrel and rhesus monkeys under fixed-ratio and fixed-interval schedules of intravenous cocaine injection were similar to previously reported rates and patterns of responding maintained in various species under fixed-ratio and fixed-interval schedules of food, water, or electric shock presentation (e.g., Kelleher and Morse, 1964, 1968; Morse and Kelleher, 1966; McKearney, 1968, 1969). Under simple fixed-ratio and fixed-interval schedules, and under multiple schedules where fixed-ratio and fixed-interval components alternated within the same session, fixed-ratio responding was more markedly affected than fixed-interval responding by changes in the dose of cocaine. Under second-order schedules, long sequences of responding comprising successive patterns of fixed-ratio or fixed-interval responding could be maintained by intermittent injections of higher doses of cocaine than under the simple fixed-ratio and fixed-interval schedules. When parameter values of the second-order schedules were chosen so that cocaine was injected only at the end of each daily session, high rates and characteristic fixed-ratio patterns of responding were maintained by doses of cocaine as high as 1.5 mg/kg. Pretreatment with this dose of cocaine almost completely suppresses responding maintained under fixed-ratio schedules of food presentation (Gonzalez and Goldberg, 1974; Woods and Tessel, 1974). Thus, the scheduling techniques described in this paper allow a complete separation of the reinforcing effects of cocaine from its other pharmacological effects. The second-order schedules also provide a valuable experimental technique for exploring the complex interrelationships between behavior, environmental stimuli, and injections of drug, which result in the maintenance of drug-seeking and drug-taking behavior.

ACKNOWLEDGMENTS

This research was supported by USPHS Research Grants MH07658, DA00499, MH02094 and Research Career Program Award 1-K5-MH22589 with facilities and services furnished in part by the New England Regional Primate Research Center, Harvard Medical School, Southborough, Massachusetts (USPHS Grant RR-00168, Division of Research Resources, National Institutes of Health).

REFERENCES

Barrett, J.E.: Effects of alcohol, chlordiazopoxide, cocaine and pentobarbital on responding maintained under fixed-interval schedules of food or shock presentation. J. Pharmacol. exp. Ther., in press.

Goldberg, S.R.: Sequences of rapid responding maintained by cocaine self-injection in squirrel monkeys (Abstract). Pharmacologist 13, 281 (1971).

Goldberg, S.R.: Comparable behavior maintained under fixed-ratio and second-order schedules of food presentation, cocaine injection or d-amphetamine injection in the squirrel monkey. J. Pharmacol. exp. Ther. 186, 18-30 (1973a).

Goldberg, S.R.: Control of behavior by stimuli associated with drug injections. In: Psychic Dependence. Goldberg, L. and Hoffmeister, F., Eds., pp. 106-109, Berlin: Springer-Verlag, 1973b.

Goldberg, S.R.: Stimuli associated with drug injections as events that control behavior. Pharmacol. Rev. (in press).

Goldberg, S.R., Hoffmeister, F., Schlichting, U.U., Wuttke, W.: A comparison of pentobarbital and cocaine self-administration in rhesus monkeys: Effects of dose and fixed-ratio parameter. J. Pharmacol. exp. Ther. 179, 277-283 (1971).

Goldberg, S.R. and Kelleher, R.T.: Behavior controlled by scheduled injections of cocaine in squirrel and rhesus monkeys. J. exp. Analysis Behav. 25, 67-78 (1976).

Goldberg, S.R., Kelleher, R.T., Morse, W.H.: Second-order schedules of drug injection. Fed. Proc. 34, 1771-1776 (1975).

Gollub, L.R.: The relations among measures of performance on fixed-interval schedules. J. exp. Analysis Behav. 7, 337-343 (1964).

Gonzalez, F.A. and Goldberg, S.R.: Behavioral effects of cocaine compared under two schedules of food presentation in the squirrel monkey (Abstract). Pharmacologist 16, 215 (1974).

Herd, J.A., Morse, W.H., Kelleher, R.T., Jones, L.G.: Arterial hypertension in the squirrel monkey during behavioral experiments. Am. J. Physiol. 217, 24-29 (1969).

Herrnstein, R.J. and Morse, W.H.: Effects of pentobarbital on intermittently reinforced behavior. Science 125, 929-931 (1957).

Kelleher, R.T.: Characteristics of behavior controlled by scheduled injections of drugs. Pharmacol. Rev. (in press).

Kelleher, R.T. and Morse, W.H.: Escape behavior and punished behavior. Fed. Proc. 23, 808-817 (1964).

Kelleher, R.T. and Morse, W.H.: Determinants of the specificity of the behavioral effects of drugs. Ergebn. Physiol. 60, 1-56 (1968).

McKearney, J.W.: Maintenance of responding under a fixed-interval schedule of electric shock presentation. Science 160, 1249-1251 (1968).

McKearney, J.W.: Fixed-interval schedules of electric shock presentation: Extinction and recovery of performance under different shock intensities and fixed-interval durations. J. exp. Analysis Behav. 12, 301-313 (1969).

Morse, W.H. and Kelleher, R.T.: Schedules using noxious stimuli. I. Multiple fixed-ratio and fixed-interval termination of schedule complexes. J. exp. Analysis Behav. 9, 267-290 (1966).

Pickens, R. and Thompson, T.: Cocaine-reinforced behavior in rats. J. Pharmacol. exp. Ther. 161, 122-129 (1968).

Smith, C.B.: Effects of d-amphetamine upon operant behavior of pigeons: enhancement by reserpine. J. Pharmacol. exp. Ther. 146, 167-174 (1964).

Wilson, M.C., Hitomi, M., Schuster, C.R.: Psychomotor stimulant self-administration as a function of dosage per injection in the rhesus monkey. Psychopharmacologia 22, 271-281 (1971).

Woods, J.H. and Tessel, R.E.: Fenfluramine: Amphetamine congener that fails to maintain drug-taking behavior in the rhesus monkey. Science 185, 1067-1069 (1974).

A COMPARISON OF COCAINE AND DIETHYLPROPION UNDER TWO DIFFERENT SCHEDULES OF DRUG PRESENTATION

Chris E. Johanson and Charles R. Schuster

Departments of Psychiatry and Pharmacological and Physiological Sciences, The University of Chicago, Pritzker School of Medicine, Chicago, Illinois 60637

Research over the last decade has demonstrated that animals repeat those responses that are followed by intravenous injections of psychomotor stimulant drugs (Schuster and Johanson, 1974). This reinforcing property is shared by a number of drugs of that class, including cocaine, the amphetamines, methylphenidate, phenmetrazine and pipradrol - to mention a few (see Schuster and Johanson, 1974, for references). With few exceptions, every stimulant tested with infrahuman animals has been shown to maintain responding under a wide variety of environmental circumstances. In addition, this phenomenon has been demonstrated in several species, including rats (Pickens and Thompson, 1968), squirrel monkeys (Goldberg, 1973; Stretch, Gerber, and Woods, 1971), rhesus monkeys (Deneau, Yanagita, and Seevers, 1969), and baboons (Findley, Robinson, and Peregrino, 1972). Although the majority of studies has utilized fixed-ratio schedules (every nth response followed by an injection) of presentation (Wilson, Hitomi, and Schuster, 1971; Balster and Schuster, 1973a), many experiments have utilized additional schedules. These include interval schedules (Balster and Schuster, 1973b; Dougherty and Pickens, 1973), concurrent schedules (Iglauer and Woods, 1974; Iglauer, Llewellyn, and Woods, 1975), multi-operant schedules (Johanson and Schuster, 1975; Johanson, 1975) and second-order schedules (Goldberg, 1973). The results from all these studies show that psychomotor stimulant drugs maintain responding regardless of the species of the experimental animal and regardless of the schedule of presentation. Therefore, it appears that one of the pharmacological properties shared by all psychomotor stimulant drugs is the ability to act as a positive reinforcer: each will initiate and maintain an increased frequency of the behavior it follows (Skinner, 1938).

The illicit use of a drug by humans is undoubtedly related to its reinforcing properties. If the drug reinforcement mechanism is common to both animals and man, it is possible to develop an animal model of human drug abuse to investigate the modification of drug-maintained behavior by pharmacological, organismic, and environmental variables (Schuster and Johanson, 1973). Evidence for the validity of this animal model is rapidly accumulating. Animals self-administer the same drugs which humans use for non-medical purposes; these include not only the psychomotor stimulants but opiates, barbiturates, and alcohol as well (Schuster and Johanson, 1974). In addition the pattern of intake of these drugs in experimental animals is very similar to the pattern of their illicit use by man. Stimulants, for instance, are taken in cycles with days of high intake alternating with days of low intake (Deneau et al., 1969; Johanson, Balster, and Bonese, 1976). This pattern is reminiscent of that reported for humans (Kramer, Fischman, and Littlefield, 1967). Finally, the physiological and behavioral consequences of the repeated self-administration of drugs is similar from animal to man (Fischman and Schuster, 1975; Ellinwood and Duarte-Escalante, 1972). This information strongly suggests that an animal model of intravenous drug self-administration can be useful in studying factors which influence the non-medical use of drugs in man.

The principal medical uses of psychomotor stimulant drugs have been for the treatment of obesity, hyperkinesis, and narcolepsy. Pharmaceutical companies are eagerly trying to develop new drugs for these applications which possess lower abuse potential than those currently available. If such drugs are developed, the production of psychomotor stimulant drugs with high abuse potential could be sharply curtailed, thus reducing the quantities available for diversion into the illicit market. If animal studies are valid predictors, it is possible to evaluate new stimulant compounds for their dependence potential during their pre-clinical testing. Although it is true that some drugs appear to lack positive reinforcing properties (e.g., chlorpromazine, fenfluramine), it is unlikely that the psychomotor stimulants can be replaced in all of their applications with drugs completely devoid of reinforcing properties. A more realistic goal is to find drugs with significantly less dependence potential than those currently available. The problem then is to develop a methodology capable of comparing the reinforcing efficacy of different drugs. In operant terms, this is comparable to assessing the strength of a positive reinforcer (Skinner, 1938). The strength of two different reinforcers can be compared by measuring the relative frequency or rate of behavior each maintains. Since this definition is operational, the strength of a positive reinforcer may change with its schedule of presentation. This point can be illustrated by comparing dose-response functions generated by different schedules of psychomotor stimulant drug injection. During fixed-ratio schedules of presentation, rate of responding was inversely related to drug dose (Wilson et al., 1971; Goldberg, 1973; Balster and Schuster, 1973a). In contrast, rate of responding maintained by fixed-interval schedules with time-outs between injections (Balster and Schuster, 1973b), concurrent schedules (Iglauer and Woods, 1974, Iglauer et al., 1975), and choice schedules (Johanson, 1971, 1975; Johanson and Schuster, 1975) increased with increases in dose. Rate of responding maintained by psychomotor stimulant drugs on a second-order schedule did not change as a function of dose (Goldberg, 1973). These differences may be due to the fact that reinforcers not only maintain behavior which they follow but modify subsequent behavior as well (Schuster and Balster, 1972; Catania, 1973). Although these elicited effects have only been studied in a limited way with non-drug reinforcers (Nevin, 1974), considerable research has been done on the effects of non-contingent injections of drugs on behavior. The results indicate that the effects of drugs, including stimulants, are largely dependent upon the schedule of presentation of the stimulus maintaining behavior, regardless of its nature (Dews, 1955; Morse and Kelleher, 1970; Kelleher and Morse, 1968). Therefore, it is likely that rates of self-administration of psychomotor stimulants are determined only partially by their reinforcing properties. It is not sufficient, then, to assess relative strength of drugs as positive reinforcers by using rates of responding generated by one schedule of presentation to predict the relative dependence potential of drugs. An alternative strategy is to test drugs by using a variety of schedules of presentation, particularly ones which minimize the non-reinforcing effects of a drug. In addition, it is important to use schedules which mimic the contingencies of presentation in effect for humans. One approach is the use of a preference procedure in which animals are given a choice between two magnitudes of a single reinforcer or between two reinforcers and in which injections are separated by relatively long periods of time (Findley et al., 1972; Johanson, 1971, 1975; Johanson and Schuster, 1975; Griffiths, Wurster, and Brady, 1975). In order to validate any new procedure such as this, it is necessary to determine its predictiveness with standard compounds for which there exists some estimate of their actual abuse in man.

In the present experiments, the relative reinforcing efficacy or strength of two different drugs, cocaine and diethylpropion, were compared using two schedules of presentation in the rhesus monkey. Diethylpropion was investigated because it is a psychomotor stimulant drug which is similar in its profile of pharmacological actions to cocaine and the amphetamines (Jonnson, 1969). Despite this similarity and its availability on the market for over 15 years, there is little evidence for non-medical use, except when more preferred stimulant drugs are unavailable (Jasinski, Nutt, and Griffith, 1974). On the basis of this data, it was predicted that diethylpropion would act as a positive reinforcer like other stimulant drugs. However, the epidemiological data further predicts that diethylpropion would not be self-administered when other stimulants such as cocaine were available.

In the first experiment, animals were initially trained to lever-press on a fixed-ratio 10 schedule of cocaine injection. Various doses of diethylpropion were then substituted in order to determine whether this drug would serve as a reinforcer when it was the only drug available. In the second experiment, rhesus monkeys were trained to choose between cocaine and diethylpropion in order to investigate their relative reinforcing properties.

EXPERIMENT 1: FIXED-RATIO SCHEDULE OF DRUG PRESENTATION

Method

Animals. The animals in this study were three male rhesus monkeys (A041, A065 and A069) weighing between 4.0 and 7.2 kg. All animals had been used in previous studies involving responding maintained by psychomotor stimulant drugs and were each equipped with a single-lumen silicon venous catheter (Ronthor Silatube, S-1125 Duro 50) at the beginning of the experiment. Each catheter had been implanted under sodium pentobarbital anesthesia (30 mg/kg i.v.). The proximal end of the catheter was inserted into a major vein for a distance calculated to terminate in the superior vena cava; the distal end was threaded subcutaneously and exited the body through an incision in the back of the animal. Since median catheter life was approximately three months, it was not always possible to maintain a single catheter for the duration of the experiment. When a catheter became dislodged, the monkey was removed from the experiment for a minimum of 10 days. At this time, a replacement catheter was surgically inserted in one of the internal jugular, external jugular, or femoral veins, and the animal was then returned to the experiment. Animal A041 kept a single catheter throughout the experiment while A065 and A069 were each recatheterized once.

All animals had continuous access to water and were given 20 Purina Monkey Chow biscuits and a sugar cube saturated with liquid vitamins every morning. In addition, their diet was frequently supplemented with fresh fruit. When necessary, antibiotics were administered intramuscularly to arrest a catheter tract infection.

Apparatus. Each monkey was housed in a sound-attenuated wooden cubicle that served as the experimental space. Mounted on the door of the cubicle were two lever boxes, each of which was 20 cm from the floor and 10 cm from the center line. The front of each box contained a response lever (PRL-001, BRS/LVE, Beltsville, Md.) and a strip of Plexiglas, which was 5 cm above the lever and could be transilluminated by stimulus lights. The door also had a one-way mirror for observing the monkey. The entire ceiling was made of Plexiglas and could be transilluminated by either white or red lights.

Each monkey wore a stainless-steel harness connected to a spring arm 46 cm in length and 1.3 cm in diameter (E & H Engineering, Chicago, Ill.) which was attached to the back of the cubicle (Schuster and Johanson, 1974). This arrangement allowed the monkey relatively unrestricted movement within the cubicle and provided protection for the catheter which was threaded through the arm. Outside the cubicle, the catheter was connected to a peristaltic infusion pump (754X, Cole-Parmer Instrument Co., Chicago, Ill.) which delivered solutions at the rate of 6 ml/min.

Cables connected the experimental cubicles to electromechanical programming and recording equipment located in an adjacent room.

Procedure. No training was required for any of the animals since each had previously been trained to press a lever for drug injections. The terminal schedule of injection was a fixed-ratio 10 (FR 10; ten responses for each injection of the right lever [lever 1]). Responding on the left lever (lever 2) had no programmed consequences in this experiment. Initially 0.2 mg/kg/inj of cocaine was available on the FR 10 schedule during a 3hr daily session. After responding became stable, saline or different doses of diethylpropion were substituted for the cocaine solution for 6 consecutive sessions. The doses of diethylpropion tested and the order of testing are given in Table 1. Following the substitution of each test dose of diethylpropion, saline was substituted for an additional six sessions. Prior to the substitution of the next dose of diethylpropion, the animals were returned to the baseline conditions of 0.2 mg/kg/inj cocaine for 3 sessions. Therefore the usual sequence of conditions was: 1) 0.2 mg/kg/inj of cocaine for three sessions, 2) a test dose of diethylpropion for six sessions, and 3) saline for six sessions. Following the testing of all seven doses, the lowest (0.01 mg/kg/inj) and the highest dose (3.0 mg/kg/inj) were repeated. However, their presentation was preceded by six saline sessions rather than 3 cocaine sessions. Following the availability of 3.0 mg/kg/inj diethylpropion, saline was again substituted for six sessions.

In order to compare extinction responding resulting from the substitution of saline following diethylpropion, saline was occasionally substituted following cocaine (Table 1). For animal A041 this was done both prior to the testing of 0.01 mg/kg/inj diethylpropion and prior to the second testing of 3.0 mg/kg/inj diethylpropion. For animal A065 this additional cocaine-saline sequence was repeated three times, twice before the testing of 0.5 mg/kg/inj diethylpropion and once before the testing of 0.2 mg/kg/inj diethylpropion. The sequence was repeated three times for animal A069

Table 1

Order of Diethylpropion Testing in Experiment 1

Animal	Dose (mg/kg/inj)						
	0.01	0.05	0.2	0.5	1.0	1.5	3.0
A041	3*	6	4	2	7	1	5
A065	5	2	4*	1**	3	6	7
A069	4	3*	1*	2	5	6*	7

*Additional cocaine - saline sequence interspersed prior to the testing of indicated dose.

prior to the testing of 0.05 mg/kg/inj, 0.2 mg/kg/inj and 1.5 mg/kg/inj diethylpropion.

During each experimental session, the number of injections delivered and the total number of responses on the operative lever were recorded every thirty minutes. Drug or saline availability was associated with an illuminated white stimulus light above the operative lever as well as a white ceiling light. These lights were extinguished during injections and a red lever light and red ceiling light were illuminated.

For each animal, the injection volume was 0.2 ml/kg of body weight. Therefore, the injection duration varied from 8 to 14.4 seconds. All the drugs were dissolved in physiological saline and doses refer to the salt. Solutions were changed at least once every two weeks.

Results

Although the mean number of cocaine injections received during a 3-day period of availability fluctuated somewhat over the entire experiment, there were no systematic trends observed for any of the animals. The overall means were 67.8, 32.6 and 45.2 injections for animals A041, A065, and A069, respectively.

Figure 1 shows the mean number of saline injections taken by each animal for each period of availability over the entire experiment. These means are calculated from the last three sessions of access. For animals A065 and A069, the mean number of saline injections was generally low throughout the experiment. The number of

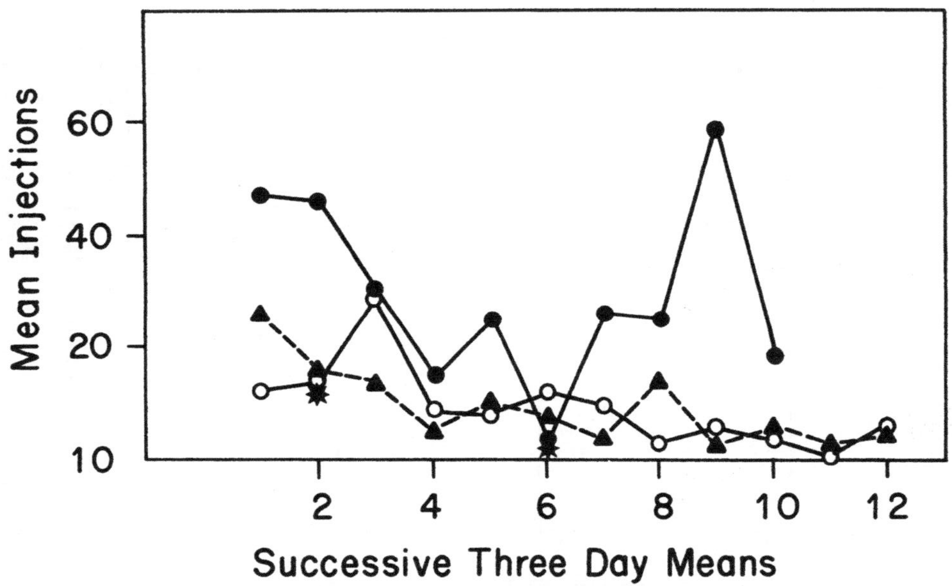

Fig. 1. Mean number of saline injections received during each successive period of availability for animals A041 (closed circles), A065 (open circles) and A069 (triangles). Each mean is based upon the last three days of access to saline. The asterisk (*) indicates catheter replacement.

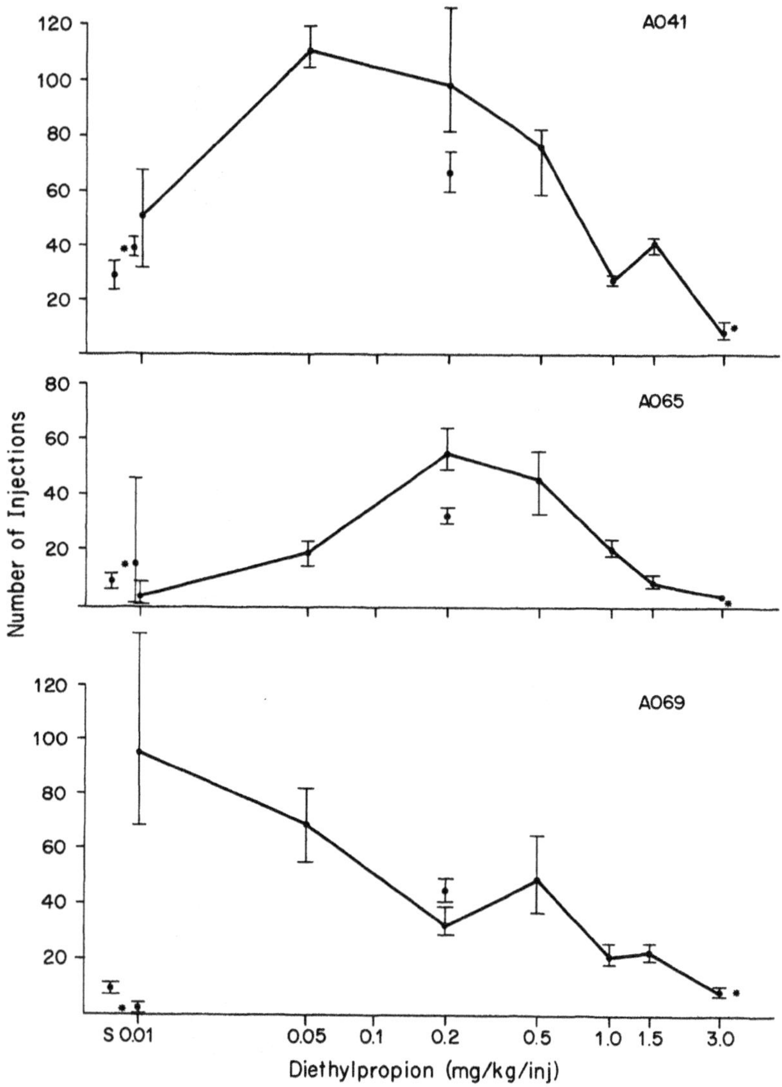

Fig. 2. Mean number of injections of each dose of diethylpropion for each animal. These means are calculated from the last three days of access. The brackets indicate the range. The mean and standard error of 0.2 mg/kg/inj and saline injections are also shown. The results of the second testing of 0.01 mg/kg/inj and 3.0 mg/kg/inj diethylpropion which followed saline availability rather than cocaine are indicated by the asterisk (*).

saline injections for A041 was higher and fluctuated to a greater degree. For each animal, responding maintained by saline tended to decrease with repeated exposures to saline extinction periods. This is reflected by the fact that overall mean number of saline injections for the first half of the experiment was higher than for the second half.

Figure 2 shows the mean and range of injections of various doses of diethylpropion for each animal. The means and ranges were calculated from the last 3 sessions of each substitution. The overall mean and standard error of 0.2 mg/kg/inj cocaine and saline injections are also shown. In general, the dose-response curve for animals A041 and A065 had an inverted U shape, but for A069, responding was inversely related to dose. Inspection of Fig. 2 shows that the mean number of injections of 0.2 mg/kg of cocaine was about the same as the number of injections obtained when testing 0.5 mg/kg of diethylpropion for all three animals.

TABLE 2

Number of Saline Injections Self-Administered on the First Day Following Cocaine or Diethylpropion in Experiment 1

	A041	A065	A069
0.01	27	1	35
0.05	55	11	36
0.2	90	17	26
0.5	63	29	27
1.0	26	27	50
1.5	88*	32	22
3.0	9	4	19
0.2 mg/kg/inj cocaine	57, 64 ($\overline{X}$=60.5)	95*, 91, 41 ($\overline{X}$=75.7)	96*, 9, 49 ($\overline{X}$=51.3)

* First Saline Substitution

Repeating the lowest dose (0.01 mg/kg/inj) following saline rather than cocaine produced mixed results. For A041 the mean number of injections was within the range of the first determination but the variability was reduced. For A065 the mean of the second determination was higher and the range was greater but totally overlapping the range of the first determination. For A069, responding maintained by 0.01 mg/kg/inj diethylpropion when it followed saline was very low. This is in contrast to the first determination when this dose was tested following cocaine and was found to maintain higher and more variable rates of responding than any other dose. The number of injections of 3.0 mg/kg/inj diethylpropion was the same following both cocaine and saline availability.

Table 2 presents the number of saline injections self-administered on the first day following each dose of diethylpropion and following 0.2 mg/kg/inj cocaine. The highest number of saline injections occurred during the first saline substitution for animals A065 and A069. For A041, it was the second highest. In addition, for A065 and A069, the mean number of saline injections following cocaine was higher than occurred following diethylpropion. The two distributions overlapped for A041. For A065, the relationship between dose of diethylpropion and number of saline injections on the first day of substitution increased to a peak at 1.5 mg/kg/inj and then decreased. There was no systematic relationship between these two variables for A041 and A069.

EXPERIMENT 2: CHOICE SCHEDULE OF DRUG PRESENTATION

Method

Animals. The animals in this study were four male rhesus monkeys (A022, 3029, 3043, and 3117) weighing between 5 and 6 kg at the beginning of the experiment. A022 had been tested previously in studies utilizing the same procedure described below but with responding maintained by cocaine or methylphenidate (Johanson and Schuster, 1975). The other three animals had no prior experimental or drug history. Each animal was prepared with a double-lumen, polyvinyl chloride catheter (#1100, U.S. Catheter and Instrument Co., Billerica, Mass.) according to the procedure described in Experiment 1. Animal A022 was catheterized in the right femoral vein prior to the beginning of the present experiment and maintained this catheter throughout the duration of the experiment. Animal 3029 remained catheterized in the right internal jugular for the entire study. However, both 3043 and 3117 required additional catheters in order to complete the experiment. These were replaced as described in Experiment 1.

All animals had continuous access to water and were given 20 Purina Monkey Chow biscuits and a sugar cube saturated with liquid vitamins every morning. In addition, their diet was frequently supplemented with fresh fruit. When necessary, antibiotics were administered intramuscularly to arrest a catheter tract infection.

Apparatus. The apparatus for this experiment was identical to that of Experiment 1.

Procedure. Training: Initially each lever-press on the right hand lever in the presence of a red stimulus light produced cocaine delivery (0.1 mg/kg). Lever responses usually occurred sufficiently often that training was unnecessary; occasionally, however, raisins were taped to the lever to encourage manipulation of it. After acquisition of the lever-press response, the requirement for cocaine delivery was gradually raised to five (FR 5). Next, responding on the FR 5 schedule was maintained by cocaine in the presence of a green stimulus light. Finally, the red or green stimulus lights randomly appeared above either lever. Total exposure to these training conditions never exceeded 2 hours.

Terminal Schedule: Each daily session consisted of two sampling periods followed by several choice trials. During the first sampling period, a red or green stimulus light (S_1) was illuminated above the left lever while the stimulus light above the right lever remained dark. At this time, the ceiling was transilluminated by the white light. Five responses on the left lever resulted in the injection of 1 ml of drug A. Responses of the right lever were recorded but had no other programmed consequences. During the injection, which lasted 10 seconds, the lever light and white ceiling light were turned off and a red ceiling light was illuminated. The position of S_1 switched to the right lever box and thereafter alternated with each injection of drug A. Five injections were permitted during the first sampling period. After the fifth injection, a 30-min time-out occurred during which only the white ceiling light was illuminated and responding was recorded but had no additional programmed consequences. After the time-out, the second sampling period began in which five opportunities were given for self-injection of drug B. The stimulus (S_2) associated with availability of drug B was different in color from S_1. If S_1 was red, S_2 was green, and vice versa. In all other respects, however, the procedures used during this second sampling period were identical to those used during the first sampling period. After the fifth injection of drug B, another 30-min time-out was initiated.

The remainder of the session consisted of choice trials during which S_1 and S_2 were simultaneously presented, one over each lever. Five responses on the lever illuminated by S_1 resulted in the injection of 1 ml of drug A, whereas five responses on the lever illuminated by S_2 resulted in the injection of 1 ml of drug B. The first response on one lever terminated the stimulus over the other lever and made responses on that lever inconsequential for the remainder of the trial. The lever lights and white ceiling light were turned off, and a red ceiling light was illuminated during the injection of either drug solution. After each injection, the white ceiling light was illuminated for 15 min and responding had no programmed consequences.

This procedure was repeated on all choice trials with the restriction that S_1 and S_2 randomly appeared above each lever on 50% of the trials. A session lasted until all choice trials were completed or until 24 hours had passed. The number of choice trials available to individual animals was 18 or 20. For any comparison the number remained constant. With the exception of A022, which had been in previous choice experiments, the initial comparison was between 0.1 mg/kg/inj of cocaine (drug A) and saline (drug B). Animals 3029 and 3043 chose the cocaine solution on over 75% of the trials in less than 10 days. Animal 3117 did not choose either solution reliably after 12 days, so the cocaine dose was raised to 0.2 mg/kg/inj. Within 3 days, this animal chose cocaine on over 75% of the trials. At this point, comparisons between diethylpropion and cocaine began.

Table 3 shows the comparisons made between the drugs for all four animals as well as the order and duration of testing. The dose of 0.5 mg/kg/inj diethylpropion (drug A) was compared to saline, 0.1 mg/kg/inj of cocaine, 0.5 mg/kg/inj of cocaine and 1.0 mg/kg/inj of diethylpropion. In each case, 0.5 mg/kg/inj diethylpropion was available during the first sampling period. In addition, a dose of 1.0 mg/kg of diethylpropion was compared to saline, 0.1 mg/kg/inj of cocaine and 0.5 mg/kg/inj of cocaine. In these comparisons, diethylpropion was available during the first sampling period. Additional comparisons not shown in Table 3 were made as follows: 1) 1.0 mg/kg/inj diethylpropion vs 0.2 mg/kg/inj cocaine for A022; 2) 1.0 mg/kg/inj diethylpropion vs 0.05 mg/kg/inj cocaine and vs 0.025 mg/kg/inj cocaine for 3029; 3) 0.025 mg/kg/inj cocaine vs saline for 3029; and 4) 0.5 mg/kg/inj cocaine vs saline for 3043.

During the initial comparison between 0.5 mg/kg/inj diethylpropion and saline, S_1 was green and S_2 was red. In order to determine that responding during choice trials was a function of its consequences (i.e., the injection of one drug solution rather than the other drug solution) and not other variables, such as color preference or prior drug solution-stimulus pairings, the predicted non-preferred drug solution (saline in comparison to drug, diethylpropion in comparison to cocaine, and 0.5 mg/kg/inj diethylpropion in comparison to 1.0 mg/kg/inj diethylpropion) was paired with the stimulus associated with the preferred drug solution in the previous comparison. A comparison was continued until: 1) the animal chose the drug solution associated with the stimulus not preferred in the

Table 3

Comparisons Between Diethylpropion and Saline, Cocaine, or Another Dose of Diethylpropion for Each Animal During Experiment 2: Duration and Order of Testing

0.5 mg/kg Diethylpropion				1.0 mg/kg Diethylpropion			
	#	Days	Order		#	Days	Order
Saline	A022	15	1	Saline	A022	19	2
	3029*	23	1				
	3043	17	1		3043	11	6
	3117	12	1				
0.1 mg/kg Cocaine	A022	28	4	0.1 mg/kg Cocaine	A022	17	3
	3029*	13	4		3029*	21	5
	3043	14	5		3043	12	8
	3117	23	2		3117*	17	3
0.5 mg/kg Cocaine	A022	12	5	0.5 mg/kg Cocaine	A022	17	6
	3029*	12	2		3029*	17	3
	3043*	23	4		3043	11	2
	3043	11	9		3117*	9	4
1.0 mg/kg Diethyl-propion	3029*	9	9				
	3043	23	7				
	3117	24	5				

* N of Choice Trials = 18, Otherwise 20.

last comparison (requiring a switch in stimulus preference) on at least 75% of the trials for at least three consecutive sessions; 2) the animal chose a drug solution between 40 and 60% of the trials for at least seven consecutive sessions, indicating no preference; or 3) the animal did not switch its choice of stimulus color for at least seven consecutive sessions. If the monkey did not change its choice of stimulus color, the stimulus lights associated with the drug solutions were reversed and the same comparison repeated. Only data from this second determination were used.

All data analyses are based on performance during the last three sessions of each comparison. Performance on choice trials is expressed in terms of the mean percent of trials in which diethylpropion was selected. Rates of responding during the first sampling period are expressed as responses per minute.

Drug Solutions: Cocaine HCl and diethylpropion HCl were dissolved in physiological saline such that all doses were delivered in a 1 ml volume. Doses refer to the salt of each drug. New drug solutions were prepared at least once every 2 weeks.

Results

Performance during sampling periods. Figure 3 shows mean rate of responding during the first sampling period of all sessions in which 0.5 mg/kg/inj or 1.0 mg/kg/inj diethylpropion was drug A and saline or cocaine was drug B for each animal. For three of the animals response rate maintained by 0.5 mg/kg/inj diethylpropion was higher than that maintained by 1.0 mg/kg/inj diethylpropion. These results are similar to Experiment 1. For animal 3029, however, rate of responding maintained by diethylpropion was directly related to dose.

Performance during choice trials. Figure 4 shows the percent of trials that the two doses of diethylpropion were chosen when compared to saline and increasing doses of cocaine for animal A022. Both doses were preferred to saline on over 75% of the trials, and as the dose of cocaine was increased, preference switched to cocaine. The results for 3029 were similar (Fig. 5). Since in the comparison between 0.025 mg/kg/inj cocaine and saline, responding was not maintained, 0.025 mg/kg/inj cocaine was not a reinforcer in this procedure. Therefore, for 3029 the comparison between this dose and 1.0 mg/kg/inj diethylpropion is functionally equivalent to comparing diethylpropion to saline.

For animal 3042 (Fig. 6), only the higher dose of diethylpropion was preferred to saline on 75% of the trials. Both doses of cocaine were preferred to 0.5 mg/kg/inj diethylpropion on 75% of the trials, but when compared to 1.0 mg/kg/inj diethylpropion, neither

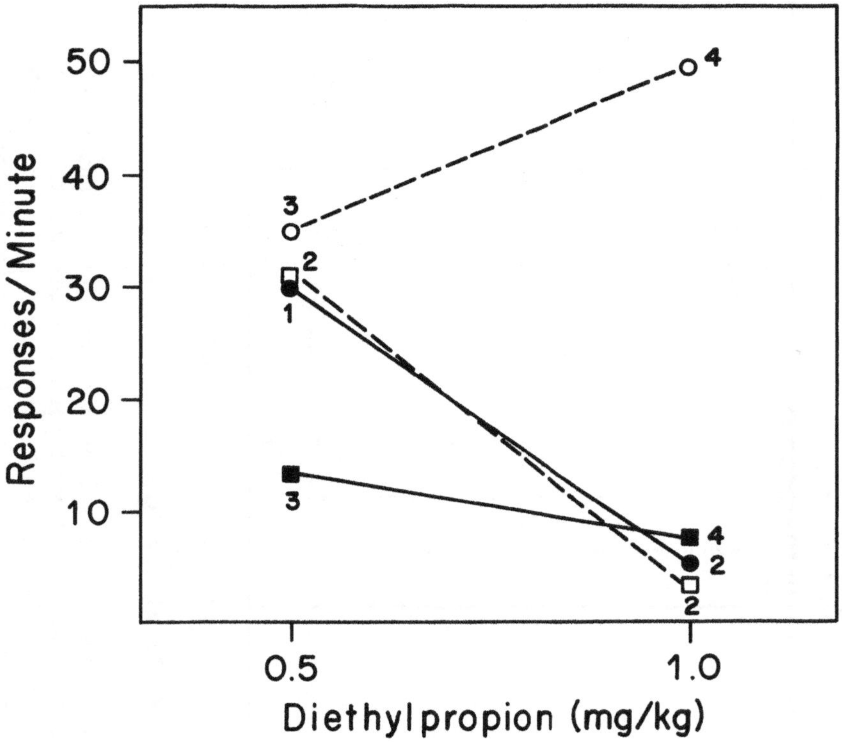

Fig. 3. Mean rates of responding expressed in responses per minute maintained by 0.5 and 1.0 mg/kg/inj diethylpropion during the first sampling period for each animal. The lines in the figure refer to the following animals: 3029 o----o ; 3117 □----□ ; A022 ●——● ; 3043 ■——■ . For every comparison for each animal the mean rate was calculated from data of the last three days of the comparison. The points shown represent the average of these means separately for the two doses. The numbers by the data points indicate the number of means used for each calculation. These numbers are small for A022 because data was not collected during the first part of the experiment for this animal.

cocaine nor diethylpropion was preferred. In a comparison between 0.5 mg/kg cocaine and saline, however, drug was preferred on over 75% of the trials.

For animal 3117 (Fig. 7) the lower dose of diethylpropion was preferred to saline on over 75% of the trials. In the comparisons between 0.1 mg/kg cocaine and both doses of diethylpropion, neither

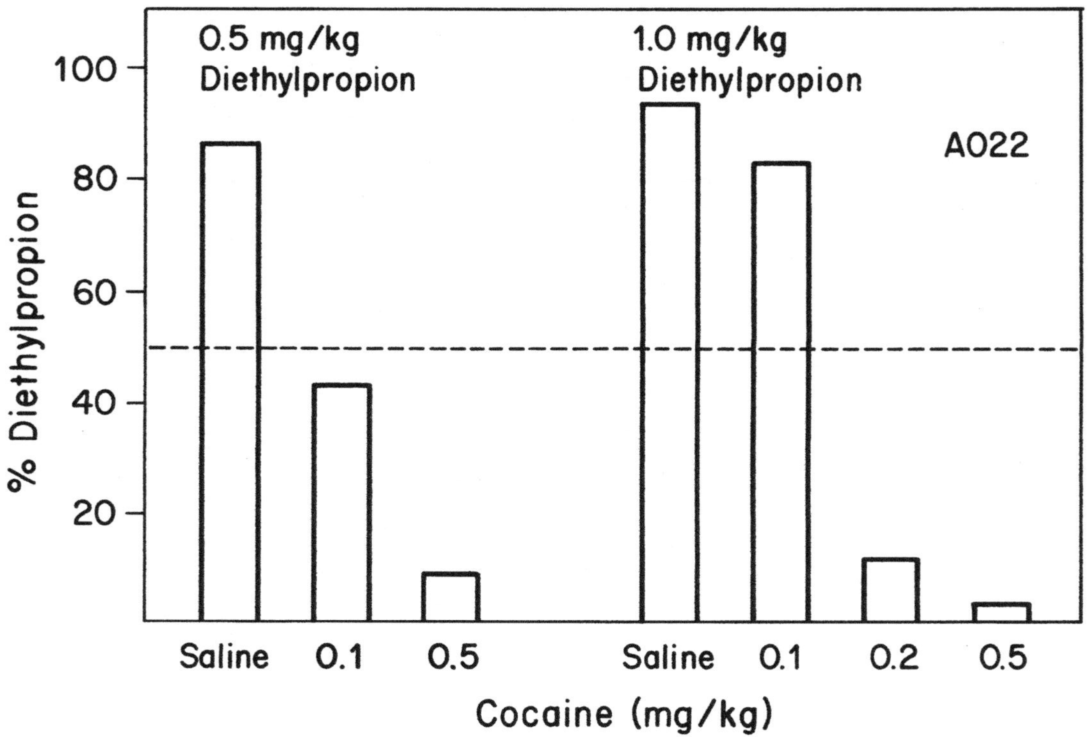

Fig. 4. Mean percent of trials diethylpropion was chosen over saline and cocaine for animal A022. Each column represents the results of a comparison between diethylpropion and the solution indicated below it. The means are calculated from the last three days of each comparison. Columns on the left are for 0.5 mg/kg/inj diethylpropion; those on the right are for 1.0 mg/kg/inj diethylpropion. The dotted line indicates 50% choice.

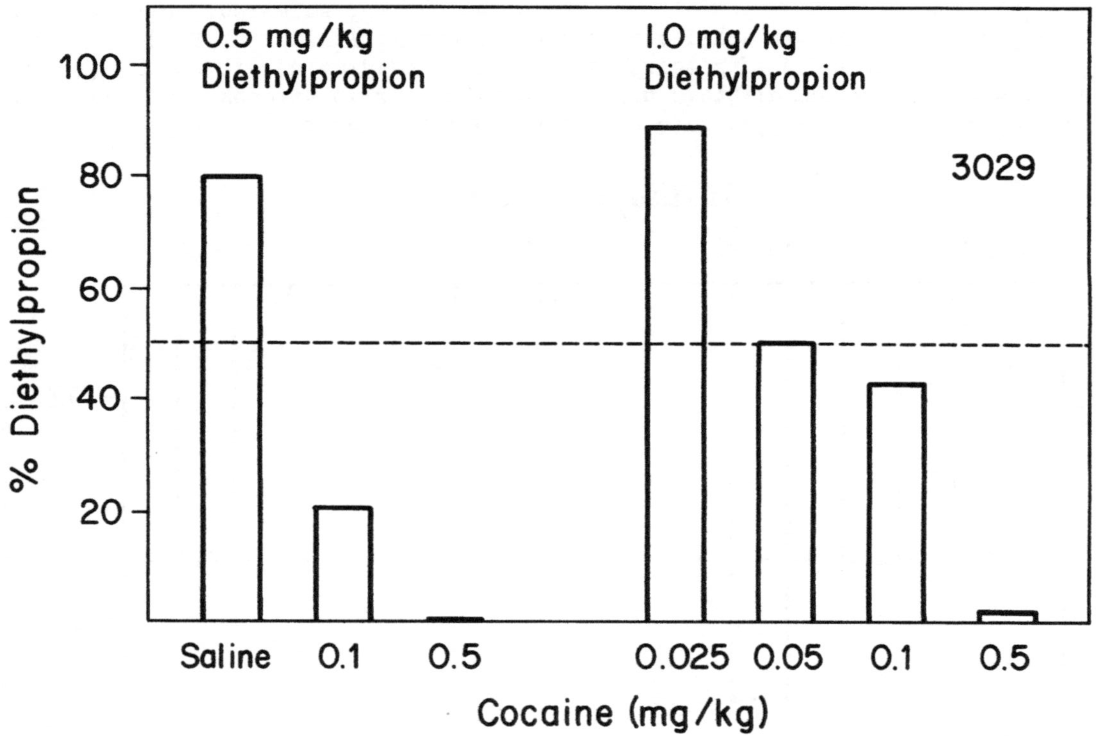

Fig. 5. Mean percent of trials diethylpropion was chosen over saline and cocaine for animal 3029. Each column represents the results of a comparison between diethylpropion and the solution indicated below it. The means are calculated from the last three days of each comparison. Columns on the left are for 0.5 mg/kg/inj diethylpropion; those on the right are for 1.0 mg/kg/inj diethylpropion. The dotted line indicates 50% choice.

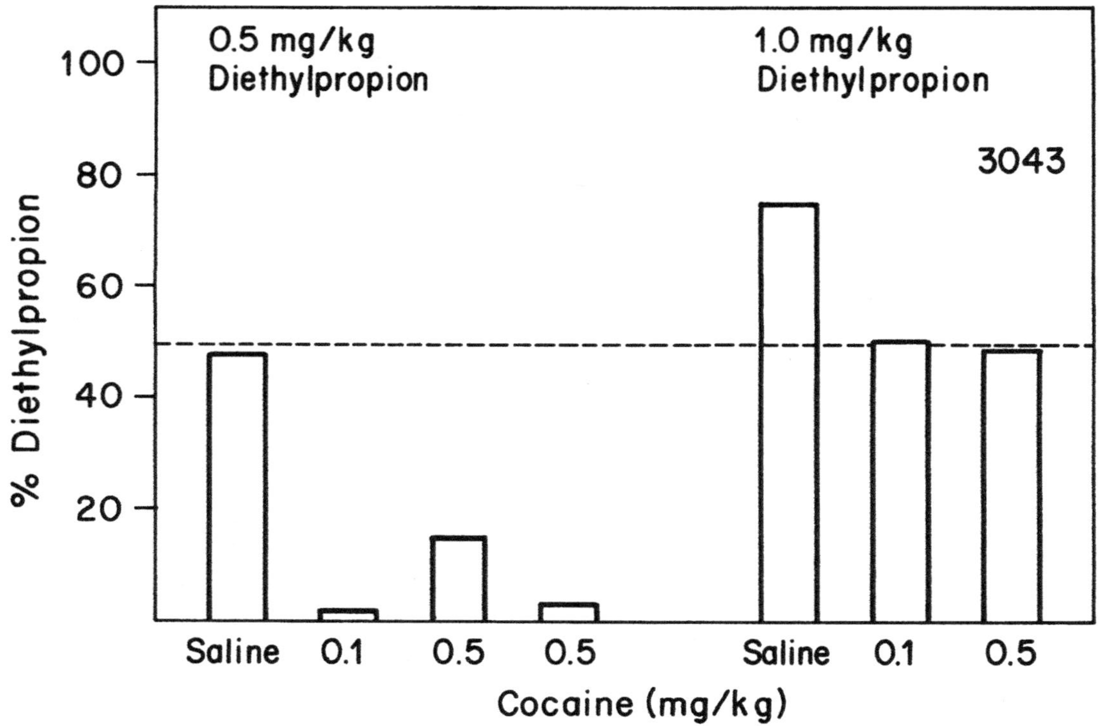

Fig. 6. Mean percent of trials diethylpropion was chosen over saline and cocaine for animal 3043. Each column represents the results of a comparison between diethylpropion and the solution indicated below it. The means are calculated from the last three days of each comparison. Columns on the left are for 0.5 mg/kg/inj diethylpropion; those on the right are for 1.0 mg/kg/inj diethylpropion. The dotted line indicates 50% choice.

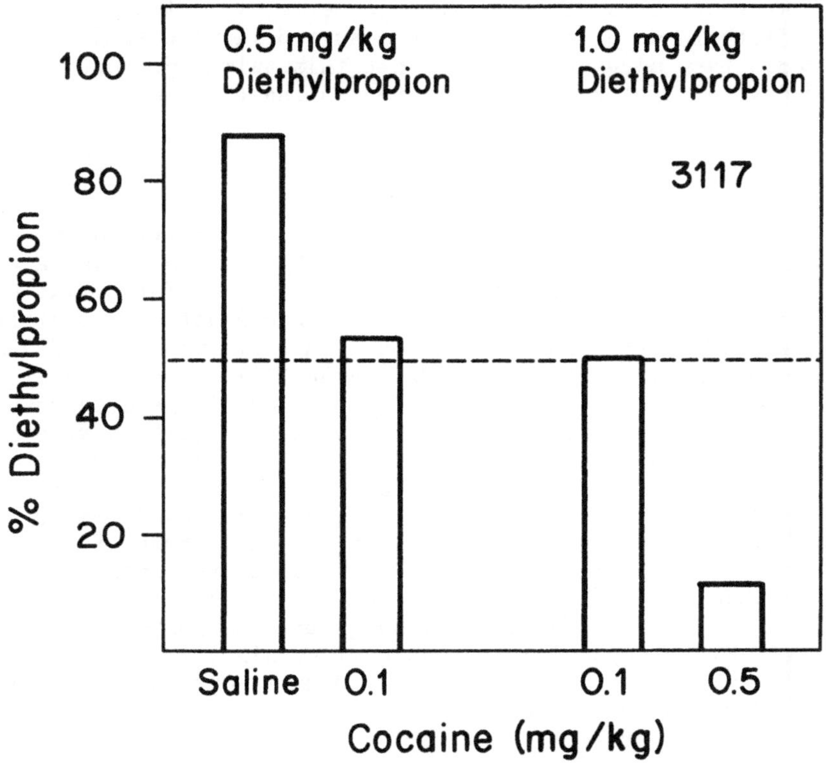

Fig. 7. Mean percent of trials diethylpropion was chosen over saline and cocaine for animal 3117. Each column represents the results of a comparison between diethylpropion and the solution indicated below it. The means are calculated from the last three days of each comparison. Columns on the left are for 0.5 mg/kg/inj diethylpropion; those on the right are for 1.0 mg/kg/inj diethylpropion. The dotted line indicates 50% choice.

drug was preferred. However, in the comparison between 1.0 mg/kg/inj diethylpropion and a higher dose of cocaine (0.5 mg/kg/inj) the latter was preferred on over 75% of the trials.

Two animals (3029 and 3117) preferred 1.0 mg/kg/inj diethylpropion over 0.5 mg/kg/inj diethylpropion on a mean of 90.7 and 81.7% of the trials, respectively. Animal 3043 showed no preference in this comparison. This is surprising since, in the comparisons between diethylpropion and cocaine, increasing the dose of diethylpropion from 0.5 mg/kg to 1.0 mg/kg modified the preference for cocaine. Compared to the low dose of diethylpropion, both 0.1 and 0.5 mg/kg cocaine were preferred on over 75% of the trials. Increasing the dose of diethylpropion to 1.0 mg/kg resulted in neither drug being preferred. Even more puzzling is that this animal did not prefer the low dose of diethylpropion to even saline (Fig. 6).

DISCUSSION

In the first experiment, responding on a fixed-ratio 10 schedule of presentation was maintained by diethylpropion across a wide range of tested doses for all three animals. Therefore, like other psychomotor stimulant drugs, diethylpropion can act as a positive reinforcer. Similar results were found when 0.5 mg/kg/inj diethylpropion was available 23 hours a day on an FR 1 schedule of presentation (Johanson et al., in press). The shape of the dose-response curve in the present study is similar to those generated with other stimulants (Wilson et al., 1971; Balster and Schuster, 1973a). Responding increased as dose was increased at the lower end of the range and then decreased as dose was further increased; daily intake remained relatively constant compared to the magnitude of the increase in dose. Cocaine is more potent than diethylpropion by a factor of 2.5 (0.5 mg/kg diethylpropion generates rates of responding similar to 0.2 mg/kg cocaine). Although this estimate of relative potencies is based upon only one dose of cocaine, it is probably generally accurate since additional studies in our laboratory indicate that the dose-response functions for cocaine and diethylpropion are roughly parallel.

If reinforcing efficacy is related to response rate, lower doses of diethylpropion seemingly are more reinforcing than higher doses. However, this inverse relationship between rate of responding maintained by drugs and dose probably reflects one or more of the drug's other effects on ongoing behavior (Johanson and Schuster, 1975). Since these other effects differ significantly between drugs, there is an inherent difficulty in utilizing rate of self-administration under single schedules for comparing the <u>relative</u> strength of drugs as positive reinforcers.

There is some evidence that the strength of a positive reinforcer can be measured by the rate of decline in responding during extinction, i.e., resistance to extinction (Nevin, 1974). Measuring strength under conditions where drug is not administered clearly avoids some of the problems discussed above (Balster and Schuster, 1976). In the present experiment, extinction responding was measured following both cocaine and various doses of diethylpropion. In general, rate of responding was higher following cocaine. However, rates during extinction did not seem to be related to dose of diethylpropion. If we assume that different doses of a drug differ in their ability to maintain responding; i.e., differ in strength, this result is puzzling. However, the present results may be confounded by repeated exposure to extinction and the unsystematic order of testing doses. Indeed, as shown in Fig. 1, extinction responding gradually decreased over the course of the experiment. Similar results have been found when food was used to maintain behavior (Bullock and Smith, 1953). Therefore, the higher rates of saline self-administration seen following cocaine availability could be due to the fact that this manipulation was performed early in the experiment rather than demonstrating that cocaine has greater reinforcing efficacy.

The second experiment was designed to avoid some of the problems encountered in the first study. Two doses of diethylpropion, 0.5 and 1.0 mg/kg/inj, were compared to saline and several doses of cocaine in a choice procedure. With one exception, both these doses of diethylpropion were reliably preferred to saline. The preference for this drug complements a previous study (Johanson et al., in press) and Experiment 1, which demonstrate that these doses can serve as positive reinforcers for lever-pressing behavior in rhesus monkeys. Preferences for cocaine as well as methylphenidate over saline have also been shown with this procedure (Johanson and Schuster, 1975).

In the comparison between 0.5 and 1.0 mg/kg of diethylpropion, two of the three animals tested preferred the higher dose to the lower dose. Although the exceptional animal is puzzling, these results are similar to those which generally demonstrate that higher doses of a particular stimulant are preferred to lower doses (Johanson and Schuster, 1975).

In the comparisons between diethylpropion and cocaine, cocaine was generally preferred. Although several comparisons resulted in neither drug being preferred, only one animal, A022, at one dose comparison, ever showed a reliable preference for diethylpropion (1.0 mg/kg) rather than cocaine (0.1 mg/kg). It is possible that raising the dose of diethylpropion would result in its being chosen by additional animals. However, rates of responding for doses above 1.0 mg/kg diethylpropion in Experiment 1 were well below saline levels, indicating relatively long rate-disrupting effects. In choice experiments comparing two doses of cocaine the higher of the two doses was usually chosen over the lower except in comparisons between high doses (e.g., 1.5 mg/kg/inj vs 0.5 mg/kg/inj) which generate low rates of responding on an FR schedule (Wilson et al., 1971). In these comparisons, neither cocaine solution was preferred (Johanson and Schuster, 1975). Since this may have been due to the relatively severe rate-disrupting effects of these doses, using higher doses of diethylpropion seemed unwarranted. It seems, then, that with one exception, regardless of the dose, cocaine was preferred to diethylpropion. This is in contrast to comparisons between cocaine and another psychomotor stimulant drug, methylphenidate, where animals prefer the higher dose regardless of the drug (Johanson and Schuster, 1975).

In comparing diethylpropion and cocaine, the differences in the rate of responding (Experiment 1) and choice measures (Experiment 2) are most likely due to the fact that in the choice trials failure to respond *per se* did not influence the evaluation of the reinforcing efficacy of each drug. Further, the time-out period following choice trials allowed the immediate suppressant actions of the injected drug some time to dissipate. Balster and Schuster (1973b) used a 15-minute time-out after each cocaine injection maintaining fixed-interval (FI) responding in order to separate the behavioral suppressant actions from the reinforcing actions of cocaine. Under these conditions, rate of responding was a direct function of dose.

That the schedule alone cannot account for this result is suggested by the fact that Dougherty and Pickens (1973) found an inverse function relating dose and rate of responding using an FI schedule of cocaine reinforcement in rats with no time-out after reinforcement. Iglauer and Woods (1974) used monkeys trained under a concurrent variable-interval, variable-interval schedule of cocaine reinforcement where the dose in each independent variable-interval schedule differed in magnitude and found that the relative rates of responding maintained by these different doses was a direct function of their magnitude. An important feature of the schedule in that study was a 5-minute time-out period after each injection to minimize the interactions of the drug's disrupting and reinforcing effects. Further, the authors conclude that the measure of relative rate was not greatly influenced by the drug's rate-decreasing effects Goldberg (1973), using monkeys trained under a second-order fixed-interval schedule of fixed-ratio components maintained by cocaine injections, found that response rate did not decrease with increments in dose as it did during a single fixed-ratio schedule. One of the common features of these studies is the use of schedules minimizing rate of reinforcement to avoid, at least in part, the interaction of the reinforcing and other behavioral actions of drugs. In addition, in the present study, the use of preference procedures provided measures of reinforcement which were minimally affected by failure to respond *per se*.

The present experiments demonstrate that although all psychomotor stimulant drugs may serve as positive reinforcers, a choice procedure allows one to distinguish between them in terms of their relative reinforcing efficacy. The results obtained with diethylpropion and cocaine in the fixed-ratio and choice procedures are those predicted from epidemiological data; diethylpropion is self-administered only when more highly reinforcing psychomotor stimulant drugs are not available. This concordance of experimental data with actual experience with these drugs in man lends additional credence to the use of choice procedures for evaluating new drugs in the hopes of finding therapeutically efficacious drugs with relatively less dependence potential.

ACKNOWLEDGMENTS

Research supported by National Institutes of Health Grants DA-00047, DA-00250, and MH-11052.

Portions of this work have been presented in: Johanson, C.E.: Pharmacological and environmental variables affecting drug preference in rhesus monkeys, Pharmac. Rev. 27 (in press).

Portions of this paper are based on a dissertation submitted to the Graduate School of The University of Chicago by C.E. Johanson in partial fulfillment of the requirements for the degree of Doctor of Philosophy.

The authors would like to thank Merrell-National Laboratories for their financial support of some aspects of this research and the supply of diethylpropion.

REFERENCES

Balster, R.L. and Schuster, C.R.: A comparison of d-amphetamine, l-amphetamine and methamphetamine self-administration in rhesus monkeys, Pharmac. Biochem. Behav. 1, 67-71 (1973a).

Balster, R.L. and Schuster, C.R.: Fixed interval schedule of cocaine reinforcement: Effect of dose and infusion duration, J. exp. Analysis Behav. 20, 119-129 (1973b).

Balster, R.L. and Schuster, C.R.: A preference procedure which compares efficacy of different intravenous drug reinforcers in the rhesus monkey. In: Cocaine and Other Stimulants. Ellinwood, E.H. and Kilbey, M.M., Eds. New York: Plenum Press, 1976.

Bullock, D.H. and Smith, W.C.: An effect of repeated conditioning-extinction upon operant strength, J. exp. Analysis Behav. 46, 349-352 (1953).

Catania, A.C.: The nature of learning. In: The Study of Behavior: Learning, Motivation, Emotion, and Instinct. Nevin, J.A. and Reynolds, G.S., Eds., pp.30-68. Glenview, Ill.: Scott, Foresman, 1973.

Deneau, G., Yanagita, T., and Seevers, M.H.: Self-administration of psychoactive substances by the monkey. A measure of psychological dependence, Psychopharmacologia 16, 30-48 (1969).

Dews, P.B.: Studies on behavior. I. Differential sensitivity to pentobarbital of pecking performance in pigeons depending. on the schedule of reward, J. Pharmac. exp. Ther. 113, 393-401 (1955).

Dougherty, J. and Pickens, R.: Fixed-interval schedules of intravenous cocaine presentation in rats, J. exp. Analysis Behav. 20, 111-118 (1973).

Ellinwood, E.H. and Duarte-Escalante, O.: Chronic methamphetamine intoxication in three species of experimental animals. In: Current Concepts on Amphetamine Abuse. Ellinwood, E.H., Ed., pp. 59-68. Washington: U.S. Government Printing Office, 1972.

Findley, J.P., Robinson, W.W., and Peregrino, L.: Addiction to secobarbital and chlordiazepoxide in the rhesus monkey by means of a self-infusion preference procedure, Psychopharmacologia 26, 93-114 (1972).

Fischman, M.W. and Schuster, C.R.: Behavioral, biochemical and morphological effects of methamphetamine in the rhesus monkey. In: Behavioral Toxicology. Weiss, B. and Laties, V.G., Eds., pp. 375-399. New York: Plenum Press, 1975.

Goldberg, S.R.: Comparable behavior maintained under fixed-ratio and second-order schedules of food presentation, cocaine injection or d-amphetamine injection in the squirrel monkey, J. Pharmac. exp. Ther. 186, 18-30 (1973).

Griffiths, R.R., Wurster, R.M., and Brady, J.V.: Discrete trial choice procedure: Effects of naloxone and methadone on choice between food and heroin, Pharmac. Rev. 27 (in press).

Iglauer, C., Llewellyn, M.E., and Woods, J.H.: Concurrent schedules of cocaine injection in rhesus monkeys: Dose variations under independent and non-independent variable-interval procedures, Pharmac. Rev. 27 (in press).

Iglauer, C. and Woods, J.H.: Concurrent performances: Reinforcement by different doses of intravenous cocaine in rhesus monkeys, J. exp. Analysis Behav. 22, 179-196 (1974).

Jasinski, D.R., Nutt, J.G., and Griffith, J.D.: Effects of diethylpropion and d-amphetamine after subcutaneous and oral administration, Clin. Pharmac. Ther. 16, 645-652 (1974).

Johanson, C.E.: Choice of cocaine by rhesus monkeys as a function of dosage. In: Proceedings of the 79th Annual Convention. American Psychological Association, pp. 751-752. Washington: American Psychological Association, 1971.

Johanson, C.E.: Pharmacological and environmental variables affecting drug preference in rhesus monkeys, Pharmac. Rev. 27 (in press).

Johanson, C.E., Balster, R.L., and Bonese, K.: Self-administration of psychomotor stimulant drugs: The effects of unlimited access, Pharmac. Biochem. Behav. 4 (in press).

Johanson, C.E. and Schuster, C.R.: A choice procedure for drug reinforcers: Cocaine and methylphenidate in the rhesus monkey, J. Pharmac. exp. Ther. 193, 676-688 (1975).

Jonsson, C.O.: Behavioral studies of deithylpropion in man. In: Abuse of Central Stimulants. Sjoquist, F. and Tottie, M., Eds., pp. 71-80. New York: Raven Press, 1969.

Kelleher, R.T. and Morse, W.H.: Determinants of the specificity of behavioral effects of drugs, Ergebn. Physiol. 60, 1-56 (1968).

Kramer, J.C., Fischman, V.S., and Littlefield, D.C.: Amphetamine abuse, J. Am. Med. Ass. 201, 89-93 (1967).

Morse, W.H. and Kelleher, R.T.: Schedules as fundamental determinants of behavior. In: The Theory of Reinforcement Schedules. Schoenfeld, W.N., Ed., pp. 139-185. New York: Appleton-Century-Crofts, 1970.

Nevin, J.A.: Response strength in multiple schedules, J. exp. Analysis Behav. 21, 389-406 (1974).

Pickens, R. and Thompson, T.: Cocaine-reinforced behavior in rats: Effects of reinforcement magnitude and fixed-ratio size, J. Pharmac. exp. Ther. 161, 122-129 (1968).

Schuster, C.R. and Balster, R.L.: Self-administration of agonists. In: Agonist and Antagonist Actions of Narcotic Analgesic Drugs. Kosterlitz, H.W., Collier, H.O.J., and Villarreal, J.E., Eds., pp. 243-254. London: MacMillan, 1973.

Schuster, C.R. and Johanson, C.E.: The use of animal models for the study of drug abuse. In: Research Advances in Alcohol and Drug Problems. Gibbins, R.J., Israel, Y., Kalant, H., Popham, R.E., Schmidt, W., and Smart, R.G., Eds., pp. 1-31. New York: John Wiley and Sons, 1974.

Schuster, C.R. and Johanson, C.E.: Behavioral analysis of opiate dependence. In: Opiate Addiction: Origins and Treatment. Fisher, S. and Friedman, A.M., Eds., pp. 77-92. Washington: V.H. Winston and Sons, 1973.

Skinner, B.F.: The Behavior of Organisms. New York: Appleton-Century-Crofts, 1938.

Stretch, R., Gerber, G.J., and Woods, J.M.: Factors affecting behavior maintained by response-contingent intravenous infusions of amphetamine in squirrel monkeys, Can. J. Physiol. Pharmac. 49, 581-589 (1971).

Wilson, M.C., Hitomi, M., and Schuster, C.R.: Psychomotor stimulant self-administration as a function of dosage per injection in the rhesus monkey, Psychopharmacologia 22, 271-281 (1971).

A PREFERENCE PROCEDURE THAT COMPARES EFFICACY OF DIFFERENT INTRAVENOUS DRUG REINFORCERS IN THE RHESUS MONKEY

Robert L. Balster and Charles R. Schuster

Departments of Psychiatry and Pharmacological and Physiological Sciences, University of Chicago, Pritzker School of Medicine

A number of animal species, including man, will perform operant responses for intravenous injections of various psychoactive drugs. The comparability between certain aspects of infrahuman drug self-administration and human drug abuse (see Schuster and Thompson, 1969; Schuster and Johanson, 1974 for reviews) has validated the use of laboratory animals as a means of studying elements of human drug-taking behavior under highly controlled conditions. One of the problems with research in this area has been that, in addition to reinforcing behavior which precede them, drug injections can also affect subsequent responding. For example, an injection of cocaine will reinforce the response which produced it but may also increase the likelihood of responding over the next few minutes because cocaine often increases response rates when given noncontingently. An important area of current research concerns the development of new dependent variables that can separate the reinforcing effects of drugs from their other behavioral effects.

One of the aspects of drug self-administration research for which these considerations are crucial concerns the measurement of the efficacy of intravenous drug reinforcers. Many important questions for the laboratory study of drug-taking behavior require a means of evaluating changes in the strength of drug reinforcement as a function of certain behavioral or pharmacological manipulations. Examples of important behavioral variables that might be expected to affect drug reinforcement efficacy are extinction, delay of reinforcement, work requirement, punishment, stress, or the concurrent availability of other reinforcers. Pretreatment with drugs (the same drug as the reinforcer, antagonists of the reinforcer, other drugs of abuse, or modifiers of brain chemistry), tolerance, physical dependence, withdrawal, or structural modifications of the molecule are examples of pharmacological variables whose effects on drug reinforcement efficacy are important to study. A second area in which the evaluation of drug reinforcement efficacy is of interest concerns the evaluation of abuse potential of psychoactive drugs. Since most drugs that are taken recreationally by man are also reinforcers in animals, one could use self-administration studies to predict this for new drugs. In addition to evaluating whether or not a drug possesses the potential for recreational use by man, it would be useful to get a quantitative estimate of the relative extent of this property. Does, for example, the abuse potential of a new anorexic compare to that of cocaine, the amphetamines, diethylpropion or fenfluramine? It has been suggested that a measure of drug reinforcement efficacy in animals would be predictive of the magnitude of this aspect of abuse liability of new drugs (Brady, Griffiths, and Winger, 1975; Schuster and Balster, 1973; Yanagita, 1973).

On first examination, it may seem reasonable that, after a particular behavioral or pharmacological manipulation, if the animal self-administers more injections, one could conclude that the manipulation made the drug more reinforcing. The potential fallacy of this conclusion becomes apparent when we consider the kinds of experimental manipulations that have been shown to increase the rate of self-administration. Lowering the dose per infusion has been shown by a number of investigators to increase the rate of self-administration of opiates (e.g., Hoffmeister and Schlichting, 1972), psychomotor stimulants (e.g., Balster and Schuster, 1973; Wilson, Hitomi, and Schuster, 1971), and pentobarbital (e.g., Goldberg, Hoffmeister, Schlichting, and Wuttke, 1971). In the case of psychomotor stimulants, over a wide dose range, the animals will adjust their response rates as a consequence of changes in dose per infusion to produce relatively constant blood levels of the drug (Yokel and Pickens, 1974). One might, therefore, posit that <u>increased total intake</u> of drug might reflect increased reinforcement efficacy. Goldberg et al. (1971), however, have shown that nalorphine pretreatment has a biphasic effect on rate of morphine self-administration. At low doses of nalorphine, morphine intake <u>increases</u>, and only at high doses does it decrease. Thus, two manipulations that might be expected to decrease reinforcement efficacy (lowering the dose per infusion and pretreatment with an antagonist) can increase rate and total amount of drug self-administration. It is clear that more sophisticated dependent variables that reflect reinforcement efficacy will have to be developed, and research in this area is ongoing in a number of laboratories.

Following the lead of investigators studying reinforcement efficacy with more conventional modalities of reinforcement such as food (Catania, 1963; Neuringer, 1967; Holland and Davison, 1971), choice procedures have been developed that allow for pairwise comparisons of different drug solutions (Findley, Robinson, and Peregrino, 1972; Iglauer and Woods, 1974; Johanson and Schuster, 1975; Brady et al., 1975). Each of these procedures differs substantially and we will not have time to describe each in detail. Some of these procedures will be discussed by other contributors to this conference (Johanson and Schuster; Brady and Griffiths). One thing that characterizes all these methods is that the animals are allowed to choose one of two available drug solutions. In all but one case (Iglauer and Woods, 1974), the choice is exclusive; i.e., the animals can get an infusion of only one of the drug solutions each trial. The intertrial interval ranges from six minutes (Iglauer and Woods, 1974) through 15 minutes (Johanson and Schuster, 1975) to three hours (Brady et al., 1975). The animals have a number of choice trials per day. The dependent variable is usually percent of choices for each drug solution. These procedures have been validated by showing that animals will generally choose high doses over low doses of the same drug and have also been used to make comparisons of different drugs.

One of the factors that may be important for the type of data collected from the use of these procedures concerns the independence of trials. Even with fairly long intertrial intervals of three hours, but especially with shorter intervals, the drug chosen on trial N might be expected to influence choices on trial N + 1 and perhaps subsequent trials due to accumulation and/or drug interactions. This problem is most easily illustrated by considering the situation if one were comparing drugs in the opiate series; for example, an agonist such as morphine with a partial agonist-antagonist such as pentazocine. A pentazocine choice on trial N would undoubtedly result in an antagonism of the pharmacological actions of subsequent morphine choices, especially with relatively short intertrial intervals (6-15 minutes). Under these conditions, the interpretation of choice responding would be hopelessly confounded by drug interactions.

In this paper, we will describe a choice procedure that avoids the difficulties of drug accumulation or drug interaction since choice trials occur during extinction, at a time sufficiently removed from drug administration to allow the drug to be metabolized.

We used this choice procedure to study two comparisons. In one animal, comparisons were made between two sets of doses of cocaine (0.02 mg/kg/inj vs. 0.025 mg/kg/inj and 0.4 mg/kg/inj vs. 0.1 mg/kg/inj); and, in two other animals, two drugs with widely different pharmacological effects and durations of action (cocaine vs. morphine) were compared at one set of doses. This comparison was made to demonstrate the feasibility of this procedure to compare drugs whose interaction would confound the interpretation of choice data. We consider the results of each of these comparisons as preliminary data. Our principal purpose here is to illustrate this choice method.

GENERAL METHODOLOGY

The following studies utilized rhesus monkeys individually housed in 1.3 x 1.3 x 1 m sound-attenuated wooden cubicles that served as the experimental space. Mounted on the door of the cubicle were two response levers 20 cm from the floor and 50 cm apart. Above each lever was a light panel which could be transilluminated by various color stimulus lights. In addition, the ceiling contained a 30 x 30 cm area which could be transilluminated with either a red or white houselight. The cubicles and electromechanical programming equipment were located in separate rooms and masking noise was provided by fans mounted to each cubicle.

Each monkey wore a stainless steel harness (Deneau, Yanagita, and Seevers, 1969) and a spring restraining arm. They were surgically prepared with venous catheters of siliconized rubber. The catheter passed subcutaneously to the animals back where it exited into the harness, through the restraining arm to a peristaltic pump, which could be switched by the experimenter to deliver either of two different drug solutions for any given experimental session. The infusion volume was 0.1 ml/kg delivered over 10 sec.

Choice Procedure Comparing Different Doses of Cocaine

Method. One male rhesus monkey weighing 6.1 kg was housed in a self-administration cubicle as described in the general methodology. Initially, during a daily one-hour session indicated by the illumination of the white houselight, the light panel over one of the levers was illuminated with a white light. Responses on that lever were followed by an injection of 0.1 mg/kg cocaine hydrochloride dissolved in physiological saline. The infusion volume was 0.1 ml/kg and the duration 10 seconds. During the 10-second infusions, the houselight switched from white to red and the light over the lever was turned off. The lever that was indicated as correct by the stimulus light changed randomly after each reinforcement. Responses on the incorrect lever at this point had no consequence.

After four sessions the animal made no incorrect responses and the response requirement on the correct lever was gradually increased to 10 consecutive correct responses (fixed ratio; FR10). Incorrect responses reset the FR requirement. The correct lever changed randomly after each completed FR as before. After the animal stabilized on FR10, the conditions were again changed such that not every completed FR was followed by a cocaine infusion, although the houselight changed from white to red for 10 seconds and the light over the lever terminated as before. An average of every five (variable ratio, VR5) completed FR's was followed by a cocaine infusion. Thus, the terminal schedule of reinforcement was a second-order VR5 (FR10).

The animal was given seven sessions of training on this schedule before discrimination training was begun. During discrimination training, the animal worked for one of two doses of cocaine each session in a random sequence. Each dose was paired with a different color stimulus light. On days when the animal was reinforced with 0.2 mg/kg/inj cocaine, a yellow light was illuminated over the correct lever. On days when the animal was reinforced with 0.025 mg/kg inj cocaine, a blue light was illuminated. The first test for preference was programmed after 30 sampling sessions, 15 with each dose-stimulus color pairing. The preference test consisted of a one-hour session during which the VR5 schedule of drug reinforcement was changed to extinction. When the session began, both levers were operative, with a blue stimulus light over one lever and a yellow stimulus light over the other lever. The FR10 portion of the schedule was retained and still produced a stimulus change in the houselights, following which the stimulus colors over the levers were randomly changed. Responses on each lever reset the FR on the other lever. The animal's preference was indicated by the number of completed FR's associated with each stimulus color.

Following the first preference test session, the drug-stimulus color pairing was reversed and the animals were retrained. Three tests for discrimination reversal were given with 20 sampling sessions between each. The entire procedure is summarized in Table 1.

After these tests were completed, two different stimulus colors were used to compare 0.4 and 0.1 mg/kg/inj cocaine. A red stimulus light was paired with the low dose and a green light with the high dose. Again, 30 sampling sessions were given before the first preference test, followed by a discrimination reversal. Two tests for reversal were programmed, each preceded by 20 sampling sessions.

Results. The results of the choice tests are presented in Fig. 1. The one-hour test session was divided into four 15 min blocks and the number of completed FR's associated with each stimulus color are shown. The FR's completed on lever 1 are represented by the dark portion of the bar, and the FR's completed on lever 2 by the open portion of the bars. The bars in Column A indicate high dose choices and in Column B low dose choices.

It can be seen that in spite of a strong lever 2 preference (more FR's completed on lever 2 regardless of stimulus color), this animal completed more FR's on the lever illuminated by the stimulus color that had been paired with the higher dose during training.

Table 1. Summary of Experimental Procedure

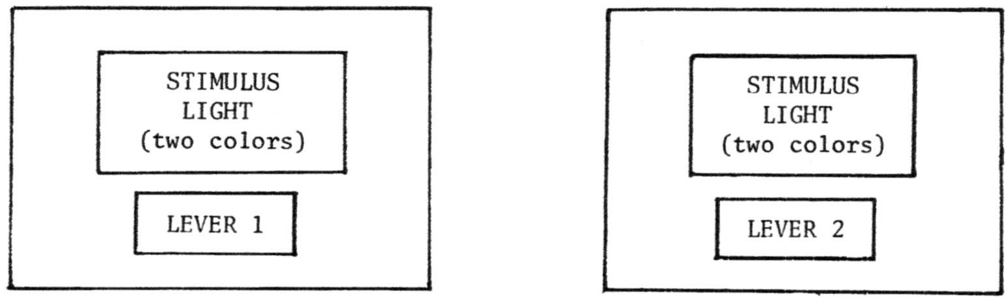

SAMPLING SESSIONS
- -Duration one hour
- -Reinforcement by only one drug solution each session
- -Correct lever indicated by illumination of drug associated stimulus light above lever
- -Correct lever switches randomly after the completion of 10 consecutive correct responses - fixed-ratio (FR) 10
- -Incorrect responses reset the FR requirement on the correct lever
- -Drug infusions after an average of 5 completed FR's - variable ratio (VR) 5

CHOICE SESSIONS
- -Duration one hour, drug infusions withheld for the entire session - extinction
- -Both levers correct with different color stimulus light over each lever
- -Stimulus lights switch randomly after the completion of each FR10
- -Responses on each lever reset the FR requirement on the other lever
- -Animal's preference indicated by number of completed FR's associated with each stimulus color

DISCRIMINATION REVERSAL
- -Light color associated with each drug solution switched to other drug solution for sampling sessions

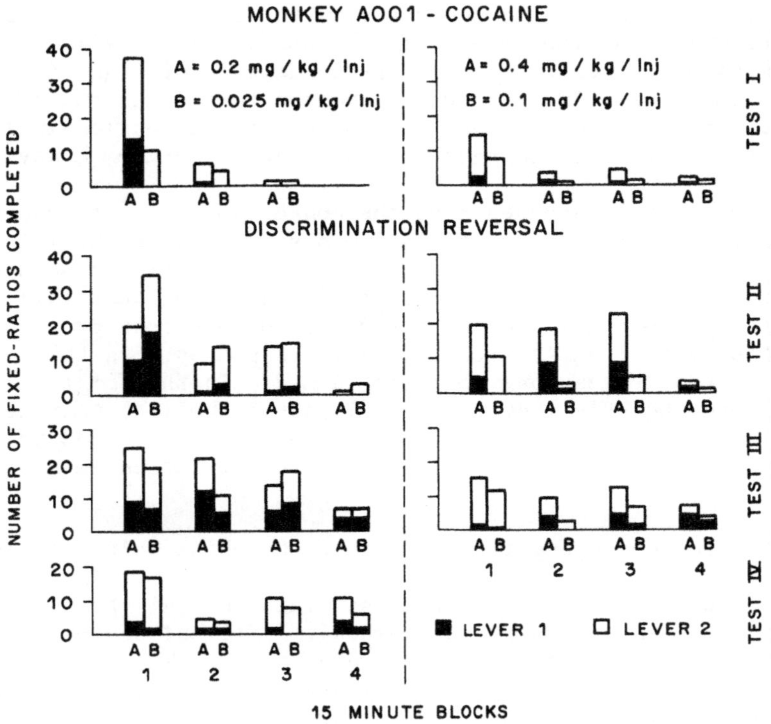

Fig. 1. Number of fixed-ratios completed associated with stimulus lights paired with a high dose (A) and a low dose (B) of cocaine during sampling sessions.

The binomial probability of at least 47 high dose choices out of 64 is significant ($z = 3.6$; $p \leq 0.0001$). The animal's lever 2 preference made the discrimination reversal difficult to attain and never quite reached significance ($z = 1.43$; $p \leq 0.08$ on Test IV).

When the light colors were changed and the animal was retrained with two other doses of cocaine (0.4 vs. 0.1 mg/kg/inj), he again chose the light associated with the high dose ($z = 1.97$; $p \leq 0.02$). In this case the discrimination reversal was obtained within 20 sessions ($z = 4.83$; $p \leq 0.00003$).

Since the animal was not reinforced with drug injections during the one-hour test session, the rate of responding decreased over the course of the session. This can be seen by comparing successive 15-minute blocks for each of the test sessions illustrated in Fig. 1. There was no consistent tendency for the animal to switch from light A choices to light B choices over the course of the test session. We were concerned that light A choices might extinguish early in the session (since there was a preponderance of light A choices at this time) resulting in light B choices toward the end of the session. This was the reason for looking at the session in 15-minute segments. This tendency did not seem to occur, however.

We were also concerned that the monkey would cease responding over the course of a number of choice sessions since the illumination of both lever lights always indicated extinction sessions. The purpose of using a second order schedule was to prevent this as much as possible by providing conditioned reinforcers (change in house-lights and lever lights) after every 10 responses. In this experiment eight choice sessions were programmed. In the first, the animal completed 64 FR's (640 responses) and in the last test session he completed 77 (770 responses). Therefore, there was no tendency for responding to decrease over successive extinction sessions.

Choice Procedure Comparing Cocaine to Morphine Reinforcement

In order to further test the usefulness of this procedure, two drugs, cocaine and morphine, of markedly different pharmacological activities and durations of action were tested. The choice of cocaine and morphine for comparison illustrates to the extreme the necessity of obtaining drug-free comparisons.

The major difficulty in comparing two different compounds is, of course, the choice of doses for comparison. There are at least four alternatives to the solution of this problem. When two drugs with similar durations of action and pharmacological activities, in addition to similar chemical structure, are compared, one can simply obtain preference data for equimolar doses. An example would be the comparison of the reinforcement efficacy of heroin, morphine, and codeine. However, the choice of dose for comparison of any of these compounds with other analgesics, such as etonitazine and dextropropoxyphene, with diverse pharmacological properties and chemical structures is more difficult.

A second alternative is to obtain dose-response curves for both drugs, comparing a wide range of dosages of both compounds. Obtaining dose-response curves for both drugs is very time-consuming. A third alternative, related to the second, is to select a single dosage of Drug A to use as a standard against which to compare different dosages of the test compound, Drug B.

A fourth alternative is to empirically equate dosages of each drug by comparing them in other experimental procedures. For example, equianorexic doses of stimulants might be compared for preference. Alternatively, doses might be chosen on their ability to disrupt operant-responding in experimental animals. A variation of this latter alternative was used in the present study. Dosages of cocaine and morphine were chosen on their ability to maintain equal rates of self-administration during the sampling sessions. Unit doses of 200 µg/kg of cocaine and 25 µg/kg of morphine resulted in each one-hour session.

Method. The subjects were one female (A018) and one male (A058) rhesus monkey, each weighing 4.0 kg. They were housed in experimental cubicles as described in the general methodology. They were trained on the FR10 schedule of reinforcement as in the cocaine dose experiment using 100 µg/kg/inj cocaine hydrochloride. At this point discrimination training began, using a dose of 200 µg/kg/inj

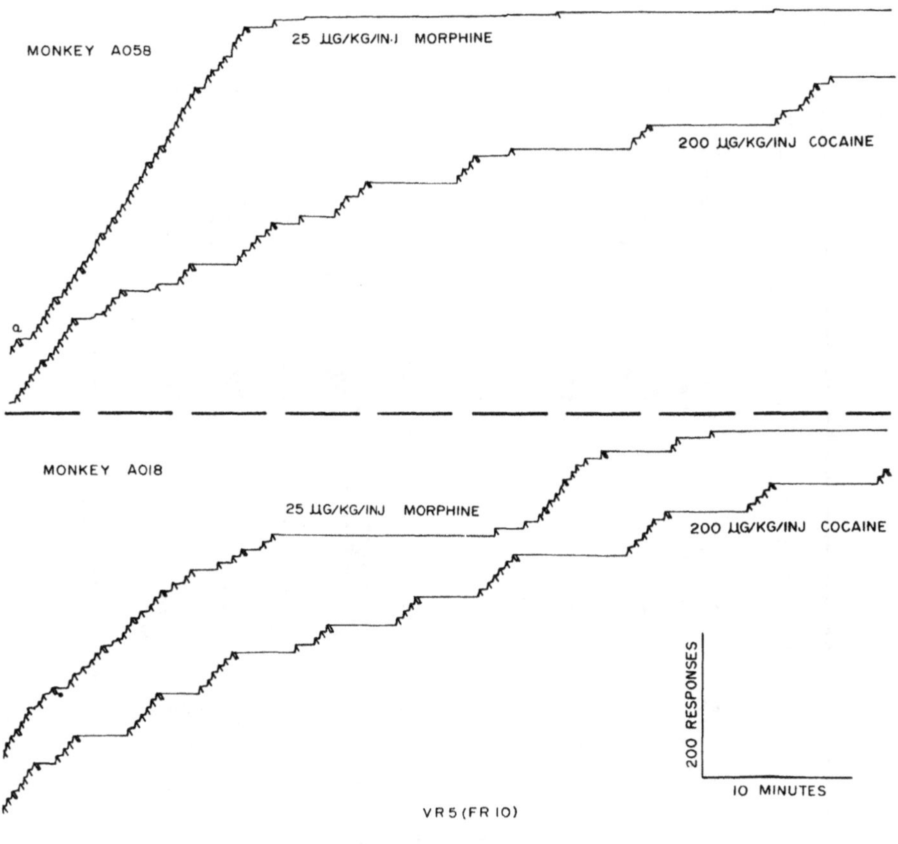

Fig. 2. Representative cumulative records for two animals during sampling sessions for cocaine and morphine reinforcement. Correct responses are recorded cumulatively. Completed fixed-ratios are indicated by a brief downward pen deflection. During infusions the pen stays down for the duration of the injection (a).

cocaine paired with one color stimulus light and 25 µg/kg/inj morphine sulfate paired with a different stimulus light. The VR5 portion of the terminal schedule was added on the first sampling session. Discrimination training was continued for 30 sessions, 15 with each drug-stimulus color pairing in a random sequence. After the preference test, the drug-stimulus color pairing was reversed and test sessions were programmed between every 20 sampling sessions.

Results. Figure 2 shows representative cumulative records for sampling sessions for both animals. These doses of cocaine and morphine result in about 45 completed FR's per session and nine drug injections. Although the overall rates are the same for both drugs, the patterns are clearly different. In the case of cocaine, with the exception of the first two or three injections, the animals

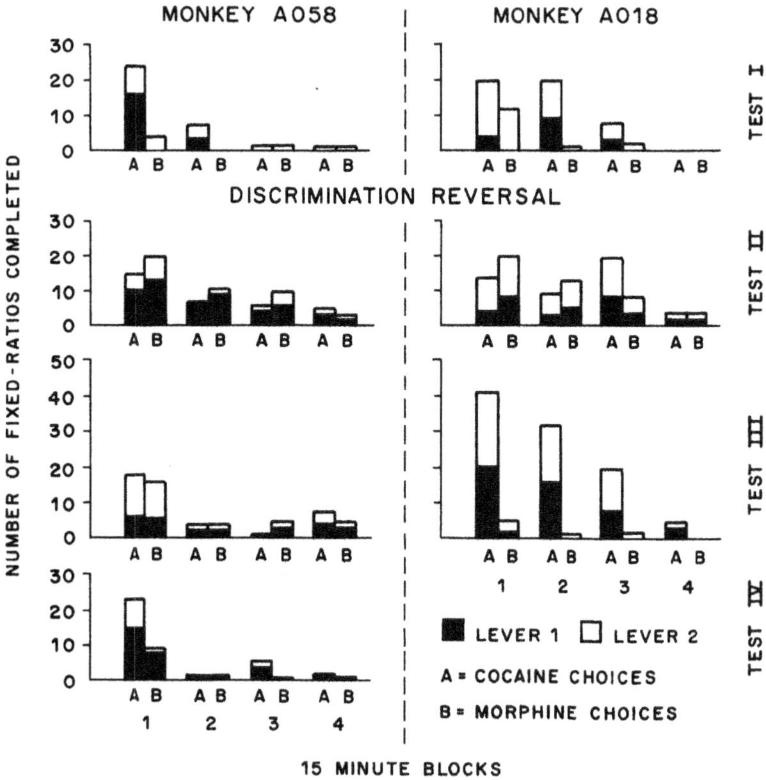

Fig. 3. Number of fixed-ratios completed associated with stimulus lights paired with 200 µg/kg/inj cocaine (A) and 25 µg/kg/inj morphine (B) during sampling sessions.

space their responses over the entire session. Most of the morphine, however, is self-administered in the first 20 minutes of the session. This points out clearly the difficulty of using an empirical means of equating drug dosage. As Fig. 2 shows, if we had chosen 30 minutes instead of one hour for the duration of the session, different dosages would have been used for comparison. However, any pharmacological potency which might serve as a means of equating drug dosage is also highly dependent upon the specific conditions under which the measures are obtained (Thompson and Schuster, 1968).

Figure 3 presents the results of the choice tests following training and discrimination reversal for both animals. Animal A058 showed a strong lever 1 preference and animal A018 a lever 2 preference. Nevertheless, both animals showed a reliable preference for cocaine over morphine at these unit doses. Monkey A058 made 34 cocaine choices out of 39 ($z = 4.48$; $p \leq 0.00003$) and monkey A018 made 48 cocaine choices out of 63 ($z = 4.03$; $p \leq 0.00003$) on the first test session. Monkey A058 required 60 sessions to demonstrate a reversal ($z = 2.62$; $p \leq 0.004$ for Test IV), whereas monkey A018 made significantly more cocaine choices in Test IV: 40 sampling sessions after the discrimination reversal ($z = 8.6$; $p \leq 0.00003$).

GENERAL DISCUSSION

As we stated at the outset, the principle purpose of this paper was to illustrate a choice procedure that allows for experimental animals to indicate drug preferences in the absence of either drug accumulation or drug interactions. This procedure, like others, has advantages and limitations.

Although the data we have collected is limited, we feel that the usefulness and validity of this procedure has been demonstrated. The observation that higher doses of cocaine were preferred over lower ones confirms results obtained in other choice procedures (Iglauer and Woods, 1975; Johanson and Schuster, 1975). In the animal we tested, preferences were always shown on Test I, after 30 sampling sessions, 15 with each dose. It might have been possible to demonstrate preferences after fewer sampling sessions, but we did not test at earlier times. The number of sessions required to make dosage comparisons in the present study is somewhat more than that required for other procedures in which doses of cocaine of comparable magnitude difference were studied (Iglauer and Woods, 1975; Johanson and Schuster, 1975). On the other hand, the session duration each day is substantially less.

Perhaps one of the major limitations of this procedure is that animals would be expected to eventually cease responding on test days since they have a stimulus (both lever lights on instead of just one) that is consistently correlated with extinction conditions. We saw no evidence for fewer test responses over eight test sessions (each separated by at least 20 sampling sessions) in the animal used to compare cocaine doses, nor was there any evidence for this in the two animals in the cocaine vs. morphine experiment over the three or four test sessions which they had. Nevertheless, with further testing extinction should take place. Additional research using this technique will be necessary to determine how many dosage comparisons can be obtained with each subject.

ACKNOWLEDGMENTS

This research was supported by NIH Grants MH-18,245 and MH-11, 042 to C.R.S. and was carried out while the first author was a post-doctoral fellow supported by NIH Training Grant MH-07,083.

The present address of Dr. Robert Balster is: Pharmacology Department, Medical College of Virginia, Virginia Commonwealth University, Richmond, Virginia.

REFERENCES

Balster, R.L. and Schuster, C.R.: A comparison of d-amphetamine, l-amphetamine, and methamphetamine self-administration in the rhesus monkey. Pharmac. Biochem. Behav. 1, 67-71 (1973).

Brady, J.V., Griffiths, R., and Winger, G.: Drug-maintained performance procedures and the evaluation of sedative hypnotic dependency potential. In: Hypnotics: Methods of Development and Evaluation. Kagan, F., Harwood, T., Rickels, K., Rudzik, A.D., and Sorer, H., Eds., pp. 221-235. Holliswood, New York: Spectrum Publications, Inc., 1975.

Catania, A.C.: Concurrent performances: A baseline for the study of reinforcement magnitude. J. exp. Analysis Behav. 6, 299-300 (1963).

Deneau, G., Yanagita, T., and Seevers, M.H.: Self-administration of psychoactive substances by the monkey: A measure of psychological dependence. Psychopharmacologia 16, 30-48 (1969).

Findley, J.P., Robinson, W.W., and Peregrino, L.: Addiction to secobarbital and chlordiazepoxide in the rhesus monkey by means of a self-infusion preference procedure. Psychopharmacologia 26, 93-114 (1972).

Goldberg, S.R., Hoffmeister, F., Schlicting, U.U., and Wuttke, W.: A comparison of pentobarbital and cocaine self-administration in rhesus monkeys: Effects of dose and fixed-ratio parameter. J. Pharmac. exp. Ther. 179, 277-283 (1971).

Hoffmeister, F. and Schlicting, U.U.: Reinforcing properties of some opiates and opioids in rhesus monkeys with histories of cocaine and codeine self-administration. Psychopharmacologia 23, 55-74 (1972).

Hollard, V. and Davison, M.C.: Preference for qualitatively different reinforcers. J. exp. Analysis Behav. 16, 375-380 (1971).

Iglauer, C. and Woods, J.H.: Concurrent performances: Reinforcement by different doses of intravenous cocaine in rhesus monkeys. J. exp. Analysis Behav. 22, 179-196 (1974).

Johanson, C.E. and Schuster, C.R.: A choice procedure for drug reinforcers: Cocaine and methylphenidate in the rhesus monkey. J. Pharmac. exp. Ther. 193, 676-687 (1975).

Neuringer, A.J.: Effects of reinforcement magnitude on choice and rate of responding. J. exp. Analysis Behav. 10, 417-424 (1967).

Schuster, C.R. and Balster, R.L.: Self-administration of agonists. In: Agonist and Antagonist Action of Narcotic Analgesic Drugs. Kosterlitz, H.W., Collier, H.O.J., and Villarreal, J.E., Eds., pp. 243-254. London: MacMillan, 1973.

Schuster, C.R. and Johanson, C.E.: The use of animal models for the study of drug abuse. In: Research Advances in Alcohol and Drug Problems. Gibbons, R.J., Israel, Y., Kalant, H., Popham, R.E., Schmidt, W., and Smart, R.G., Eds., Vol. 1, pp. 1-31. New York: John Wiley, 1974.

Schuster, C.R. and Thompson, T.: Self-administration of and behavioral dependence on drugs. Ann. Rev. Pharmacol. 9, 483-502 (1969).

Thompson, T. and Schuster, C.R.: Behavioral Pharmacology. Englewood Cliffs, N.J.: Prentice-Hall, 1968.

Yanagita, T.: An experimental framework for evaluation of dependence liability of various types of drugs in monkeys. Bull. Narcotics 25, 7-17 (1973).

Yokel, R.A. and Pickens, R.: Drug level of d- and l-amphetamine during intravenous self-administration. Psychopharmacologia 34, 255-264 (1974).

Wilson, M.C., Hitomi, M., and Schuster, C.R.: Psychomotor stimulant self-administration as a function of dosage in the rhesus monkey. Psychopharmacologia 22, 271-281 (1971).

THE EFFECTS OF RESPONSE CONTINGENT AND NON-CONTINGENT SHOCK ON DRUG SELF-ADMINISTRATION IN RHESUS MONKEYS

David M. McLendon and Robert T. Harris

Department of Physiology, Baylor College of Medicine, Houston, Texas

Suppression of ongoing positively reinforced behavior by the presentation of aversive stimuli has been reported in some cases while facilitation of such behavior has been noted in other instances. A major variable in these studies is the contingency of the aversive stimulus upon the response of the animal. The majority of these investigations have been concerned with the effects of aversive stimuli on food reinforced responding. Azrin (1956) found that response contingent punishment had a greater effect on responding than did shock delivered on a non-contingent basis. Hunt and Brady (1955) also demonstrated the importance of response contingency in a punishment situation. These investigations reported greater suppression of the punished response when the punishment was response contingent. In a review of the area, Church (1963) concluded that if the aversive stimulus is contingent upon the response of the animal, greater suppression, or less facilitation, will occur than if the shock is not contingent upon the response. Facilitation of responding has been found to occur under certain conditions. Holz and Azrin (1962) found that punishment can facilitate responding under conditions where low intensity punishment has been correlated with positive reinforcement.

The effects of shock on operant responding maintained by drug reinforcers also have been reported. In man, punishment by electric shock has been found to suppress alcohol drinking (Millo, Sobell, and Schaefer, 1971) and cigarette smoking (Powell and Azrin, 1968). Grove and Schuster (1974) found cocaine self-administration in rhesus monkeys to be suppressed by punishment as a function of shock intensity. However, the suppressant effects of the shock were attenuated by increasing delays in the response-shock interval. Smith and

Davis (1974) also found suppression of amphetamine and morphine self-administration in rats by response contingent shock.

Although responding for cocaine and morphine has been found to be suppressed by response contingent shock, it has not been established that responding for all drugs that function as reinforcers in monkeys is suppressed in the same manner or if the degree of suppression can be considered as a measure of relative reinforcing strength. To test this, Experiment I of this investigation compared the effects of three intensities of response-contingent shock (punishment) on responding for intravenous infusions of cocaine, morphine, and pentobarbital in rhesus monkeys. Experiment II was concerned with the same comparisons except that in this condition, the shock was non-contingent upon the response of the animal.

METHODS

Eight male rhesus monkeys weighing between 4 and 6kg were used as subjects. Four of the animals had been used previously in other drug self-administration studies and four were naive. No animal had previous shock experience. The monkeys were divided into two groups of four with two naive animals in each group. Using the method of Deneau, Yanagita, and Seevers (1969), each was fitted with a tubular stainless steel harness and a hollow, flexible restraining arm. Each was housed individually with ad lib access to water. Animals were fed once daily in the evening.

After adaptation, the animals were surgically prepared under sodium pentobarbital anesthesia with a chronic indwelling Silastic catheter implanted into the jugular or femoral vein. The catheter exited from the animal through an interscapular stab wound. The catheter passed out the restraining arm where it connected to a Cole-Parmer peristatic infusion pump. Electrodes consisted of two stainless steel wire loops affixed to the animal's back inside the harness. The manipulanda consisted of a panel which replaced the door of the cage and contained one microswitch lever and one jeweled light. The onset of the light signaled the beginning of the drug access period which lasted four hours each day. Animals ran seven days a week. Drug infusions were contingent upon an FR-1 response by the animal in all cases and consisted of a 10-second, 0.5ml infusion of the drug. Cocaine and pentobarbital unit doses were 200 μg/kg/infusion and morphine was 75μg/kg/infusion. In an effort to maintain relatively comparable daily response rates across drugs for each animal, pentobarbital and morphine doses were adjusted for two animals to alter their response rate.

To control for order effects, each of the four animals in each group was presented the three drugs in a different order. Generally, each animal was allowed to self-administer the drug for 15 to 20 days before the beginning of the shock even though stable response rates were attained much earlier in some cases. Shocks were administered in an ascending order with intensities at 4ma, 8ma, and 10ma for a duration of 500msec. Each monkey was exposed to each intensity level for at least seven days or until a stable rate of responding was achieved. In no case was this more than 12 days. Stability was defined as ± 15% variation in infusion rate over a three day period. This of course could not be achieved at low response rates of 3-4 infusions/day and suppression to these levels was accepted as stability. The animal was transferred directly from one intensity level to the next. The animals in Experiment I received one shock with each third infusion while the animals in Experiment II received one shock every 10 minutes regardless of responding. Using this procedure, the animals in each condition would receive approximately the same number of shocks had they continued to self-administer at their baseline rates under the shock conditions.

The experimental conditions were programmed with silent solid state equipment housed in the experimental room. Responses were recorded on digital counters and cumulative recorders. Shock was delivered from a constant current shock source (BRS/LVE SG-903). Electrode resistance at the shock source varied between 30k and 50k ohms.

RESULTS

The results are presented individually for each monkey. Figure 1 shows the results for monkey 6367 of Experiment I. The effects of the response contingent shock are presented in three separate bar graphs, one for each drug. The number of infusions self-administered over the four-hour access period is plotted on the vertical axis. The levels plotted in all cases represent stable performance. In some cases, responding would drop to near zero levels upon the introduction of the shock or when the shock level was increased, and then rise on the following days. In these cases, the graphs represent the level of stable responding over at least a three-day period and do not reflect the transient suppression of responding. For animal 6367, it can be seen that all levels of shock suppressed responding for all three drugs. For pentobarbital, the 4ma shock resulted in suppression to 27% of baseline performance with suppression increasing to 2% of baseline at 10ma. At this intensity the monkey would make 2-3 responses, sometimes receiving one shock. No responses occurred on some days. With removal of the shock, infusions returned to 91% of baseline levels. In cases such as this, where responding was completely suppressed, the removal of the shock was not discriminable to the animal, so re-shaping the animal was

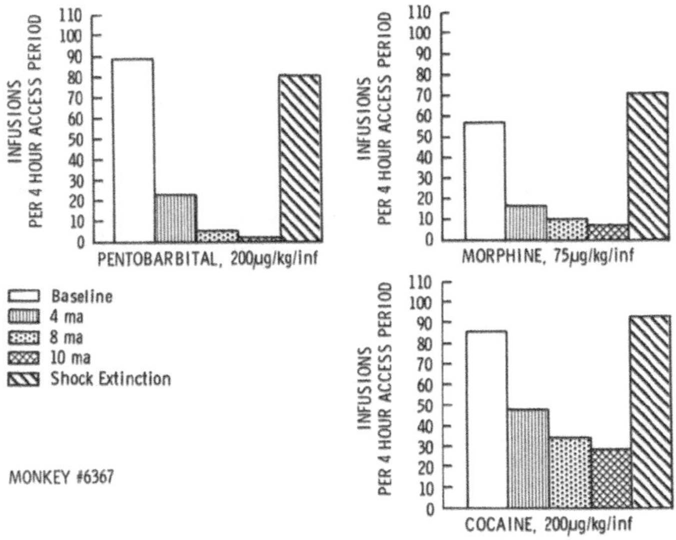

Fig. 1. Effects of response contingent shock on drug self-administration.

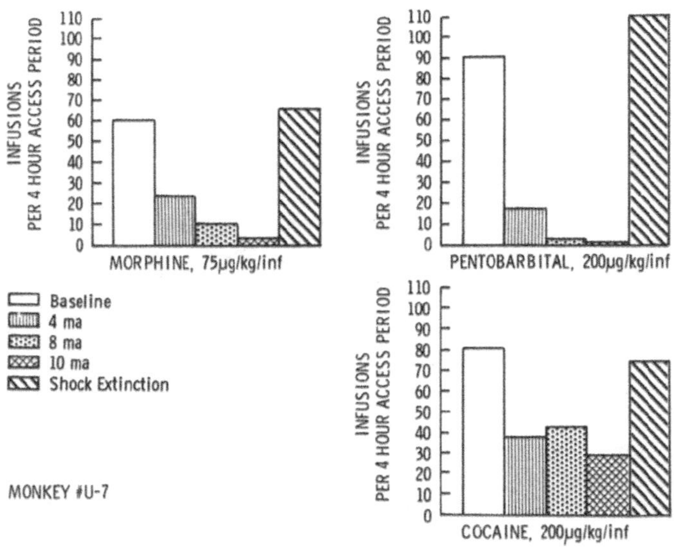

Fig. 2. Effects of response contingent shock on drug self-administration.

necessary. A similar suppression of responding can be seen for morphine self-administration. Suppression at 4ma was to 29% of baseline levels. Response suppression increased with increasing shock intensity to 12% of baseline at 10ma. Cocaine suppression was also directly related to shock intensity, but the degree of suppression was not as great as with morphine or pentobarbital. At 4ma, cocaine suppression was to 56% of baseline level. At 10ma, suppression was to 34% of baseline.

Figure 2 shows that for monkey U-7, the effect of shock on morphine and pentobarbital self-administration was suppression that increased with shock intensity. Almost complete suppression of responding occurred at 10ma for both drugs. At 4ma, morphine suppression was to 42% of baseline levels and pentobarbital was to 20% of baseline. Responding for cocaine was suppressed to 46% of baseline at 4ma, to 55% at 8ma, and to 35% of baseline at 10ma. Although the degree of suppression appeared to be related to shock intensity, the relationship was not linear. Again, cocaine self-administration was suppressed less than was responding for morphine or pentobarbital.

Figure 3 shows the data for monkey 5931. In this case, pentobarbital responding was almost completely suppressed at all three shock intensities. Because of the degree of suppression, the animal required re-shaping after the removal of the shock. For cocaine self-administration, suppression was inversely related to shock intensity. The animal responded at 35% of his baseline level at 4ma and at 55% at 10ma. Suppression of morphine self-administration increased with the intensity of the shock with suppression to 35% of baseline levels at 4ma and to 10% at 10ma.

Figure 4 shows the data for the last animal in this group. Again, response suppression was greater for morphine and pentobarbital than for cocaine. For cocaine, at 4ma, responding was suppressed to 47% of baseline levels. At 8ma, suppression was to 41% of baseline, and 10ma to 24%. With pentobarbital, responding was suppressed to 7% of baseline levels at 4ma, and almost total suppression occurred at 8 and 10ma. On many days at these intensities, the animal made no response for pentobarbital and generally received no shocks after receiving one or two on the first days at the higher intensities. Morphine responding was suppressed to 17% of baseline at 4ma with almost complete suppression at 8 and 10ma.

The data for Experiment I indicate that all intensities of shock suppressed responding for all three drugs. However, in each case, cocaine responding was suppressed less than responding for morphine or pentobarbital. When the data for these four animals were combined, the mean percentage of baseline responding for pentobarbital was 14% at 4ma, 4% at 8ma, and 2% at 10ma. Morphine was 31% at 4ma, 13% at 8ma, and 8% at 10ma. For cocaine,

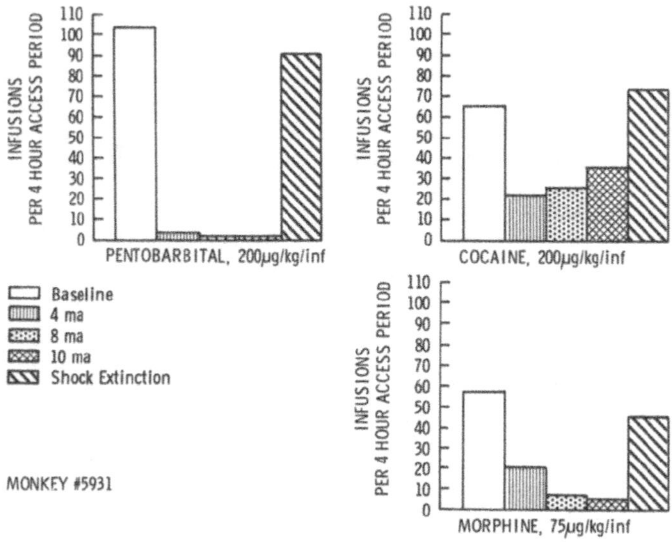

Fig. 3. Effects of response contingent shock on drug self-administration.

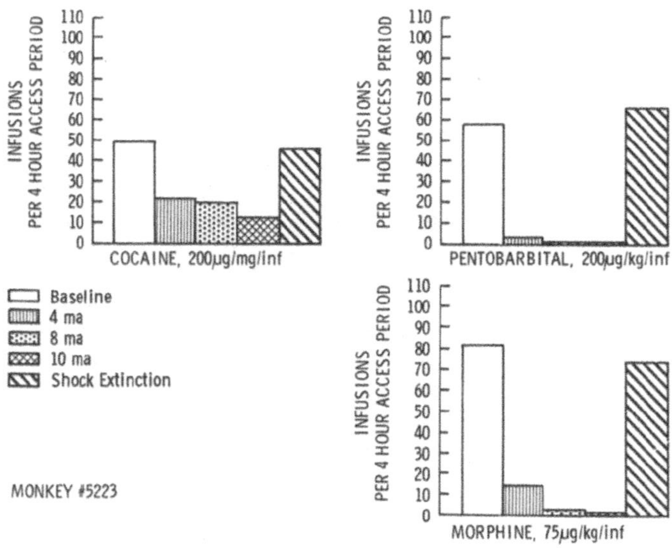

Fig. 4. Effects of response contingent shock on drug self-administration.

suppression was 46% at 4ma, 44% at 8ma, and 37% of baseline at 10ma. With each animal, suppression of pentobarbital and morphine self-administration increased with shock intensity. This relationship was also observed for cocaine for two of the monkeys. Responding for cocaine was inversely related to shock intensity for one animal and, in another animal, varied with shock as an inverted-U function. No clear order effects were observed in this experiment.

Experiment II consisted of self-administration of the same three drugs; but, in this condition, shock was administered every 10 minutes regardless of the animal's behavior. Figure 5 shows the results for monkey 4811. It can be seen that suppression by shock was not observed for any of the drugs except for pentobarbital at the 4ma intensity. However, there was no suppression at 8 or 10ma. In this case, responding was suppressed to near zero levels on the first day of shock for this animal, but responding increased on the following days and was maintained at a suppressed level until shock intensity was increased to 8 ma.

Figure 6 shows that the responding of this animal was similar to the previous monkey. Upon introduction of the shock in the pentobarbital condition, responding increased to 112% of baseline then decreased to 56% of baseline at 8ma. Other than this, no suppression or facilitation of drug intake was noted as a function of shock intensity. Generally, responding was maintained at a steady rate and was not changed or disrupted by the shock.

Figure 7 shows that the shock had a greater effect on self-administration for this animal than for the previous two. It can be seen that, for cocaine, self-administration increased as the shock level increased and even increased to the highest levels upon removal of the shock. An analysis of the cumulative records and observation of the animal disclosed that the shock induced the animal to press or attack the lever. As the intensity of the shock increased, the animal seemed to attack the lever immediately after the shock with increasing aggression. The animal hit the lever after each shock and post-shock bursts of responding were noted in many cases. The 10-second infusion period prevented the animal from receiving more infusions since these bursts of responding during the infusion were not reinforced. This behavior was not noted for pentobarbital or morphine for this animal. For this animal, pentobarbital self-administration was suppressed to 26% of baseline at 4ma. After this, pentobarbital responding increased with shock intensity and returned to baseline levels. No change in morphine responding was observed.

Figure 8 shows the results for animal 6369. Morphine self-administration remained relatively stable over the treatment period. For pentobarbital, a slight suppression of responding occured at 4ma

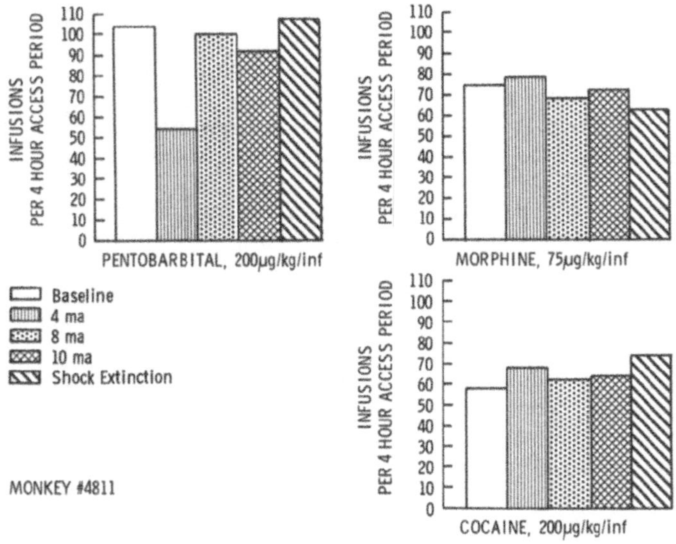

Fig. 5. Effects of response non-contingent shock on drug self-administration.

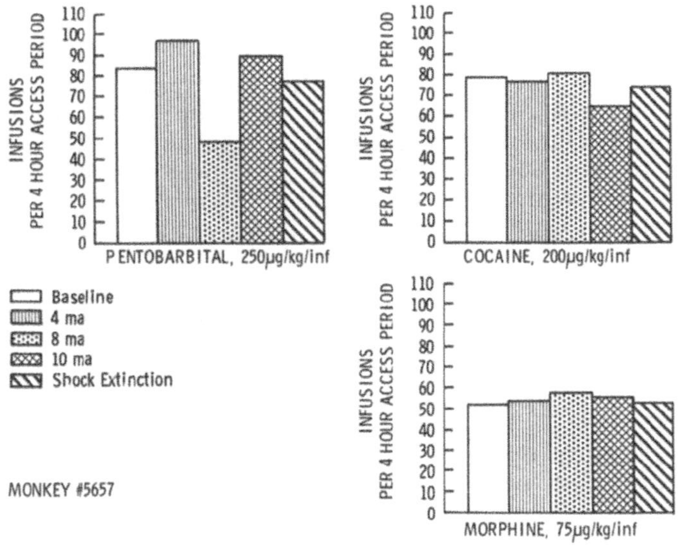

Fig. 6. Effects of response non-contingent shock on drug self-administration.

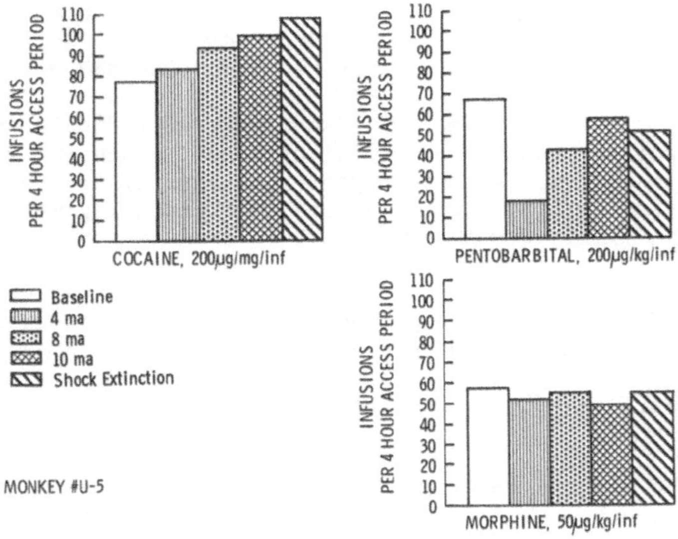

Fig. 7. Effects of response non-contingent shock on drug self-administration.

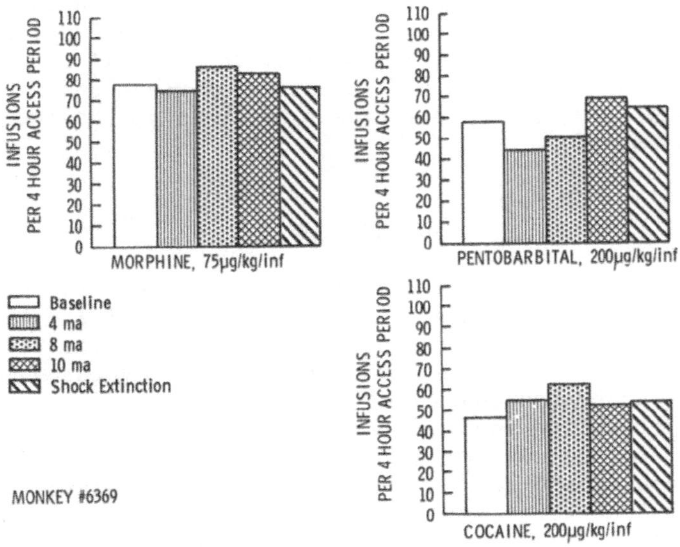

Fig. 8. Effects of response non-contingent shock on drug self-administration.

and a slight facilitation at 10ma. These changes are only minor and are not clearly related to shock. Responding for cocaine increased slightly at 4 and 8ma, but the increase was not noted at 10ma, and the removal of the shock had no noticeable effect.

The data for the animals in Experiment II indicate that, although slight suppression or facilitation of responding for these drugs can result from non-contingent shock administration, these effects are transitory and inconsistent. Responding was found to generally be maintained at baseline levels and responding did not vary in any systematic manner as a function of shock or shock intensity. Nor were there any notable changes in patterns of drug self-administration resulting from the non-contingent shock. An analysis of the cumulative records for the animals in Experiment II showed that the patterning of responding present during the baseline performance was preserved under all intensity levels of shock.

For the monkeys in Experiment I, the response-contingent shock disrupted the typical patterning of self-administration of morphine and pentobarbital because of response suppression. Because of the extreme suppression of pentobarbital responding, the characteristic patterning of spaced groups of infusions was obviated. Generally, the responding that did occur was at the beginning of the access period and there was not a tendency to continue to self-administer the drug after one or two shocks were received. A similar finding characterizes morphine self-administration under these conditions, especially at the 8 and 10ma intensities. At 4ma, there was a tendency to self-administer the drug over the access period although responding was suppressed. For cocaine, the typical patterning of spaced infusions was maintained across the three shock intensities. However, generally, as shock intensity increased, the inter-infusion interval increased.

DISCUSSION

The effects of response contingent and non-contingent shock on responding for cocaine, morphine, and pentobarbital are consistent with results obtained with non-drug reinforcers. Food reinforced responding has been found to be suppressed more by response contingent shock than by non-contingent shock (Church, 1963). Azrin (1956) found that increasing the response-shock interval attenuated the suppression of food responding, and Grove and Schuster (1974) found a similar result with cocaine responding. The results of the present investigation agree with these findings in that, if the shock were contingent upon the animal's response, suppression of responding occurred. Suppression did not occur if there were no shock-response contingency. The results of this study also support the findings of other investigators concerning the relationship between response rate and shock intensity. This present study found that as shock intensity increased, response suppression increased. This was observed in all cases for morphine and pentobarbital responding and for two of the monkeys self-administering cocaine. Of the other two monkeys self-administering cocaine, response suppression was inversely related to shock intensity in one case and varied as an inverted U-shaped function in another. This suppression occurred only if the shock was contingent upon the response and, in Experiment II where the shock was non-contingent, no consistent suppression or facilitation was observed. One animal which did show facilitation of cocaine responding exhibited lever press attack behavior resembling that reported by Weiss and Strongman (1969) and by Azrin, Hutchinson, and Hake (1967). Although this occurred in only one animal, it could be explained by the notion of Azrin et al. (1967) that attack behavior occurs only if escape or avoidance does not eliminate the shock, since in this experiment the animal could not escape or avoid the shock.

Rachlin (1966) studied the effects of mild punishment with electric shock on food reinforced responding in pigeons and noted transient emotional effects as a result of the introduction of the shock. This effect subsided with repeated shocks. Similar transient alterations in response rate were observed in both of the present experiments. These effects were most apparent in the response contingent situation where the monkeys, in effect, had the option of avoiding the shock. These effects were usually characterized by large drops in response rates with recovery on the following days. In some cases, the animals increased their response rates, thereby obtaining a large number of shocks. After one or two days, the monkeys' performance generally stabilized. These transient effects were also observed with the response non-contingent group and were usually characterized by response suppression which returned to baseline levels after one or two days. In many instances, no disruption of responding was noted for animals in this group.

Of particular interest in this study was the observation that, in the response contingent group, the magnitude of suppression by shock was different for the three drugs. Consistently, the monkeys' responding for cocaine was much less attenuated, relative to baseline, than for morphine or pentobarbital. Pentobarbital responding at 4ma was at 14% of baseline performance and 2% of baseline performance at 10ma. At these same intensities cocaine was self-administered at 46% of baseline level at 4ma and 37% at 10ma. Morphine appeared to fall somewhere between these two levels and was self-administered at 31% of baseline level at 4ma and 8% at 10ma.

Rachlin (1966) considered that punishment of a positively reinforced response somehow subtracts from the strength of the reinforcer. The findings of the present investigation agree with the results of others that indicate that, by increasing the intensity of the punishment, the strength of the reinforcer is reduced. The response then varies as a function of the intensity of punishment. The results of this study seem to indicate that, in operant behavior maintained by drug reinforcers, the nature of the reinforcer may be a variable related to the drug. To the extent that reinforcer strength may be equated with resistance to suppression by shock punishment, cocaine would appear to be more reinforcing under these conditions. By these standards, pentobarbital would seem to be the least reinforcing of the drugs used in this study. This, then, appears to suggest that the relative reinforcing efficacy of drugs may be indexed by their sensitivity to shock punishment.

An alternative explanation is that the drug interacts with perception of pain or with the threshold of the aversive stimulus. There is some evidence to support the notion that such an interaction exists. For example, Houser and Houser (1973) found that amphetamine increased the aversive threshold using a titration technique in an avoidance/escape experiment. The effect was lost, however, upon continued administration of the drug. Morphine, a true analgesic, was able to reliably increase the aversive threshold. The results of Experiment II, however, argue against a drug and aversive threshold interaction explanation. If cocaine possessed the property of altering the aversive threshold, and morphine is known to have this property, then alterations in infusion intake could attenuate the aversive stimulus. An increase in morphine self-infusion rate would certainly argue for this explanation, but this was not observed to occur. No systematic changes in the amount of any drug self-administered were observed under conditions of unavoidable shock - suggesting that the drug effect itself did not interact with the painful stimulus.

Drug dose could also be an influential variable. Grove and Schuster (1974) found that the suppressant effect of the shock on cocaine self-administration was independent of drug dose for the two unit doses of 100 and 200μg/kg/infusion used. However, the relevance of drug dose, particularly when comparing different drugs in a punished self-administration paradigm, cannot be ruled out. Another possible explanation of the data is that the reinforcement from cocaine may have faster onset and, therefore, provide quicker positive reinforcement for the animal's responding. Pentobarbital was self-administered in bursts of infusions, and morphine responding was characterized by most infusions occurring at the beginning of the access period. It is possible, then, that the animal would have to obtain more shocks for pentobarbital and morphine than cocaine in order to obtain the positive reinforcement from the drug.

The results of the present investigation appear to indicate that punishment of drug self-administration in monkeys could be a useful technique to compare the reinforcing strengths of drugs that function as reinforcers. However, other drug comparisons and additional variables must be considered in order to determine the relationship between punishment and the reinforcing efficacy of drugs.

ACKNOWLEDGMENT

This research was supported in part by a National Institutes of Health Fellowship (F22 DA 01667) from the National Institute on Drug Abuse to David McLendon and in part by NIDA grant (DA 00667) to Robert Harris.

REFERENCES

Azrin, N.H.: Some effects of two intermittent schedules of immediate and non-immediate punishment, J. Psychol. 42, 3-21 (1956).

Azrin, N.H. and Holz, W.C.: Punishment. In: Operant Behavior: Areas of Research and Application. Honig, W.K., Ed., pp. 380-447. New York: Appleton-Century-Crofts, 1966.

Azrin, N.H., Hutchinson and R.R., and Hake, D.F.: Attack, avoidance, and escape reactions to aversive shock, J. exp. Analysis Behav. 10, 131-148 (1967).

Church, R.M.: The varied effects of punishment on behavior, Psychol. Rev. 70, 369-402 (1963).

Deneau, G., Yanagita, T., and Seevers, M.H.: Self-administration of psychoactive substances by the monkey, Psychopharmacologia (Berl.) 16, 30-48 (1969).

Grove, R.N. and Schuster, C.R.: Suppression of cocaine self-administration by extinction and punishment, Pharmac. Biochem. Behav. 2, 199-208 (1974).

Holz, W.C. and Azrin, N.H.: Interactions between the discriminative and aversive properties of punishment, J. exp. Analysis Behav. 5, 229-234 (1962).

Houser, V.P. and Houser, F.L.: The alteration of aversive thresholds with cholinergic and adrenergic agents, Pharmac. Biochem. Behav. 1, 433-444 (1973).

Hunt, H.F. and Brady, J.V.: Some effects of punishment and intercurrent "anxiety" on a simple operant, J. comp. Physiol. Psychol. 48, 305-310 (1955).

Millo, K.C., Sobell, M.B., and Schaefer, H.H.: Training social drinking as an alternative to abstinence in alcoholics, Behav. Ther. 2, 18-27 (1971).

Powell, J.R. and Azrin, N.H.: The effects of shock as a punisher for cigarette smoking, J. appl. Behav. Analysis 1, 63-71 (1968.

Rachlin, H.: Recovery of responses during mild punishment, J. exp. Analysis Behav. 9, 251-263 (1966).

Smith, S.G. and Davis, W.M.: Punishment of amphetamine and morphine self-administration behavior, Psychol. Rec. 24, 477-480 (1974).

Weiss, K.M. and Strongman, K.T.: Shock-induced response bursts and suppression, Psychon. Sci. 15, 238-240 (1969).

DRUG-MAINTAINED PERFORMANCE AND THE ANALYSIS OF STIMULANT REINFORCING EFFECTS

Joseph V. Brady and Roland R. Griffiths

The Johns Hopkins University School of Medicine

Baltimore, Maryland 21205

Research over the past decade involving drug-maintained performance procedures has demonstrated a good correspondence between compounds self-administered by laboratory animals and those abused by man (Schuster and Thompson, 1969; Deneau, Yanagita, and Seevers, 1969; Woods and Tessel, 1974). More recently, experimental attention has been directed toward the rank ordering of such compounds with respect to their abuse liability relative to the range of drugs self-administered by animal preparations (Yanagita, 1974; Brady, Griffiths, and Winger, 1975). Behavioral procedures for the assessment of comparative dependency potential have been based upon research evaluating the performance-maintenance potential (e.g., reinforcing properties) of a variety of environmental stimuli (e.g., food, water, drugs, etc.). Observed variation in this performance-maintenance potency has been assumed to reflect the "strength" (Hodos, 1961) or "efficacy" (Johanson and Schuster, 1975) of stimuli as response-contingent reinforcers, though the hypothetical status of such intervening processes requires interpretative caution (and healthy skepticism) in comparative assessments of drug abuse liability. Behavioral procedures for measuring the differential reinforcing effects of stimuli may provide, nonetheless, useful information about the relative reinforcing efficacy of various doses of a single drug as well as the rank ordering of different drugs for their abuse potential. The application of these procedures to the analysis of drug self-administration in laboratory animals has generally involved four methodological approaches emphasizing: (1) progressive-ratio measures, (2) rates of drug maintained responding, (3) concurrent schedules of drug reinforcement, and (4) discrete-trial choice procedures.

Progressive-ratio procedures for evaluating relative reinforcing properties between drugs involve establishing a performance baseline that provides for drug self-administration contingent upon emission of a specified operant response. The number of responses required for each reinforcement is then systematically increased until the subject's responding falls below some criterion level. The response requirement at which the criterion is met is referred to as the "breaking point." Orderly increasing relationships have been reported between breaking point and such variables as degree of food deprivation (Hodos, 1961), the concentration or volume of a liquid reinforcer (Hodos and Kalman, 1963), and the intensity or train duration of reinforcing electrical intracranial stimulation (Keesey and Goldstein, 1968; Hodos, 1965). Since the breaking point varies systematically as a function of these several "motivational" conditions, it has been argued that it provides an index of the relative strength of a reinforcer (Hodos, 1961; Hodos and Kalman, 1963).

Yanagita (1973) first reported on the use of such a progressive ratio procedure for comparative evaluation of several different reinforcing drugs including cocaine at various doses. Monkeys were first permitted to self-administer a compound intravenously on a fixed-ratio 100 schedule. Free access to drug self-administration under these conditions was allowed on a 24-hour per day basis. During the progressive-ratio test, the response requirement was doubled after a fixed number of injections beginning at 100 responses. A test was terminated when the time interval since the last injection exceeded 24 hours. Using this procedure, it was demonstrated that generally larger units of cocaine (0.03, 0.12, and 0.48mg/kg/injection) maintained higher progressive-ratio performance than lower doses of this drug.

A related series of experiments using a somewhat modified progressive-ratio procedure for assessing breaking point values of different compounds at various doses have recently been reported by the present authors (Brady, Griffiths, and Winger, 1975; Griffiths, Findley, Brady, Gutcher, and Robinson, 1975). The procedure featured an extended time-out period (3 hours) between trials which were scheduled on a 24-hour a day basis. During a trial, responding on a ratio schedule was reinforced with a single infusion of drug. The ratio requirement in each trial was increased only once each week. Data obtained using this procedure with a series of five chair-restrained, individually-housed baboons, surgically prepared with intravenous catheters, compared breaking point values for different self-administered compounds including cocaine at several doses. The sequence of ratio values involved was 160, 320, 640, 1280, 4800, and 9600. The breaking point determinations for all subjects, drugs, and doses are summarized in Fig. 1 with the number of determinations under each condition indicated above each bar.

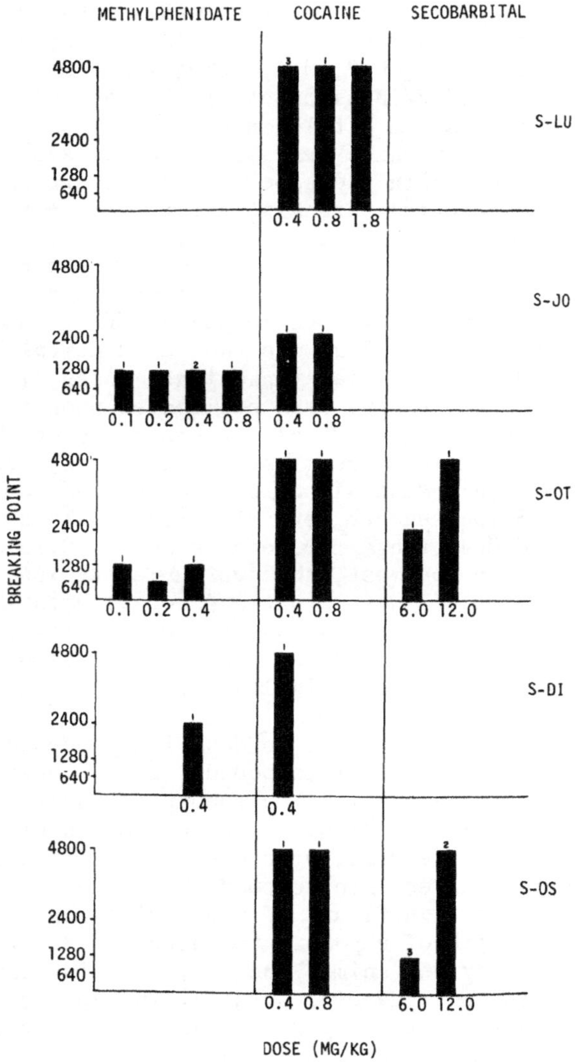

Fig. 1. Breaking point values for doses of methylphenidate, cocaine and secobarbital in five subjects. Each bar represents breaking point obtained at indicated dose of drug. Numeral above bar indicates the number of determinations at that dose. In all cases, multiple determinations resulted in identical breaking point values. Absence of bar indicates subject was not exposed to that condition. (From Griffiths et al., 1975.)

Of particular interest for the analysis of stimulant reinforcing effects are the 12 breaking point determinations obtained with cocaine in a total of five subjects as well as the 9 breaking points obtained with methylphenidate in a total of 3 subjects. Over the dose ranges studied (0.1, 0.2, 0.4, 0.8mg/kg/infusion methylphenidate; 0.4, 0.8, 1.6mg/kg/infusion cocaine), manipulation of doses of these two compounds had little or no effect on breaking points. Of the six occasions on which multiple doses of a stimulant compound were examined within the same subject, there was only one instance in which identical breaking points were not obtained. In that instance, S-OT showed breaking point values of 1280, 640, and 1280 at doses of 0.1, 0.2, and 0.4mg/kg of methylphenidate, respectively. Given that the intermediate dose produced the lowest breaking point value (an unlikely dose-response effect) and that the effect was not obtained in S-JO who showed identical breaking points over a wide range of methylphenidate doses, it seems likely that this difference may have been eliminated upon further replication. In any case, in five out of six occasions on which subjects were exposed to multiple doses of stimulant drugs, identical breaking points were obtained at all doses studied and for all replications (a total of 19 separate determinations). These observations involved a 4-fold dose range for cocaine and an 8-fold range for methylphenidate. In contrast, the two subjects exposed to two doses of secobarbital (7 determinations total) both showed increases in breaking points when the dose was increased from 6.0 to 12.0 mg/kg. Furthermore, both of these subjects had demonstrated dose independence with respect to stimulant drugs.

These findings with respect to dose independence of breaking point values for the stimulant compounds (i.e., cocaine and methylphenidate) are at variance with the reported results of Yanagita's study (1973) demonstrating higher breaking points with increasing doses of cocaine. There were, of course, major procedural differences which must be taken into account when comparing the two studies. Among the most significant of these differences (e.g., intertrial interval, length of exposure to successive ratio increments, breaking point criterion, animal species), cocaine dose range would seem to require the most careful scrutiny in the light of more recent findings with other comparative assessment procedures to be described in subsequent sections of this paper.

<u>Response-rate measures</u> have enjoyed long-standing theoretical and experimental popularity as critical variables in the evaluation of behavioral assessment techniques (Kelleher and Morse, 1968; Skinner, 1938). Despite this traditional emphasis, response rates have proven of questionable reliability as measures for determining reinforcement strength. When the behavioral performance is

maintained by intravenous drug administration, for example, there is frequently a negative correlation between the reinforcement magnitude (i.e., drug dose) and the response rate (e.g., Goldberg, Hoffmeister, Schlichting, and Wuttke, 1971). This has been shown to be particularly true when a continuous schedule of drug reinforcement (CRF) is used with psychomotor stimulant drugs like d-amphetamine (Pickens and Harris, 1968), methylphenidate (Wilson, Hitomi, and Schuster, 1971), and cocaine (Pickens and Thompson, 1971; Woods and Schuster, 1968). Where the schedule of reinforcement does not involve such a close relationship between response rate increases and elevations in drug intake, however, the rate of responding may reflect differential reinforcement magnitude independently of reinforcement frequency. With fixed interval (FI) schedules, for example, Stebbins, Mead, and Martin (1959), using sucrose concentration, and Meltzer and Brahlek (1968, 1970), using number of food pellets, found response rate to be positively related to reinforcement magnitude.

More recently, Balster and Schuster (1973) reported a series of experiments relating response rate on an FI schedule of cocaine reinforcement to dose and infusion duration. Rhesus monkeys were maintained on a multiple schedule consisting of fixed interval components (FI 9 min, limited-hold 3 min) of food or drug reinforcement alternating with 15 min time-out periods following each reinforcement or limited-hold expiration. Daily sessions began with a single FI food component followed by 3 cocaine components with the sequence repeated 10 times for a total of 10 food reinforcements and 30 drug reinforcements. Under such conditions, response rate maintained by cocaine was generally shown to be a positive function of dose magnitude over the range from 0 to 800 μg/kg/infusion though there was little differential effect on food reinforced responding over most of the indicated dose range. At the higher cocaine doses (e.g., 800 μg/kg/infusion), however, increasing rate relationships were not uniformly discernible in the drug-maintained FI performances and the food-maintained FI rates decreased significantly. In addition, FI response rates maintained by cocaine were found to be inversely related to infusion rates for unit doses of both 200 and 400 μg/kg/infusion over a range of infusion durations from 5 to 200 secs. Increasing the duration of the cocaine infusion produced a change in response rate similar to decreasing unit dose although the FI response rate change for a given increase in infusion duration was less at a unit dose of 400 μg/kg than at 200 μg/kg.

In the present volume, McLendon and Harris (in press) have described a somewhat different response rate measure for comparing different drug reinforcers. Based upon a punishment technique which provided for the delivery of electric shock contingent upon drug self-infusion, cocaine self-administration was found to be more resistant to suppression than either morphine or pentobarbital. Though pentobarbital self-infusion appeared to be the most easily suppressed of the three drugs, dose-effect relationships were not reported.

Concurrent schedule procedures for evaluating the relative reinforcing properties of drugs bear a close relationship to the relative rate measures upon which they are both experimentally and theoretically based. When two concurrently available, equally valued variable interval (VI) schedules (on two separate operanda) produce different reinforcing stimuli, relative response rates appear to reflect reinforcer magnitude or reinforcer strength with reasonable reliability. Response rates on concurrent VI schedules of different durations of food reinforcement, for example, have been shown to correspond to the magnitude of the reinforcer (Catania, 1963). And a similar procedure has been used to measure relative preference between qualitatively different reinforcers (Hollard and Davison, 1971). Most recently, Iglauer and Woods (1974) have reported a study of such concurrent schedules maintained by intravenous drug delivery in which comparisons were made between different doses of cocaine with rhesus monkeys. Variable interval response rates for a dose of 0.1 mg/kg/infusion cocaine were found to be higher than response rates on equally valued, concurrently available VI schedules maintained by either 0.025 or 0.05 mg/kg/infusion of the same drug. When the concurrent VI schedule was maintained by 0.2 or 0.4 mg/kg/infusion cocaine, however, the 0.1 mg/kg/infusion cocaine dose maintained lower comparative response rates.

Discrete-trial choice procedures for assessing the relative reinforcing properties of stimulus events have been reported to effectively discriminate between various food presentation durations (Neuringer, 1967), and were subsequently explored by Findley, Robinson, and Peregrino (1972) for comparing different self-administered drugs. Johanson and Schuster (1975) and Johanson (in press) have also described such a drug-choice procedure with monkeys which involved self-administration of a compound under one stimulus condition and then introducing a second self-administered dose or compound under a different stimulus condition. When both stimulus conditions were presented simulataneously, the animal's choice or preference was indicated simply by the number of times the response associated with one stimulus-drug condition was selected compared to the other. These studies have shown that animals prefer (more than 75% of the choices) all self-administered doses of cocaine, diethylpropion, and methylphenidate over saline. In addition, high doses of both cocaine and methylphenidate were selected over lower doses of each drug, respectively. Dose-dependent effects were also observed when comparisons between cocaine and methylphenidate were made using this preference procedure. A similar procedure for assessing cocaine dose preferences as well as drug choices (e.g., cocaine vs. morphine) based upon stimulus-controlled extinction performance is described in the present volume by Balster and Schuster.

A variant of this choice procedure for evaluating preference with baboons has been described by the present authors (Brady, Griffiths, and Winger, 1975; Griffiths, Wurster, and Brady, in press), using a discrete trial methodology which required a minimum 3-hour time-out between intravenous drug self-administration opportunities. At the beginning of each trial, the animal was presented with one of two or three differently colored stimulus lights and a switching lever which changed the light colors. In order to proceed with the trial, the baboon was required to switch colors so that each stimulus light appeared at least twice. The animal was then permitted to continue changing colors or proceed with the trial in the color of his choice by completing a response requirement on a second lever (15 responses on a shock-avoidance schedule). Each of the light colors was associated with the delivery of a specific consequence (e.g., food or drug). Responding on the second lever eventuated in delivery of the compound appropriate to the particular light color present when the response requirement was completed. Using this procedure with heroin-dependent baboons maintaining a stable choice baseline between exclusive food (75% preference) and heroin (25% preference) options, Griffiths, Wurster, and Brady (in press) have shown that non-contingent naloxone administration superimposed upon the choice baseline produces dose-dependent increases in the percent of trials in which heroin is selected over food. In contrast, non-contingent methadone administration superimposed upon this same choice baseline produced consistent decreases in the percent trials on which heroin was selected over food.

Brady, Griffiths, and Winger (1975) have also described the application of this discrete trial choice procedure in the analysis of a preference performance with a baboon involving three drug self-administration options. Responses on the switching lever changed the color of the light stimulus from red to green to yellow. Fifteen responses on the second lever in the presence of the red light produced an infusion of heroin; responses during the yellow light condition resulted in a saline infusion; and responses in the presence of the green light produced a naloxone infusion. Under these conditions, selections of the green light stimulus quickly decreased to zero while choice of the red light approached 100%. When the colors associated with heroin and saline conditions were reversed so that 15 responses in the presence of the yellow light resulted in a heroin infusion, the frequency of yellow light selection increased while that of the red light decreased.

A modification of the choice procedure described above and reported by Griffiths, Wurster, and Brady (in press) has been used in a recent preference study involving different doses of cocaine with two baboons. The animals were initially trained on a variant of the choice procedure that involved 30-trials each day with a 10 min time-out period following each trial. The choice schedule also differed from the procedure described above in that the shock-avoidance requirement was eliminated. Following initial food training, the baboons were surgically prepared with intravenous catheters, as described by Deneau et al. (1969), and infusions of different doses of cocaine were associated with two differently colored stimulus lights. Figure 2 shows the results of seven consecutive choice determinations with a range of cocaine doses in one of the baboons (S-HR). Prior to drug introduction, S-HR showed a strong bias toward the blue stimulus, as indicated by the low rate of red choices during the first three days plotted on the graph. When an infusion of 0.1 mg/kg cocaine was associated with the red stimulus on day 4, while an infusion of saline was associated with selection of blue, there was a clear shift in preference toward the red color over the next 5 days. Reversal of the options on day 9 so that the 0.1 cocaine dose was associated with selection of the blue stimulus and saline was associated with selection of red produced a clear shift in preference toward the blue stimulus. Subsequent choice determinations, as shown in Fig. 2, involved options associated with several different doses of cocaine (i.e., 0.1 vs. 0.1 mg/kg/infusion; 0.05 vs. 0.1 mg/kg/infusion; 0.075 vs. 0.1 mg/kg/infusion); and on each of these determinations the higher dose of cocaine (0.1 mg/kg) was preferred to the lower doses.

Figure 3 summarizes the results obtained with the second baboon (S-HE) in the course of a similar choice experiment involving different doses of cocaine. The first 5 choice determinations replicated the findings with S-HR demonstrating that a cocaine dose of 0.1 mg/kg was consistently selected over the lower doses of cocaine (0.03; 0.056; and 0.075 mg/kg). The subsequent determinations involved comparison of higher doses of cocaine. Starting on day 67, S-HE was exposed to successive determinations involving 0.1 vs. 0.133 mg/kg, 0.1 vs. 0.17 mg/kg, 0.1 vs. 0.3 mg/kg, and 0.1 vs. 0.4 mg/kg. As shown in Fig. 3, the baboon did not demonstrate a clear preference for either option during any of these preference determinations. When cocaine doses were again reduced to levels at which discriminative choice determinations had previously been made by this animal, no preference between doses of 0.056 and 0.1 mg/kg/infusion could be discerned over a 7-day period (i.e., experimental days 108 to 114), though the baboon did subsequently show a preference for 0.2 mg/kg/infusion cocaine over saline (days 115 through 124). Finally, three successive choice determinations between 0.1 and 0.3 mg/kg/infusion cocaine with baboon S-HE are shown in Fig. 3 for experimental days 125 through 143. While a preference for the 0.3 dose was evident on the first determination (i.e., days 125 through 129), the results obtained with two subsequent reversal determinations showed no clear preference for either option.

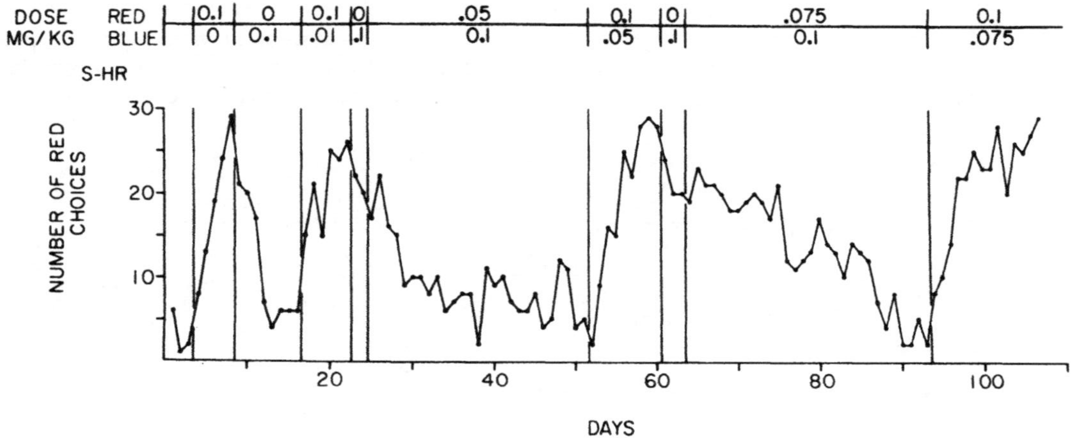

Fig. 2. Daily choice performance for S-HR. Trials involved choosing between two options (red or blue) each associated with a different dose of cocaine. Thirty trials were scheduled daily, each followed by a 10 min time-out.

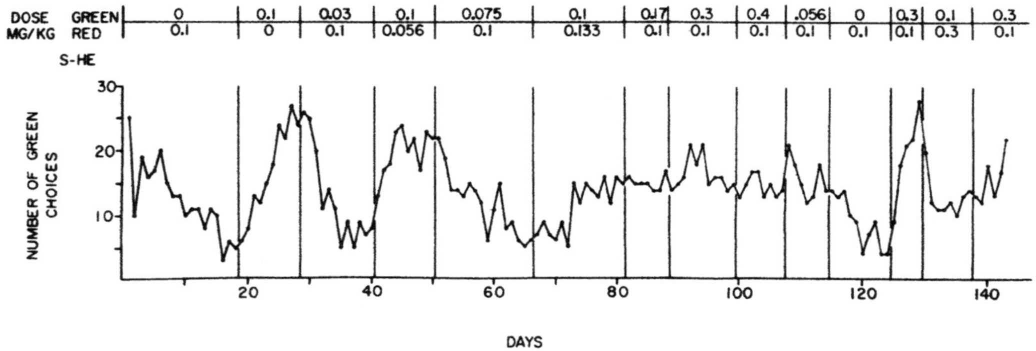

Fig. 3. Daily choice performance for S-HE. Trials involved choosing between two options (green or red) each associated with a different dose of cocaine. Thirty trials were scheduled daily, each followed by a 10 min time-out.

The results of this experiment show clearly that a dose of 0.1 mg/kg cocaine can be preferentially discriminated by baboons from a range of lower doses, including alternatives as close as 0.075 mg/kg. The unique finding that the relative reinforcing properties of different cocaine doses can be discriminated with such small magnitude variations suggests that the slope of the dose-effect curve may be quite steep over this lower range of doses. At higher doses (i.e., above 0.1 mg/kg), in contrast, choice determinations were less reliable (though higher dose preferences can be demonstrated under some conditions), and the results point to a more shallow dose-response curve at cocaine dose levels above 0.1 mg/kg.

DISCUSSION AND CONCLUSIONS

The sigmoidal characterization of the cocaine reinforcement dose-effect curve described above is consistent with the results of other studies (e.g., Balster and Schuster, 1973) showing a breakdown of dose-dependent preference and discriminability functions at high cocaine dose levels. Moreover, the infusion rate effects described by Balster and Schuster (1973) in this same study (i.e., the effect of increasing cocaine infusion duration resembled the effect of decreasing unit dose) were less evident at a dose of 400 μg/kg than at 200 μg/kg. These convergent findings from several different methodological approaches to the analysis of stimulant effects suggest that the reinforcing efficacy of such compounds may be more closely related to the initial infusion-produced "rush" than to the magnitude or duration of more delayed pharmacological consequences.

The relationships suggested by these findings also provide a basis for reconciling the apparent discrepancy between the fixed ratio breaking points for cocaine reported by Yanagita (1973), on the one hand, and by Griffiths et al. (1975), on the other. The latter investigators reported that cocaine breaking point determinations were not affected by dose manipulations in the range of 0.4 - 1.6 mg/kg/infusion. This range is well above the differential discriminability threshold (i.e., the shallow section of the dose-response curve) suggested on the basis of results obtained with discrete trial choice procedures. In contrast, the study by Yanagita (1973) demonstrated a direct relationship between dose and breaking point; however, the study focused on a lower dose range (i.e., 0.03; 0.12; 0.48 mg/kg/infusion) at which preferential discriminability has been confirmed with discrete-trial choice procedures.

Despite the persistent skepticism which continues to surround laboratory research efforts to evaluate the relative reinforcing properties of drugs (Kelleher and Goldberg, in press), robust findings from the array of self-infusion studies summarized in this review reveal a degree of correspondence across animal species, procedural approaches, and pharmacological agents which is indeed impressive. When considered in the somewhat ephemeral light that characterizes most psychopharmacological effects, the emergent experimental analyses of drug-maintained performances would appear to hold considerable promise for the development of a potentially useful behavioral-pharmacological technology for the assessment of drug reinforcement efficacy.

ACKNOWLEDGMENT

This research was supported by NIDA Grant DA 01147 and DEA Contract J-69-15.

REFERENCES

Balster, R.L., Schuster, C.R.: Fixed-interval schedule of cocaine reinforcement: effect of dose and infusion duration. J.exp. Analysis Behav. 20, 119-129 (1973).

Balster, R.L., Schuster, C.R.: A preference procedure which compares efficacy of different intravenous drug reinforcers in the rhesus monkey. In: Cocaine and Other Stimulants. Ellinwood, E.H., Kilbey, M.M., Eds. New York: Plenum Press, 1976.

Brady, J.V., Griffiths, R.R., Winger, G.: Drug-maintained performance procedures and the evaluation of sedative hypnotic dependency potential. In: Hypnotics: Methods of Development and Evaluation. Kagan, F., Harwood, T., Rickels, K., Rudzik, A., Sorer, H., Eds., pp. 221-235. New York: Spectrum Publications, Inc., 1975.

Catania, A.C.: Concurrent performance: A baseline for the study of reinforcement magnitude. J.exp.Analysis Behav. 6, 299-300 (1963).

Deneau, G.A., Yanagita, T., Seevers, M.H.: Self-administration of psychoactive substances by the monkey. Psychopharmacologia 16, 30-48 (1969).

Findley, J.D., Robinson, W.W., Peregrino, L.: Addiction to secobarbital and chlordiazepoxide in the rhesus monkey by means of a self-infusion preference procedure. Psychopharmacologia 26, 93-144 (1972).

Goldberg, S.R., Hoffmeister, R., Schlicting, U.V., Wuttke, W.: A comparison of pentobarbital and cocaine self-administration in rhesus monkeys: Effects of dose and fixed ratio parameters. J.Pharmac.exp.Ther. 179, 277-283 (1971).

Griffiths, R.R., Findley, J.D., Brady, J.V., Gutcher, K., Robinson, W.W.: Comparison of progressive-ratio performance maintained by cocaine, methylphenidate and secobarbital. Psychopharmacologia 43, 81-83 (1975).

Griffiths, R.R., Wurster, R., Brady, J.V.: Discrete-trial choice procedure: Effects of naloxone and methadone on choice between food and heroin. In: Control of Drug-Taking by Schedules of Reinforcement. Kelleher, R., Goldberg, S., Krasnegor, N., Eds. Pharmac.Rev. (in press).

Hodos, W.: Progressive ratio as a measure of reward strength. Science 134, 943-944 (1961).

Hodos, W.: Motivational properties of long durations of rewarding brain stimulation. J.comp.Physiol.Psychol. 59, 219-224 (1965).

Hodos, W., Kalman, J.: Effects of increment size and reinforcer volume on progressive-ratio performance. J.exp.Analysis Behav. 6, 387-392 (1963).

Hollard, V., Davison, M.C.: Preference for qualitatively different reinforcers. J.exp.Analysis Behav. 16, 375-380 (1971).

Iglauer, C., Woods, J.H.: Concurrent performances: Reinforcement of different doses of intravenous cocaine in the rhesus monkey. J.exp.Analysis Behav. 22, 179-196 (1974).

Johanson, C.: Several pharmacological and environmental variables affecting drug preference in rhesus monkeys. In: Control of Drug-Taking by Schedules of Reinforcement. Kelleher, R., Goldberg, S., Krasnegor, N., Eds. Pharmac.Rev. (in press).

Johanson, C., Schuster, C.R.: Choice procedure for comparing drug reinforcers: Cocaine and methylphenidate in the rhesus monkey. J.Pharmac.exp.Ther. (in press).

Keesey, R.E., Goldstein, M.D.: Use of progressive fixed-ratio procedures in the assessment of intracranial reinforcement. J.exp.Analysis Behav. 11, 293-301 (1968).

Kelleher, R., Goldberg, S.: General introduction. In: Control of Drug-Taking by Schedules of Reinforcement. Kelleher, R., Goldberg, S., Krasnegor, N., Eds. Pharmac.Rev. (in press).

Kelleher, R., Morse, W.: Determinants of the specificity of behavioral effects of drugs. Ergebn.Physiol. 60, 1-56 (1968).

McLendon, D.M., Harris, R.T.: The effects of response contingent and non-contingent shock on drug self-administration in rhesus monkeys. In: Cocaine and Other Stimulants. Ellinwood, E.H., Kilbey, M.M., Eds. New York: Plenum Press, 1976.

Meltzer, D., Brahlek, J.A.: Conditioned suppression and conditioned enhancement with the same positive UCS: An effect of CS duration. J.exp.Analysis Behav. 13, 67-73 (1970).

Meltzer, D, Brahlek, J.A.: Quantity of reinforcement and fixed-interval performance. Psychonom.Sci. 12, 207-208 (1968).

Neuringer, A.J.: Effects of reinforcement magnitude on choice and rate of responding. J.exp.Analysis Behav. 10, 417-424 (1967).

Pickens, R., Harris, W.: Self-administration of d-amphetamine by rats. Psychopharmacologia 12, 158-163 (1968).

Pickens, R., Thompson, T.: Characteristics of stimulant drug reinforcement. In: Stimulus Properties of Drugs. Thompson, T., Pickens, R., Eds., 177-192. New York: Appleton-Century-Crofts, 1971.

Schuster, C.R., Thompson, T.: Self-administration of and behavioral dependence on drugs. Ann.Rev.Pharmac. 9, 483-502 (1969).

Skinner, B.F.: The Behavior of Organisms. New York: Appleton-Century-Crofts, 1938.

Stebbins, W.C., Mead, P.B., Martin, J.M.: The relation of amount of reinforcement to performance under a fixed-interval schedule. J.exp.Analysis Behav. 2, 351-355 (1959).

Wilson, M.C., Hitomi, M., Schuster, C.R.: Psychomotor stimulant self-administration as a function of dosage per injection in the rhesus monkey. Psychopharmacologia 22, 271-281 (1971).

Woods, J.H., Schuster, C.R.: Reinforcement properties of morphine, cocaine, and SPA as a function of unit dose. Int.J.Addictions 3, 231-237 (1968).

Woods, J.H., Tessel, R.E.: Fenfluramine: amphetamine congener that fails to maintain drug-taking behavior in the rhesus monkey. Science 185, 1068-1069 (1974).

Yanagita, T.: An experimental framework for evaluation of dependence liability in various types of drugs in monkeys. Bull.Narcot. 1, 25-57 (1973).

ACUTE SYSTEMIC EFFECTS OF COCAINE IN MAN: A CONTROLLED STUDY OF INTRANASAL AND INTRAVENOUS ROUTES OF ADMINISTRATION

Richard B. Resnick, Richard S. Kestenbaum,
and Lee K. Schwartz
Department of Psychiatry, New York Medical College
5 East 102nd Street, New York, New York 10029

An upsurge in cocaine use has been anticipated by workers in the drug abuse field for some time (Ellinwood, 1973), and the popular press recently has been reporting major nationwide increases in the non-medical use of the drug. The increase is apparently occurring both in opiate users and the general population. For example, out of 55,745 students in the seventh through twelfth grades in Dallas, Texas, 2,108, or 4%, reported using cocaine; and 1,250 of them reported they had used it at least one time during the week the questionnaire was answered (Gossett, Lewis, and Phillips, 1971). A series of surveys have indicated that up to 84% of regular heroin users also use cocaine (Chambers, Taylor, and Moffet, 1972; Edmundson, Davies, Acker, and Myer, 1972). The New York State Narcotic Addiction Control Commission reported 81.7% of 180 randomly selected, certified narcotic addicts during 1969-1970 abused cocaine. The Clinical Research Center at Lexington found that, of 1,096 opiate addicts, 72.9% reported cocaine abuse during 1968-1969; and a 10% increase in cocaine use among heroin addicts in San Francisco between 1971 and 1972 has been reported (Gay, Sheppard, Inaba, and Newmeyer, 1973).

Although the basic systemic action of cocaine is known to be sympathomimetic, the magnitude and duration of its effects at different doses have not been systematically studied. There have been no controlled studies of the physiologic or behavioral effects of cocaine in individuals who are free of serious organic disease or psychopathology. The literature describing systemic effects of cocaine in man is contradictory and largely anecdotal. Several texts state that the approximate fatal dose of cocaine is 1.2 gm and severe toxic effects or death due to "idiosyncrasy" have been reported from doses as low as 20 mg (Goodman and Gilman, 1970; Sollman, 1948). Others state that the minimal lethal dose is 30 mg (Krupp and Chatton, 1974). These assertions are not documented and the pre-morbid conditions, route, and rate of administration are not specified. Some anesthesia texts state that the topical dose of cocaine must never exceed 100 mg (Gray and Nunn, 1971; Wood-Smith and Stewart, 1962; Mayer, 1924), whereas others state that the maximum dosage on mucous membranes of the respiratory tract should be 200 mg (Smith, 1973; Lee, 1960).

The present study was undertaken to assess physiologic and subjective effects over a thirty-minute observation period of single doses of 10 mg and 25 mg cocaine by intranasal and intravenous administration.

METHOD

Nineteen volunteer subjects between 21 and 42 years of age who had a history of frequent and regular use of cocaine during the preceding six months and who had taken no medication for the previous 24 hr participated in the study. Any volunteer who had a serious illness or history of a condition that contraindicated use of cocaine was not accepted.

A repeated-measures design in which each subject served as his own control was employed. Subjects' responses were measured before receiving medication and then at 2, 5, 10, 15, 20, 25, and 30 min after. Each subject received placebo, 10 mg, and 25 mg cocaine. Twelve subjects received the three dosages intranasally and twelve subjects received the dosages intravenously. Five of the subjects participated in trials using both routes of administration. The order in which the doses were administered was counterbalanced across subjects.

Subjects were seated in a comfortable chair and EKG leads were attached. They were allowed to relax for five to ten minutes, during which baseline measurements were obtained. The subjects were told that they would receive an injection or nose drops containing cocaine and that the purpose of the experiment was to evaluate the effects of the drug by measuring their responses. In addition to making each of the judgments requested, they were encouraged to report spontaneous observations.

A solution of 0.5 cc cocaine in water was instilled into the nostrils or 1.5 cc was injected intravenously over 90 seconds. Intravenous placebo consisted of 1.5 cc water and intranasal placebo was 0.5 cc 1% lidocaine. A minimum of two days intervened between dosages for each subject.

The physiologic parameters measured were: heart rate, blood pressure, respiration, oral temperature, and handgrip strength. Heart rate was recorded by means of an electrocardiogram. Blood pressure was measured with a sphygmostat or a mercury sphygmomanometer. Respiratory rate was determined by using a stethoscope. Temperature was taken by oral thermometer. Hand grip strength was assessed by means of a hand dynamometer that measures kilograms of force.

Subjective effects that were measured consisted of: "high," pleasantness, speeding, hunger, strength, and acute effects. Subjects reported sensations of "high" and speeding on a five-point scale from zero to five. Feelings of physical strength and pleasantness were reported on a twelve point scale from -6 to +6. Degree of hunger was reported on a ten point scale from -5 to +5. Acute effects were assessed by the number of statements rated "true" on a thirty-six item modified Addiction Research Center Inventory for acute amphetamine effects (Hill, Haertzen, Wolbach, and Miner, 1963).

RESULTS

Heart rate, systolic blood pressure, and diastolic blood pressure dose-response curves for placebo, 10 mg, and 25 mg cocaine administered intravenously and intranasally are shown in Fig. 1. The peak responses after cocaine are compared to the peak responses after placebo. The mean time-course curves for the physiologic and subjective measures are shown in Fig. 2 and Fig. 3 respectively.

Intranasal cocaine produced physiologic and subjective effects only at the 25 mg dosage. When administered intranasally, 10 mg cocaine showed no difference from placebo on any of the measurements. Intravenously, both 10 mg and 25 mg cocaine produced significant dose-related effects on the physiologic and the subjective measures. Paired t-tests were used to estimate levels of statistical significance. All differences are significant at the 0.01 level unless otherwise stated. The details of these results are described below.

Physiological Measurements (Figures 1 & 2)

Intranasal Route. A significant mean increase of 7 mm systolic pressure ($p < 0.02$) was observed ten minutes following 25 mg cocaine. Measurements taken up to thirty minutes showed decreases, but still not to baseline level. There were no changes after 25 mg compared to placebo on any of the other measures. No significant differences from placebo after 10 mg cocaine were obtained.

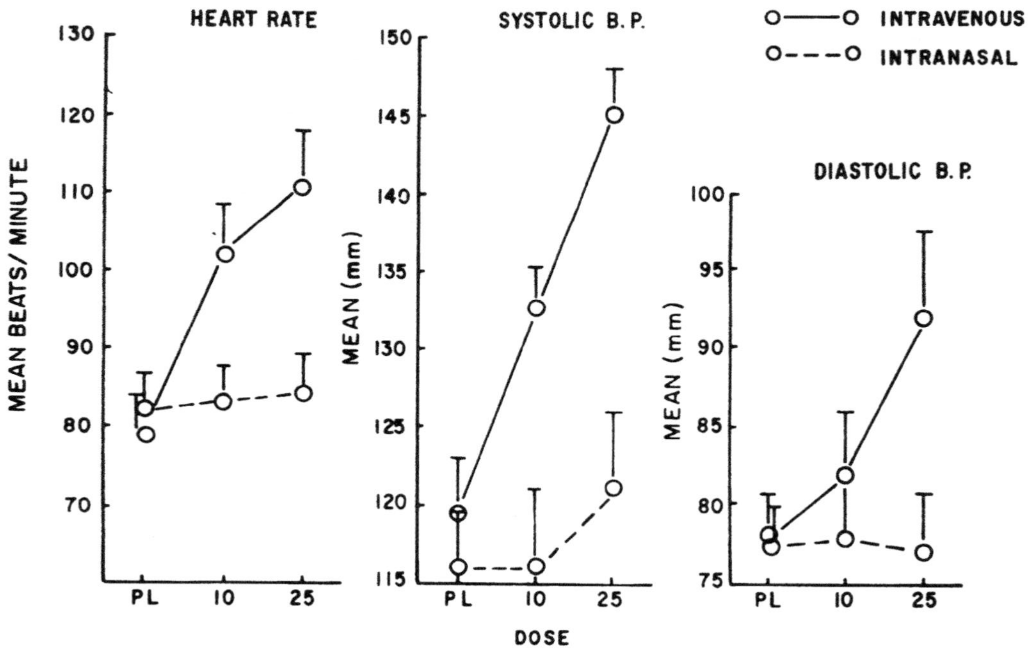

Fig. 1. Dose-response curves for the effects of placebo (Pl), 10 mg cocaine (10), and 25 mg cocaine (25) administered intravenously and intranasally on heart rate, systolic blood pressure, and diastolic blood pressure. Each point represents the mean of the peak responses after drug administration for 12 subjects. Vertical bars indicate the standard error of the mean.

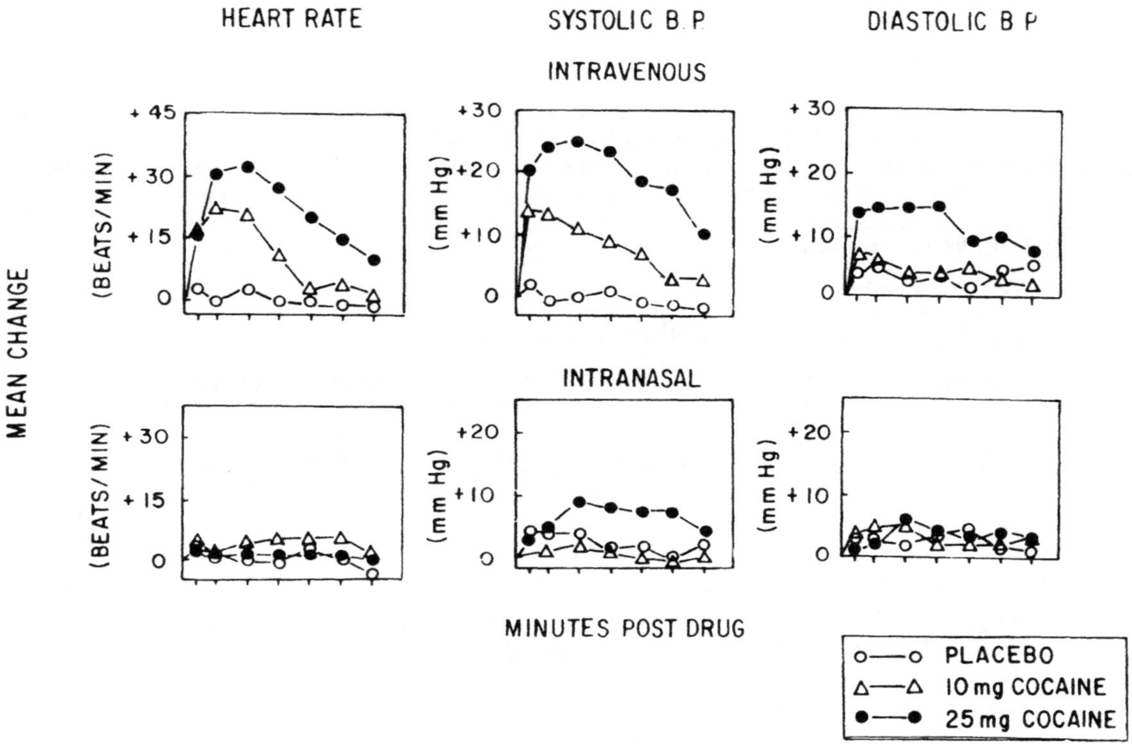

Fig. 2a. Time-course curves over a 30-min observation period for the psychologic effects of placebo, 10 mg, and 25 mg cocaine administered intravenously and intranasally. Each point represents the mean of 12 subjects, except for hand grip strength where each point represents the mean of four subjects.

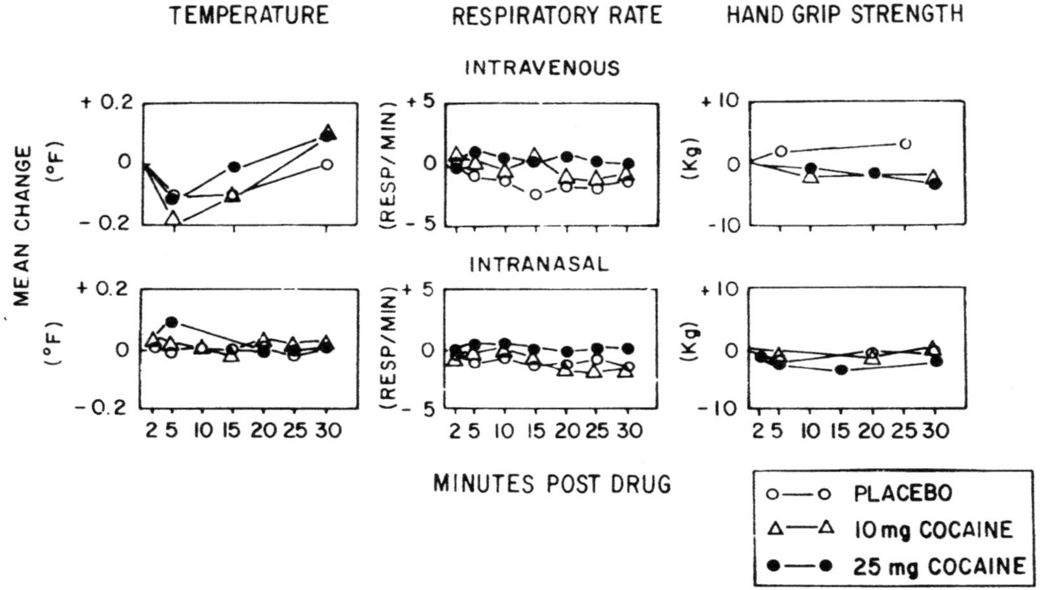

Fig. 2b. Time-course curves over a 30-min observation period for the psychologic effects of placebo, 10 mg, and 25 mg cocaine administered intravenously and intranasally. Each point represents the mean of 12 subjects, except for hand grip strength where each point represents the mean of four subjects.

Intravenous Route. Following intravenous cocaine, the following average increases compared to placebo occurred for 10 mg cocaine and 25 mg cocaine respectively: heart rate (+23 beats/min and +32 beats/min), systolic blood pressure (+13 mm and +26 mm), diastolic blood pressure (+5 mm and +14 mm). The 5 mm diastolic increase was not significant. There were no significant changes in respiratory rate, oral temperature, or hand grip strength following either dose of cocaine.

The onset of intravenous effects occurred within 2 min following the injection. Whereas the effects of 10 mg cocaine peaked at 2 to 5 min, 25 mg cocaine effects peaked somewhat later, 10 to 15 min following the injection.

Although 10 mg cocaine effects returned virtually to baseline within 20 to 25 min, 25 mg cocaine effects were still evident at 23% to 54% of their strength at the end of the 30-min observation period. Measurements taken on some subjects at 35 and 40 min showed decreasing effects that had not, however, returned to baseline levels.

The largest effects for individual subjects were as follows: at 10 mg, one subject's heart rate increased from 70 beats to 135 beats per min and another subject's blood pressure rose from 114/68 to 142/116; at 25 mg, one subject's heart rate went from 66 beats to 156 beats per min and another's blood pressure increased from 114/78 to 176/140.

Subjective Measurements (Figure 3)

Intranasal Route. Significant changes were observed following the 25 mg cocaine dose on the acute effects scale ($p < 0.02$), the scale of "high" ($p < 0.02$), and the scale of pleasantness ($p < 0.05$). These subjective effects peaked within 10 min and 54% to 68% of the effects were still evident at the end of the 30-min observation period. Subjects' reports indicated that the 25 mg dosage provided a very mild and somewhat pleasant experience. There were no significant changes following 25 mg on the scales measuring speeding, hunger, or strength. No significant differences were obtained after 10 mg cocaine.

Intravenous Route. Intravenous cocaine produced significant dose-related increases compared to placebo on each of the subjective measures except strength. The onset of these effects occurred within 2 min and peaked within 10 min.

Effects from the 10 mg dose returned to baseline within 15 min for the pleasantness scale and within 25 min for the "high," speeding, and hunger scales. Effects from 25 mg cocaine virtually

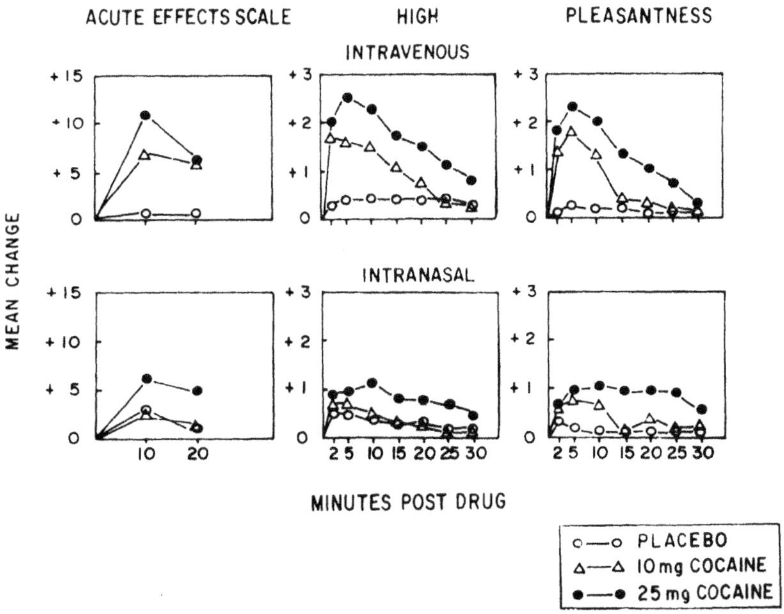

Fig. 3a. Time-course curves over a 30-min observation period for the subjective effects of placebo, 10 mg, and 25 mg cocaine administered intravenously and intranasally. Each point represents the mean of 12 subjects.

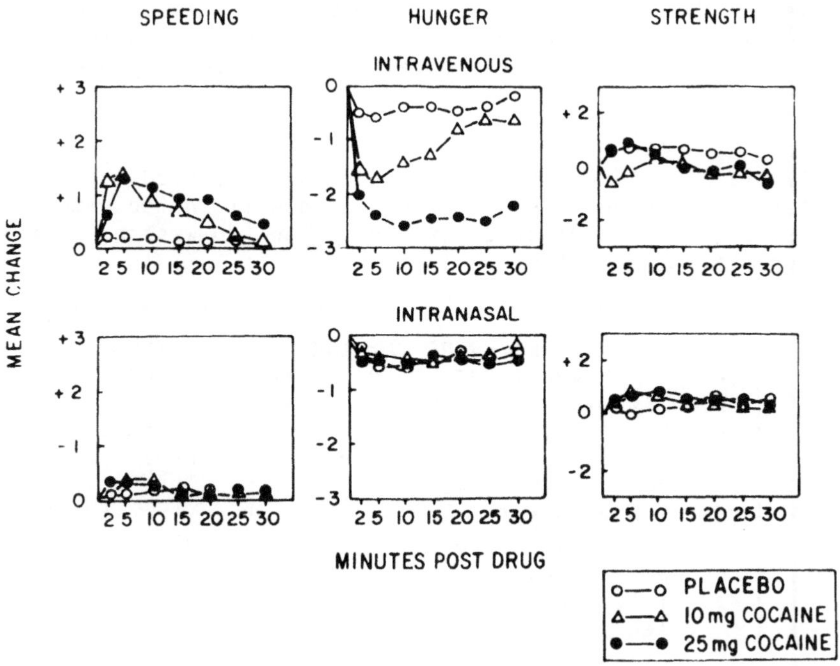

Fig. 3b. Time-course curves over a 30-min observation period for the subjective effects of placebo, 10 mg, and 25 mg cocaine administered intravenously and intranasally. Each point represents the mean of 12 subjects.

returned to baseline levels within 30 min on all scales except hunger. Anorexia persisted throughout the entire observation period. At 20 min after the larger dose of cocaine, the acute effects scale still showed 50% of the ratings obtained at 10 min.

Acute Effects Scale. Each of the 36 items on the Acute Effects Scale discriminated between placebo and at least one dosage of cocaine by one of the routes of administration. The nine items that were the best dose-related indicators of cocaine effects and also discriminated between the two routes of administration are listed in Table 1. The tenth item on the table was the most frequent spontaneous report of subjects. The four items that were most frequently rated "true" following cocaine are listed in Table 2, but

Table 1. Items 1 through 9 are the best dose-related Acute Effects indicators of cocaine effects which also discriminated between intravenous and intranasal adminstration. Item 10 was the most frequent spontaneous report of subjects.

1.	I have a pleasant feeling in my stomach.
2.	My thoughts come more easily than usual.
3.	I feel less discouraged than usual.
4.	My memory seems sharper to me than usual.
5.	I fear that I will lose the contentment that I have now.
6.	I have a weird feeling.
7.	Right now I feel as if all my needs are satisfied.
8.	I feel an increasing awareness of bodily sensations.
9.	I have a floating feeling.
10.	I feel more relaxed.

Table 2. Statements on the Acute Effects Scale that were rated "true" most frequently after administration of cocaine.

1.	I feel as if something pleasant had just happened to me.
2.	I am in the mood to talk about the feeling I have.
3.	A thrill has gone through me one or more times since I started the test.
4.	I feel like joking with someone.

Table 3. Statements on the Acute Effects Scale that were more frequently rated "true" following 10 mg than 25 mg intravenous cocaine.

1. I feel as if something pleasant had just happened to me.
2. I am in the mood to talk about the feeling I have.
3. I can completely appreciate what others are saying when I am in this mood.
4. I feel a very pleasant emptiness.
5. I feel so good that I know other people can tell it.
6. I feel like joking with someone.
7. I would be happy all the time if I felt as I feel now.

these did not show dose-related differences. A subset of seven statements from the original 36 were more frequently rated "true" following 10 mg than 25 mg intravenous cocaine (Table 3).

COMMENTS

The results of this study were that by the intranasal route 10 mg cocaine produced no changes different from placebo and 25 mg dose produced minimal changes only in systolic blood pressure and feelings of "high." When intravenously administered, however, both dosages of cocaine produced significant dose-related physiological and subjective responses.

We chose to administer the intranasal cocaine by solution because we believed this technique would be more likely to insure absorption of the doses administered. However, some subjects reported feeling the solution go down their throats; it is possible, therefore, that directly "snuffing" cocaine flakes would have resulted in a greater response at the same dosages.

The mean increase in systolic blood pressure after 25 mg intravenous cocaine was approximately the same as that observed after 20 mg oral d-amphetamine (Jasinski, Griffith, Carr, Gorodetzky, and Kullberg, 1974). The variablity between subjects was also similar: increases in systolic blood pressure after amphetamine ranged from +6 mm to +47 mm and after cocaine from +10 mm to +56 mm (Jasinski, personal communication).

There was a positive relationship between the mean magnitude and time-course of changes in blood pressure and heart rate and changes in subjective effects. This relationship, however, was not consistently found in each subject. Some individuals, particularly the more experienced cocaine users, rated subjective effects lower than others who had equally large physiologic changes.

Although the mean curves for pleasantness showed a marked increase following cocaine, one of the subjects reported an unpleasant experience together with a strong "high" after the 25 mg intravenous dose. This individual entered the experimental session feeling depressed. The observation of a dysphoric reaction after cocaine in a depressed subject is consistent with a report on the effects of cocaine in depressed patients (Post, Kotin, and Goodwin, 1974).

Four subjects reported that they felt mildly uncomfortable from symptoms of anxiety and depression 20 to 30 min after the 25 mg intravenous dose. One of these subjects had a similar feeling after the 10 mg intravenous dose. These effects persisted beyond the period of observation and were stated to be characteristic of "crashing" after cocaine.

Although mean ratings of pleasantness were higher after the larger dose of intravenous cocaine, the reverse was true for two out of the twelve subjects. Their experience was explained by the pronounced tachycardia following the higher dose which they did not like. The seven statements that were more frequently rated "true" on the Acute Effects Scale after the 10 mg than after the 25 mg dose appear to be items that reflect an increased interpersonal awareness and general pleasantness.

We found no evidence for the common belief that cocaine increases muscular strength; our measurements tended to show decreased strength after cocaine. The anorexia following cocaine persisted for a longer time than any of the other effects.

Systolic blood pressure appears to be the most sensitive correlate of subjective cocaine effects. The ten items listed in Table 1 best discriminate between dosages and routes of administration and may be a useful scale for further study of cocaine. It is hoped that the dose-response and time-course curves will provide information for additional explorations of systemic cocaine in man.

REFERENCES

Chambers, C.D., Taylor, W.J.R., and Moffet, A.D.: The incidence of cocaine abuse among methadone maintenance patients. Int. J. Addictions 7, 427-441 (1972).

Edmundson, W.T., Davies, J.E., Acker, J.D., and Myer, R.: Patterns of drug abuse epidemiology in prisoners, Ind. Med. Surg. 41, 15-19 (1972).

Ellinwood, E.H.: Amphetamine and stimulant drugs. In: Drug Use in America: Problem in Perspective (Second Report of the National Commission on Marijuana and Drug Abuse). Pp. 140-157. Washington: U.S. Government Printing Office, 1973.

Gay, G.R., Sheppard, C.W., Inaba, D.S., and Newmeyer, J.: An old girl: Flyin' low, dyin' slow, blinded by snow. Cocaine in perspective, Int. J. Addict. 8, 1027-1042 (1973).

Goodman, L.S. and Gilman, A.: The Pharmacological Basis of Therapeutics, 4th ed. New York: MacMillan, 1970.

Gossett, J.T., Lewis, J.M., and Phillips, V.A.: Extent and prevalence of illicit drug use as reported by 56,745 students, J. Am. med. Ass. 216, 1464-1470 (1971).

Gray, T.C. and Nunn, J.F., Eds.: General Anesthesia, 3rd ed. New York: Appleton-Century-Crofts, 1971.

Hill, E.H., Haertzen, C.A., Wolbach, A.B., and Miner, E.F.: The Addiction Research Center Inventory: Appendix, Psychopharmacologia 4, 184-205 (1963).

Jasinski, D.R., Griffith, J.D., Carr, C., Gorodetzky, C.W., and Kullberg, M.P.: Progress report from the Clinical Pharmacology Section of the Addiction Research Center. In: Committee on Problems of Drug Dependence. Pp. 88-115. Washington: National Research Council of the National Academy of Sciences, 1974.

Krupp, M.A. and Chatton, M.J.: Current Medical Diagnosis and Treatment. Los Altos, Calif.: Lange Medical Publications, 1974.

Lee, J.A.: Synopsis of Anesthesiology, 4th ed. Bristol, Great Britain: John Wright and Son, 1960.

Mayer, E.: The toxic effects following the use of local anesthetics: An analysis of 4 deaths submitted to the Committee for the Study of the Effects of Local Anesthetics of the A.M.A., J. Am. med. Ass. 82, 876-885 (1924).

Post, R.M., Kotin, J., and Goodwin, F.K.: The effects of cocaine on depressed patients, Am. J. Psychiat. 131, 511-517 (1974).

Smith, R.B.: Cocaine and catecholamine interaction, Arch. Otolar. 98, 139-141 (1973).

Sollman, T.: A Manual of Pharmacology and its Applications to Therapeutics and Toxicology, 7th ed., pp. 262-279. Philadelphia: W.B. Saunders, 1948.

Wood-Smith, F.G. and Stewart, H.C.: Drugs in Anaesthetic Practice. Washington: Butterworths, 1962.

COCAINE: BLOOD CONCENTRATION AND PHYSIOLOGICAL EFFECT AFTER INTRANASAL APPLICATION IN MAN

Robert Byck, Peter Jatlow, Paul Barash, and Craig Van Dyke

Yale University School of Medicine

333 Cedar Street, New Haven, Connecticut 06510

This paper reports preliminary results from a multidisciplinary study of the actions of cocaine in man. We are in the process of evaluating the relationship of blood concentrations of drug to physiological effect after intranasal application to man. This communication is divided into three parts. The first is a report of a method that allows determination of cocaine plasma concentrations reached after clinically effective doses in man (Jatlow and Bailey, 1975). The second part of the study is the presentation of the results of work with surgical patients who received cocaine as part of their ordinary clinical care (Van Dyke, Barash, Jatlow, and Byck, 1975). In these patients blood concentrations were determined after intranasal application of cocaine for anesthetic purposes. The third section of the paper reports blood concentrations found in normal subjects given cocaine as part of an experimental procedure in which a multiplicity of physiological measures are compared with the amount of cocaine present in the blood. Only preliminary physiological results are presented in this section. In addition we have studied the excretion of cocaine metabolites after intranasal application of various doses in surgical patients and experimental subjects and report the sensitivity of the EMIT method for detecting cocaine metabolites.

The study of a drug's actions ideally should consider these actions in relationship to available drug at the receptor site. In the past pharmacologists have used the dose of the drug administered as an indication of the relative amount of available drug. Recently, methods for determination of blood concentrations in animals and man have allowed a second approximation of the desired number. Estimation of plasma concentration of drug allows an investigator a more accurate method of determining the relationships of available drug to effect. Plasma concentration is nonetheless still one step removed from the final site of action. Diffusional barriers, plasma binding, plasma breakdown, receptor affinity, and other variables still remain as obstacles to the ideal.

Studies of the action of cocaine after its intranasal application are most useful if they can be related to plasma concentration of the drug. Because of its intense vasoconstrictor effect, cocaine is probably slowly absorbed from vascularized sites. Since cocaine is used both clinically and illicitly by intranasal application, it becomes pertinent to trace the sojourn of cocaine in the blood after administration by this route. The pattern of cocaine blood concentrations is important also because surgical procedures often are performed immediately after the application of cocaine. The actions of cocaine, if prolonged, may modify the physiological response to surgical procedures.

Cocaine has always been considered to be an evanescent drug. Street reports indicate that the "high" is intense, rapid in onset, and brief in duration. We know, however, from biochemical studies, that cocaine has other actions beyond its immediate intense sympathomimetic effects (Van Dyke and Byck, 1975). For example, cocaine blocks reuptake of amines in the periphery and perhaps in the central nervous system. What, then, can account for the pattern of effects of cocaine? Is the drug brief in its actions because its sojourn in the blood is short; or, alternatively, does it have a long action because its effects, after binding to receptor sites, are prolonged even though the blood concentrations are high for only a short period? In order to investigate these questions, we first developed a method for determination of plasma concentrations of cocaine. In the past plasma assays of low concentrations of cocaine could be accomplished only by gas-liquid chromatography - mass fragmentography (see Hawkes, quoted in Post, 1974). The following method utilizes a sensitive nitrogen detector in conjunction with gas-liquid chromatography.

ANALYTIC METHOD

Plasma concentrations of cocaine were determined by gas chromatography. Since it is difficult to measure drug concentrations of less than 100 ng/ml with a conventional flame ionization detector, we used a selective nitrogen (alkali flame) detector which allowed a significant increase in sensitivity and selectivity and permitted the analysis of cocaine in plasma at concentrations as low as 5 ng/ml.

Materials and Methods

We used a model 3920 Perkin Elmer Gas Chromatograph with a nitrogen phosphorous detector. The operating conditions used were as follows: a 1.8 meter by 2 mm ID glass column was packed with 3% OV-17 on 100-120 mesh gas chrome Q. The carrier gas was helium and air flow rates were 20 ml/min, 400 ml/min, and 1 ml/min, respectively. The injector, column, and detector temperatures were 280, 260, and 300°C, respectively. The rubidium silicate glass bead detector temperature was approximately 350-400°C. Low hydrogen flow rates were required for the nitrogen detector. All glassware was soaked overnight in HCl and rinsed with heptane/isoamyl alcohol before use.

All reagents were AR grade. Methanol, isoamyl alcohol, and heptane were redistilled in glass and the heptane was subsequently passed through alumina. After purification 5 ml of heptane containing 2% isoamyl alcohol was evaporated and the residue, dissolved in methanol, was chromatographed to check for interfering peaks. Solid sodium carbonate-sodium bicarbonate buffer mixture was prepared by combining 20 parts of sodium carbonate with 17½ parts of sodium bicarbonate. Seven hundred mg of this mixture was added to 10 ml of water to prepare the aqueous buffer. Stock standards of 10 ml of cocaine base dissolved in 10 ml of methanol were prepared and found to be stable indefinitely. Plasma standards were made by adding diluted stock standards of drug-free plasma in various concentrations to establish the linearity of the technique. In all studies standards were prepared in the subjects' own zero time (pre-drug) plasma. The n-propyl ester of benzoylecgonine was used as the internal standard. This cocaine homologue (cocaine is the methyl ester of benzoylecgonine) was synthesized in our laboratory (Jatlow and Bailey, 1975). The internal standard was diluted with n-propanol to provide a concentration corresponding in peak area to a cocaine concentration of about 100 mg/liter, and stored in dilute form at -15°C. Forty µcl of dilute internal standard was added to each 100 ml of heptane/isoamyl alcohol prepared for the initial extraction. This provided approximately 200 ng of internal standard per ml of plasma extracted.

The heparinized specimens were collected in glass syringes and placed on ice immediately. In later experiments sodium fluoride in a final plasma concentration of 0.129 w/v was added to the samples in order to prevent esterase breakdown of the cocaine present in plasma. Two ml of plasma, 0.5 ml of carbonate buffer, and 10 ml heptane/isoamyl alcohol (50/1) containing internal standard were placed into 15 ml glass-stoppered centrifuge tubes. After an extraction for 2-3 min and centrifugation at 2000 rpm, the upper solvent layer was transferred to a clean 15 ml centrifuge tube. One ml of 0.1N H_2SO_4 was added and extraction for 2-3 min was carried out. After centrifugation the solvent was aspirated and discarded. After washing with heptane/isoamyl alcohol (without internal standard), the solvent was discarded. Solid buffer was added to the aqueous phase which was re-extracted with 2 ml of heptane/isoamyl alcohol. The aqueous phase was discarded after centrifugation, and the solvent was dried over sodium sulphate and evaporated under nitrogen at room temperature. The residue was then dissolved in 10 ml of ethanol and 2 ml of this sample was chromatographed. The coefficient of variation (standard deviation/mean) of the procedure at 100 ng/ml cocaine concentration was 3%. Measurements on drug-free plasma showed background levels corresponding to cocaine concentrations of 0.5 - 2.0 ng/ml. In order to rule out the possibility of interfering peaks from other drugs, we tested the benzodiazepines, common antihistamines, chlorpromazine, morphine, methadone, propoxyphine, codeine, amphetamine, caffeine, nicotine, and commonly used local anesthetics (procaine, lidocaine, and carbocaine), all of which showed no interference. Methaqualone had the same relative retention time as cocaine. Pentazocaine, desipramine, nortriptyline, and atropine had retention times close to that of cocaine but could be resolved from it. Norcocaine also could be resolved from the cocaine peak.

It is particularly important in using this procedure to use glassware that is free of contaminants. For example, plasma in contact with rubber stoppers, such as those found with Vacutainers (Becton-Dickinson), showed one or more nonspecific interfering peaks. Reagent-grade and even "chromatographic-grade" solvents yielded interfering peaks of varying size. For this reason the heptane was redistilled and passed through alumina before use, and all specimens were collected with heparinized glass syringes. We found that Coca Cola (R) ("the real thing") did not interfere with the assay even if it was chromatographed.

Preliminary studies have indicated that the same analytic procedures can be applied to urine without alteration. However, one should note that the concentration of benzoylecgonine, the principal cocaine metabolite in urine, is far greater than that of the parent drug. Benzoylecgonine is not extracted by this procedure.

SURGICAL PATIENTS

The first application of this technique for determination of plasma concentrations was to use two groups of surgical patients and evaluate in them the concentrations reached after intranasal application for therapeutic purposes of intubation. Cocaine is by no means an outmoded drug in surgery. It is used both for its local anesthetic action and for its intense vasoconstrictor action. It is advantageous to be able to pass intratracheal tubes without excessive bleeding and the vasoconstrictor effect assists in this procedure. Operations in the area of the nasal mucosa are often done with cocaine because of its prolonged duration of action and its ability to minimize bleeding. Nonetheless, restrictions on investigation of cocaine, which have largely been psychological rather than legal, have prevented us from learning very much about its actions even under circumstances of surgery. The following study presents data from two groups of patients who were later given general anesthetics; and the data, although pertinent clinically, may represent a net effect of pathological processes, drug interaction, and surgical manipulations as well as the normal uptake and distribution of cocaine in the blood after intranasal application.

Methods

Subjects were 9 patients undergoing cardiovascular surgery (CV patients) and 4 patients undergoing dental surgery (dental patients) who were informed about the study and agreed to participate. A 10% solution of cocaine hydrochloride (1.5 mg/kg) was applied topically to their nasal mucosa prior to nasal intubation. All patients received diazepam (10 mg/70 kg) and morphine sulfate (10 mg/70 kg) intramuscularly 1 hour prior to general anesthesia. The CV patients were given intravenous (i.v.) diazepam or sodium pentothal and either succinylcholine or pancuronium bromide for muscle relaxation, while the dental patients were given i.v. sodium pentothal and succinylcholine. Both groups received nitrous oxide and halothane as maintenance anesthetics.

In all patients we obtained 10 ml blood samples before application and at 10, 15, 20, and 60 minutes after application of cocaine. We obtained additional blood samples at 3 and 6 minutes in 8 patients to detect any early peak values, which otherwise might have been missed. No samples were collected from CV patients after they were placed on cardio-pulmonary bypass since this markedly increased their blood volume and would have rendered subsequent plasma levels invalid. For this reason we do not have plasma levels in these patients beyond 4 hours after cocaine application. We obtained samples from dental patients for as long as 6 hours after drug application. All blood samples were immediately placed in ice and transported to the laboratory where the plasma was separated and analyzed with minimal delay.

Results

Plasma concentrations of cocaine increased rapidly for 15-20 minutes, peaked at 15-60 minutes, and then decreased gradually over the next 3-5 hours (Figs. 1 and 2). Cocaine was measurable in the

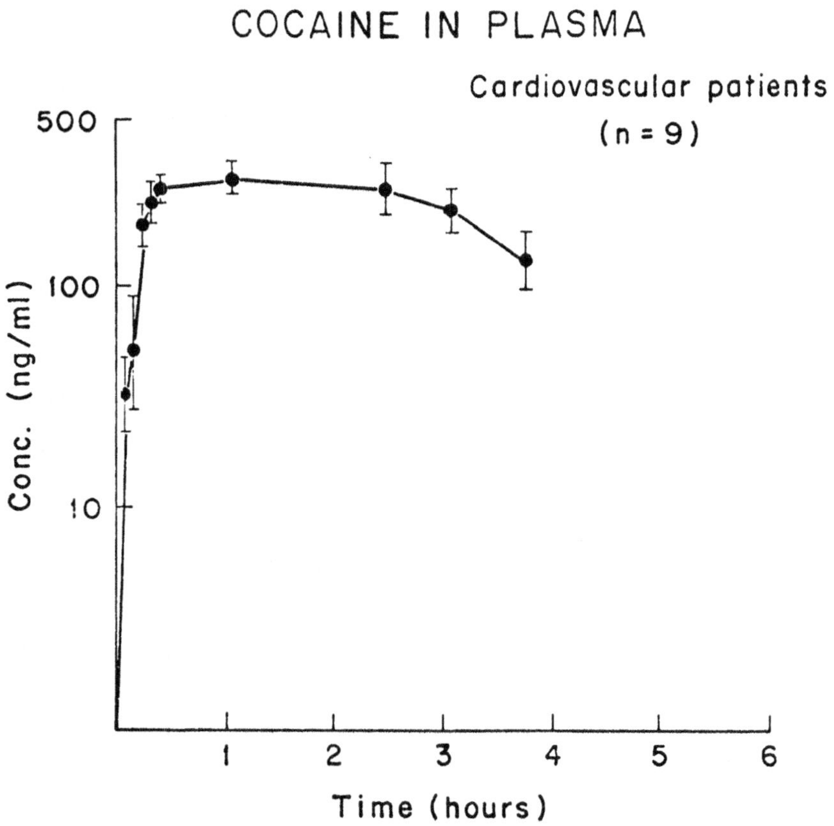

Fig. 1. Semi-logarithmic representation of cocaine hydrochloride plasma concentration time-course for cardiovascular patients. Values at 10, 15, 20, and 60 minutes are the mean for 9 patients ± SE. Values at other times are based on fewer patients.

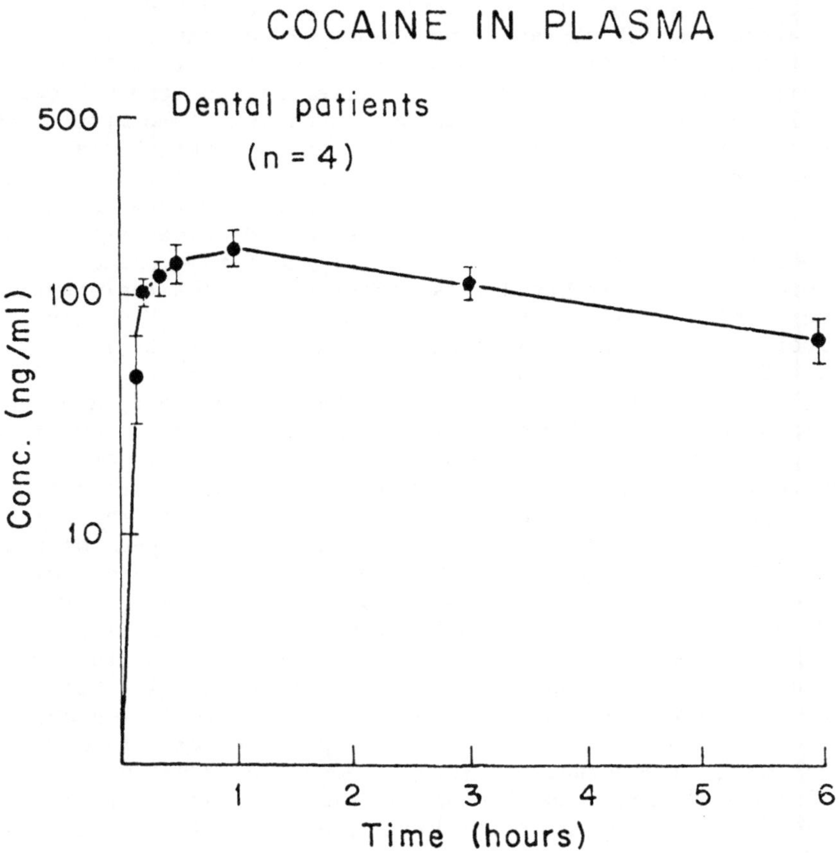

Fig. 2. Semi-logarithmic representation of cocaine hydrochloride plasma concentration time-course for dental patients. Values at 10, 15, 20, and 60 minutes are the mean for 4 patients ± SE. Values at other times are based on 3 patients.

blood within 3 minutes and for as long as 6 hours after application. Maximum plasma concentrations ranged from 120 ng/ml to 474 ng/ml calculated as the free base.

The maximum plasma concentrations of CV patients were significantly greater than the maximum plasma concentrations of dental patients ($p = 0.001$ Mann-Whitney two sample test). A number of factors could explain this difference. Arterial blood samples were obtained from CV patients and venous blood samples were obtained from dental patients. To ascertain whether this affected our results, we compared simultaneous arterial and venous blood samples in cardiovascular patients on 2 occasions (a 3-minute sample and a 60-minute sample) and found a venous-arterial plasma level ratio of 0.84 and 0.98, respectively. Other investigators (E. Erikssen, S. Englessen, S. Wahlquist, and B. Ortengren, 1966) found that the peripheral venous-arterial blood concentration ratio for lidocaine was 0.73 ± 0.03 (mean ± SE) and for priolocaine was 0.47 ± 0.03. They attributed this difference to the rapid uptake of these local anesthetics by skeletal muscle. The CV patients were older (52.1 ± 2.9 years, mean ± standard error [SE]) and heavier (76.1 ± 4.9 kg) than the dental patients (33.2 ± 11.4 years, 66.5 ± 2.0 kg). Similarly, Berkowitz, Ngai, Yang, Hempstead, and Spector (1975) reported that older patients had higher plasma concentrations following the same dosage of morphine sulfate. The CV patients also had abnormal cardiovascular function with lowered cardiac output. In fact 4 patients were in congestive heart failure at the time of surgery, and 3 of these 4 patients had the 3 highest peak plasma levels. Other investigators (Halkin, Meffin, Melmon, and Rowland, 1975; Stenson, Constantino, and Harrison, 1971; Thomson, Melmon, Richardson, Cohn, Steinbrunn, Cudihee, and Rowland, 1973) reported that peak plasma levels of lidocaine following i.v. administration were significantly increased in patients with congestive heart failure. This was attributed to decreased liver perfusion and a slower rate of lidocaine metabolism. CV patients also received different drugs preoperatively (e.g., isosorbide dinitrate and digitalis) and during induction of anesthesia. These agents might alter the distribution, protein binding, or metabolism of cocaine. The *in vitro* half life of cocaine in human plasma at 37°C was about 30 minutes. Our preliminary data suggest that plasma cholinesterase is responsible for the observed rapid hydrolysis of cocaine. Both neostigmine and physostigmine (eserine) prevented the *in vitro* hydrolysis of cocaine in human plasma. Plasma from a patient with a history of succinylcholine sensitivity, with low serum cholinesterase activity and a low dibucaine number, also failed to hydrolyze cocaine. Any drugs (e.g., succinylcholine) or chronic clinical conditions that alter the activity of this enzyme might, theoretically, affect the rate of cocaine metabolism.

Our finding that cocaine persisted in the plasma for 4-6 hours was unexpected in view of the reports by street users and by Adriani and Campbell (1956, 1958; Adriani, 1960) but was consistent with the reports of Woods, Cochin, Fornefeld, McMahon, and Seevers (1951) and Woods, McMahon, and Seevers (1951). To ascertain whether this might be caused by prolonged absorption, we obtained swabs (cotton wetted with normal saline) of the nasal mucosa from 5 patients 1, 2, and 3 hours after cocaine application. These swabs were then eluted and analyzed by thin-layer chromatography (TLC). The swabs were eluted with 0.1N H_2SO_4. The aqueous phase was adjusted to pH 9.6-9.8 with carbonate buffer, and extracted with ether. The ether was evaporated and the residue was analyzed by the use of thin-layer chromatography using ethyl acetate:methanol: ammonia (85:10:5) and sprayed with potassium iodoplatinate. Compounds with the same Rf as cocaine were identified in the 1, 2, and 3 hour nasal swabs from these patients. In 2 patients the spots were eluted from the TLC plates, submitted to GLC, and yielded a single peak with the same relative retention time as cocaine. The presence of cocaine on the nasal mucosa for 3 hours after application suggested that prolonged absorption of cocaine, perhaps as a result of its vasoconstrictive action, might explain its persistence in plasma. This was consistent with the results of Nayak, Misra, and Mulé (1974 and 1975) and Misra, Nayak, Patel, Vadlamani, and Mulé (1974), who found in rats that, after a 20 mg/kg s.c. dose, there was 27.7% of the dose remaining at the site 1 hour after injection and 8.8% remaining after 4 hours.

The cocaine plasma concentrations in dental patien s (Fig. 2) peaked at approximately 60 minutes and then decreased in a log-. linear fashion over the next 5 hours with an apparent plasma half-life of 3.8 hours. Since cocaine remained on the nasal mucosa for 3 hours, this probably did not represent a true biologic half-life but rather represented a combination of absorption and elimination Similarly, Nayak et al. (1974 and 1975) and Misra et al. (1974) found the plasma half-life of cocaine in rats was 4.99 hours following a 20 mg/kg SC dose.

The peak plasma concentrations occurred later than the time of maximum euphoria reported by street users. These reports indicated peak psychological highs within 3-5 minutes of application and almost no effect 15 minutes after application. In fact, individuals who abuse cocaine may repeat the dosages every 15 minutes to maintain the psychological effect. In our study, the peak plasma concentrations occurred about 60 minutes after application and it is possible that the intense euphoria from cocaine may be related to the rapidly increasing plasma levels of cocaine and not to peak values. Alternatively, since cocaine is highly lipid soluble, the euphoria may better correlate with concentrations at brain receptor sites than peak plasma concentrations. Nayak et al. (1974 and 1975) and Misra et al. (1974) found significant concentrations of cocaine and its active metabolite, norcocaine, in the brains of rats following i.v. (8 mg/kg) and s.c. (20 mg/kg) injections.

NORMAL SUBJECTS

The purpose of the experiment was to correlate blood concentrations with physiological changes after intranasal drug administration. Since, at this time, we are in the middle of a series of experiments based on a Latin square design, we present here the blood concentration data from only a single dose in 4 individuals. We will comment on our impressions of the physiological effects without presenting statistically analyzed data.

Methods

The subjects were normal individuals with a moderately heavy prior use of cocaine. All were male and over 21. Their weights were all close to 70 kg so that the dosages, although expressed on a mg/kg basis, were quite similar in all individuals. They had been previously screened and demonstrated to be in good health. All had normal electrocardiograms and electroencephalograms. Their psychological status was evaluated by 2 psychiatrists and by a psychiatric nurse clinician as well as by the Minnesota Multiphasic Personality Inventory. The subjects were selected by recruiting volunteers who had no knowledge of the purposes of the study but knew only that it was involved with "illicit drugs." It was not until the entire medical and psychological screening procedure was completed that the subjects were informed the experiment would be with intranasal cocaine. Each subject had a one-hour session with the principal investigator during which the consent form was explained to them. The possible complications involved in the use of cocaine were explained and the subjects were encouraged to question all portions of the experiment. Only after the consent form was fully understood and the general principles of the experiment were recognized was the subject permitted to sign the consent form.

The problem of informed consent to an experiment such as this is a very serious one. It is clear that both agencies and institutional committees look with extreme caution at experiments involved with drugs of abuse. Cocaine, because of its reputation as a dangerous drug and because of the legal problems involved with its use (it is classified as a narcotic under law), is perhaps one of the trickiest drugs to work with in terms of human experimentation. We spent approximately one year clearing the permissions and various consent forms through the requisite committees. Problems in maintaining confidentiality in subjects in such an experiment are also immense. Although our subjects have used cocaine, they were generally middle class and college educated. They were not from a group of drug abusers in constant trouble with the law. Because of this, we felt the major risk to our subjects was the possibility of their being recognized by peers from their social group, who were unaware of the subjects' illicit drug usage. Precautions had to be taken to maintain their anonymity and to minimize the number of people knowing the study's purpose. Various procedures to be detailed elsewhere (Byck, unpublished data) were used to insure that they could not be identified either by their hospital records or by any of the normal methods of tracking down the identity of patients.

The subjects were admitted to the General Clinical Research Unit of Yale-New Haven Hospital for an overnight stay. This in itself represented many difficulties. They were the only "normal" subjects on the floor that is largely devoted to the treatment of cancer by experimental chemotherapy. Subjects were informed that the maintenance of their anonymity was to a great extent dependent on themselves. The nursing staff knew the purpose of the experiment but was not informed about the screening criteria necessary to admit subjects to the study.

The following physiological variables were measured in the first 6 hours of each experiment: eight lead electroencephalogram, five lead electrocardiogram, temperature via the auricular canal (core body temperature), heart rate, blood pressure via an ultra sound monitoring device, and pupillary size by means of an infrared pupillography device. Electrocardiograms were taken for the next 16 hours by a portable ECG recorder (Hitman Medcraft). During the course of the experiment urine was collected for measurement of MHPG and steroid excretion. Various blood samples for cocaine blood concentration MHPG, serum prolactin, growth hormone, and cortisol were drawn during the course of the experiment and urine was collected for 48 hours following the experiment in order to examine the excretion of cocaine as detectable by the EMIT method. The physiological and chemical measures will be reported elsewhere. Mood Adjective (Zuckerman, Lubin, Vogel, and Valerius, 1964) check lists, "high scales", and the amphetamine, barbiturate, and morphine scales of the Addiction Research Center Inventory (Hill, Haertzen, Wolbach, and Miner, 1963) were administered at set intervals. Cocaine was analyzed by the method described above and results were as follows.

Results

Cocaine was given by instillation into the nose in a 10% solution in doses of 0.19, 0.38, 0.75, and 1.5 mg/kg. Data from 4 subjects who received a dose of 0.38 mg/kg are shown in Fig. 3. Individual curves are presented to show both the similarities in these curves and the relationship in excretion time to that of the surgical patients. It is obvious that the concentrations reached were not as high as those in the patients in whom a considerably higher dose had been administered. The drop-off rate of the cocaine plasma concentrations after the peak is somewhat more rapid than that seen in the surgical patients. In the few subjects for whom we have analyzed concentration curves after doses equivalent to those given in the surgical patients, there does appear to be a difference both in the peak concentration reached and in the drop-off rate although the estimated plasma half-lives are still consistent. At the lower dosages, peak concentrations were obtained between 15-60 minutes after administration of cocaine. Subjects reported highs somewhat earlier than the onset of the peak plasma concentration and the "high" (measured on a 7 point scale) for the 0.38 mg/kg dose never achieved a rating higher than "as good as usual" (subject's usual dose of cocaine).

All doses of cocaine failed to produce a discernible effect on measures of cardiovascular function. Occasionally, the blood pressure or heart rate increased, but this seemed to be related more to the psychological events accompanying the experiment than to the action of the drug. Our preliminary impression is that pupillary size changed when cocaine was administered in doses of 0.75 or 1.5 mg/kg but not at the lower dosages. It is clear that any statistically significant changes seen after intranasal application of cocaine in the doses used were of such a small degree as to be clinically insignificant. One observation which is worth noting was that many subjects fell asleep approximately 2 to 3 hours after drug administration. Whether this is a reliable finding will have to await computer analysis of the power spectrum of electroencephalographic records.

On all subjects the urinary excretion of benzoylecgonine, the major metabolite of cocaine, was monitored with the EMIT system. Preliminary results indicated that benzoylecgonine excretion may be detectable for as long as 36 hours after intranasal administration. There was an indication that the duration of excretion was dose dependent. The results from both the normal subject study and the surgical patient study will be reported separately.

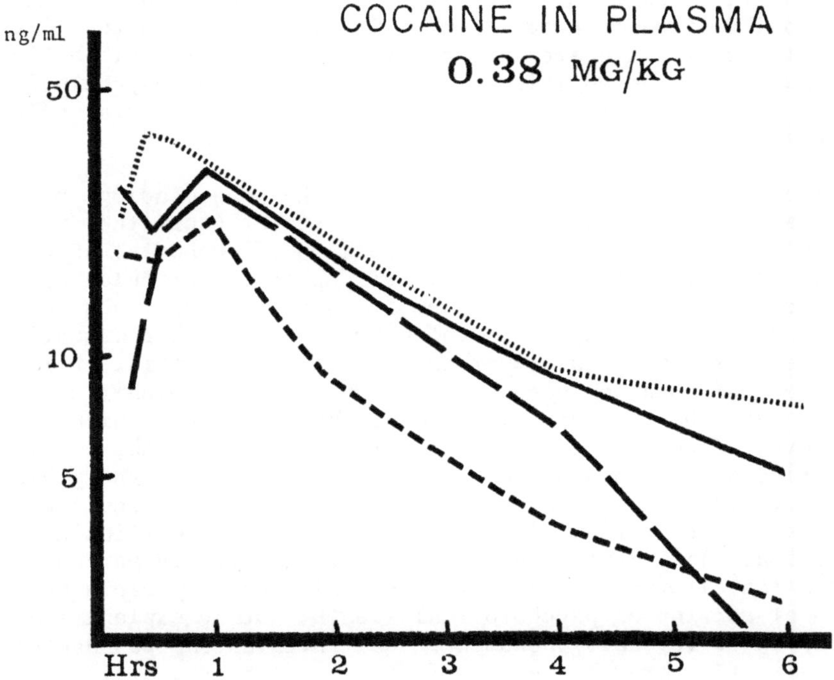

Fig. 3. Concentration of cocaine in plasma of four normal volunteers after intranasal administration of 0.38 mg/kg. Time in hours.

Discussion

The primary findings in this study indicate that, after a single intranasal dose, cocaine reached its peak plasma concentration between 15 to 60 minutes after administration, then had a prolonged sojourn in the blood before it was finally eliminated. We find that it is a drug that is absorbed more slowly than expected and eliminated for several hours after administration. In these dosages cocaine did not appear to have any major physiological effect. Onset of the psychological high preceded peak concentrations in the plasma. Cocaine may be hydrolyzed in the plasma by pseudocholinesterase in addition to its metabolism in the liver. All of these findings are in opposition to commonly held beliefs about cocaine. The addition of other, unanalyzed, psychological and physiological data may shed further light on the real effects of cocaine.

The pertinence of these studies to the phenomenology of drug abuse is somewhat limited. Frequently, street users take repeated doses of cocaine to sustain their feelings of euphoria. From our data we would expect a sequential buildup in the circulating blood concentration of cocaine and it is surprising to us that street users do not report a continuous high but keep reporting evanescent psychological experiences. In view of this, it is possible that cocaine, because of its high lipid solubility, is rapidly taken up by brain tissue, thereby providing a high effective level of cocaine to the receptors. Initially, the concentration of cocaine at brain receptor sites might exceed the plasma cocaine concentration. Over the next 1-2 hours, cocaine concentrations in the brain would fall as they reached equilibrium with the plasma. This cannot be tested experimentally in man but remains a tantalizing possibility to explain the very rapid and short action of cocaine on psychological events. Other explanations have been advanced for this phenomena: one involves the passage of cocaine directly through the cribiform plate into the brain. Another possibility is that the effect is secondary to rate of change rather than the absolute blood concentration of cocaine. Which of these, in fact, accounts for the phenomena remains to be determined. In the course of these experiments, we have seen a longer effect of cocaine on psychological functions than we expected. The subjective "high" extends for a longer period than is ordinarily described. Whether this is peculiar to our experimental conditions is yet to be determined.

IMPLICATIONS FOR FUTURE RESEARCH

It is clear that additional research must be undertaken. Repeat doses by the intranasal route should be studied to determine whether there is a significant buildup in the plasma concentrations of cocaine and whether this higher concentration of cocaine, if it does occur, is related to psychological effect. There is a possibility that the persistent vasoconstriction following the initial application of cocaine will limit the absorption and effect of subsequent applications. This remains to be investigated. Here we have reported the preliminary results for one part of the study. The report of the entire study perhaps will shed a greater light on the clinical pharmacology of cocaine.

The characterization of cocaine in relation to amphetamine and other drugs is a necessary next step. Our observation of a sedative effect must be dispelled or confirmed. The characterization of the central nervous system effects of other local anesthetics is also necessary for our understanding of cocaine.

Knowledge of the pharmacokinetics of cocaine by other routes of administration is needed. These data will give us a better idea of the *in vivo* metabolism of cocaine and may provide a more effective treatment of adverse reactions.

ACKNOWLEDGMENTS

This research was supported in part by Burroughs-Wellcome Fund, National Institute on Drug Abuse contract ADM 45-74-164, Clinical Research Center Grant FR 00125 from USPHS, and by a Research Support Grant from Yale University.

We thank Ms. Barbara Clinton, R.N., project coordinator, for her invaluable aid; Mr. Steven Record and Barry Margolin, Ph.D., for their assistance in data processing; Mr. Joel Radding for his technical assistance; and G.L. Hammond, M.D., V.B. Khachane, M.D., C.T. Sasake, M.D., and H.R. Sleeper, D.D.S., for their cooperation.

REFERENCES

Adriani, J.: The clinical pharmacology of local anesthetics, Clin. Pharmacol. Therap. 1, 645-673 (1960).

Adriani, J. and Campbell, D.: The absorption of topically applied tetracaine and cocaine, Laryncoscope, St. Louis 68, 65-72 (1958).

Adriani, J. and Campbell, D.: Fatalities following topical application of local anesthetics to mucous membranes, J. Am. med. Ass. 162, 1527-1530 (1956).

Berkowitz, B.A., Nagai, S.H., Yang, J.C., Hempstead, J., and Spector, S.: The disposition of morphine in surgical patients, Clin. Pharmacol. Therap. 17, 629-635 (1975).

Campbell, D. and Adriani, J.: Absorption of local anesthetics, J. Am. med. Ass. 168, 873-877 (1958).

Erikssen, E., Englessen, S., Wahlquist, S., and Ortengren, B.: Study of the intravenous toxicity [of prilocaine] in man and some *in vitro* studies on the distribution and absorbability, Acta Chir. Scand. 358, Suppl. 25 (1966).

Halkin, H., Meffin, P., Melmon, K.L., and Rowland, M.: Influence of congestive heart failure on blood levels of lidocaine and its active monodeethylated metabolite, Clin. Pharmacol. Therap. 17, 669-676 (1975).

Hill, E.H., Haertz, C.A., Wolbach, A.B., and Miner, E.J.: The Addiction Research Center Inventory: Appendix, Psychopharmacologia Berl. 4, 184-205 (1963).

Jatlow, P.I. and Bailey, D.N.: Gas-chromatographic analysis for cocaine in human plasma with use of a nitrogen detector, Clin. Chem. 21, 1918-1921 (1975).

Misra, A.L., Nayak, P.K., Patel, M.N., Vadlamini, N.L., and Mulé, S.J.: Identification of norcocaine as a metabolite of [^{3}H]-cocaine in rat brain, Experientia 30, 1312-1314 (1974).

Nayak, P.K., Misra, A.L., and Mulé, S.J.: Physiologic disposition and metabolism of [^{3}H]-cocaine in the rat, Fed. Proc. 33, 527 (1974).

Nayak, P.K., Misra, A.L., and Mulé, S.J.: Physiological disposition and biotransformation of [^{3}H]-cocaine in acute and chronically-treated rats, Fed. Proc. 34, 781 (1975).

Post, R.M., Kotin, J., and Goodwin, F.K.: The effects of cocaine on depressed patients, Am. J. Psychiat. 131(5), 511-517 (1974).

Stenson, R.E., Constantino, R.T., and Harrison, D.C.: Interrelationships of hepatic blood flow, cardiac output, and blood levels of lidocaine in man, Circulation 43, 205-211 (1971).

Thomson, P.D., Melmon, K.L., Richardson, J.A., Cohn, K., Steinbrunn, W., Cudihee, R., and Rowland, M.: Lidocaine pharmacokinetics in advanced heart failure, liver disease and renal failure in humans, Ann. intern. Med. 78, 499-508 (1973).

Van Dyke, C., Barash, P., Jatlow, P., and Byck, R.: Cocaine: Plasma concentrations after intranasal application in man, Science, in press.

Van Dyke, C. and Byck, R.: Cocaine: 1884 - 1974. In: Cocaine and Other Stimulants. Ellinwood, E.H., Jr. and Kilbey, M.M., Eds. New York: Plenum Press, 1976.

Woods, L.A., Cochin, J., Fornefeld, E.J., McMahon, F.G., and Seevers, M.H.: The estimation of amines in biological materials with critical data for cocaine and mescaline, J. Pharmac. exp. Ther. 101, 188-199 (1951).

Woods, L.A., McMahon, F.G., and Seevers, M.H.: Distribution and metabolism of cocaine in the dog and rabbit, J. Pharmac. exp. Ther. 101, 200-204 (1951).

Zuckerman, M., Lubin, B., Vogel, L., and Valerius, E.: Measurement of experimentally induced effects, J. Cons. Psychol. 28, 418-425 (1964).

PHYSIOLOGICAL AND BEHAVIORAL EFFECTS OF INTRAVENOUS COCAINE IN MAN

Marian W. Fischman, Charles R. Schuster, and Norman A. Krasnegor*

Departments of Psychiatry and Pharmacological and Physiological Sciences, Pritzker School of Medicine, The University of Chicago, Chicago, IL 60637

*National Institute on Drug Abuse, Rockville, MD 20852

Although the pharmacology of cocaine has been studied in infra-human organisms, there have been few studies of its physiological effects in humans, and no systematic studies of its behavioral effects in man. This is true despite the fact that over the past few years there has been an increase in the incidence of abuse of cocaine in this country. Most of the information we now have about the effects of cocaine in man is anecdotal in nature and not based upon scientific investigations.

Cocaine is a unique drug in that it is both a local anesthetic and a sympathomimetic with powerful central nervous system stimulant effects. Like other psychomotor stimulant drugs, such as the amphetamines, it can produce psychological dependence, but does not appear to cause any physical dependence. Unlike those drugs, however, there does not seem to be a development of tolerance to any of its effects and, in fact, it was suggested by Tatum and Seevers (1929) that rabbits, dogs, monkeys, and man all develop a supersensitivity to the behavioral and physiological effects of cocaine. Recent research with monkeys (Matsuzaki, Misra, and Mulé, 1975; Post and Kopanda, in press) and cats (Teeters, Koppanyi, and Cowan, 1963) as well as evidence from the street (Gay, Sheppard, Inaba, and Newmeyer, 1973) support the possibility of an increased sensitivity to some of the physiological and euphoric effects of cocaine after repeated use. On the other hand, both Hatch and Fischer (1972), measuring gross behavioral changes in dogs after 10 weekly cocaine injections, and Gunne and Johnsson (1964), measuring both gross behavior and urinary catecholamine levels in rats, failed to find evidence for the development of either tolerance or supersensitivity.

Cocaine and d-amphetamine appear to share many of the same characteristics, and, in fact, are frequently considered as being in the same drug class, with amphetamine discussed as the prototype (Jaffe, 1975). The toxic syndrome seen after prolonged use of cocaine is clinically similar to that seen after long-term amphetamine use (Kramer, Fischman, and Littlefield, 1967; Jaffe, 1975). It includes bruxism, enhanced sense of physical and mental capacity, anorexia, picking on the face and extremities, stereotyped repetitious behavior patterns and mild paranoia. The similarity of these two drugs has been supported also by data collected from infrahumans that indicate that both cocaine and d-amphetamine can serve as reinforcers to maintain lever press responding (Balster and Schuster, 1973; Wilson, Hitomi, and Schuster, 1971). In addition, rhesus monkeys given free access to these drugs self-inject them with similar patterns of intake (Johanson, Balster, and Bonese, in press), and similar toxic syndromes are produced by high doses of either of these drugs (Deneau, Yanagita, and Seevers, 1969; Fischman and Schuster, 1975). The similarities in physiological and subjective effects, gross behavioral changes, and patterns of intake lend credence to the idea that cocaine and the amphetamines may similarly affect behavior.

The data presented in this report were collected in the first of a series of studies in which physiological, behavioral, and subjective effects of intravenous cocaine in man will be compared with those seen after intravenous d-amphetamine. The present study investigated some of the physiological and subjective effects of cocaine at doses ranging from 4 to 32 mg and compared these effects to those seen after 10 mg of d-amphetamine.

METHOD

Subjects. Nine male volunteers, each with a long history of illicit intravenous cocaine use, were the subjects in this experiment. They ranged in age from 21-35. Prior to acceptance, each subject was given an extensive drug history interview and a thorough psychiatric and physical examination. All subjects were admitted to the Clinical Research Ward of Billings Hospital 24 hours prior to the first test day, and were maintained in the hospital for the duration of the two week experiment. They all signed a consent form which indicated that psychomotor stimulant drugs would be administered, possibly on a daily basis, during the two-week period of hospitalization. When not participating in a behavioral or physiological test session, subjects were free to engage in recreational activities of their own choice on the ward. Five subjects (Group I) were tested while prone on an examination table; physiological and subjective data were collected. Four other subjects (Group II) were tested while sitting up and engaged in an auditory signal detection task.

GENERAL PROCEDURE

Physiological Measures. All physiological measuring and recording equipment were located in a room adjacent to the experimental room. The following measures were taken, recorded on a dynograph recorder, type 504A (Offner Electronics), and stored for PDP8/E computer analysis.

1. Blood pressure. For each subject a blood pressure cuff, with an ultrasonic flow transducer over the brachial artery, was placed on the arm not being used for intravenous injections. Systolic and diastolic blood pressure were monitored on an Arteriosonde 1216 Automatic Blood Pressure Monitor (Roche). This monitor could be programmed to sample blood pressure at intervals of 1, 2, or 5 minutes during each session.

2. Heart rate and ECG. Three pregelled monitoring electrodes (American Hospital Supply) were placed on the subject's chest. These were connected to a Datascope Monitor/Defibrillator 2 where a digital read-out of heart rate and an ECG wave form were always available. In addition, beat to beat time was recorded by a PDP8/E computer (Digital Equipment Corporation).

3. Temperature. a. Skin. For each subject, a small thermistor probe was attached to the index finger of the arm into which intravenous injections were not made. This probe was connected to a Digital Temperature Monitor (Biofeedback Systems) so that a digital read-out was always available.

b. Core. A rectal thermistor probe, also connected to a Digital Temperature Monitor, was used to measure core body temperature in two subjects.

4. Respiration. Each subject wore a pair of Manning bellows tied around the chest. Air pressure inside the bellows was compared to the ambient air pressure by a pressure transducer which amplified and filtered the respiration wave form. This was represented graphically on the Beckman dynograph and stored for later computer analysis.

Experimental Procedure. Group I: Each subject was prone on a medical examination table during sessions. Two scalp vein butterfly infusion sets attached to saline drip bags were inserted into separate veins in one arm. A 23 g needle was used for drug injection and a 19 g needle for blood withdrawal. Thermistor probes, blood pressure cuff, Manning bellows, and monitoring electrodes were all appropriately attached to the subject. He was then allowed to lie quietly for 30-45 minutes prior to baseline recording. Heart rate, blood pressure, ECG, and temperature were then recorded. After at least 30 minutes had elapsed, a modified Addiction Research Center Inventory and the Profile of Mood Scales questionnaire were administered (see below) and a blood sample was taken. Approximately 5-15 minutes later, either saline or drug was administered in a 1 ml volume over 60 sec. If saline was administered, a second infusion of either drug or saline of the same volume and duration was administered approximately 15 minutes later. If the initial injection was drug, an infusion of 1 ml of saline was administered after all physiological measures had returned to pre-drug levels.

Cocaine was administered three or four times per week, never more than once daily (with the exception of subject 9) and always in an ascending dose series. The doses used were 4, 8, 12, 16, 20, and 24 mg for all five subjects. Three subjects received 28 mg in addition, and one subject, 32 mg. Ten mg of d-amphetamine was administered once to two subjects. All other days were used as saline control sessions.

Blood samples (10 ml/sample for subject 1, 20 ml/sample for all others) were collected at 5, 10, 20, 30, and 60 minutes post saline or drug. These samples were used to develop a procedure for measuring the presence of cocaine and its metabolites in plasma. Details of this procedure have been reported elsewhere (Javaid, Dekirmenjian, Brunngraber, and Davis, 1975).

Subjective Measures. Two questionnaires were administered twice each during every drug or placebo (saline) session. Forty-nine questions from the 550 item Addiction Research Center Inventory (ARCI, Haertzen, 1966) were used. This series of scales was designed to measure the subjective effects of drugs. The specific items used were compiled by Martin et al. (1971) in their study of some effects of a variety of psychomotor stimulant drugs in man. They were taken from the Morphine-Amphetamine (MBG), Pentobarbital, Chlorpromazine, Alcohol (PCAG), LSD, and Benzedrine (BG) scales. These are described (Martin et al., 1971) as including measures of sedation and euphoria, an estimate of dysphoric and psychotomimetic changes, and an empiric amphetamine scale. The second questionnaire administered was a stimulant form of the Profile of Mood Scales (POMS). In this test, a 75 item four-point adjective rating scale, six scale categories can be distinguished for scoring purposes.

One hour after drug or saline was administered, subjects were required to fill out a drug effects questionnaire. They were asked to identify the drug they had been given that day and to compare it on a scale from 0-10 (0 = placebo, 5 = the same, 10 = the highest ever taken) with the illegally acquired stimulants that they were accustomed to self-injecting for recreational purposes.

Group II: Subjects were tested while sitting up engaged in an auditory signal detection task. Those behavioral data will be reported in a future publication . The same procedures and measures were used in assessing the effects of intravenous cocaine; the drug schedule, however, was changed. Subjects 6 and 7 received only 12 and 24 mg cocaine, each dose twice. Subject 8 received 12 mg, 16 mg, and 2 doses of 32 mg cocaine; and subject 9 received 3 doses of 16 mg and 5 doses of 32 mg. All subjects received two injections of 10 mg d-amphetamine.

Drug Preparation. Cocaine HCl and d-amphetamine SO_4 were both weighed and dissolved in physiological saline in the hospital pharmacy. All doses are expressed in terms of the salt. After manufacture, all solutions were cultured to test for sterility prior to their use in this study.

RESULTS

Physiological Effects

Intravenous cocaine produced a dose-related increase in heart rate in all subjects tested. Mean heart rate averaged 74 beats/min prior to drug, and peaked at 100 beats/min after 16 mg and 112 beats/min after 32 mg cocaine (Fig. 1). Four and 8 mg cocaine did not cause an increase in absolute heart rate. Because of the variability in pre-drug heart rate, the heart rate data were also analyzed using a measure of percent change from the thirty minute baseline (Fig. 2). Four mg of cocaine did not differ in effect from saline; 8 mg had an intermediate effect, with a median peak change in heart rate of 21%; while 16 and 32 mg had very similar effects, with median peak changes of 32-34%. In general, increases in heart rate began 2-5 minutes after the drug injection and peaked at 10 minutes regardless of the dose administered. Heart rate had returned to pre-drug baseline by 46 minutes following all doses of cocaine. Figure 3 shows that median peak percent change in heart rate increased in a generally linear fashion with dose. These two measures (dose and peak heart rate) are significantly correlated (F test, $p < 0.05$).

A dose-related increase in blood pressure after intravenously administered cocaine was also observed. The effects of cocaine and

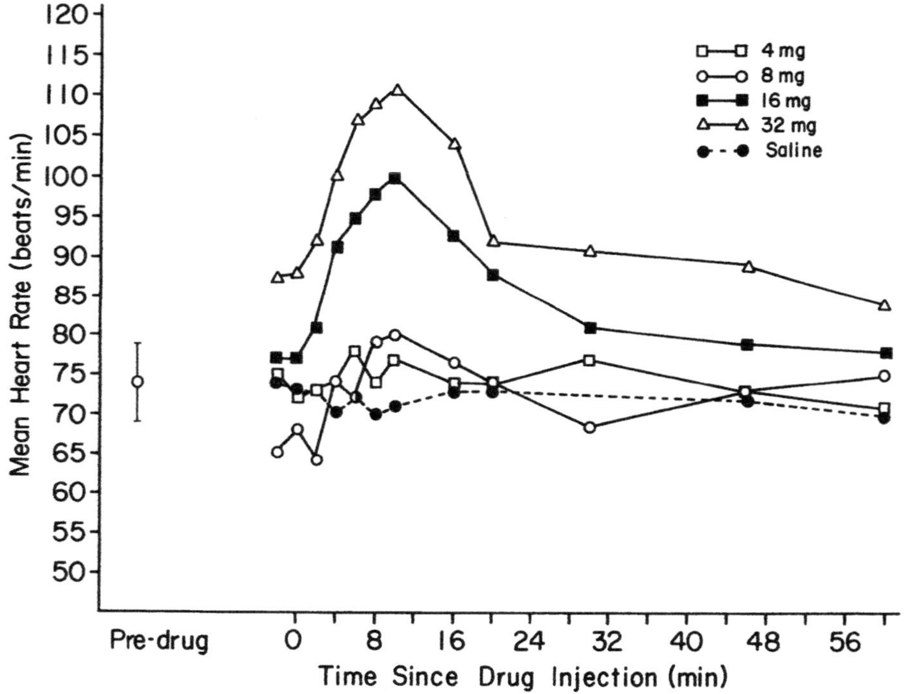

Fig. 1. Mean heart rate (beats/min) for one hour after intravenous injection of saline and doses of 4-32 mg of cocaine. The mean of all thirty minute pre-drug baseline heart rate means is indicated with its standard error bracketed around it. Heart rate was recorded every two minutes; each data point was computed from four separate measures of beat-to-beat time, taken once every thirty seconds. The saline function represents data collected on day 8 of the 10 day experimental series.

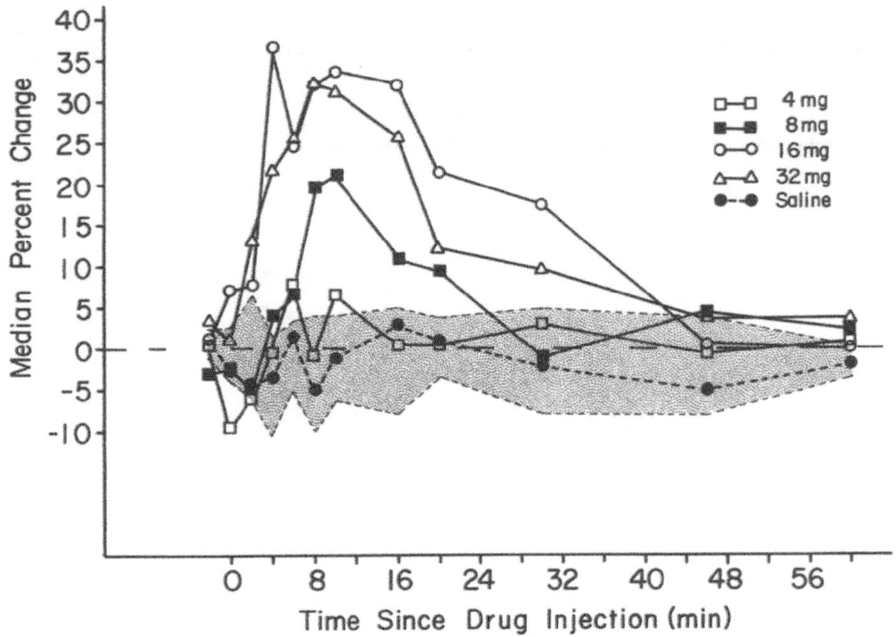

Fig. 2. Median percent change in heart rate for one hour after saline or 4-32 mg cocaine. Percent change was calculated for each dose of cocaine with reference to its own thirty minute pre-drug baseline. The saline function represents data collected on day 8 of the experimental series; the shaded area around it indicates the semi-interquartile range of those data.

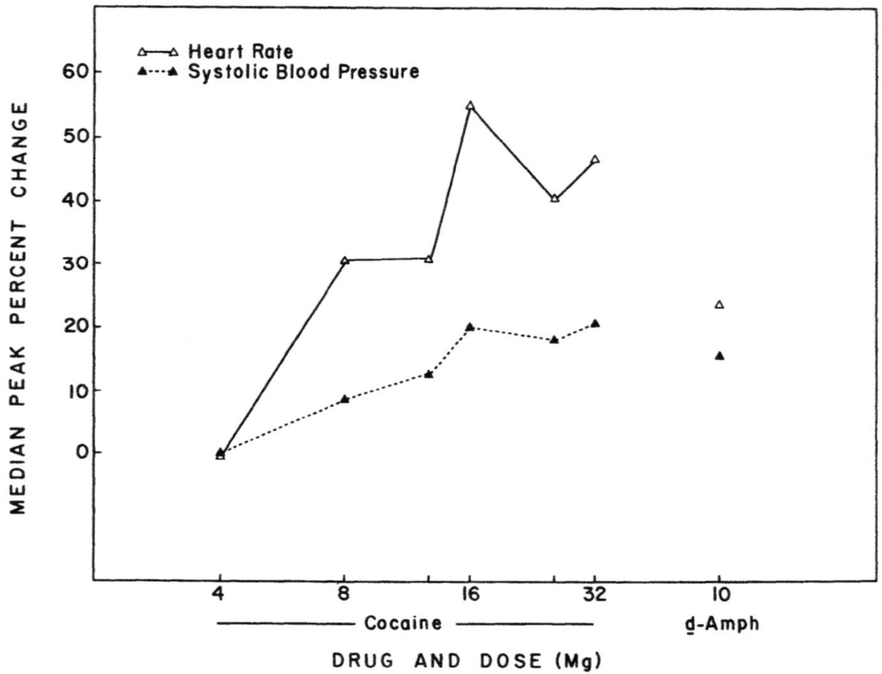

Fig. 3. Median peak percent change in heart rate and systolic blood pressure after saline, 4-32 mg cocaine and 10 mg d-amphetamine. Percent change was calculated for each dose and drug with reference to baseline data collected for 30 min prior to injection of that dose or drug.

d-amphetamine on diastolic and systolic effects were highly correlated. Because of this only systolic blood pressure changes are shown. in Figs. 3 and 4. The median percent change in systolic blood pressure was no different from placebo after 4 and 8 mg of cocaine (Fig. 4). Both 16 and 32 mg caused a peak change of 10-15% (130-140 mm Hg) which generally occurred 10 minutes after drug administration. There was a monotonic linear relationship (F test, $p < 0.01$) between dose and peak systolic blood pressure. This is shown in Fig. 3.

The effects of intravenous cocaine and d-amphetamine on blood pressure and heart rate are compared in Fig. 5. There was a median increase in both heart rate and systolic blood pressure of 10-15% after d-amphetamine. This effect on blood pressure was closely similar to that seen after 24 mg of cocaine, both in terms of peak and duration of effect. There was no dose of cocaine that closely resembled the d-amphetamine effect on heart rate. The effects of 8 mg of cocaine were similar, but it caused a greater median peak percent change and had a shorter duration of action. Neither heart rate nor systolic blood pressure returned to baseline levels at sixty minutes after injection of 10 mg of d-amphetamine.

Respiration and temperature data are not presented in this paper. Both respiration and skin temperature showed great intrasubject variability after administration of placebo as well as during pre-drug baseline determinations. Possible effects of drug, therefore, may have been obscured by this variability. Core temperature remained constant during all phases of this study.

Subjective Effects

Subjects were able to accurately discriminate all doses of cocaine above 4 mg as well as 10 mg of d-amphetamine from placebo. They were less able to discriminate between cocaine and amphetamine. Cocaine was incorrectly identified as amphetamine on three separate occasions (twice at 16 mg and once at 32 mg); d-amphetamine was identified incorrectly as cocaine five times and correctly only twice. Subjects were asked to rate their drug effect on a scale of 0-10 (0 = no drug; 5 = same as average drug on the street; 10 = highest ever taken) as compared to the stimulant drugs they were accustomed to using outside of the experimental situation. Those data are shown in Figure 6. Sixteen mg cocaine was generally rated as similar to the average dose that subjects were self-injecting on the street. Doses of 24 and 32 mg of cocaine were rated as among the highest these subjects had ever taken. There was a generally dose related increase in subjective rating, with d-amphetamine rated as having a subjective effect comparable to 12 to 16 mg of cocaine.

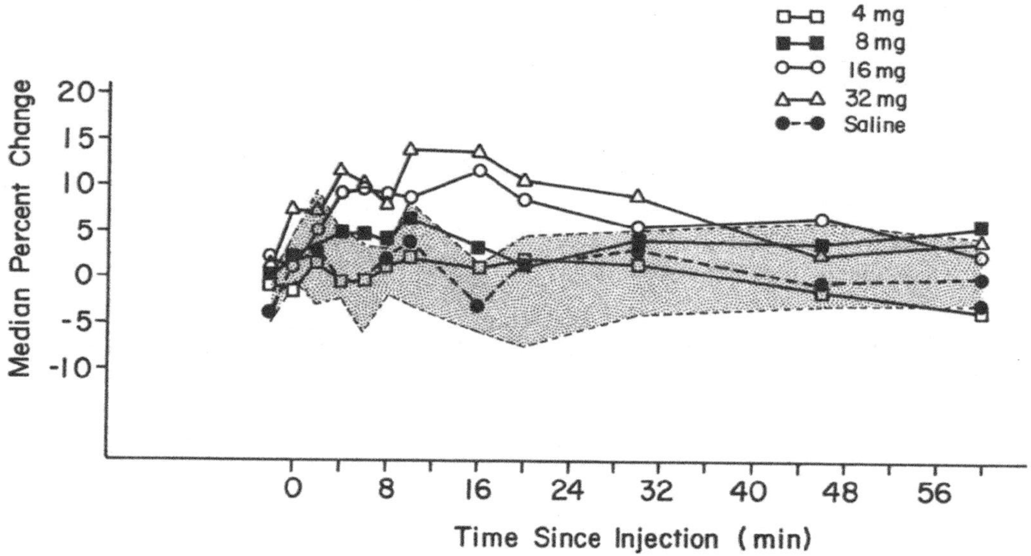

Fig. 4. Median percent change in systolic blood pressure for one hour after intravenous injection of saline or 4-32 mg cocaine. Percent change was calculated for each dose of cocaine from the pre-drug baseline measured during the 30 min prior to injection of that dose. The saline function represents data collected on day 8 of the experimental series; the shaded area indicates the semi-interquartile range for those data.

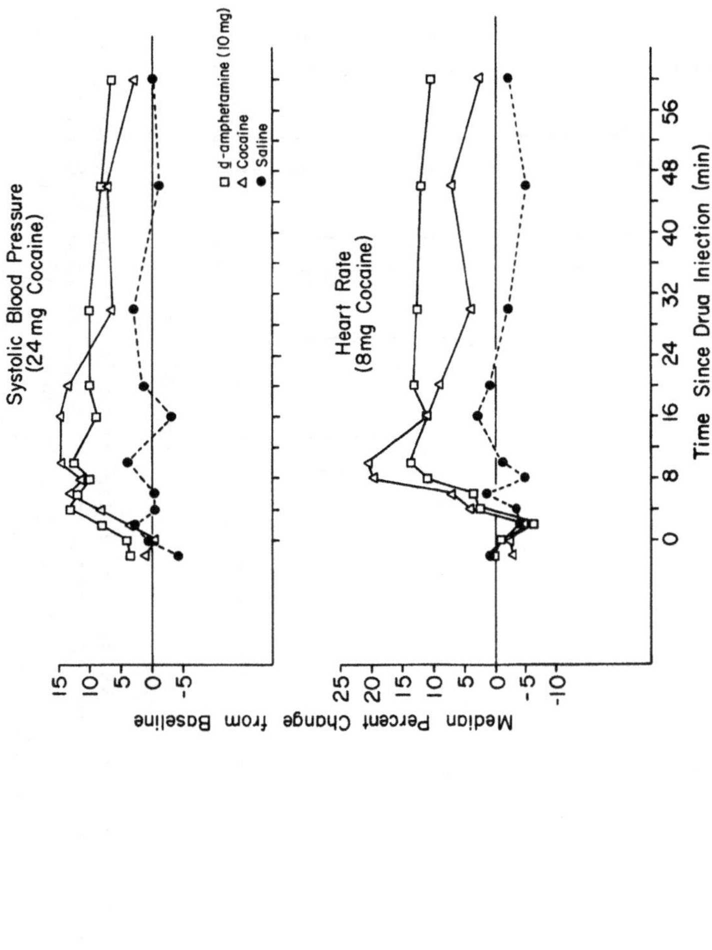

Fig. 5. A comparison of the effects of intravenous cocaine and d-amphetamine on heart rate and systolic blood pressure. Median percent change is shown after 10 mg d-amphetamine compared with 8 mg cocaine for heart rate effects and 24 mg cocaine for blood pressure effects.

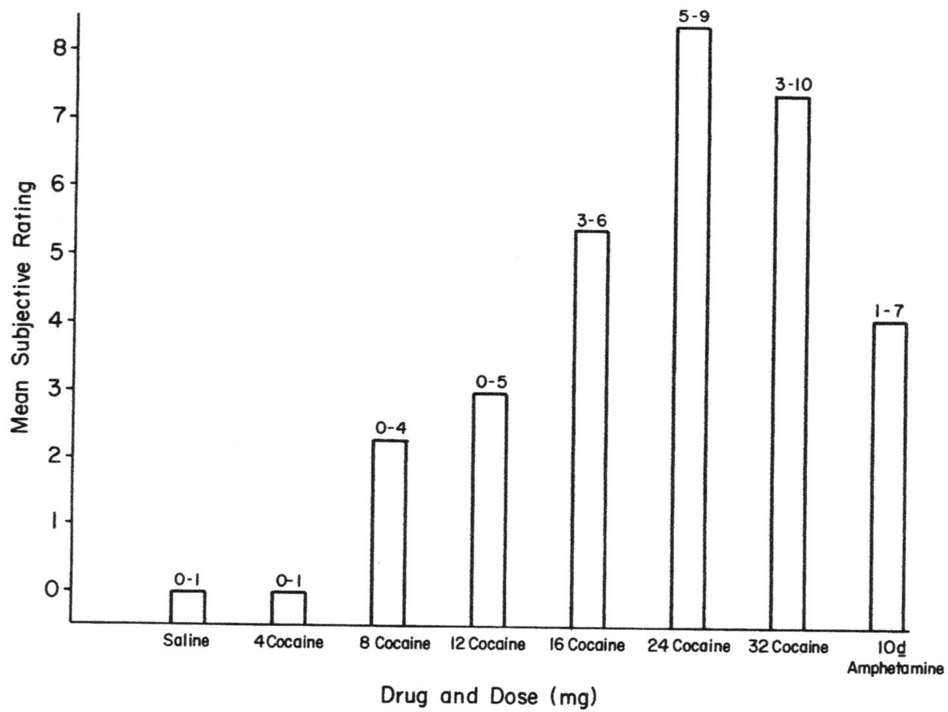

Fig. 6. Mean subjective ratings for intravenous injections of saline, cocaine, and d-amphetamine. Subjects were asked to rate each intravenous injection on a 0-10 scale (0 = no drug, 5 = the same, 10 = the highest ever taken), comparing it to the dose of stimulant drug they are accustomed to self-administer when the drug is acquired illicitly. The numbers above each bar indicate the range of ratings obtained from all subjects tested.

A short form of the Addiction Research Center Inventory was administered prior to and fifteen minutes after each drug or saline administration. Five separate scales were represented in this inventory, each defined in terms of the items comprising that scale. A difference score (post-drug minus pre-drug) was computed for each. scale at each drug or saline condition. These scores are shown in Fig. 7. Scores on these scales were very stable when saline was administered; virtually no change was measured after injection. However, scores on the five separate scales were consistently related to drug dose. Amphetamine (A), Morphine-Amphetamine (MBG) and Benzedrine (BG) scale scores all increased after cocaine injection in a dose-related fashion. The LSD scale scores remained relatively unchanged except at doses of 24 mg or higher. PCAG scores decreased at all doses of cocaine except 4 mg. Ten mg of d-amphetamine caused similar, although not identical, effects on these scores (Fig. 7). All three of the stimulant scale scores increased; their relative rate of change was different from that seen after cocaine.

Analysis of the Profile of Mood Scales data indicated that increasing doses of cocaine were found to have a statistically reliable positive effect ($p < 0.05$) on three mood clusters: friendliness, amphetamine-like feelings, and vigor. When the mood-change scores after 10 mg of d-amphetamine were compared to those seen after cocaine administration, they were found to be equivalent to the scores following a dose of 8 mg cocaine.

DISCUSSION

Intravenous cocaine, administered to human subjects in doses ranging from 4-32 mg, caused significant dose-related increases in blood pressure and heart rate. There was also a positive relationship between dose and duration of action but no apparent interaction of dose with onset of action. Ten mg of d-amphetamine had effects similar to those seen after cocaine. Depending on the physiological measure used in the comparison, that dose of d-amphetamine was comparable in effect to 8-24 mg of cocaine. The dose-related vasopressor action of cocaine in man has also been reported by Post, Kotin, and Goodwin (1974). The pressor effect and tachycardia seen after d-amphetamine replicate data reported by Martin et al. (1971) and Griffith, Cavanaugh, Held, and Oates (1972).

The variability seen in respiration rate was probably due to equipment inadequacies. Therefore, it is not clear at this time whether or not cocaine, in the doses tested, has any effect on respiration rate. In addition, finger temperature was highly correlated with ambient room temperature which was, unfortunately, impossible to maintain at a constant level. This may have obscured an anticipated fall in fingertip temperature due to the vaso-

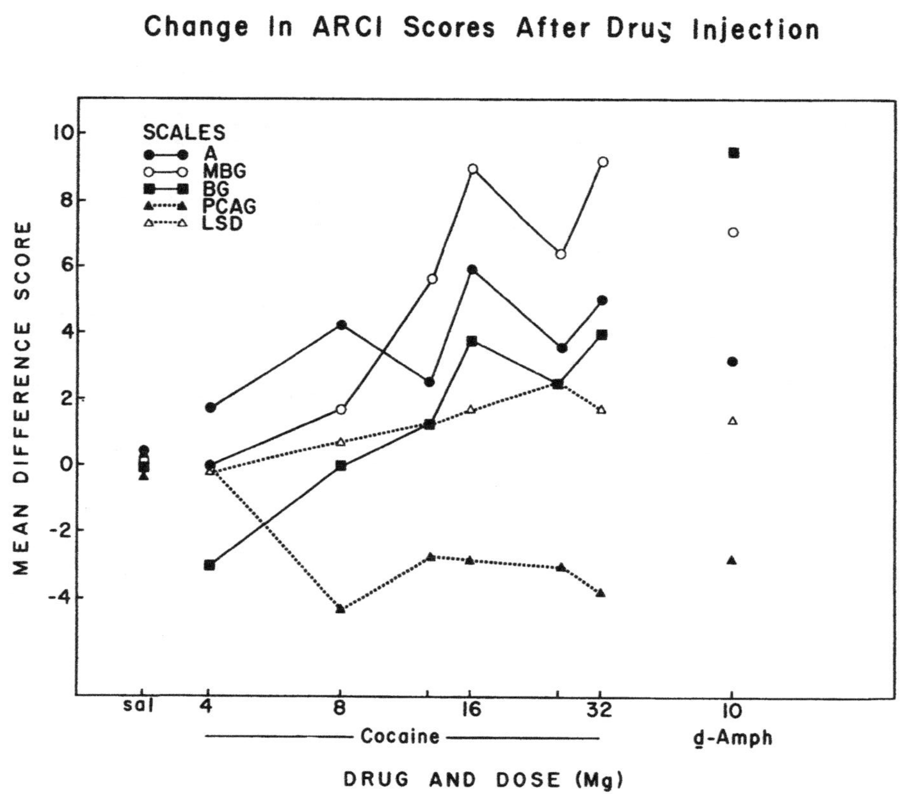

Fig. 7. Mean change in scores on five separate scales of the Addiction Research Center Inventory. A short form of the Inventory was answered prior to drug or saline injection and again fifteen min after injection. The scales were: Amphetamine (A), Morphine-Amphetamine (MBG), Benzedrine (BG), Lysergic Acid (LSD), and Pentobarbital, Chlorpromazine, Alcohol (PCAG).

constriction that is caused by intravenous injections of other sympathomimetic drugs. Neither cocaine nor 10 mg of d-amphetamine caused any change in core body temperature. Ten mg of d-amphetamine was probably too low a dose to produce a temperature change, since increased body temperature has been reported after amphetamine (Ellinwood, 1974; Griffith et al., 1972). Although 32 mg of cocaine appeared to be a moderately high dose according to the subjective ratings and other physiological data collected in this study, it was by no means the "sublethal overdose" that has been described as causing either amphetamine hyperthermia (Ellinwood, 1974) or the pyrexia accompanying cocaine poisoning in animals (Richie and Cohen, 1975). It is therefore not surprising that no changes in body temperature were recorded after any of the doses of cocaine, since none caused any of the toxic effects that appear to be associated with its hyperthermic effect.

In general, 10 mg of d-amphetamine appeared to have a potency comparable to 8-16 mg cocaine. Heart rate peak effect and changes on the POMS were similar to those produced by 8 mg of cocaine, while measures of blood pressure peak effect, most of the ARCI stimulant scale scores, and subjective ratings were similar to those produced by 16 mg of cocaine. In addition, the time course of the pressor effect appeared most similar to that seen after 24 mg cocaine.

Prior to beginning this study, all subjects were informed that they would receive intravenous stimulant drugs. Their decisiòn as to what drug they received on any particular day may, however, have been influenced by the fact that cocaine was administered more frequently than either d-amphetamine or saline. Thus, in general, if a subject guessed cocaine on all drug days, he would have been correct approximately 70% of the time; if he guessed cocaine on all drug or placebo days, he would have been correct 50% of the time. When cocaine was the drug administered, subjects identified it correctly on 94% of the trials; d-amphetamine, however, was correctly identified on only 29% of the trials. This is interesting because it has been suggested (Kramer et al., 1967) on the basis of anecdotal evidence that, although the immediate effects of intravenous amphetamine and cocaine may be indistinguishable, a distinction can be made by experienced users because the effects of cocaine are dissipated more rapidly. However, it was not always true that the effects of cocaine dissipated more rapidly than those of d-amphetamine. The cues that people use in discriminating these drugs are not known; but, perhaps, if subjects were allowed to wait longer than sixty minutes after drug administration, thus given time for the effects of cocaine but not d-amphetamine to dissipate, their drug discriminations would have been better.

Parallel dose-related functions were obtained with cocaine over a wide range of physiological and subjective measures. It is impressive how closely these measures follow each other considering the broad spectrum of variables measured. Heart rate, blood pressure, ARCI stimulant scale scores, and subject rating of each injection all exhibited similarly shaped dose response relationships. In general, 8 mg of cocaine produced a substantial increase in each of the measures. The increase continued and peaked at approximately 16 mg cocaine. With the exception of the subjective ratings, which peaked at 24 mg, decreases in effect were found at 24 mg, with a return to, or close to, the 16 mg value after 32 mg cocaine.

Results on the POMS questionnaire indicate that increasing doses of cocaine cause increases in amphetamine-like feelings, friendliness, and vigor. These results are consistent with verbal reports obtained through interviews with habitual cocaine users as well as descriptions of the cocaine "high" in literature (Freud, 1963; Byck, 1975).

The data presented in this paper have clearly indicated that, although cocaine has local anesthetic as well as psychomotor stimulant actions, its stimulant actions clearly mimic those reported for other stimulant drugs, such as the amphetamines, diethylpropion, and methylphenidate (Griffith et al., 1972; Jasinski, Nutt, and Griffith, 1974; Martin et al., 1971; Jonsson, 1969). All of these drugs have been reported to produce pressor effects, tachycardia, increased scores on various stimulant-correlated subjective effects questionnaire scales, and general reports of "euphoria" in the subjects using them. In addition, preliminary evidence from our laboratory suggests that this similarity of effect may also extend to measures of performance. Clearly, further research is needed to fully delineate the spectrum of behavioral actions of cocaine.

ACKNOWLEDGMENTS

This research was supported by National Institute on Drug Abuse, Contract ADM-45-74-165, and National Institute of Mental Health Grant MH-11052.

Portions of this paper were presented in Cardiovascular and Subjective Effects of Intravenous Cocaine in Man by Fischman, M.W.. Schuster, C.R., Krasnegor, N., Shick, J.F.E., Resnekov, L., and Freedman, D.X.; Archives of General Psychiatry (in press).

REFERENCES

Balster, R.L. and Schuster, C.R.: A comparison of d-amphetamine, 1-amphetamine and methamphetamine self-administration in rhesus monkeys, Pharmac. Biochem. Behav. 1, 67-71 (1973).

Byck, R.: Introduction. In: Cocaine Papers: Sigmund Freud by R. Byck. New York: Stonehill Publishing Co., 1975.

Deneau, G., Yanagita, T., and Seevers, M.H.: Self-administration of psychoactive substances by the monkey. A measure of psychological dependence, Psychopharmacologia 16, 30-48 (1969).

Ellinwood, E.H.: Emergency treatment of acute adverse reactions to CNS stimulants. In: A Treatment Manual for Acute Drug Abuse Emergencies. Bourne, P.G., Ed., pp. 63-67. Washington: U.S. Government Printing Office, 1974.

Fischman, M.W. and Schuster, C.R.: Behavioral, biochemical and morphological effects of methamphetamine in the rhesus monkey. In: Behavioral Toxicology. Weiss, B. and Laties, V., Eds., pp. 375-394. New York: Plenum Press, 1975.

Freud, S.: The Cocaine Papers. Donoghue, A.K. and Hillman, J., Eds. Vienna, Zurich: Dunquin Press, 1963.

Gay, G.R., Sheppard, C.W., Inaba, D.S., and Newmeyer, J.A.: An old girl: Flyin' low, dyin' slow, blinded by snow. Cocaine in perspective, Int. J. Addict. 8, 1027-1042 (1973).

Griffith, J.D., Cavanaugh, J., Held, J., and Oates, J.A.: Dextroamphetamine: Evaluation of psychomimetic properties in man, Archs gen. Psychiat. 26, 97-100 (1972).

Gunne, L.M. and Johnsson, J.: Effects of cocaine administration on brain, adrenal and urinary adrenaline and noradrenaline in rats, Psychopharmacologia 6, 125-129 (1964).

Hatch, R.C. and Fischer, R.: Cocaine-elicited behavior and toxicity in dogs pretreated with synaptic blocking agents, morphine, or diphenylhydantoin, Pharmac. Res. Commun. 4, 383-392 (1972).

Jaffe, J.H.: Drug addiction and drug abuse. In: The Pharmacological Basis of Therapeutics. Goodman, L.S. and Gilman, A., Eds., pp. 282-324. New York: MacMillan, 1975.

Jasinski, D.R., Nutt, J.G., and Griffith, J.D.: Effects of diethylpropion and d-amphetamine after subcutaneous and oral administration, Clin. Pharmacol. Therap. 16, 645-652 (1974).

Javaid, J.I., Dekermenjian, H., Brunngraber, E.G., and Davis, J.M.: Quantitative determination of cocaine and its metabolites benzoylecgonine and ecgonine by gas-liquid chromatography, J. Chromat. 110, 141-149 (1975).

Johanson, C.E., Balster, R., and Bonese, K.: Self-administration of psychomotor stimulant drugs: The effects of unlimited access, Pharmac. Biochem. Behav. (in press).

Kramer, J.C., Fischman, V.S., and Littlefield, D.C.: Amphetamine abuse, J. Am. med. Ass. 201, 305-309 (1967).

Martin, W.R., Sloan, J.W., Sapira, J.D., and Jasinski, D.R.: Physiologic, subjective and behavioral effects of amphetamine, methamphetamine, ephedrine, phenmetrazine and methylphenidate in man, Clin. Pharmacol. Therap. 12, 245-258 (1971).

Matsuzaki, M., Misra, A.L., and Mulé, S.J.: Development of acute tolerance to cardio-respiratory functions and EEG activities of cocaine and pseudo-cocaine in the monkey, The Pharmacologist 17, 190 (1975).

Post, R.M. and Kopanda, R.T.: Cocaine, kindling, psychosis, Am. J. Psychiat. (in press).

Post, R.M., Kotin, J., and Goodwin, F.K.: The effects of cocaine on depressed patients, Am. J. Psychiat. 131, 511-517 (1974).

Richie, J.M. and Cohen, P.J.: Cocaine, procaine and other synthetic local anesthetics. In: The Pharmacological Basis of Therapeutics. Goodman, L.S. and Gilman, A., Eds., pp. 379-403. New York: MacMillan, 1975.

Tatum, A.L. and Seevers, M.H.: Experimental cocaine addiction, J. Pharmac. exp. Ther. 36, 401-410 (1929).

Teeters, W.R., Koppanyi, T., and Cowan, F.F.: Cocaine tachphylaxis, Life Sci. 7, 509-518 (1963).

Wilson, M.C., Hitomi, M., and Schuster, C.R.: Psychomotor stimulant self-administration as a function of dosage per injection in the rhesus monkey, Psychopharmacologia 22, 271-281 (1971).

EFFECTS OF INTRAVENOUS COCAINE ON MHPG EXCRETION IN MAN

Javaid I. Javaid, Haroutune Dekirmenjian
and John M. Davis
Illinois State Psychiatric Institute, 1601 W. Taylor
Street, Chicago, Illinois 60612

Although there is a substantial body of evidence on the behavioral and pharmacological effects of cocaine in animals, the clinical effects of this drug in man have only been described anecdotally. There are virtually no systematic studies of cocaine's behavioral effects on man when given under controlled experimental conditions nor are there any studies of the biological mechanism by which cocaine produces these effects. Clinically, it is an agent that produces euphoria and in this respect is similar to amphetamine. Moreover, like amphetamine or methylphenidate, when taken in larger amounts, it can produce a paranoid psychosis. It is also abused in a manner similar to amphetamine. This paper is a collaborative work between the research unit at the Illinois State Psychiatric Institute and Drs. Fischman and Schuster at the University of Chicago. The latter workers report in this volume (Fischman, Schuster, and Krasnegor, 1976) the experimental protocol that they prepared when they administered injections of cocaine or placebo. Their work primarily concerns the subjective effects of cocaine and also its effects on cardiovascular measures and cognitive performance. The present paper is a companion report and presents our preliminary results on the pharmacological evidence concerning how cocaine produces its behavioral effects on a biochemical level.

Fröhlich and Loewi (1910) showed that cocaine increased the sensitivity of different tissues to epinephrine. Since then many studies have shown that cocaine potentiates the effects of catecholamines in a variety of adrenergically innervated systems, probably by blocking the reuptake into adrenergic tissue of catecholamines, thus making more neurotransmitter available at the receptor site (Whitby, Hertting, and Axelrod, 1960; Dengler, 1965; Trendelenburg, 1968; Axelrod, 1971; Fekete and Borsy, 1971). Cocaine may also release norepinephrine (NE) (Teeters, Koppanyi, and Cowan, 1963; Maengwyn-Davis and Koppanyi, 1966). The role of dopamine-containing neurons and the behavioral effects of cocaine have been discussed by Christie and Crow (1971). In this volume there has been additional discussion by several authors. Particular attention should be drawn to the work of Scheel-Krüger (1976) who investigated the effects of cocaine on dopamine and norepinephrine at a biochemical and a behavioral level.

It has been shown that cocaine alters both the uptake of tryptophan and the activity of tryptophan hydroxylase (Knapp and Mandell, 1972). Thus, the serotonergic system may be directly affected by cocaine. Several workers in this volume have presented papers on the effects of cocaine on serotonin.

Animal studies of cocaine's properties help us to work out the mechanism by which cocaine produces its behavioral effects in man. Direct methods cannot be applied to man, so indirect methods must be used to gain clues as to how cocaine affects amines in this species. The evidence from animals and man, when taken together, may eventually allow us to piece together the pharmacological mechanism of action in the human. The proposed investigation is designed to gather information on the effects of cocaine on NE in man.

Since the initial identification of 3-methoxy-4-hydroxyphenethyleneglycol (MHPG) as a naturally occurring O-methylated metabolite of NE (Axelrod, Kopin, and Mann, 1959), there have been reports that indicate that MHPG is the major metabolite of brain NE in a wide variety of mammalian species (Rutledge and Jonason, 1967; Maas and Landis, 1968). In the dog 25-30% of the urinary MHPG reflects the brain NE metabolism to a greater extent than any other NE metabolite. Thus, the assay for urinary MHPG could be an indirect "marker" for central NE turnover. Urinary MHPG has been shown to be low in depressed patients (Maas, Dekirmenjian, and Fawcett, 1974) a disease for which it is hypothesized that low levels of brain NE may play a causative role. It has also been found to be elevated in manic patients in whom high NE levels have been postulated as a causative agent (Jones, Maas, Dekirmenjian, and Fawcett, 1973). The strategy of our investigation is to use urinary MHPG as a marker for brain NE turnover.

Although the effects of cocaine on release and blockade of reuptake cannot be clearly separated and quantitated, there is certainly some suggestion that perhaps the effect on reuptake would be the more predominant one. If the reuptake pump is blocked, NE cannot be taken up and hence exposed to monoamine oxidase inside the nerve ending for the initial conversion of NE to the dihydroxyphenethylene. This aldehyde is then converted to MHPG. Hence, if cocaine has a primary action on blocking NE uptake at the doses that produce euphoric effects in our experimental subjects, our hypothesis would be that this would be reflected in decreased levels of MHPG formation in the brain and hence decreased levels of MHPG excretion in urine.

In previous studies, the effects of 25 mg of amphetamine given orally to patients have been investigated (Fawcett, Maas, and Dekirmenjian, 1972). These doses of amphetamine cause a clear-cut euphoric effect and markedly lower 24 hour urinary MHPG levels. On an animal level, there is, of course, evidence that amphetamine and cocaine inhibit the reuptake of NE. If uptake of NE is inhibited and more NE is available at the receptor site, it is possible that, through a feedback inhibition, synthesis may be decreased. This also would act in such a way that cocaine would lower MHPG. In our judgement, however, the predominant pharmacologic property probably is uptake inhibition; hence our prediction that cocaine would decrease MHPG levels in urine.

METHOD

Clinical. The clinical methodology is described in detail elsewhere in this volume (Fischman et al., 1976). Briefly, 9 male volunteers, each with a long history of cocaine use, ranging in age from 21-35, were maintained in the hospital for a period of two weeks. After signing a consent form, all 9 volunteers were administered i.v. cocaine 3-4 times per week in doses of 4, 8, 12, 15, and 20 mg. All other days were used as saline control periods. The following physiological measures were checked routinely: blood pressure, heart rate, temperature, respiration, and subjective measures.

Biochemical. Just before the administration of the drug or placebo, all patients were asked to void and then three consecutive urines were collected at three-hour intervals. Sodium metabisulfite (0.5 mg/ml of urines) was added as preservative and volumes were recorded and frozen at -16°C until analysis. 3-Methoxy-4-hydroxyphenethyleneglycol was determined by the method of Dekirmenjian and Maas (1970) by gas-liquid chromatography using an electron capture detector. Creatinine was determined by the colorimetric method of Bonsnes and Taussky (1945).

TABLE 1

DOSE RESPONSE CURVE OF I.V. COCAINE
ON EXCRETION OF MHPG

Time Period of Urine Collection	Dose Cocaine 4 mg	8 mg	12 mg	16 mg	20 mg
0-3	101* ± 8**	99 ± 11	96 ± 15	123 ± 12[1]	146 ± 28[4]
3-6	91 ± 4	102 ± 11	105 ± 11	128 ± 11[2]	118 ± 29
6-9	110 ± 4	131 ± 29	81 ± 14	132 ± 22[3]	150 ± 31[5]

*Percent of control MHPG/mg creatinine, placebo MHPG/mg creatinine for 0-3, 3-6, 6-9 was 0.75 ± 0.11, 0.75 ±.13, 0.84 ± 0.10, respectively.

**Standard error of mean difference expressed as percent of control mean value.

[1]p = 0.15
[2]p = 0.10
[3]p = 0.25
[4]p = 0.22
[5]p = 0.25

Paired T-Test - each drug injection paired with matched saline injection.

RESULTS

Three urine samples were collected in successive three-hour periods. If there was a sudden change in MHPG coincident with the cocaine injection, it could be most clearly seen in the initial collection (see Table 1). We could not exclude the possibility that the inhibition of metabolism mediated through the blocking of the membrane pump would be carried on for a slightly longer period so that this decrease could possibly be observed in the second or third period. In Table 1 the data are presented comparing MHPG excreted during saline infusions with MPHG excreted at the various doses of i.v. cocaine. The data are expressed as percentage of control for each of the three successive collections. With 4, 8, and 12 mg of cocaine there was no change in MHPG levels. The observed values essentially formed a normal distribution around 100%. At 16 and 20 mg, there was a slight but statistically nonsignificant increase in MHPG. Since our prediction was that MHPG would decrease after

TABLE 2

DOSE RESPONSE CURVE OF I.V. COCAINE
ON NINE-HOUR URINARY MHPG

Dose Cocaine				
4 mg	8 mg	12 mg	16 mg	18 mg
95[x] ± 4[t]	115 ± 13	98 ± 10	128* ± 17	148** ± 22

[x]Expressed as percent of control MHPG/mg creatinine. Placebo was 0.74 ± 0.09 mg MHPG/mg creatinine.

[t]Standard error of mean difference expressed as percent of control mean value.

*p = 0.17 Paired T-Test - each drug injection
**p = 0.11 paired will match saline injection.

cocaine administration, this apparent change is in the opposite direction. However, the increase of MHPG was not significant statistically. Since this is an ongoing study, the series of experiments are continuing. In addition, the urinary MHPG determinations have not been done on all the patients tested so that the present data are clearly preliminary. The present data represent 3-6 infusions at each dosage level. It is possible that there might be slight changes in MHPG at each time point but their magnitude is not sufficient to reach statistical significance. For this reason the MHPG for the 0-3, 3-6 and 6-9 hour periods were combined to give the total MHPG for the nine-hour period. These results are presented in Table 2. Again there were no significant changes for 4, 8, and 12 mg doses of cocaine, as was expected from the fractional collections. There was a modest increase in combined nine-hour MHPG values for 16 mg and 20 mg doses of cocaine; however, neither of these increases was statistically significant. Thus, we would conclude that cocaine does not alter urinary MHPG in the first 9 hours after cocaine administration. Since the direction of the changes in urinary MHPG are opposite to the prediction, we feel that the weight of this evidence does not confirm or disprove our initial hypothesis that cocaine inhibits the reuptake of norepinephrine.

DISCUSSION

We would emphasize that, since this is a preliminary report of an experiment still in progress, we do not yet have complete biochemical data even for those patients who have completed the clinical phase. For this reason and also because of the small sample size (about 5-6 measurements at each dose level), these results must be considered as tentative.

Considering the animal evidence, we would expect cocaine to inhibit the reuptake of NE, thus preventing NE from reaching intracellular sites of metabolism and hence, resulting in less brain MHPG formed and a concomitantly diminished urinary excretion. However, no statistically significant change in MHPG was observed. Indeed the changes for the higher doses tended to be in the opposite direction. Although these are preliminary results, we cannot exclude the possibility of slight increase in MHPG at 16 and 20 mg even though this was not statistically significant. Note also that Fischman et al. (1976) found a dose-related increase in heart rate with clear-cut increases observed in the range of 16 and 20 mg. Subjective effects also showed a peak at 16 mg. Additionally, 16 mg of cocaine was generally rated by the subjects as similar to the dose they self-administered while on the street. If the slight increase in urinary MHPG at higher cocaine doses is found to be significant after further experimentation, one may suspect an increase in NE release rather than an inhibition of reuptake of NE after cocaine administration. Electrical stimulation of the locus coeruleus in rat brain induces NE release as shown by increase in MHPG sulfate levels (Korf, Aghajanian, and Roth, 1973). Since we expected that the predominant effect of cocaine would be inhibition of NE reuptake, thus lowering MHPG values, the data presented in this report would disprove our previous hypothesis.

Since animal studies indicate that cocaine has effects on both dopamine and serotonin as well as NE, studies on the effect of cocaine on dopamine and serotonin metabolism should be carried out to explore the relationship between behavioral and pharmacological effects of cocaine on cerebrospinal fluid HVA and 5HIAA after probenecid administration. The role of acetylcholine in modulating the effects of cocaine in man is one area that deserves investigation. Our group has previously shown that the administration of physostigmine, a drug that increases brain acetylcholine, counteracts the exacerbation of the psychosis by amphetamine and methylphenidate in schizophrenics (Davis and Janowsky, 1975). Therefore, like these two drugs, cocaine's behavioral and biochemical effects may also be sensitive to modulations of central cholinergic systems. Thus, studies are needed to assess the pharmacologic properties of cocaine in man on dopamine, serotonin, and acetylcholine.

SUMMARY

Drs. Fischman, Schuster, and Krasnegor (1976) report results of an experiment in which small doses of i.v. cocaine were compared to placebo with respect to cardiovascular and subjective effects. The experiment reported here is the biochemical companion paper that assesses the alterations of NE metabolism in the brain by use of urinary 3-Methoxy-4-hydroxy-phenethyleneglycol as a marker for brain norepinephrine. It was predicted that, if cocaine effects NE, it would be by inhibition of the reuptake pump. Uptake of NE would cease; hence, NE would not be available for intracellular metabolism. This would lead to lowered brain MHPG levels reflected by lower urinary MHPG levels. The observed MHPG values following the various doses of cocaine indicated that cocaine failed to produce a drop in urine MHPG values.

ACKNOWLEDGMENT

This research was partially supported by National Institute on Drug Abuse Contract ADM-45-74-165, and National Institute of Mental Health Grant MH-11052.

REFERENCES

Axelrod, J., Kopin, I.J., and Mann, J.D.: 3-Methoxy-4-hydroxyphenylglycol sulfate, new metabolite of epinephrine and norepinephrine, Biochim. biophys. Acta. 36, 576 (1959).

Axelrod, J.: Noradrenaline: Fate and control of its biosynthesis, Science 173, 598-606 (1971).

Bonsnes, R.W. and Taussky, H.H.: On the colorimetric determination of creatinine by Jaffe reaction, J. biol. Chem. 158, 581 (1945).

Christie, J.E. and Crow, T.J.: Turning behavior as an index of the action of amphetamines and ephedrines on central dopamine neurones, Br. J. Pharmacol. 42, 658-667 (1971).

Davis, J.M. and Janowsky, D.: Cholinergic and adrenergic balance in mania and schizophrenia. In: Neurotransmitter Balances Regulating Behavior. Domino, E.F. and Davis, J.M., Eds., pp. 135-148. Ann Arbor, Mich.: Edwards Brothers, Inc., 1975.

Dekirmenjian, H. and Maas, J.W.: An improved procedure of 3-Methoxy-4-hydroxyphenylethyleneglycol determination by gas liquid chromatography, Anal. Biochem. 35, 113-122 (1970).

Dengler, H.J.: The effect of drugs on monoamine uptake in isolated tissue. In: Pharmacology of Cholinergic and Adrenergic Transmission. Roelle, G.B., Douglas, W.W., and Carlsson, A., Eds., p. 261. New York: Macmillan, 1965.

Fawcett, J.A., Maas, J.W., and Dekirmenjian, H.: Depression and MHPG excretion: Response to dextroamphetamine and tricyclic antidepressants, Arch. gen. Psychiat. 26, 246-251 (1972).

Fekete, M. and Borsy, J.: Chlorpromazine-cocaine antagonism: Its relation to changes in dopamine metabolism in the brain. Eur. J. Pharmacol. 16, 171-175 (1971).

Fischman, M.W., Schuster, C.R., and Krasnegor, N.A.: Physiological and behavioral effects of intravenous cocaine in man. In: Cocaine and Other Stimulants. Ellinwood, E.H. and Kilbey, M. M., Eds. New York: Plenum Press, 1976.

Fröhlich, A. and Loewi, O.: Über eine Steigerung der Adrenalinempfindlichkeit durch Cocaïn, Arch. exp. Path. Pharmak. 62, 159-169 (1910).

Jones, F.D., Maas, J.W., Dekirmenjian, H., and Fawcett, J.A.: Urinary catecholamine metabolism during behavioral changes in a patient with manic depressive cycles, Science 179, 300-302 (1973).

Knapp, S. and Mandell, A.J.: Narcotic drugs: Effects on the serotonin biosynthetic system of the brain, Science 177, 1209-1211 (1972).

Korf, J., Aghajanian, G.K., and Roth, R.H.: Increased turnover of norepinephrine in the rat cerebral cortex during stress: Role of the locus coeruleus, Neuropharmacol. 12, 933-938 (1973).

Maas, J.W. and Landis, D.H.: In vivo studies of metabolism of norepinephrine in central nervous system, J. Pharmac. exp. Ther. 163, 147-162 (1968).

Maas, J.W., Dekirmenjian, H., and Fawcett, J.A.: MHPG excretion by patients with affective disorders, Int. Pharmacopsychiat. 9, 14-26 (1974).

Maengwyn-Davis, G.D. and Koppanyi, T.: Cocaine tachyphylaxis and effects on indirectly acting sympathomimetic drugs in the rabbit aortic strip and in splenic tissue, J. Pharmac. exp. Ther. 154, 481-492 (1966).

Rutledge, C.O. and Jonason, J.: Metabolic pathways of dopamine and norepinephrine in rabbit brain *in vitro*, J. Pharmac. exp. Ther. 157, 943-502 (1967).

Scheel-Krüger, J.: Cocaine: Discussion on the role of dopamine in the biochemical mechanism of action. In: Cocaine and Other Stimulants. Ellinwood, E.H. and Kilbey, M.M., Eds. New York: Plenum Press, 1976.

Teeters, W.R., Koppanyi, T., and Cowan, F.F.: Cocaine tachyphylaxis, Life Science 7, 509-518 (1963).

Trendelenburg, U.: The effect of cocaine on the pacemaker of isolated guinea pig atria, J. Pharmac. exp. Ther. 161, 222-231 (1968).

Whitby, L.G., Hertting, G., and Axelrod, J.: Effect of cocaine on the disposition of noradrenaline labelled with tritium, Nature, Lond., 187, 604-605 (1960).

PSYCHOLOGIC TEST RESPONSES AND METHYLPHENIDATE

D.S. Janowsky, L. Huey, and L. Storms

Department of Psychiatry, University of California

at San Diego School of Medicine, La Jolla, California

92037

Janowsky, El-Yousef and Davis (1973a) have previously described the immediate activation or worsening of pre-existing psychotic symptoms in actively psychotic schizophrenics by a small (0.5 mg/kg) dose of methylphenidate. This phenomena differs from the predominantly paranoid psychosis occurring in normals, as well as psychotics, which follows chronic high dose amphetamine administration (Griffith, Cavanaugh, Held and Oates, 1972). Methylphenidate-induced psychosis activation does not occur in patients receiving placebo injections, in remitted schizophrenic patients, or in normals (Janowsky et al., 1973a). Also, intravenous methylphenidate has been found by Janowsky and Davis (1974) to be about 1.5 times as effective as d-amphetamine and 3 times as effective as l-amphetamine in activating psychotic symptoms. Due to these interrelationships, and methylphenidate's specific biochemical effects on brain dopamine in rats (Ferris, Tang, and Maxwell, 1972; Snyder, Taylor, Coyle and Meyerhoff, 1970; Yaryura-Tobias, Diamond and Merlis, 1970; Angrist, Sathananthan and Gershon, 1973; Scheel-Kruger, 1971), Janowsky et al. (1973a; 1974) have implied a dopaminergic etiology to the phenomena of psychostimulant-induced psychosis activation in schizophrenics.

Although the effects of methylphenidate, d- and l-amphetamine are quite dramatic in activating such schizophrenic symptoms as delusions and hallucinations (Janowsky et al., 1973a), some uncertainty exists as to how to interpret the meaning of this observation. Since patients who receive psychostimulants generally feel more talkative and trusting, it is at least possible that the apparent increase in psychotic symptoms induced by a psychostimulant merely represents an increase in friendliness and trust. Word association tests and proverb interpretation tests were utilized to help make the above distinction.

METHODS

Subjects

The two groups of subjects consisted of 16 actively psychotic schizophrenic inpatients and 18 non-psychotic inpatients. All patients were diagnosed by the patients' psychiatric resident and the psychiatric ward chief according to the criteria of the Diagnostic and Statistical Manual of the American Psychiatric Association (DSM II). All subjects were in good health without evidence of cardiovascular disease, organic brain dysfunction, or other physical illness. No subject had received electroshock therapy during the previous year. All subjects utilized in the study were voluntarily admitted to the inpatient unit and a fully-informed consent was obtained from each patient, in compliance with the University of California at San Diego Human Use Committee.

Procedure

Each subject received 0.5 mg/kg methylphenidate IV in two divided doses 5 minutes apart or one single dose given over a 30 second period of time. Pulse and blood pressure were monitored every 10 minutes beginning 20 minutes before and ending 1 hour after methylphenidate infusion. Using a five point rating scale as described previously (Janowsky, El-Yousef, Davis and Sekerke, 1973b), each subject was rated on: 1) talkativeness; 2) amount of interaction; 3) Global psychosis, as well as other variables. Each also was rated using the Brief Psychiatric Rating Scale (BPRS) prior to methylphenidate infusion and every 10 minutes for 1 hour after the infusion.

In addition, 20 minutes before infusion, 20 minutes after infusion, and 24 hours after methylphenidate infusion, 15 of the 16 schizophrenics and 17 of the 18 non-psychotic subjects were given the Kent-Rosanoff word association test (Palermo and Jenkins, 1964). Specifically, each patient was asked to give the first response which came to mind for each of the same 50 words on the Kent-Rosanoff word association test (Palermo and Jenkins, 1964). The Kent-Rosanoff word association test was scored for the number of common responses, defined as one of the five most frequent responses according to published norms (Palermo and Jenkins, 1964).

At 20 minutes before, 20 minutes after, and 24 hours after methylphenidate infusion, each subject also was given a different set of projective tests each consisting of 5 Holtzman ink blots (Holtzman, 1961). Each subject was randomly assigned one of 6 possible orders of the set of ink blots, so that the number of subjects who received a given set of 5 cards first, second, or third was approximately equal. For each Holtzman card, each patient was asked to give one response telling what the blot looked like. The responses to the Holtzman ink blots were rated by a clinical psychologist (L.S.) on four dimensions using a 0-7 point scale. The dimensions were: paranoid trends, autism, inappropriateness to the blot, and thought disorder. The total number of responses given a rating of 6 or 7 (in the pathological range) was used as the pathological response score. Since each ink blot response was separately coded and the responses for all patients and all cards scrambled, the psychologist-rater was unaware of the diagnosis of the patient who produced a given response and the condition under which the response was given.

The proverb interpretations were obtained using standardized criteria (Gorham, 1961), and a total proverb score attained for each of the 3 phases of the experiment.

All data for the schizophrenic and non-psychotic groups were separately analyzed by comparison of the average scores before, during and after methylphenidate intoxication with the use of the student's one-tailed t-test for paired observations. Differences between the schizophrenic and non-psychotic groups were analyzed with the use of the student's one-tailed t-test.

Analysis of the data revealed that, consistent with previous work, methylphenidate 0.5 mg/kg significantly increased over baseline the Global mean psychosis ratings and BPRS scores at 20 minutes and 1 hour after methylphenidate infusion in the schizophrenic group but not in the non-psychotic group. The non-psychotic patients showed a very small, statistically insignificant, increase in the psychosis scores after methylphenidate infusion. Methylphenidate caused significant increases in the diastolic and systolic blood pressure and pulse in both the schizophrenic and non-psychotic patients. These findings are summarized in Table 1.

The psychosis ratings of the schizophrenic patients were statistically significantly higher at baseline ($p < .001$), 20 minutes after ($p < .001$), and 24 hours after ($p < .001$) methylphenidate infusion than were those of the non-psychotics at comparable experimental phases. For all the above times, the BPRS scores paralleled the Global psychosis ratings. The average baseline and 20 minutes post-methylphenidate infusion observations did not significantly differ for diastolic and systolic blood pressure when

TABLE 1

Effect of Methylphenidate on Mean Psychosis Ratings, Pulse and Blood Pressure in 16 Schizophrenic and 18 Non-Schizophrenic Patients Before and 20 Minutes after Administration of Methylphenidate 0.5 mg/kg

	Schizophrenics		Non-Schizophrenics	
	Baseline	+20 Min	Baseline	+20 Min
PSYCHOSIS RATINGS	1.9 ± 0.3	3.0 ± 0.3*	0.1 ± 0.1	0.4 ± 0.2
BLOOD PRESSURE				
Systolic	123 ± 3.3	145 ± 3.4**	126 ± 4.1	143 ± 5.0**
Diastolic	75 ± 3.3	83 ± 3.8*	79 ± 1.9	86 ± 3.5*
PULSE (Beats/Min)	90 ± 2.5	122 ± 5.3**	89 ± 3.2	103 ± 4.4*

* $p < .05$--student's t-test for paired results comparing baseline with +20 minutes scores; results expressed as average ± standard error of the mean.

** $p < .001$

the schizophrenic and non-psychotic patients were compared. However, 20 minutes and one hour after methylphenidate intoxication, the schizophrenic patient group showed a significantly greater increase in pulse rate than did the non-psychotic patient group ($p < .001$).

As shown in Table 2, a significant increase in abnormal pathologic projective test responses occurred in the schizophrenic group 20 minutes after, but not 24 hours after, methylphenidate intoxication. This statistically significant increase did not occur in the non-psychotic group of patients although a slight increase in pathologic responses did occur. Furthermore, the number of pathologic responses was significantly less in the non-psychotic group than in the schizophrenic group before ($p < .02$), during ($p < .01$), and 24 hours after ($p < .01$) methylphenidate intoxication, thus demonstrating that, in our hands, the Holtzman projective test can distinguish between schizophrenic and non-psychotic patients.

Table 3 indicates that the majority of schizophrenic and non-psychotic subjects displaying projective pathologic test responses prior to infusion showed an increase, rather than a decrease, in pathologic responses after methylphenidate infusion. Significantly, more non-psychotic than schizophrenic patients (N=7 vs N=1) showed

TABLE 2

Mean Number of Pathologic Holtzman Card Responses in 16 Schizophrenic and 18 Non-Psychotic Patients Before, 20 Minutes After and 24 Hours After Administration of Intravenous Methylphenidate 0.5 mg/kg

	Schizophrenics		Non-Schizophrenics	
BASELINE	2.3 ± 0.5		0.8 ± 0.3	
		p <.05*		p=NS
+20 MINUTES	4.4 ± 0.9		1.6 ± 0.5	
		p <.05		p=NS
+24 HOURS	2.2 ± 0.4		0.6 ± 0.4	

* significance determined using student's t-test for paired results comparing baseline and +20 minute values and +20 minute and +24 hour values. Results expressed as group average ± standard error of the mean.

TABLE 3

Number of Schizophrenic and Non-Schizophrenic Patients Giving Pathologic Responses to Holtzman Ink Blots Following Intravenous Infusion of Methylphenidate 0.5 mg/kg

	Non-Pathologic Responders*	Pathologic Responses--Change from Baseline to +20 Minutes			
		Unchanged	Decreased	Increased	Total
SCHIZOPHRENICS (N=16)	1	2	4	9	15
NON-SCHIZOPHRENICS (N=18)	7	0	2	9	11
TOTAL SUBJECTS (N=34)	8	2	6	18	26

* patients showed no pathologic response throughout test phases

no pathologic responses at all (scores of 6 or 7) throughout the experiment.

Table 4 demonstrates that, similar to the results using projective tests, a significant decrease over baseline in common word associations occurred 20 minutes after, but not 24 hours after, methylphenidate infusion in schizophrenics but not in non-psychotic patients. A significantly lower number of common word associations occurred in the schizophrenics as compared to the non-psychotic patients during all phases of the experiment ($p < .001$ before, $p < .001$ 20 minutes after, $p < .001$ 24 hours after methylphenidate infusion), demonstrating that the Kent-Rosanoff word association test can distinguish between schizophrenic and non-schizophrenic patients.

TABLE 4

Mean Number of Kent-Rosanoff Word Association Test Scores in 15 Schizophrenic and 17 Non-Schizophrenic Patients Before, 20 Minutes After and 24 Hours After Administration of Intravenous Methylphenidate 0.5 mg/kg

	Mean Number of Appropriate Responses			
	Schizophrenics		Non-Schizophrenics	
BASELINE	23.8 ± 2.1		32.9 ± 1.7	
		p <.05		p=NS
+20 MINUTES	18.3 ± 3.0		32.6 ± 2.1	
		p=NS		p=NS
+24 HOURS	22.2 ± 2.0		34.0 ± 1.9	

significance determined using student's t-test for paired results comparing baseline and +20 minute values and +20 minute and +24 hour values. Results expressed as group average ± standard error of the mean

Table 5 demonstrates that in both the schizophrenic and non-psychotic groups, the number of schizophrenic and non-psychotic patients showing a decrease in common word associations was greater following methylphenidate infusion than the number showing an increase.

TABLE 5

Number of Schizophrenic and Non-Schizophrenic Patients Showing Changes on the Kent-Rosanoff Word Association Test,* Following Infusion of Intravenous Methylphenidate 0.5 mg/kg

	Direction of Change--Baseline to +20 Minutes			
	Unchanged	Negative	Positive	Total
SCHIZOPHRENICS	3	11	1	15
NON-SCHIZOPHRENICS	5	8	4	17
TOTAL SUBJECTS	8	19	5	32

*a difference of at least 3 appropriate responses is considered a change in a given patient

DISCUSSION

The above data are consistent with the assumption that methylphenidate significantly activates the schizophrenic thought process in actively ill, schizophrenic patients, but not in non-psychotic, non-schizophrenic subjects. It supports previous reported observations (Janowsky et al., 1973a), showing an intensification of hallucinations and delusions in actively ill schizophrenic patients. The fact that the schizophrenic patient group's word association test scores showed less commonality after methylphenidate infusion would strongly suggest that methylphenidate infusion causes a loosening of associations in schizophrenic patients. The fact that such a decrease in word association commonality did not occur to a significant degree in the non-psychotic group would suggest that the schizophrenic patient's associative process is relatively more sensitive to methylphenidate's psychostimulant effects. However, it should be noted that methylphenidate caused more of the non-psychotic patients to show decreased commonality than to show increased commonality. This suggests that the effect of methylphenidate on word associations is not entirely specific to schizophrenics. Nevertheless, since loosening of associations is considered a major primary symptom of schizophrenia (Bleuler, 1950), it would appear that methylphenidate affects the schizophrenic thought process, as such, rather than affecting only such "secondary" symptoms as delusions and hallucinations (Storms and Broen, 1969). The projective test results parallel the above observations and indicate that the autistic and projective components of schizophrenia are increased by methylphenidate.

The above study does not give direct information about the biochemical basis of psychostimulant-induced increases in psychotic symptoms, bizarre projective responses, and decreased common word associations. However, a clue may be offered by the fact that a significantly greater increase in heart rate occurred after methylphenidate administration in the schizophrenic patients as compared to the non-psychotic patients. Although this increase in heart rate may have reflected increased anxiety, or the fact that many of the schizophrenic patients were receiving antipsychotic agents, it is also possible that schizophrenics have a greater receptor activity and/or sensitivity to stimulation by catecholamines released by methylphenidate. Other possibilities are that available catecholamine stores of schizophrenics exceed those of non-schizophrenics or that they lack adequate catabolizing enzymes (MAO or COMT) to decrease released catecholamines.

Assuming a catecholaminergic etiology to the phenomena of psycho-stimulant-induced psychosis activation, the question as to whether the psychologic effects of methylphenidate are due predominantly to noradrenergic or dopaminergic influences is unanswered. The following information outlines the evidence that methylphenidate predominantly effects: dopamine, norepinephrine, dopamine and norepinephrine, or either dopamine or norepinephrine.

The following evidence implicates norepinephrine and dopamine equally in causing psychosis activation. Janowsky et al. (1974) found that methylphenidate, d-amphetamine, and l-amphetamine were effective in activating psychotic symptoms in a ratio of 3:2:1 respectively. Analysis of the work of Ferris et al. (1972) likewise shows that methylphenidate is more potent than d-amphetamine, which in turn is more potent than l-amphetamine, in blocking the uptake of norepinephrine and dopamine into rat brain synaptosomes derived from cortex, hypothalamus, and striatum. Generally, with the exception of the findings of Coyle, Taylor and Synder (1969; 1970) studies of the relative effects of d- and l-amphetamine show that d-amphetamine is about 3 times as potent as l-amphetamine in inhibiting dopamine <u>and</u> norepinephrine uptake from striatum and that d-amphetamine and l-amphetamine are equipotent in blocking the uptake of these neurotransmitters in cortex and hypothalamus. Also, d-amphetamine appears to be about 3 times as effective as l-amphetamine in releasing dopamine and norepinephrine from striatum and into ventricular fluid and equipotent in releasing these neurotransmitters from cortex and hypothalamus (Ferris et al., 1972; Heikkila, Orlansky, Mytilineou and Cohen, 1975; Ziance, Azzaro and Rutledge, 1972; Von Voigtlander and Moore, 1973; Moore, Carr, and Dominic, 1970; Thornburg and Moore, 1973; Harris and Baldessarini, 1973). Thus, the above studies indicate that the potency ratios of methylphenidate, d-amphetamine and l-amphetamine appear to exhibit parallel effects on both dopamine and norepinephrine and on psychosis activation.

Supporting a dopaminergic etiology for psychostimulant-induced psychosis activation, is evidence that methylphenidate appears to selectively release dopamine from striatal synaptosomes in contrast to its negligible effect on striatal norepinephrine (Ferris et al., 1972). Also, the dopamine agonist, ET484 and L-DOPA (a predominantly dopamine elevating precursor) activate psychotic symptoms in schizophrenia (Yaryura et al., 1970; Angrist et al., 1973; Angrist, personal communication). These facts would argue for a dopaminergic etiology to the phenomena of psychostimulant-induced psychosis activation.

In contrast, in support of a noradrenergic etiology for psychostimulant induced psychosis action, d-amphetamine is approximately twice as effective as l-amphetamine in activating intracranial self-stimulation (ICS) when infused into a predominantly noradrenergic ICS brain area, whereas d- and l-amphetamine are equipotent in activating ICS when infused into a dopaminergic ICS brain area (Phillips, Brooke and Fibiger, 1975). Also, Janowsky et al. have recently found that methylphenidate causes a consistent increase in human serum growth hormone, but no effect on serum prolactin (Janowsky, unpublished observations). Since evidence exists that prolactin secretion may be regulated by dopamine, while growth hormone may be regulated most predominantly by norepinephrine, these findings tentatively would suggest that methylphenidate selectively effects the noradrenergic system in man.

Other neurotransmitters, such as acetylcholine, also may regulate psychosis activation. The cholinomimetic agent, physostigmine, a cholinesterase inhibitor, antagonizes methylphenidate-induced psychosis activation in man (Janowsky et al., 1973a), and stereotyped gnawing behavior in rats (Janowsky, El-Yousef, Davis and Sekerke, 1972). Anticholinergic agents antagonize the therapeutic effects of the dopamine blocking antipsychotic agents (Singh and Kay, 1975) and increase amphetamine-induced stereotyped behaviors in mice (Scheel-Kruger, 1970). Also biochemical evidence suggests that central catecholaminergic and cholinergic neurotransmitters may be mutually inhibiting with respect to turnover. Thus, dopaminergic agonists decrease acetylcholine turnover and dopamine blocking agents increase acetylcholine turnover (Ladinsky, Consolo, Bianchi, Samanin and Ghezzi, 1975; Trabucchi, Cheney, Racagni and Costa, 1975). Furthermore, evidence recently has been reviewed indicating existence of a striatal dopamine-acetylcholine-GABA feedback loop. Here, dopamine is said to inhibit acetylcholine neurons; acetylcholine stimulates GABA neurons; and GABA inhibits dopaminergic neurons (Trabucchi et al., 1975). Such circuitry could exist with regard to the phenomena of psychostimulant-induced psychosis activation in which a psychostimulant, by increasing dopaminergic activity, would inhibit cholinergic activation, thus decreasing GABA activity and causing further release of dopamine (Trabucchi et al., 1975).

There are certain clinical and ethical implications of using psychostimulants as interviewing or psychodiagnostic agents. Although an increase in pathologic Holtzman responses and decrease in common word associations did not occur in 100% of the schizophrenics tested, the use of methylphenidate in combination with clinical observations, projective tests, and a word association test did reveal diagnostically-relevant information in virtually all cases in which it was utilized by us. The combination of administration of psychologic tests and a psychostimulant may thus have potential clinical usefulness in the rapid differential diagnosis of the schizophrenic patient. We have previously noted that psychostimulant interviews, as such, can be contributory in the making of a differential psychiatric diagnosis and in the understanding of intrapsychic dynamics in the majority of instances in which we have used them (Janowsky et al., 1973a; 1974). We have seldom felt, or been told by patients or staff, that the experience was disagreeable. When done with the sympathy and support of attending psychiatric personnel, the interviews have often been considered psychotherapeutic by patients and staff alike due to the insights gained by the patients while they experience an encapsulated and time-limited increase in psychotic symptoms. However, we believe psychostimulant interviews should not be performed with patients who are fearful of the procedure or who have not given informed consent. Although we often did find the test to be clinically useful, we are certain that similar information and benefits could be obtained in most cases by the use of perceptive clinical interviewing techniques and/or psychologic tests alone--a more conservative strategy.

REFERENCES

Angrist, B., Sathananthan, G., and Gershon, S.: Behavioral effects of L-Dopa in schizophrenic patients, Psychopharmacologia 31, 1-12 (1973).

Bleuler, E.: Dementia Praecox or the Group of Schizophrenias (Monograph Series on Schizophrenia Number 1). New York: International University Press, 1950.

Coyle, J.T. and Snyder, S.H.: Catecholamine uptake by synaptosomes in homogenates of rat brain: Stereospecificity in different areas, J. Pharmac. exp. Ther. 170, 221-231 (1969).

Ferris, R., Tang, F., and Maxwell, R.: A comparison of the capacities of isomers of amphetamine, deoxypiradrol and methylphenidate to inhibit the uptake of tritiated catecholamines into rat cerebral cortex slices, synaptosomal preparations of rat cerebral cortex, hypothalamus and striatum and into adrenergic nerves of rabbit aorta, J. Pharmac. exp. Ther. 181, 407-416 (1972).

Gorham, D.: Verbal abstraction in psychiatric patients: Assay of impairment utilizing proverbs, J. ment. Sci. 107, 52-59 (1961).

Griffith, J., Cavanaugh, J., Held, J., and Oates, J.: Dextroamphetamine: Evaluation of psychotomimetic properties in man, Archs gen. Psychiat. 26, 97-100 (1972).

Harris, J. and Baldessarini, R.: Uptake of (^{3}H)-catecholamines by homogenates of rat corpus striatum and cerebral cortex: Effects of amphetamine analogues, Neuropharmacology 12, 669-679 (1973).

Heikkila, R.E., Orlansky, H., Mytilineou, C., and Cohen, G.: Amphetamine: Evaluation of d- and l-isomers as releasing agents and uptake inhibitors for ^{3}H-dopamine and ^{3}H-norepinephrine in slices of rat neostriatum and cerebral cortex, J. Pharmac. exp. Ther. 194, 47-56 (1975).

Holtzman, W.: Ink Blot Technique: Administration and Scoring Guide. Minneapolis: University of Minnesota Press, 1964.

Janowsky, D.S., El-Yousef, M.K., Davis, J.M., and Sekerke, H.J.: Cholinergic antagonism of methylphenidate-induced stereotyped behavior, Psychopharmacologia 27, 295-303 (1972).

Janowsky, D.S., El-Yousef, M.K., and Davis, J.M.: Provocation of schizophrenic symptoms by intravenous administration of methylphenidate, Archs gen. Psychiat. 28, 185-191 (1973a).

Janowsky, D.S., El-Yousef, M.K., and Davis, J.: Antagonistic effects of physostigmine and methylphenidate in man, Am. J. Psychiat. 130, 1370-1376 (1973b).

Janowsky, D.S. and Davis, J.M.: Dopamine, psychomotor stimulants, and schizophrenia: Effects of methylphenidate and the stereoisomers of amphetamine in schizophrenics. In: Neuropsychopharmacology of Monoamines and Their Regulatory Enzymes. Usdin, E., Ed., pp. 317-323. New York: Raven Press, 1974.

Ladinsky, H., Consolo, S., Bianchi, S., Samanin, R., and Ghezzi, D.: Cholinergic-dopaminergic interaction in the striatum: The effect of 6-hydroxydopamine or pimozide treatment on the increased striatal acetylcholine levels induced by apomorphine, piribedil and d-amphetamine, Brain Res. 84, 221-226 (1975).

Moore, K., Carr, L., and Dominic, J.: Functional significance of amphetamine induced release of brain catecholamines. In: Amphetamines and Related Compounds. Costa, E. and Garattini, S., Eds., pp. 371-384. New York: Raven Press, 1970.

Palermo, D. and Jenkins, J.: Word Association Norms: Grade School Through College. Minneapolis: University of Minnesota Press, 1974.

Phillips, A.G., Brooke, S.M., and Fibiger, H.C.: Effects of amphetamine isomers and neuroleptics on self-stimulation from the nucleus accumbens and dorsal noradrenergic bundle, Brain Res. 85, 13-22 (1975).

Scheel-Krüger, J.: Central effects of anticholinergic drugs measured by the apomorphine gnawing test in mice, Acta pharmac. 28, 1-16 (1970).

Scheel-Krüger, J.: Comparative studies of various amphetamine analogues demonstrating different interactions with the metabolism of the catecholamines in the brain, Eur. J. Pharmacol. 14, 47-59 (1971).

Singh, M.M. and Kay, S.R.: A comparative study of haloperidol and chlorpromazine in terms of clinical effects and therapeutic reversal with benztropine in schizophrenia: Theoretical implications for potency differences among neuroleptics, Psychopharmacologia 43, 103-113 (1975).

Snyder, S., Taylor, J., Coyle, J., and Meyerhoff, B.: The role of brain dopamine in behavioral regulation and the actions of psychotropic drugs, Am. J. Psychiat. 127, 199-207 (1970).

Storms, L. and Broen, W.: A theory of schizophrenic behavioral disorganization, Archs gen. Psychiat. 20, 129-144 (1969).

Thornburg, J. and Moore, K.: Dopamine and norepinephrine uptake by rat brain synaptosomes: Relative inhibitory potencies of l- and d-amphetamine and amantadine, Res. Commun. Chem. Path. Pharmac. 5, 81-89 (1973).

Trabucchi, M., Cheney, D.S., Racagni, G., and Costa, E.: In vivo inhibition of striatal acetylcholine turnover by L-Dopa, apomorphine and (+)-amphetamine, Brain Res. 85, 130-134 (1975).

Von Voightlander, P. and Moore, K.: Involvement of nigro-striatal neurons in the in vivo release of dopamine by amphetamine, amantadine and tyramine, J. Pharmac. exp. Ther. 184, 542-552 (1975).

Yaryura-Tobias, J., Diamond, B., and Merlis, S.: The action of L-Dopa on schizophrenic patients, Curr. ther. Res. 12, 528-531 (1970).

Ziance, R.J., Azzaro, A.J., and Rutledge, C.O.: Characteristics of amphetamine-induced release of norepinephrine from rat cerebral cortex in vitro, J. Pharmac. exp. Ther. 182, 284-294 (1972).

THE COMPARATIVE PSYCHOTOGENIC EFFECTS OF L-DOPA AND ET-495

Burton Angrist, Gregory Sathananthan,

Baron Shopsin, and Sam Gershon

Neuropsychopharmacology Research Unit, Department of Psychiatry, New York University Medical Center, 550 First Avenue, New York, New York 10016

The ability of amphetamine and methylphenidate to cause a schizophreniform psychosis in non-schizophrenic individuals is one of the bases for the hypothesized relationship between dopaminergic hyperactivity and some psychotic states (Connell, 1958; Griffith, Cavanaugh, and Oates, 1970; Angrist and Gershon, 1970; Spensley and Rockwell, 1972; Bell, 1973). The demonstration that these same drugs caused florid exacerbation of symptomatology when administered to schizophrenics (Janowsky, El-Yousef, Davis, and Sekerke, 1973; Janowsky and Davis, 1974) gave impetus to this concept. However, amphetamine and methylphenidate clearly affect both norepinephrine and dopamine (Lewander, 1974; Scheel-Krüger, 1971; Ferris, Tang, and Maxwell, 1972) thereby making it difficult to specifically implicate dopaminergic mechanisms in their psychotogenic effects with certainty.

Accordingly it appeared to be an appropriate research strategy to assess the psychotogenic effects of drugs that promised to be somewhat more specific as dopaminergic agonists than amphetamine and methylphenidate. The antiparkinsonian drugs L-DOPA and ET-495 theoretically qualified as such.

The occurrence of psychiatric side effects in parkinsonian patients treated with L-DOPA suggested that the drug might prove psychotogenic in neurologically intact subjects. The possibly greater dopaminergic specificity of L-DOPA was suggested by

Everett and Borcherding's report (1970) that it increases consistently brain dopamine levels while having only slight or inconsistent effects on brain norepinephrine.

Lieberman (1974) reported that 2 of 8 parkinsonian patients treated with ET-495 showed both increased confusion and disorientation and grossly psychotic deterioration, suggesting psychotogenic potential. The pharmacologic effects of ET-495 reported by Corrodi, Fuxe, and Ungerstedt (1971) include decreased dopamine turnover and induction of rotation toward the intact side in rodents with unilateral 6-hydroxydopamine-induced nigrostriatal lesions. These imply direct dopamine receptor stimulation. Creese's (1974) demonstration that rats treated as neonates with 6-hydroxydopamine respond behaviorally to both ET-495 and apomorphine but not to amphetamine further suggests direct stimulation of dopamine receptors. These findings were important to our theoretic framework since a receptor stimulant, if devoid of other effects, would constitute a specific agonist indeed.

METHODS

Patients giving consent to participate in these studies were transferred to the Neuropsychopharmacology Research Unit. All medications were discontinued with the exception of chloral hydrate or sodium Amytal for agitation or insomnia, and the subjects were observed for 4 days to 3 weeks (further specified below). In the studies with L-DOPA, matched placebo was used. None was used in studies of ET-495, as none was available. Before starting either drug all patients had a physical examination, clinical laboratory tests, including CBC, urinalysis, BUN and liver function profile, and an EKG. Laboratory studies and EKGs were repeated weekly. Patients receiving over 5 gm L-DOPA per day had EKGs done twice weekly. L-DOPA was initiated at 750 mg per day. Initial ET-495 dosage was 60 mg per day. Both were increased until behavioral effects or side effects required discontinuation. All patients received a standard hospital diet without vitamin supplements.

Schizophrenics were dropped from the study and treated with standard neuroleptics if they showed clinical deterioration during the observation period before L-DOPA or ET-495 was administered. Behavioral ratings consisted of the Brief Psychiatric Rating Scales (BPRS), the Clinical Global Impression (CGI), and the Dosage Record and Treatment Emergent Symptoms (DOTES). These were administered prior to drugs, weekly, and at termination. Non-schizophrenics' behavioral change was documented by ward observations and daily interviews. Rating scales were not used in this group.

RESULTS

Schizophrenic Patients - L-DOPA

Ten patients received placebo for a mean of 6.1 days (range 5-10 days). L-DOPA was administered for a mean of 21.2 days (range 11-29 days). The mean maximal daily dose attained was 5,050 mg (range 3-6 gm). Rating scale analysis showed significant deterioration on two raters' BPRS scores for conceptual disorganization, emotional withdrawal and agitation-excitement, and significant diminuation of motor retardation. Hostility and blunted affect were scored as worsened by both raters but only one's scores attained statistical significance. Similarly both measures showed worsening on the CGI with only one attaining statistical significance.

All patients showed clinical deterioration. Descriptively, two response patterns were evident. Three patients showed stimulant effects, psychomotor activation, increased talkativeness, freer expression of psychopathology, intrusiveness (to the point of becoming socially inappropriate), and irritability.

A second response pattern was shown by the remaining seven patients. This consisted of the stimulant effects noted in the first group and a dose related increase in the individual symptom pattern present at baseline. Two patients showed the emergence of *de novo* symptoms: auditory hallucinations in one case and mannerisms in the second. These data are summarized in Table 1. Examples of these various response patterns are as follows.

Psychomotor Activation. Patient No. 1 was a 50 year-old ex-postal worker diagnosed as suffering from schizophrenia. At baseline he was depressed, hopeless, showed severe motor retardation, and expressed somatic delusions to the effect that he had been made impotent when a physician had performed a rectal examination during his adolescence and "done something to the gland." He stated his stomach "didn't work," denied bowel movements, sleeping or appetite although he was objectively hyperphagic and hypersomnic. On L-DOPA he developed drowsiness and anorexia at 2000 mg/day. The dose was diminished and then increased without these effects recurring. At 2750 mg/day he showed activation. Motor activity was increased and pressure of speech was evident. Whereas before he tended to "fade into the background" of the ward, his presence now became ubiquitous and attention demanding. He initiated conversations in a socially inappropriate fashion and repetitiously and intrusively voiced the same somatic delusions which previously had to be elicited by questioning. Mood was unchanged during this time: his hopelessness, anhedonia, and pessimism were unaltered. This psychomotor stimulation disappeared 72 hours after L-DOPA was discontinued.

Table 1 Behavioral Effects of L-DOPA in 10 Schizophrenic Patients

Pt No./Age/Sex/Diagnosis	Behavioral Changes After L-DOPA
1. 50, male, Schizo-affective, Depressed	Activation, increased expression of somatic delusions, depression unchanged
2. 33, female, Chronic Paranoid Schizophrenia (acute exacerbation)	Pressure of speech, increased thought disorder, emotional lability and agitation; development of auditory hallucinations
3. 49, male, Schizo-affective Depressed	Depression, pressure of speech, hypersensitivity, suspiciousness, questionably increased auditory hallucinations
4. 49, male, Schizo-affective Depressed	Impulsiveness, restlessness, irritability, hostility, fights
5. 37, female, Chronic Undifferentiated Schizophrenia	Increased thought disorder, hostility, emotional lability, more frequent and severe outbursts, pacing
6. 22, male, Acute Undifferentiated Schizophrenia	Increased hostility, agitation, emotional lability
7. 35, male, Chronic Undifferentiated Schizophrenia	Increased hostility, agitation, grandiosity and bizarre behavior
8. 46, male, Chronic Undifferentiated Schizophrenia	Increased somatic delusions, thought disorder, hostility, uncooperativeness and demandingness

Table 1, continued

Pt No./Age/Sex/Diagnosis	Behavioral Changes After L-DOPA
9. 30, male, Chronic Undifferentiated Schizophrenia	Irritability, hyperactivity, disorganization of thought, verbal and motoric "stereotypes"
10. 28, female, Acute Schizophrenic episode	Hyperactivity, increased autistic behavior, development of symbolic manneristic behavior, hypersexuality, stripping, ripping pajamas bizarrely

Psychomotor activation, plus worsening of baseline symptoms. Patient No. 5 was a 37 year-old female with chronic undifferentiated schizophrenia. Her baseline status showed withdrawn behavior with superimposed emotional lability which led to intermittent episodes of agitation and screaming. Thought disorder and pressure of speech were also present. She was preoccupied with diffuse paranoid ideas about Jews, and became agitated in response to perceived sexual advances by male patients on the ward. On L-DOPA she showed a dose related deterioration particularly with regard to thought disorder, hostility, emotional lability and agitation. Her outbursts became more frequent and severe, and paranoid ideas were expressed more frequently. Motor activation led to continuous pacing at 4500 mg/day. This behavior subsided 96 hours after L-DOPA was discontinued.

Psychomotor activation, worsening of baseline symptoms, and the development of new symptoms. Patient No. 2 was a 33 year-old female diagnosed as suffering from an acute exacerbation of chronic paranoid schizophrenia. At baseline she was hyperactive, socially inappropriate (loudly demanding contraceptive pills), and showed prominent formal thought disorder. She appeared anxious, diffusely suspicious, and expressed ideas of being able to predict peoples' deaths. On L-DOPA she showed progressive deterioration in all these areas. Pressure of speech was apparent at 1500 mg/day. Thought disorder, paranoid ideation, emotional lability, and agitation were increased at a daily dosage of 5000 mg; and auditory hallucinations were reported at this dosage where none had previously been noted. When L-DOPA was discontinued, these symptoms began to remit after 48 hours.

Schizophrenic Patients - ET-495

Seven schizophrenics were observed off neuroleptics for a mean of 9.3 days (range 4-21 days). ET-495 was administered for a mean duration of 11 days (range 6-18 days). The mean maximal daily dose obtained was just over 205 mg. Changes of BPRS scores did not attain statistical significance; side effects were encountered in all patients. Five out of seven developed nausea or nausea and vomiting. One patient suddenly developed a severe choreo-athetoid syndrome resulting in nearly continuous involuntary movement. This cleared completely 48 hours after ET-495 was discontinued. One patient, the only one in this series to show psychomotor activation, developed insomnia as a result of ET-495. She received the highest dose attained: 320 mg daily. In spite of the lack of stimulant effects that were so prominent with L-DOPA, 4 of seven patients' conditions were considered to show definite deterioration after ET-495. One (the patient who developed the choreo-athetotic syndrome) might have worsened somewhat, with respect to autism and decreased contact;

but the severity of her baseline status (diffuse paranoid ideation and almost constant giggling in response to acknowledged auditory hallucinations which were said to be sexual and which she refused to discuss further) made this difficult to document. In order to err in the direction of conservatism, the reporter scored her as "unchanged." One patient showed no psychological effects whatsoever; and another who originally was quite psychotic (she had been admitted after trying to grab a policeman's gun in response to auditory hallucinations commanding her to kill herself) showed complete clearing of all psychotic symptomatology during the eleven days that ET-495 was administered. These data are summarized in Table 2.

Non-Schizophrenics - L-DOPA

Six non-schizophrenic psychiatric inpatients received placebo for 7-10 days. Active L-DOPA was given for a mean of 22 days (range 19-28 days). The mean maximum daily dose attained was 8.83 gm. The behavioral effects of L-DOPA, side effects, and maximal dose attained are indicated in Table 3.

Non-Schizophrenics - ET-495

ET-495 was administered to 3 non-schizophrenic patients. One was an alcoholic with severe depression who was admitted because of incipient D.T.s. At 280 mg/day of ET-495 his depression cleared and he noted subjective irritability (that he concealed from examiners). The second, a detoxified glutathamide addict (who had had seizures during detoxification and was given Dilantin 400 mg/day along with ET-495), received 400 mg/day of ET-495 and developed dose related nausea, anorexia, 5 pounds weight loss, hyperactivity, dysphoria, palpitations, ideas of reference, and occasional auditory hallucinations. Although this symptomatology is technically "psychotic," he never lost insight into the fact that he was under the influence of a drug (possibly because of his familiarity with amphetamines and cocaine which he had taken in the past). The third patient was a 53 year-old male manic depressive, depressive phase, who, after receiving ET-495, developed a psychotic syndrome of auditory hallucinations about homosexuality, the reality of which he absolutely believed. These data are given both in Table 4 and the following text.

Patient No. 3 was a 53 year-old male manic depressive. His first psychiatric illness was a manic episode at age 44. In a subsequent hospitalization in the same year he was treated for depression with ECT. Since that time he has had 3 manic episodes during which he was not hospitalized and 2 periods of depression during which he

Table 2 Personal Data, Dose, Side Effects and Behavioral Effects of ET-495 Administration in Schizophrenic Patients

Pt No./Age/Sex/Diagnosis	Maximum Daily Dose ET-495	Side Effects	Behavioral Effects
1. 30, male, Chronic Undifferentiated Schizophrenia	200 mg	Nausea	Increased ideas of reference and ideas that others "knew" of past child molesting, increased irritability and somatic preoccupation, fearful of eye contact
2. 26, female, Schizo-Affective	80 mg	Vomiting	Irritable, hostile, laughing to self autistically and more frequently and openly, although auditory hallucinations were explicitly denied
3. 37, male, Acute Paranoid Schizophrenia	120 mg	Vomiting	Public praying with verbal response to auditory hallucinations, assaultive, no emotional contact
4. 38, female, Chronic Undifferentiated Schizophrenia	320 mg	Insomnia	Increased disorganization of speech, and agitation, appearance dilapidated
5. 42, male, Schizo-Affective Schizophrenia, Depressed Type	240 mg	Nausea and Vomiting	None

Table 2, continued

Pt No./Age/Sex/Diagnosis	Maximum Daily Dose ET-495	Side Effects	Behavioral Effects
6. 25, female, Hebrephrenic, Schizophrenia (or Chronic Undifferentiated) (?)	240 mg	Chorea althetosis	Some increased autism and diminished "contact" (?)
7. 24, female, Chronic Undifferentiated Schizophrenia	240 mg	Nausea and Vomiting	Complete clearing of psychosis

Table 3 Age, Sex, Diagnosis, Dose and Behavioral Effects of L-DOPA in six Non-Schizophrenic Inpatients

Pt No./Age/Sex/Diagnosis	Daily Dose L-DOPA	Behavioral Effects
1. 26, male, depression, passive-aggressive personality disorder (Homosexual orientation)	9 gm	Hypersexuality (masturbating 4-5x one day rather than 4-5x/week)
2. 37, male, chronic alcoholic	10 gm	Spontaneous and unexpected erections (while playing ping-pong with female nurse)
3. 25, male, chronic alcoholic and ex-amphetamine abuser	9 gm	Irritability, insomnia, increased motor activity, ideas of reference (understood as drug related), nausea, diaphoresis, palpitations; "Like an amphetamine crash"
4. 32, male, chronic alcoholic	10 gm	Toxic confusional state, dysarthria, dystonia mouth and tongue
5. 38, male, chronic alcoholic with depression	6 gm	Irritability, erections for the first time in several years, nausea, diaphoresis, palpitations
6. 39, male, depression and heavy drinker 2 years after gastrectomy	9 gm	Paranoid psychosis*

*Patient No. 6 developed mild pressure of speech at 9 gm/day which intensified over the next two days. At the time of termination his status had changed dramatically. He was talkative, intrusive, and socially inappropriate. He would not permit conversations to be terminated and compulsively dwelt on past injustices done to him by a brother-in-law who, he claimed, had unjustly accused him

Table 3, continued

of interstate narcotics sales and had dealings with the Mafia. He states that his own lawyer had tried to have him sent to jail because of vaguely described "big business interests." He could not explain the connection between his lawyer and brother-in-law, but alleged that they were both part of a "web" his brother-in-law had created to ruin his life. Changes in formal aspects of speech were striking at this time as well. He was compulsively circumstantial, unable to give an abbreviated "focused" account, and constantly introduced irrelevant details so that his line of thought became so rambling it could not be followed. His speech showed occasional blocking during this time, and his affect appeared incongruously blunted when compared to the content of his speech.

He also showed slight tremor, dysarthria, and dystonic movements of the face and lips at this time. His social inappropriateness, mildly blunted affect, thought disorder, and paranoid preoccupations were such that a psychiatrist "blind" to his drug intake would almost certainly have diagnosed him as a chronic paranoid schizophrenic. These signs resolved after L-DOPA was discontinued for 24 hours and 5 mg Haldol was administered intramuscularly.

Table 4 Personal Data, Dose, Behavioral and Side Effects of ET-495 Administration in Non-Schizophrenics

Pt No./Age/Sex/Diagnosis	Dose	Behavioral and Side Effects
1. 47, male, endogenous depression, alcoholism, incipient D.T.s	280 mg	Decreased depression, subjectively noticed irritability (Concealed from observer)
2. 33, male, detoxified glutethimide addict*	400 mg	Nausea, anorexia, 5 lb. weight loss, palpitations, overactivity, insomnia, dysphoria, ideas of reference, auditory hallucinations, emotional detachment (see text)
3. 53, male, manic depressive, depressed	160 mg	Hallucinatory, psychosis with preoccupation about homosexuality

*on Dilantin 100 mg q.i.d. during study

stayed at home and was unable to work, but was not hospitalized. In August 1974, he became depressed and was treated as an inpatient on our Unit. From that time until March 1975, he was an inpatient and refractory to antidepressant treatment. It was decided to administer ET-495 for possible antidepressant effect. He received ET-495 for 16 days and attained a maximum dose of 240 mg daily. This caused palpitations, irritability, and insomnia and the drug was discontinued. A second trial of ET-495 was undertaken later (after a 10-day period off all medication except h.s. chloral hydrate). The dosage was increased more gradually over the next 16 days to a maximum of 160 mg daily. At this point he became intensely upset by voices (which he stated he had been hearing for 5-6 days) and rapidly became severely agitated.

The voices consisted of another patient's, particularly, as well as voices of a psychiatrist and a male nurse on the ward. All centered around accusations of homosexuality. He heard "He's a faggot" all day long. At the window he heard "There's that cock-sucker" from the street. When alone in a ward day room, he continued to hear "Look at that cock-sucker" and "He's definitely a faggot." He was apprehensive and appeared almost tearful when he asked if he was kidding himself; i.e., was he "really" a homosexual. He absolutely refused to believe that the voices were drug-induced. Although frightened of the one patient whose voice he heard, he was not diffusely referential with regard to other patients. No formal thought disorder was appreciated. Affect was congruent but somewhat constricted. Sensoria were clear. He was oriented to day and date and able to do serial substraction of 7's from 100 fluently.

ET-495 was discontinued and Haloperidol 5 mg given intramuscularly. After 15 minutes the voices stopped for 1 1/2 hr and then reappeared. Administration of Haloperidol 10 mg orally 3x daily for 2 days led to suppression of the voices which did not recur after Haloperidol was discontinued.

DISCUSSION

Both L-DOPA and ET-495 were found to cause worsening of schizophrenic psychopathology. In addition, both were demonstrated to be capable of causing a *de novo* schizophreniform psychosis in non-schizophrenics. These findings certainly constitute support for the hypothesized role of dopamine in schizophrenia. Indeed, if either drug was completely specific as a dopaminergic agonist, these findings could be interpreted as "proof" of this hypothesis.

Unfortunately, neither drug is absolutely specific in its effects. Administration of L-DOPA, particularly in large doses, is almost certainly not without effect on other CNS systems; and certain effects considered "dopaminergic" may indirectly be mediated by these other systems. Friedman and Gershon (1972), for example, have shown that the centrally mediated emission of seminal fluid in male rats in response to L-DOPA administration is antagonized by 5-hydroxytryptamine receptor blockers but not by adrenergic, dopaminergic, or cholinergic blockers. Dunkley, Sanghvi, Friedman, and Gershon (1972) have shown that, in dogs, 5-HTP can completely block or significantly attenuate the emetic response produced by L-DOPA while PCPA can block its behavioral effects. Janowsky, El-Yousef, Davis, and Sekerke (1972) have shown that physostigmine can both block and abolish the stereotypy in rats induced by the administration of methylphenidate. Thus, both serotonergic and cholinergic mechanisms undoubtedly either affect or may indirectly mediate responses considered specifically "dopaminergic."

Similarly, ET-495 probably has actions other than stimulating dopamine receptors. Both Goldstein, Battista, Ohmoto, Anagnoste, and Fuxe (1973) and Fuxe, Agnate, Corrodi, Everitt, Hokfelt, Lofstrom, and Ungerstedt (1975) have reported findings suggesting the possible involvement of presynaptic mechanisms in the actions of ET-495. Even more important, Garattini, Barreggi, Marc, Calderini and Marsella (1974) have demonstrated that ET-495 affects brain norepinephrine. Thus, caution must still be exercised in interpreting these findings.

While the role of dopamine in the pathogenesis of schizophrenia cannot be considered "proven," the capacity of L-DOPA and ET-495, in addition to amphetamine and methylphenidate, to cause schizophreniform psychoses *de novo* and make schizophrenic psychopathology worse makes this role more likely. Although none of these drugs is specifically and exclusively a dopamine agonist, all have dopaminergic facilitation as a common denominator.

REFERENCES

Angrist, B.M. and Gershon, S.: The phenomenology of experimentally induced amphetamine psychosis. Preliminary observations, Biol. Psychiat. 2, 95-107 (1970).

Bell, D.S.: The experimental reproduction of amphetamine psychosis, Archs gen. Psychiat. 29, 35-40 (1973).

Connell, P.H.: Amphetamine Psychosis. Maudsley Monographs No. 5. London: Oxford University Press, 1958.

Corrodi, H., Fuxe, K., and Ungerstedt, U.: Evidence for a new type of dopamine receptor stimulating agent, J. Pharm. Pharmac. 23, 989-991 (1971).

Creese, I.: Behavioral evidence of dopamine receptor stimulation by piribedil (ET-495) and its metabolite S 584, Eur. J. Pharmacol. 28, 55-58 (1974).

Dunkley, B., Sanghvi, I., Friedman, E., and Gershon, S.: Comparison of behavioral and cardiovascular effects of L-DOPA and 5-HTP in conscious dogs, Psychopharmacologia 26, 161-172 (1972).

Everett, G.M. and Borcherding, J.W.: L-DOPA: Effect on concentrations of dopamine, norepinephrine and serotonin in brains of mice, Science 168, 849-850 (1970).

Ferris, R.M., Tang, F.L.M., and Maxwell, R.A.: A comparison of the capacities of isomers of amphetamine, deoxypiperadol and methylphenidate to inhibit the uptake of tritiated catecholamines into rat cerebral cortex, hypothalamus and striatum and into adrenergic nerves of the rabbit aorta, J. Pharmac. exp. Ther. 181, 407-416 (1972).

Friedman, E. and Gershon, S.: L-DOPA: Centrally mediated emission of seminal fluid in male rats, Life Sci. 11, 435-440 (1972).

Fuxe, K., Agnate, L.F., Corrodi, H., Everitt, B.J., Hökfelt, T., Lofstrom, J., and Ungerstedt, U.: Action of dopamine receptor agonists in forebrain and hypothalamus: Rotational behavior, ovulation and dopamine turnover, Adv. Neurol. 9, 223-242 (1975).

Garattini, S., Barreggi, S., Marc, V., Calderini, G., and Marsella, P.L.: Effects of piribedil on noradrenaline and MOPEG-SO_4 levels in the rat brain, Eur. J. Pharmacol. 28, 214-216 (1974).

Goldstein, M., Battista, A.F., Ohmoto, T., Anagnoste, B., and Fuxe, K.: Tremor and involuntary movements in monkeys: Effects of L-DOPA and of a dopamine receptor stimulating agent, Science 179, 816-817 (1973).

Griffith, J.J., Cavanaugh, J., and Oates, J.: Psychosis induced by the administration of d-amphetamine to human volunteers. In: Psychotomimetic Drugs. Efron, D.H., Ed., pp. 287-294. New York: Raven Press, 1970.

Janowsky, D.S. and Davis, J.M.: Dopamine, psychomotor stimulants and schizophrenia: Effects of methylphenidate and the stereoisomers of amphetamine in schizophrenics. In: Neuropsychopharmacology of Monoamines and Their Regulatory Enzymes. Usdin, E., Ed., pp. 317-323. New York: Raven Press, 1974.

Janowsky, D.S., El-Yousef, M.K., Davis, J.M., and Sekerke, H.J.: Cholinergic antagonism of methylphenidate induced stereotyped behavior, Psychopharmacologia 27, 295-303 (1972).

Janowsky, D.S., El-Yousef, M.K., Davis, J.M., and Sekerke, H.J.: Provocation of schizophrenic symptoms by intravenous administration of methylphenidate, Archs gen. Psychiat. 28, 185-191 (1973).

Leiberman, A., Le Brun, Y., Dinkar, B., and Zolfaghari, M.: The use of a dopaminergic receptor stimulating agent (piribedil, ET-495) in parkinson's disease. In: Neuropsychopharmacology of Monoamines and Their Regulatory Enzymes. Usdin, E., Ed., pp. 415-425. New York: Raven Press, 1974.

Lewander, T.: Effect of chronic-treatment with central stimulants on brain monoamines and some behavioral and physiological functions in rats, guinea pigs and rabbits. In: Neuropsychopharmacology of Monoamines and Their Regulatory Enzymes. Usdin, E., Ed., pp. 221-239. New York: Raven Press, 1974.

Scheel-Krüger, J.: Comparative studies of various amphetamine analogues demonstrating different interactions with the metabolism of the catecholamines in the brain, Eur. J. Pharmacol. 14, 47-59 (1971).

Spensley, J. and Rockwell, D.A.: Psychosis during methylphenidate abuse, New Engl. J. Med. 286, 880-881 (1972).

STRUCTURE-ACTIVITY RELATIONSHIPS OF SEVERAL AMPHETAMINE DRUGS IN MAN

John D. Griffith

NIDA Addiction Research Center

P. O. Box 12390, Lexington, Kentucky 40511

In this chapter we shall consider a series of amphetamine studies in man which were conducted at the Addiction Research Center by several investigators. A reason these studies were done was to develop and validate methods that will predict the abuse potential of amphetamine congeners. Another reason was to understand amphetamine "euphoria" in terms of phenethylamine structure.

Drug psychoactivity is influenced by factors other than drug structure; however, amphetamines are notorious for having varied subjective effects among different individuals in a group and among different groups of individuals: "...pharmacopathogenicity recapitulates psychopathogenicity...," as Post (1975) puts it, and individual subjective effects evolve along a continuum. Moreover, the subjective effects of amphetamine during chronic amphetamine administration can vary qualitatively depending on whether the dose is rapidly (Angrist and Gershon, 1970) or slowly (Griffith, Cavanaugh, Held, and Oates, 1970) escalated. These studies, therefore, should be interpreted only as single dose comparisons of amphetamine congeners in a selected population. An attempt was made to reproduce a dose-response curve corresponding to $\leq$ 30 mg of dextroamphetamine.

There is evidence that amphetamine and cocaine have similar effects in man (Bejerot, 1970). Whether these drugs have a "similar structure" is an interesting question worth exploring. Cocaine obviously does not have a phenethylamine segment, but the phenyl and amine moieties of both structures may be superimposed using flexible models. Whether these configurations are thermodynamically stable at the same receptor site is another issue (Patil, Miller, Trendelenburg, 1975).

METHODS

The studies cited here are single-dose, randomly assigned, double-blind crossover studies following methods developed by Martin, Sloan, Sapira, and Jasinski (1971). (This reference also details the questionnaire used to measure subjective effects.) A seven-day wash-out is imposed between each dose. Subjects involved may be described as prisoner-addicts with long histories of drug use, age 25-49, and in good health. Informed consent was obtained after the nature of the experiments had been fully explained.

A typical experiment involves the administration of a drug or a placebo to fasting subjects at 8:00 a.m. Physiological observations (duplicate supine systolic and diastolic blood pressures, pulse rate, respiratory rate, pupil size [determined photographically; bright target, near accommodation], and rectal temperature) are obtained 1½ hours before drug or placebo and at intervals afterwards: ½, 1, 2, 3, 4, 5, 6, 12, and 24 hours. Hunger is measured by estimating the caloric content of food eaten at the noon and subsequent meals and appetite, by a mark made on a 10 cm line indicating extremes of hunger and satiety. Sleep time is both observed sleep time (6:00 p.m. - 6:00 a.m.) and a self-estimate made by the subject the following morning.

Some of the subjective tests employed were derived from the Addiction Research Center Inventory (ARCI) by Haertzen (1966). These may be thought of as <u>drug specific</u> group scales and are so named: The MBG (Morphine-Benzedrine Group Scale), is a general measure of drug-induced euphoria; the BG (Benzedrine Group Scale), a more specific indicator of an amphetamine "high"; the PCAG (Pentobarbital-Chlorpromazine-Alcohol Group Scale), a measure of apathetic sedation; and the LSD (Lysergic Acid Diethylamide Group). The LSD Scale is more a measure of somatic symptomatology than psychotomimetic symptomatology. Martin has also developed an Amphetamine Scale which is <u>dose-specific</u> for amphetamine and contains items related principally to self-assertiveness. The Single Dose Opiate Questionnaire allows the patient to <u>categorize</u> the drug among different groups and to indicate his perceived "liking" of its overall effects. Dose-response curves are constructed from the mean 6-hour response for each measure (usually). In addition, mean placebo responses and the 95% confidence limits of mean placebo response are calculated for each measure as illustrated.

A number of studies done elsewhere often compare the blood level of a drug to its physiological and psychological effects. An alternative design used at the ARC is to identify a reliable "physiological marker" which is reliably dose-responsive. For opiate research, pupil diameter is a reliable marker; for amphetamine, supine blood pressure.

STRUCTURE-ACTIVITY

Side Chain Modified Amphetamines

Pharmacologists have recognized for several decades that a modification of the isopropylamine side-chain tends to reduce the CNS, appetite suppressing, and cardiovascular activity of amphetamine. A selective effect on appetite has been observed for some of these amphetamine congeners, especially in animal studies. Others (tranylcypromine, pheniprazine) are potent monoamine oxidase inhibitors.

Whether these side-chain modified derivatives demonstrate selectivity of action in man, however, is a moot point. Using d-amphetamine as a reference, Martin et al. (1971) initially reported on the subjective effects of four congeners (Fig. 1, #2-5). As may be noted in Table 1, methamphetamine was approximately equipotent to amphetamine and the remaining drugs differed considerably in mg-for-mg potency. None, however, seemed to have a selective effect on mood, blood pressure, or appetite relative to d-amphetamine.

Martin proposed the term "amphetamine-like" to describe this tracking of subjective and physiologic effects across potency for various amphetamine congeners in man for the purpose of assaying abuse potential. Since Martin's original study, two other side-chain modified congeners, diethylpropion and benzphetamine (Fig. 1, #6-7), have been assayed (Jasinski, Nutt, and Griffith, 1974). Both drugs are amphetamine-like and relatively weak as indicated in Table 1. Diethylpropion is also considerably less potent if administered subcutaneously than orally, suggesting the possibility of an active metabolite. This absence of parenteral potency may inhibit intravenous abuse of diethylpropion.

It is somewhat logical to presume that addicts would not be influenced by mg potency so long as the drug produced a significant "high" -- equivalent to 40 mg of amphetamine in these studies. Nonetheless, the less potent derivatives are widely prescribed and rarely abused, to date at least. Ephedrine and l-amphetamine are examples sold outside prescription controls. The reason for this relationship between potency and abuse incidence is not known.

Ring-Substituted Amphetamines

A number of psychedelic drugs have been derived from amphetamine but their effects on mood, appetite, perception, and alertness are quite variable, both among subjects and within the same subject over time. Parahydroxylation is also a minor metabolic pathway for

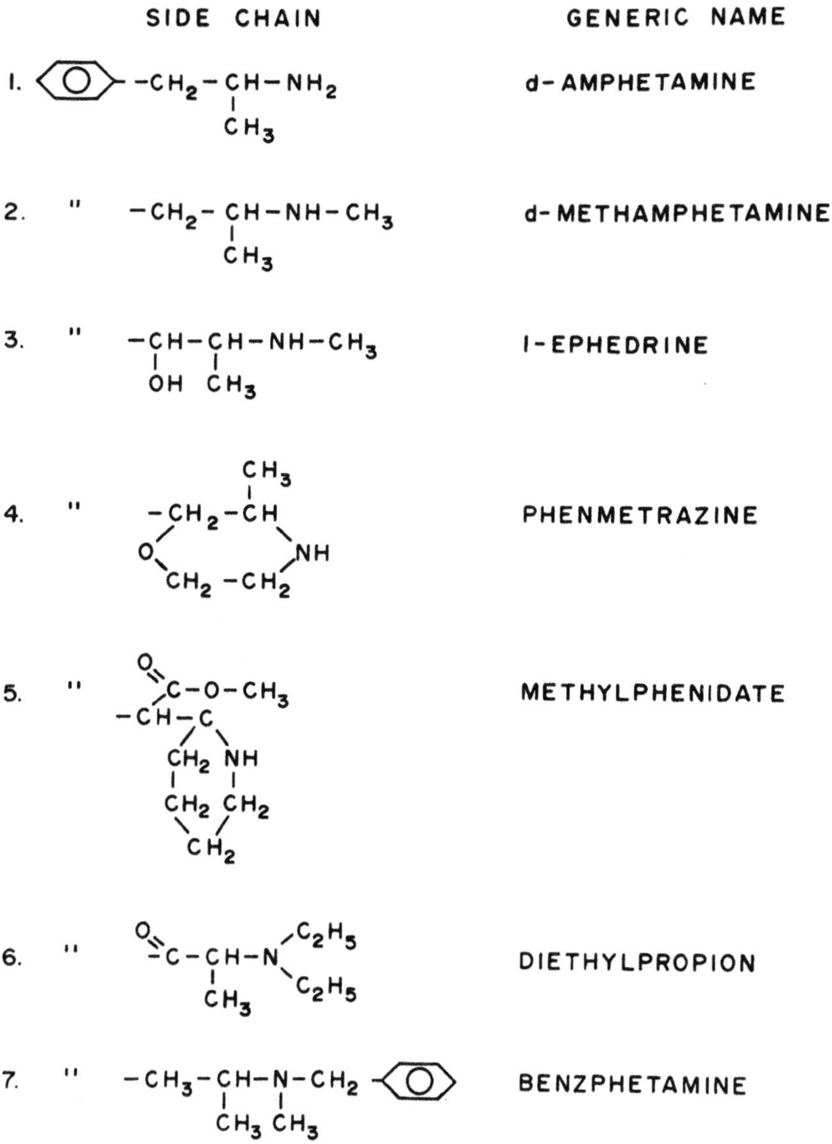

Fig. 1. Structure diagrams of side-chain modified amphetamine congeners.

TABLE 1

Relative potencies for the ability of benzphetamine to produce amphetamine-like subjective effects and comparison with relative potencies from previous studies (Expressed as mg of d-amphetamine equivalent to 1 mg of the test drug)

	MBG SCALE	AMPHETAMINE SCALE	BENZEDRINE SCALE	SYSTOLIC B.P.	DIASTOLIC B.P.	CALORIC INTAKE
d-Amphetamine	1	1	1	1	1	1
d-Methamphetamine+	----	0.93	1.68	0.92	1.49	1.19
Methylphenidate+	----	0.48	0.58	0.31	0.57	1.05
Phenmetrazine+	----	0.21	0.31	0.26	0.41	0.43
Ephedrine+	----	0.17	0.17	0.27	0.11	0.19
Diethylpropion†	0.15	0.15	0.18	0.09	0.12	0.16
Benzphetamine†	0.20	0.22	0.24	0.13	0.13	0.17

+Comparison by the subcutaneous route

†Comparison by the oral route

the inactivation of amphetamine in man. Of interest here are two ring-substituted amphetamine analogues, fenfluramine and chlorphentermine. Their structures are diagrammed in Fig. 2.

Fenfluramine (60, 120, 240 mg orally) was observed to have little effect on blood pressure or temperature and was not particularly euphorigenic as indicated by modest MBG and "Liking" Scales (Fig. 3). Unlike amphetamine, however, fenfluramine caused a marked dilation of pupils and elevation of the LSD Scale. Both drugs interfered with sleep and appetite. Fenfluramine was more often identified as an "LSD" or "barbiturate-like" substance.

An unexpected response, despite the precaution of a preliminary dose run-up, was observed among 3 subjects who manifested hallucinatory states characterized by visual and olfactory hallucinations, rapid and polar changes of mood, distorted time sense, fleeting paranoia, and sexual hallucinations. For these symptoms, diazepam was a prompt and effective antidote. The remaining five subjects receiving the largest dose of fenfluramine experienced a chlorpromazine-like sedation without hallucinations or other psychedelic effects (Griffith, Nutt, and Jasinski, 1975).

Chlorphentermine (50, 100, 200 mg) was similarly assessed. In certain respects, chlorphentermine resembles fenfluramine (Fig. 4), especially in terms of its mydriatic and sedative effects and the relative absence of vasopressor activity. On the other hand, chlorphentermine has a very minimal amphetamine-like effect, even in large doses, as compared to fenfluramine and, moreover, is not hallucinogenic.

Thus it appears that aromatic ring substitution may yield amphetamine congeners that have an anorexigenic effect without significant psychostimulant or sympathomimetic effects. However, the utility of this approach may be limited by the emergence of certain side-effects not usually associated with amphetamine, e.g., dysphoria, sedation, and/or psychedelic properties. The last may not be significant in the usual clinical application of fenfluramine, both because of dose and because tolerance to psychedelic drug effects is often observed among hallucinatory drugs.

Time-Course Effects of Amphetamine

Martin et al. (1971) further observed that the duration of amphetamine-like euphoria was paralleled by the duration of its effect on blood pressure over time. With most drugs in the doses used, this effect lasted about six hours. As may be noted in the various figures, however, sleep (attempted 16 or more hours later) was significantly impaired. Furthermore, patients were often

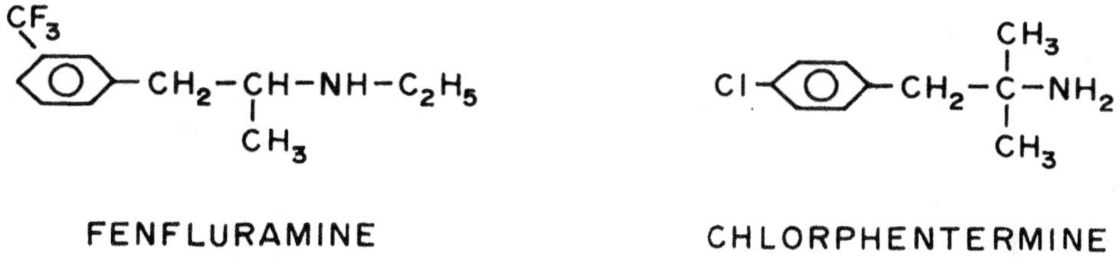

Fig. 2. Structure diagrams of fenfluramine and chlorphentermine.

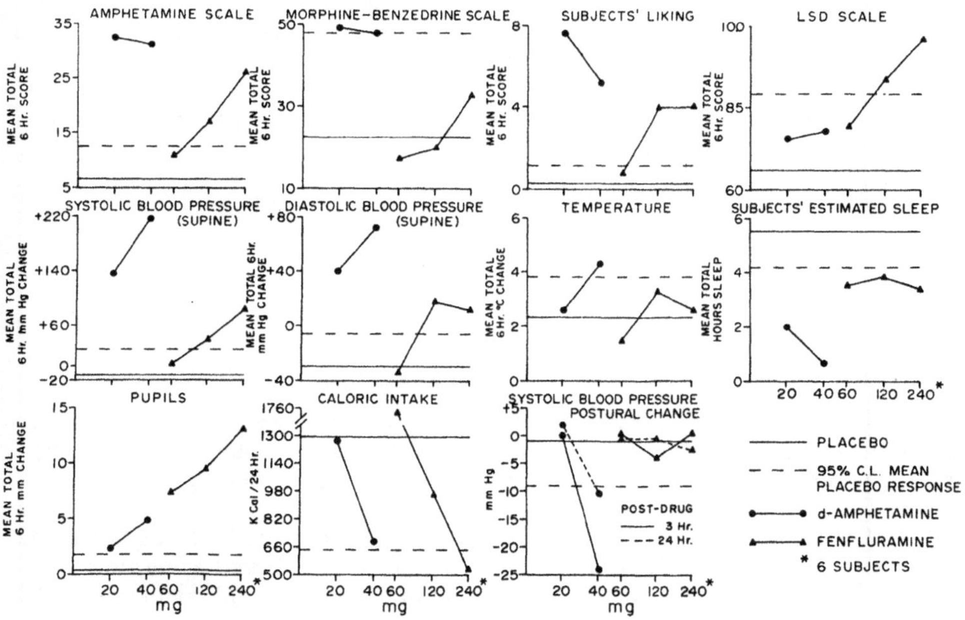

Fig. 3. Dose response curves from the comparison of fenfluramine, d-amphetamine, and placebo.

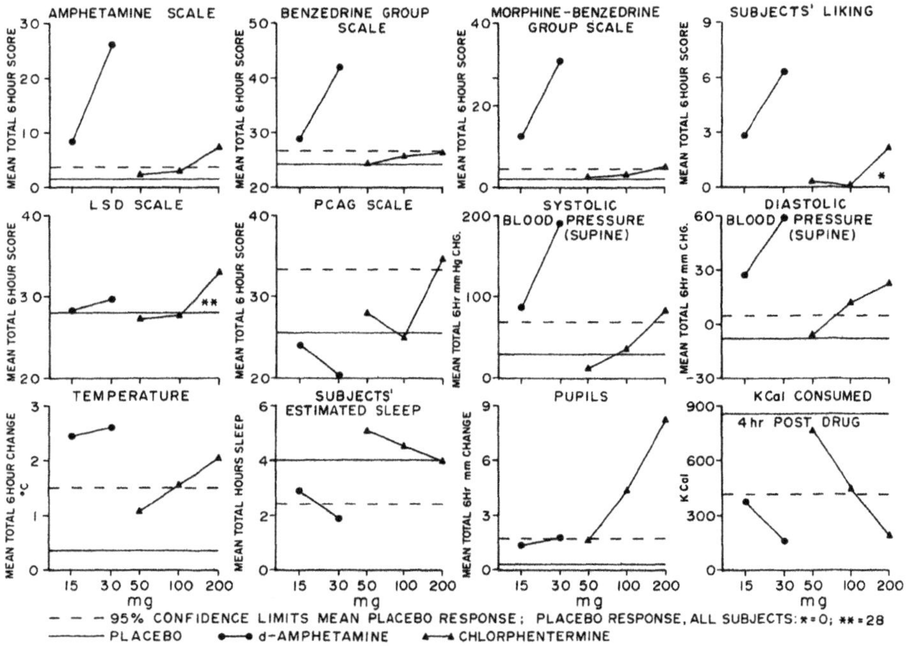

Fig. 4. Dose response curves from the comparison of chlorphentermine, d-amphetamine, and placebo.

irritable, dysphoric, hypochondriacal, and anorectic. We have observed in later studies that mydriasis (modest at best during the first 6 hours) is more prominent 24 hours after amphetamine.

The persistent dysphoric and mydriatic effects of amphetamine and its effects on sleep relative to the short-lived euphoric syndrome suggest that rather complex and perhaps independent mechanisms are involved. As mentioned in the introduction, early dysphoric effects are not uncommon in selected subjects, some of whom become tearful. Too, some of the late effects of amphetamine mimic the early effects of the ring-substituted amphetamines, previously described, which, in turn, are not unlike idiopathic states of emotional depression. Therefore, unraveling this pharmacology may be clinically relevant.

Differentiating Effects of d-Amphetamine on Supine and Standing Blood Pressure and Pulse Rate

To illustrate how experimental design can modify one's impression of amphetamine, we shall now consider a concrete example; i.e., amphetamine as a sympathomimetic pressor agent.

In the studies cited before, blood pressure and pulse rate were measured in the supine position (10 minutes bed rest). In previous studies related to the chronic effects of amphetamine (Cavanaugh, Griffith, and Oates, 1970), my colleagues and I at Vanderbilt University observed that while supine blood pressures might be elevated with chronic amphetamine, standing blood pressures were not--a response we attributed to the depletion of peripheral stores of norepinephrine by chronic amphetamine.

During amphetamine studies conducted at the ARC, however, a similar difference in blood pressure was observed 3 hours following amphetamine. This could hardly be interpreted as a chronic depleting effect.

Therefore, a study involving 5 patients was performed, each receiving 30 mg of amphetamine (subcutaneously) or a saline placebo in the crossover, 7 days apart. Supine (10 min.) and standing (2 min. erect) blood pressures and pulse rate were measured at 1 and 0.5 hours predrug and at intervals as indicated in Fig. 5 A-C.

As shown in Fig. 5A, the supine systolic blood pressures are considerably elevated over placebo values (paralleled by diastolic pressures, not illustrated). Standing pressures, conversely, are not significantly different from placebo (5B). Accompanying this fall in blood pressure with erect posture is a marked increase in pulse rate lasting > 13 hours (Fig. 5C).

To look at this reponse over the short term a separate experiment was conducted. Amphetamine was administered to two subjects (one illustrated, 5d) who were asked to remain standing for 3 minutes, one hour post-amphetamine. In the upper section of the graph (5d), we observe that standing blood pressure and pulse rate compare with supine values after placebo. Notice, however, that 1 hour post-drug, postural pulse and blood pressure changes are not a postural "bounce" but increase gradually over a period of several minutes.

These differences in blood pressure with posture are not easily explained along the lines of an indirect release of norepinephrine from adrenergic neurons leading to peripheral vasoconstriction. Whether a CNS loop is involved is a question that is especially interesting.

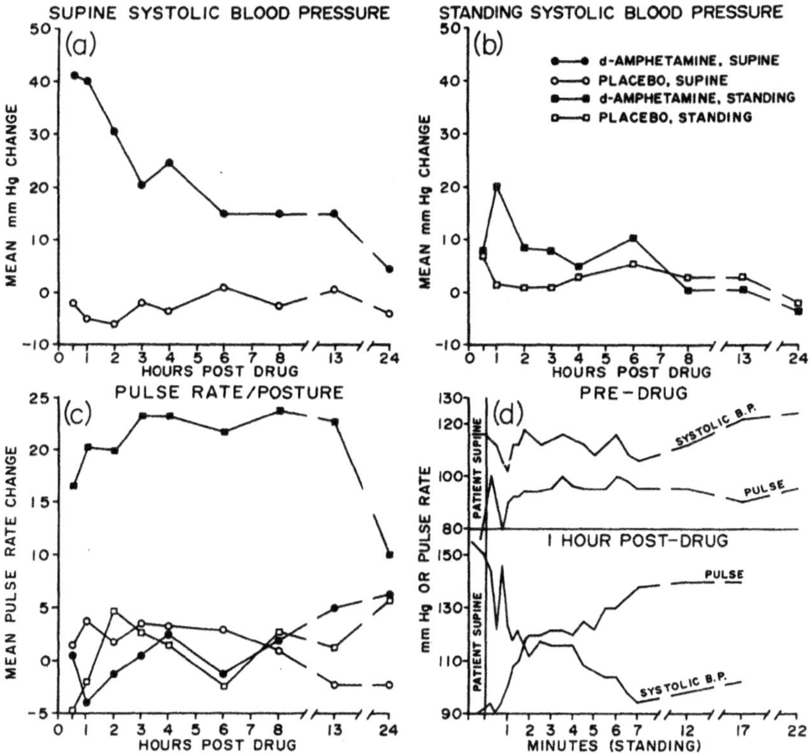

Fig. 5. Changes in supine and standing systolic blood pressure and pulse rates following d-amphetamine and placebo administration. (A) Change in supine systolic blood pressure, (B) change in standing systolic blood pressure, (C) changes in supine and standing pulse rates, and (D) lower graph illustrates time course of decrease in blood pressure and increase in pulse rate following standing from the supine position in one patient receiving d-amphetamine. Pre-drug changes are shown in upper half.

REFERENCES

Angrist, B. and Gershon, S.: Some recent studies on amphetamine psychosis--unresolved issues. In: Current Concepts on Amphetamine Abuse. Ellinwood, E.H., Jr. and Cohen, S., Eds., Washington: U.S. Government Printing Office, 1972.

Bejerot, N.: A comparison of the effects of cocaine and central stimulants, Br. J. Addict. 65, 35-37 (1970).

Cavanaugh, J.H., Griffith, J.D., and Oates, J.A.: Effect of amphetamine on the pressor response to tyramine: Formation of p-hydroxynorephedrine from amphetamine in man, Clin. Pharmacol. Therap. 11, 656-664 (1970).

Cavanaugh, J.H., Griffith, J.D., and Oates, J.A.: The effect of acute and chronic amphetamine administration on the adrenergic neuron in man. In: Amphetamines and Related Compounds. Costa, E. and Garattini, S., Eds., New York: Raven Press, 1970.

Griffith, J.D., Cavanaugh, J.H., Held, J., and Oates, J.A.: Experimental psychosis induced by the administration of d-amphetamine. In: Amphetamines and Related Compounds. Costa, E. and Garattini, S., Eds., New York: Raven Press, 1970.

Griffith, J.D., Nutt, J.G., and Jasinski, D.R.: A comparison of fenfluramine and amphetamine in man, Clin. Pharmacol. Therap. 18, 563-570 (1975).

Haertzen, C.A.: Development of scales based on patterns of drug effects, using the Addiction Research Center Inventory (ARCI), Psychol. Rep. 18, 163-194 (1966).

Jasinski, D.R., Nutt, J.G., and Griffith, J.D.: Effects of diethylpropion and d-amphetamine after oral administration, Clin. Pharmacol. Therap. 16, 645-652 (1974).

Martin, W.R., Sloan, J.W., Sapira, J.D., and Jasinski, D.R.: Physiological, subjective and behavioral effects of amphetamine, methamphetamine, ephedrine, phenmetrazine and methylphenidate in man, Clin. Pharmacol. Therap. 12, 245-248 (1971).

Patil, P.N., Miller, D.D., and Trendelenburg, U.: Molecular geometry and adrenergic drug activity, Pharmac. Rev. 26, 323-392 (1975).

Post, R.M.: Cocaine psychoses: A continuum model, Am. J. Psychiat. 132, 225-230 (1975).

AUTHOR INDEX

SUBJECT INDEX

GPSR Compliance

The European Union's (EU) General Product Safety Regulation (GPSR) is a set of rules that requires consumer products to be safe and our obligations to ensure this.

If you have any concerns about our products, you can contact us on ProductSafety@springernature.com

In case Publisher is established outside the EU, the EU authorized representative is:

Springer Nature Customer Service Center GmbH
Europaplatz 3
69115 Heidelberg, Germany

Batch number: 10723365

Printed by Printforce, the Netherlands